Neurosurgical Intensive Care

Second Edition

Javed Siddiqi, HBSc, MD, DPhil (Oxon), FRCSC, FAANS, FACS
Chair of Neurosurgery
Riverside University Health System Medical Center
Moreno Valley, California
Chief of Neurosurgery
Arrowhead Regional Medical Center
Colton, California
Neurosurgery Residency Program Director
Desert Regional Medical Center
Palm Springs, California

31 illustrations

Thieme
New York • Stuttgart • Delhi • Rio de Janeiro

Executive Editor: Timothy Hiscock
Managing Editor: Sarah Landis
Editorial Assistant: Nikole Connors
Director, Editorial Services: Mary Jo Casey
Production Editor: Torsten Scheihagen
International Production Director: Andreas Schabert
International Marketing Director: Fiona Henderson
International Sales Director: Louisa Turrell
Director of Sales, North America: Mike Roseman
Senior Vice President and Chief Operating
 Officer: Sarah Vanderbilt
President: Brian D. Scanlan
Printer: Sheridan Books, Inc.

Library of Congress Cataloging-in-Publication Data

Names: Siddiqi, Javed, 1962- editor.
Title: Neurosurgical intensive care / [edited by] Javed
 Siddiqi.
Other titles: Neurosurgical intensive care (Siddiqi)
Description: Second edition. | New York : Thieme,
 [2017] | Includes bibliographical references and
 index.
Identifiers: LCCN 2016057427| ISBN 9781626232341
 (softcover) | ISBN 9781626232358 (ebook)
Subjects: | MESH: Critical Care | Neurosurgical
 Procedures
Classification: LCC RC350.N49 | NLM WL 368 |
 DDC 616.8/0428–dc23 LC record available at
 https://lccn.loc.gov/2016057427

This second edition of Neurosurgical Intensive Care is dedicated to my wife, Seema, and to my children Amman and Saira, who inspire me to keep doing my best. It is also dedicated to my sisters, Shahina and Zarina, who always kept me on track, and represent the earliest and most enduring source of support in my life.

Contents

Contents

Foreword

Neurosurgical intensive care is a multispecialty and multidisciplinary field dedicated to improving the care and outcomes of patients with neurologic conditions. Over the past 20 years I have watched the field grow in terms of perceived need, knowledge, and acceptance across a growing number of medical specialties and disciplines. It is clearly evident in this text, which includes contributors from the specialties of neurology, vascular neurology, neurosurgery, interventional neuroradiology, anesthesiology, and critical care as well as the disciplines of nutrition and advanced practice nursing. This change has been driven as much by advances in medical knowledge and techniques as by the vision of its practitioners, such as the editor and contributors to this second edition of *Neurosurgical Intensive Care*.

By bringing together this breadth of expertise to update this concise and focused handbook, Javed Siddiqi has created a tool for practitioners from a wide range of specialties and disciplines who take care of critical neurological patients.

The format of this handbook lends itself to being easy to read, concise, and to the point. While it is not meant to be comprehensive, it captures the most important key points that are necessary for thoughtful clinical decision making. The tables and figures provide easy-to-use tools that facilitate rapid evaluation and decision making, both for trainees in neurocritical care as well as for experienced practitioners in related fields.

Dr. Siddiqi's *Neurosurgical Intensive Care* is a succinct and highly practical handbook for understanding the basics of patient management in the neurosurgical intensive care unit setting. Whether the reader is a nurse, medical student, resident, fellow or an attending physician, it is the best quick reference for managing critically ill neurosurgical patients.

Yan Qu, MD, PhD
Professor
Director of the Division of Neurosurgery
The Fourth Military Medical University
Xi'an, Shaan Xi, China

Preface

With the obvious exception of primary brain trauma, cerebral ischemia appears to be the final common pathway for most brain damage, whether from stroke, vasospasm, secondary brain injury, or tumor proliferation. Interestingly, the cornu ammonis 1 (CA1) pyramidal neurons of the hippocampus appear to be the most vulnerable to global cerebral ischemia, being the first to die, whereas motor cortex neurons appear to be relatively resistant to the same ischemia.[1] The fact that CA 1 neurons are essential for cognitive ("higher") functions, such as spatial learning and memory, versus motor cortex neurons serving movement, raises interesting questions about the evolutionary priority of memory over muscle, and learning over locomotion. While evolutionary biologists theorize about the fragility of higher brain functions over gross motor ability, the neurointensivist understands very clearly what is at stake—the patient who is physically intact, but cannot formulate new memories, concentrate, or analyze complex situations is also devastated in a way not always clinically self-evident. In short, if we can rescue CA1 neurons from the shadow of death, perhaps we stand a chance to preserve all other brain functions.[2]

The critical care of neurosurgical patients has evolved also over the recent two decades from an emphasis on pulmonary care (ventilation and oxygenation) to a more nuanced understanding of cerebral protection measures necessary to manage a disrupted blood–brain barrier. The advances in neuromonitoring methods are leading the way toward a more directed and individualized care plan for the neurocritical care patient. For example, the use of intracranial pressure monitors, external ventricular devices, brain tissue oxygen monitoring devices, and cerebral microdialysis are opening up a new frontier for tailoring interventions to the uniqueness of each patient's condition; the increasing use of continuous electroencephalography in the intensive care unit (ICU) has also rendered the invisible, silent status epilepticus, visible. Now, the traditional ICU management of fluid and electrolyte correction, as well as ventilator manipulation, has become dramatically more complex.

For the neurosurgeon involved in neurocritical care, decompression is still the mainstay of surgical intervention. For example, we still evacuate traumatic hematomas, perform hemicraniectomies for malignant edema from ischemic stroke, and resect malignant brain tumors causing mass effect; however, decompression is often insufficient as a stand-alone measure, and a large proportion of neurocritical care patients never go to the operating room. Whether our patients need open surgery or not, a nuanced understanding of neurophysiology is the best approach to neuron rescue. An evolution away from a mechanistic approach has rendered neurocritical care a multidisciplinary effort.

In this age of cerebral monitoring, after the ABCs of resuscitation, the key principles to neurocritical care follow age-old maxims of sound clinical practice: prompt diagnosis; compassionate communication with the patient and family; frequent neurologic exams to guide care; high-quality nursing; multidisciplinary collaboration; titration of therapies to avoid over- or undershooting desired goals; prudent use of blood work and neuroimaging to determine etiology of any neurological fluctuation or decline; and aggressive and early use of surgical intervention when necessary.

Finally, there is an ongoing debate among intensivists whether, when compared to general medical intensive care units, dedicated neurocritical care units improve outcomes for typical neurologic and neurosurgical patients with head injury, hydrocephalus, ischemic or hemorrhagic stroke, status epilepticus, intracranial hypertension, and the like. Although the answer to this question may be intuitive to neurointensivists, the evidence for this conclusion is becoming increasingly clear if we consider individual categories of diseases or conditions treated in a typical neurocritical care unit. For example, in their study of outcome after intracerebral hemorrhage, Diringer and Edwards reported that treatment in dedicated neurocritical care units was associated with a 3.4-fold reduction in hospital mortality rate compared with management of similar patients in general ICUs.[3] Other authors have shown similar findings for traumatic brain injury.[4,5] Perhaps the best example of the advantage of dedicated neurocritical care units comes from the management of ischemic stroke in the United States, where the highest level of national stroke accreditation for any hospital, "comprehensive stroke center," is not permitted without a dedicated neurocritical care unit. Certainly, the neurocritical care unit is the hub of stroke care in any comprehensive stroke center, involving real-time collaboration between stroke neurologists, neurointerventionalists, neurosurgeons, and neurointensivists.

Every credible trauma or stroke center should aspire to establishing a high-caliber neurocritical care unit, which is the ideal place for protocol-driven treatment of neurologic and neurosurgical diseases and conditions that may otherwise suffer from "ad hocery"; they are also uniquely equipped with specialty trained neurospecialists who can work and learn together. Another clear value of dedicated neurocritical care units is their ability to advance the frontiers of clinical neuroscience research and training in a way not hitherto possible in other venues. The presence of dedicated neurocritical care units attracts talented neurosurgeons and neurologists interested in advancing the frontiers of this expanding specialty. Luckily for the neurologic and neurosurgical patients who are their greatest beneficiaries, neurocritical care units are here to stay.

Javed Siddiqi, MD, DPhil (Oxon)

1. Zhu H, Yoshimoto T, Imajo-Ohmi S, Dazortsava M, Mathivanan A, Yamashima T. Why are hippocampal CA1 neurons vulnerable but motor cortex neurons resistant to transient ischemia? J Neurochem 2012;120(4):574–585

2. Bendel O, Bueters T, von Euler M, Ove Ogren S, Sandin J, von Euler G. Reappearance of hippocampal CA1 neurons after ischemia is associated with recovery of learning and memory. J Cereb Blood Flow Metab 2005;25(12):1586–1595

3. Diringer MN, Edwards DF. Admission to a neurologic/neurosurgical intensive care unit is associated with reduced mortality rate after intracerebral hemorrhage. Crit Care Med 2001;29(3):635–640

4. Patel HC, Menon DK, Tebbs S, Hawker R, Hutchinson PJ, Kirkpatrick PJ. Specialist neurocritical care and outcome from head injury. Intensive Care Med 2002;28 (5):547–553

5. Clayton TJ, Nelson RJ, Manara AR. Reduction in mortality from severe head injury following introduction of a protocol for intensive care management. Br J Anaesth 2004;93(6):761–767

Acknowledgments

First and foremost, I want to thank all the patients and families who have inspired this second edition of *Neurosurgical Intensive Care*, and the pursuit of life-long learning and improvement it represents. I want to express my immense gratitude to Dr. Dan Miulli, who has been my right hand in this venture, and whose fingerprints are on every part of this book. Thanks also to all my residents, fellows, colleagues, and other contributors to this second edition for an outstanding job, as well as to my staff (Dr. Fadi Andraos, Madeline Castorena, Maryann Duran), who assisted with various critical logistics. I am eternally grateful to my Thieme editors, Sarah Landis and Timothy Hiscock, who patiently kept me on track despite multiple detours.

Contributors

Daniella Abrams-Alexandru, MD
Neurosurgeon
Cape Fear Valley Medical Center
Fayetteville, North Carolina

Luis T. Arangua, MD
Stroke Neurologist and NeuroInterventionalist
Desert Regional Medical Center
Palm Springs, California

Yancey Beamer, MD
Neurosurgeon
Riverside University Health System Medical
    Center
Moreno Valley, California

Blake Berman, DO
Neurosurgeon
Desert Regional Medical Center
Palm Springs, California

Jacob Bernstein, DO, MS
Neurosurgery Resident
Riverside University Health System Medical
    Center
Moreno Valley, California

James Berry, DO
Neurosurgery Resident
Riverside University Health System Medical
    Center
Moreno Valley, California

Marc Billings, DO
Neurosurgery Resident
Riverside University Health System Medical
    Center
Moreno Valley, California

Marc Cabanne, DO
Neurosurgery Resident
Riverside University Health System Medical
    Center
Moreno Valley, California

John D. Cantando, DO
Neurosurgeon
Jupiter Medical Center
Jupiter, Florida

Tyler Carson, DO
Neurosurgery Resident
Riverside University Health System Medical
    Center
Moreno Valley, California

Jeff W. Chen, MD
Neurosurgeon, Associate Clinical Professor
Department of Neurological Surgery
UC Irvine Health
Irvine, California

Robert J. Claycomb, MD, PhD
Stroke Neurologist
Desert Regional Medical Center
Palm Springs, California

Vladimir Adriano Cortez, DO
Neurosurgeon and NeuroInterventionalist
Desert Regional Medical Center
Palm Springs, California

Dennis Cramer, DO
Neurosurgeon
Riverside University Health System Medical
    Center
Moreno Valley, California

Robert Dahlin, DO
Neurosurgery Resident
Riverside University Health System Medical
    Center
Moreno Valley, California

Jason Duong, DO
Neurosurgery Resident
Riverside University Health System Medical
    Center
Moreno Valley, California

Christopher Elia, DO
Neurosurgery Resident
Riverside University Health System Medical
  Center
Moreno Valley, California

Glenn Fischberg, MD
Stroke Neurologist and Neurointensivist
Desert Regional Medical Center
Palm Springs, California

Hammad Ghanchi, DO, MS
Neurosurgery Resident
Riverside University Health System Medical
  Center
Moreno Valley, California

Todd M. Goldenberg, MD
Chief of Neurosurgery
Kaiser Permanente
Fontana, California

Omid R. Hariri, DO, MS
Neurosurgery Resident
Riverside University Health System Medical
  Center
Moreno Valley, California

Silvio Hoshek, MD
Neurosurgeon
Arrowhead Regional Medical Center
Colton, California

Jeffery M. Jones, DO
Neurosurgeon
Memorial Hospital of Carbondale
Carbondale, Illinois

Samir Kashyap, DO
Neurosurgery Resident
Riverside University Health System Medical
  Center
Moreno Valley, California

Mark Krel, DO
Neurosurgery Resident
Riverside University Health System Medical
  Center
Moreno Valley, California

Shokry Lawandy, DO
Neurosurgeon
Riverside University Health System Medical
  Center
Moreno Valley, California

Bo-Lin Liu, MD, PhD
Neurosurgeon
Department of Neurosurgery
Tangdu Hospital, Fourth Military Medical
  University
Xi'an, China

Deependra Mahato, DO, MS
Neurosurgery Fellow
Mayo Clinic
Jacksonville, Forida

Gohar Majeed, DO, MS
Neurosurgery Resident
Riverside University Health System Medical
  Center
Moreno Valley, California

Rosalinda Menoni, MD
Neurosurgeon
Desert Regional Medical Center
Palm Springs, California

Tanya Minasian, DO
Pediatric Neurosurgery Fellow
Children's Hospital
Los Angeles, California

Dan E. Miulli, DO, MSc, FACOS
Neurosurgeon & Residency Program Director
Riverside University Health System Medical
  Center
Moreno Valley, California

Jerry Noel, DO
Neurosurgeon
Desert Regional Medical Center
Palm Springs, California

John Ogunlade, DO
Neurosurgery Resident
Riverside University Health System Medical
    Center
Moreno Valley, California

Nicholas Qandah, DO
Neurosurgeon
Mohawk Valley Health System Medical Group
New Hartford, New York

Vivek Ramakrishnan, DO
Spine Fellow
UC San Diego
San Diego, California

Kevin Ray, DO
Neurosurgery Resident
Riverside University Health System Medical
    Center
Moreno Valley, California

**Colleen Rose, RN, BSN, MS, CNRN, SCRN,
    APRN, NP-C**
Neurosurgery & Neurocritical Care Nurse
    Practitioner
Desert Regional Medical Center
Palm Springs, California

**Javed Siddiqi, HBSc, MD, DPhil (Oxon),
    FRCSC, FAANS, FACS**
Chair of Neurosurgery
Riverside University Health System Medical
    Center
Moreno Valley, California
Chief of Neurosurgery
Arrowhead Regional Medical Center
Colton, California
Neurosurgery Residency Program Director
Desert Regional Medical Center
Palm Springs, California

Paula Snyder, RN, CCRN
ICU Nurse Manager
Riverside University Health System Medical
    Center
Moreno Valley, California

John Spitalieri, DO
Neurosurgeon
NC Neurosurgery and Spine Clinic
Fayetteville, North Carolina

Gayatri Sonti, DO, MS, PhD
Neurosurgeon
Neuro & Headache Center
Rockford, Illinois

Raed Sweiss, DO
Skull Base Neurosurgery Fellow
Oregon Health and Science University
Portland, Oregon

Jon Taveau, DO
Neurosurgeon
Mount Vernon, Illinois

Margaret Wacker, MD, MS
Neurosurgeon
Arrowhead Regional Medical Center
Colton, California

Justen Watkins, DO
Neurosurgery Resident
Riverside University Health System Medical
    Center
Moreno Valley, California

Daniel J. Won, MD
Neurosurgeon
Kaiser Permanente
Fontana, California

David T. Wong, MD, FACS
Chief of Trauma and Critical Care Services
Arrowhead Regional Medical Center
Colton, California

Bailey Zampella, DO
Neurosurgery Resident
Riverside University Health System Medical
    Center
Moreno Valley, California

1 Bedside Neurologic Exam

Robert Dahlin, Dan E. Miulli, and Javed Siddiqi

Abstract
The bedside neurologic exam is the most sensitive test to determine the condition of the patient in the neurosurgical intensive care unit. It should be conducted frequently and consistently, whether the person is in a coma or not. Each part of the neurologic exam, from higher mentation to the cranial nerve exam and motor, sensory, and reflex exam, pinpoints the astute clinician to a specific pathology and anatomy.

Keywords: aphasia, coma, cortical exam, cranial nerve exam, eye exam, Glasgow Coma Scale, motor testing, verbal testing

Case Presentation

A 46-year-old woman presented to the emergency room with a spontaneous unilateral third nerve palsy manifested as a large, nonreactive pupil and minimal or no eye movement abnormalities. The patient had had a severe, and uncharacteristic, headache 2 days earlier, and she came to the emergency room only because of blurred vision. Other than the eye finding, the patient was awake and alert and in no acute distress, with a normal neurologic exam.
See end of chapter for Case Management.

1.1 Introduction

Patients admitted to the neurosurgical intensive care unit (NICU) are among the most critically ill and unstable. Many are admitted for traumatic brain injury, aneurysmal subarachnoid hemorrhage, spinal cord injury, postoperative craniotomies, stroke, and much more. With the advent of improved laboratory data and advanced imaging techniques, the physical examination has become less emphasized in training. While imaging and laboratory data augment our clinical decision making, the decision to order these tests and their interpretation should be influenced by the patient's physical exam. A detailed physical examination, with attention to all of the subtleties, is necessary to guide the treatment of a patient and the decision to order tests. Knowledge of the physical examination and its terminology also allows for more effective communication among health care workers whose clinical decision making will rely on the information passed down to them.

1.2 The Power of Observation

In the NICU, as elsewhere, the art of medicine should never be underestimated. While in many NICU patients, the neurologic exam is rendered more difficult by sedation, intubation, and paralytics, leaving the neurosurgeon and his or her team to rely on invasive monitoring data, serial neuroimaging, and intermittently withholding sedation to assess the patient, observation is still an important component of the patient's examination. For example, the obtunded or comatose patient breathing rhythmically in a specific pattern offers important lesion-localizing clues to the astute neurosurgeon (▶ Table 1.1). Observation of asymmetric spontaneous movements of the extremities, or change in their frequency, can be another clue to evolving brain or spinal cord lesions.

In the smaller number of awake patients in the NICU, the neurosurgeon has greater leeway to observe and converse with the patient. In these patients, observing whether they show any subtle localizing signs may betray early and enlarging focal lesions in the brain. For example, the patient who complains of

Table 1.1 Breathing patterns in brain injury

Breathing with rostral to caudal progression of lesions	Pattern	Location of lesion
Cheyne–Stokes	Periodic crescendo–decrescendo amplitude longer than variable pause, then repeat, yielding respiratory alkalosis	Generalized cerebral forebrain or midbrain lesion, metabolic encephalopathy without brainstem injury; impending herniation, congestive heart failure
Reflex hyperventilation	Hyperventilation with hypocapnia	Pons tegmentum, midbrain, reticular formation; psychiatric, metabolic acidosis, pulmonary congestion, hepatic encephalopathy
Apneustic	Irregular full inspiration then irregular pause	Pons, dorsal medulla, metabolic coma, transtentorial herniation
Cluster	Rapid irregular then pause	Pons, upper medulla, posterior fossa lesion; greatly increased intracranial pressure
Ataxic	No pattern	Medulla, acute posterior fossa lesion
No autonomic respiration (Ondine's curse)	Loss of autonomic respirations—awake normal breathing, no breathing during sleep or distraction	Reticular nucleus of medulla (respiratory center)
Apnea	No breathing	Bilateral damage to caudal medulla reticular nucleus
Kussmaul	Deep regular inspiration	Metabolic acidosis

a focal headache and who holds his hand over his head in the same area repeatedly, and on request is able to point to a specific area of his head as the site of most discomfort, may be helping the neurosurgeon with localization of an existent or developing lesion (tumor, hematoma, abscess, edema, etc.). This ability of the awake patient to localize the lesion for the neurosurgeon by effectively putting a finger on where it hurts the most, or showing the "Siddiqi sign," constitutes an observation and communication component of the neurologic exam with significant interobserver reliability (in patients without the confounding variables of recent soft tissue bruising or incision on the head). The value of focality of the Siddiqi sign is lost when the patient complains of a global headache, or pain "all over." A conscious attempt should be made in the NICU to not dismiss the initial observation of the patient in favor of exhaustive analyses of numerous data sets generated by an ever-increasing number of invasive monitoring techniques.

1.3 Coma

1.3.1 Glasgow Coma Scale

First published in 1974 by Graham Teasdale and Bryan Jennett, the Glasgow Coma Scale (GCS) has become a universally used tool for measuring a patient's overall state of alertness. Its score often guides medical decision making in neurointensive care. Despite its seeming simplicity there exists significant interrater variability. In an attempt to decrease this variability, a discussion will follow detailing the subtleties of this scale.

The GCS is calculated by adding up the points from each category, with motor receiving 6 points, verbal receiving 5, and eyes receiving 4. During an examination, the best scores for all three categories will be added together (▶ Table 1.2, ▶ Table 1.3). Patients are considered to be in a coma with a GCS of 8 or less.

Table 1.2 Glasgow Coma Scale (age 4 or more)

Points	Motor best response	Verbal/speech best response	Eyes best response
6	Obeys commands	–	–
5	Localizes to pain	Oriented conversation	–
4	Withdraws from pain	Confused conversation	Opens spontaneous
3	Decorticate—flexes abnormally	Inappropriate words	Opens to name or verbal stimuli
2	Decerebrate—rigid extension	Incomprehensible sounds	Opens to pressure/pain
1	No movement	No speech response	No eye opening
3–15	Add the totals of best responses from each column		

Table 1.3 Children's Coma Scale (age less than 4)

Points	Motor best response	Verbal/speech best response	Eyes best response
6	Obeys commands	–	–
5	Localizes to pain	Oriented, smiles, follows objects	–
4	Withdraws from pain	Confused but consolable	Opens spontaneous
3	Decorticate—flexes abnormally	Inappropriate, moaning	Opens to name or verbal stimuli
2	Decerebrate—rigid extension	Incomprehensible sounds, inconsolable	Opens to pressure/pain
1	No movement	No speech response	No eye opening
3–15	Add the totals of best responses from each column		

1.3.2 Motor Score

The motor score is measured out of a total of 6 points. A score of 6 points is given when a patient follows commands. Standard commands include asking patients to give a thumbs up, show two fingers, stick out their tongue, or wiggle their toes. Caution should be given when asking a patient to squeeze the examiner's hand during this part of the exam because this can often represent a frontal release sign in patients with lesions of the frontal lobe and may not indicate true command following.[1] Because of this, it is not recommended to use hand squeeze as a command. A score of 5 is given for localization. This can be interpreted as any purposeful movement performed by the patient, such as a limb crossing the midline to reach for painful stimuli or an endotracheal tube, to scratch an itch, or to fix the blanket. A score of 4 is given for withdrawal from painful stimuli. This can be given for a patient who tries to move away from a painful stimulus or who grimaces with pain. It is important not to confuse withdrawal with a spinal reflex. Withdrawal is held, whereas spinal reflexes return to a normal position while the stimulus is still being applied. The best location to perform a painful stimulus to determine withdrawal versus reflex is on the inner aspect of the upper arm. In withdrawal, the patient will move the arm away from the torso, or abduct the arm. In a reflex response, the patient will bring the arm closer to the torso, or adduct the arm. A score of 3 is given for abnormal flexion in response to painful stimuli. This is called the decorticate response and can include flexion at the biceps, wrist, or thighs or dorsiflexion without localizing to the stimuli. Decorticate posturing localizes the lesion in the brain to be above the red nucleus. Special attention should be given to the triple flexion response, which is often misinterpreted. It occurs in response to painful stimuli of the toes when a patient will dorsiflex the foot, flex at the knee, and flex at the thigh and is a form of decorticate posturing. A score of 2 is given for extensor posturing, also known as decerebrate posturing. In decerebrate posturing, there is disruption between the superior colliculi or the decussation of the rubrospinal pathway and the rostral portion of the vestibular nuclei. Decerebrate posturing consists of extension of the upper or lower extremities in response to painful stimuli. A score of 1 is given for no motor response to stimulation.

1.3.3 Verbal Score

The verbal score is measured with a total of 5 points. A score of 5 is given to patients who are oriented to name, where they are at, the date or year, and the reason they are in the hospital. Inability to answer these questions reliably constitutes a disoriented patient. A score of 4 is given when a patient is unable to answer all questions regarding orientation. However, the patient must be able to attempt to answer questions with a response that is appropriate to the question being asked. A score of 3 is given when a patient's response to a question is inappropriate to what was asked. A score of 2 is given when a patient's verbal responses are inaudible. This is constituted by mumbling, grunts, or other produced sounds. A score of 1 is given when a patient is nonverbal despite stimulation or questioning. All intubated patients receive a score of 1. However, to signify that their poor GCS score is a reflection of intubation and not neurologic injury a *T* will be placed at the end of the score to signify the patient cannot receive those points.

1.3.4 Eye Score

The eye score is measured with a total of 4 points. A score of 4 is given to patients who can open their eyes spontaneously or who, after being awakened, continue to keep their eyes open. It is important that patient not be given a score of 4 if the patient's eyes are stuck open. A score of 3 is given to patients who are able to open their eyes to voice or their name. A score of 2 is given to patients who are able to open their eyes only when stimulated with pain. A score of 1 is given to patients who do not open their eyes despite the level of stimulation given.

1.4 Cranial Nerves

The neurosurgical patient's cranial nerves may be examined quickly at bedside. Cranial nerve examination is important in identifying and localizing lesions. Multiple pathologies result in cranial neuropathies, including stroke, Chiari malformations with or without syringobulbia, fungal meningitis, posterior fossa surgery, cerebellopontine angle surgery, microvascular decompression of the trigeminal nerve, glomus jugulare tumors, and leptomeningeal carcinomatosis.

1.4.1 Cranial Nerve I: Olfactory Nerve

Olfaction is tested by supplying the patient with different odors and asking the patient to identify them. Each nostril should be tested individually. Allergic rhinitis is the most common cause of a loss or a decrease in smelling capacity. The most common neurologic cause results from significant head trauma that causes shearing of the olfactory bulb/fibers off the cribriform plate. Other causes include congenital diseases, such as Kallman syndrome, or tumors causing local compression.

1.4.2 Cranial Nerve II: Optic Nerve

Pupillary Light Reflex

The pupillary light reflex is perhaps the single most important neurologic reflex and the quickest way to get a neurosurgeon's attention. The reflex arc involved in the pupillary light reflex starts as light enters the retina and is transmitted along the optic nerve and synapses in the pretectal nucleus. Fibers from the pretectal nucleus then travel bilaterally to each Edinger–Westphal nucleus. From there, preganglionic parasympathetic fibers arise and travel with the oculomotor nerve and synapse in the ciliary ganglion and then travel in the short ciliary nerve to the sphincter muscle of the iris, leading to constriction of the pupil.

Afferent Pupillary Defect: Marcus Gunn Pupil

Afferent pupillary defect is caused by damage to the optic nerve. It can be identified by using the swinging light test. When light is directed toward the functional optic nerve the contralateral pupil will constrict normally. However, when the light is switched to the affected optic nerve, the pupil will dilate due to the pretectal nucleus receiving less light input from the damaged optic nerve.

Anisocoria

Differing pupillary diameters is termed anisocoria and is defined as a difference in pupillary size of at least 0.4 mm.[2] Anisocoria is present in 20% of the population and is generally not pathological until the difference is greater than 1 mm.[3]

Papilledema

Papilledema can be best viewed by funduscopic exam with pupillary dilation and is graded from 0 to 5 using the Frisen scale. Papilledema is characterized by haloing around the optic disc, elevation of the borders of the optic disc, and, at more severe stages, obscuration of the vessels at the optic disc. In studies it has been found to have a sensitivity of 100% and specificity of 98% for elevated intracranial pressure. However, this finding is age dependent, and in patients younger than 8 years old it indicates increased intracranial pressure in only 22% of patients.[4]

Visual Fields

Checking the visual fields is part and parcel of the cranial nerve II examination (see the discussion later in this chapter on this topic).

1.4.3 Cranial Nerve III: Oculomotor Nerve

The oculomotor nerve originates in the midbrain just anterior to the periaqueductal gray matter. The oculomotor nerve is responsible for innervation of the levator palpebrae superioris, medial rectus, inferior rectus, superior rectus, inferior oblique, and iris sphincter muscles. Loss of function of the oculomotor nerve can lead to pupillary dilation and an eye that deviates downward and laterally.

Pupil-Sparing Third Nerve Palsy

The nerve fibers that innervate the extraocular muscles travel on the periphery of the nerve and are subject to damage by microvascular pathology, such as hypertension, diabetes, or dyslipidemia. These palsies are typically incomplete and temporary, usually resolving within 3 months.[5]

Non-Pupil-Sparing Third Nerve Palsy

Multiple etiologies exist that result in unilateral dilation of a pupil, ranging from benign to life threatening and requiring emergent intervention. Although it is more typical of a neurocritical care patient to have malignant underlying pathologies, knowledge of the other causes is important to keep in mind when composing a differential diagnosis.

Mass Lesion

A mass lesion that results in uncal herniation and compression of the oculomotor nerve will lead first to a dilated pupil, followed by a nonreactive pupil.

Causes include intracerebral hemorrhage, cytotoxic edema from a stroke, subdural or epidural hematomas, and tumor. A special circumstance involving unilateral pupil dilation includes a posterior communicating artery aneurysm exerting local pressure on the oculomotor nerve.

Traumatic Mydriasis

Traumatic mydriasis arises from traumatic injury to the globe and results from either tearing of the iris sphincter muscle fibers or its nerve fibers innervating it.

Horner's Syndrome

Horner's syndrome consists of unilateral miosis, ptosis, enophthalmos, and anhidrosis. This is caused by a disruption at any point in the sympathetic innervation to the eye. Ptosis and enophthalmos are due to paralysis of Müller's muscles of the tarsal plates. Anhidrosis is due to sympathetic chain disruption in the carotid sheath.[6] Etiologies are numerous, but include Pancoast's tumor, lower cervical cord lesion, carotid injury/dissection, posterior inferior cerebellar artery occlusion (as a part of Wallenberg's syndrome), syringobulbia, and others.[7]

Adie's Pupil

Adie's pupil presents as a dilated pupil that is slow to react with light, but with almost normal response to accommodation. Adie's tonic pupil is thought to be caused by either a viral or a bacterial infection that leads to damage of the ciliary ganglion. Because patients with an Adie's pupil have damage only to the ciliary ganglion, the pupil will respond to parasympathomimetics, such as pilocarpine.

1.4.4 Cranial Nerve IV: The Trochlear Nerve

The trochlear nerve (CN IV) supplies the superior oblique muscle of the eyeball. It completely decussates in the superior medullary velum at the level of the inferior colliculus before exiting the brainstem posteriorly. Patients with trochlear nerve palsy will complain of double vision with downward gaze. On exam, the patient's pathological eye will be slightly more superior on downward medial gaze. Asking the patient to tilt the head to the contralateral side will improve the diplopia, whereas tilting the head to the ipsilateral side will worsen the diplopia.[8]

1.4.5 Cranial Nerve V: Trigeminal Nerve

The trigeminal nerve (CN V) is the largest nerve and exits the midlateral pons to supply sensation to the face and dura of the anterior and middle fossae (portio major nervi trigemini). Motor function is subserved by the motor root (portio minor nervi trigemini) supplying the muscles of mastication, tensor veli palatini, tensor tympani, and anterior belly of the digastric and mylohyoid muscles.

Corneal Reflex

The corneal reflex is elicited by stimulation of the cornea or eyelid with reflexive blinking of the eye. The afferent limb is conducted by the trigeminal nerve to the spinal trigeminal nucleus. The efferent limb is conducted by the facial nerve to elicit blinking. The V1 distribution of the trigeminal nerve can be tested by brushing either the upper eyelid or the sclera. The V2 distribution can be tested by brushing the lower eyelid.

Sensation

To test sensation each distribution of the trigeminal nerve should be checked for intact light touch, pinprick, and temperature. Each side should be compared to the patient's contralateral side because this can elucidate subtle deficiencies in sensation.

Motor

Motor can be tested by touching the cheeks and asking the patient to bite down and the examiner feels for the strength of the muscles of mastication.

1.4.6 Cranial Nerve VI: Abducens Nerve

The abducens nerve (CN VI) supplies the lateral rectus muscle of the eye. Malfunction of this cranial nerve can lead to double vision for the patient, with the affected eye being incapable of moving laterally past midline, resulting in the two eyes becoming dysconjugate.

1.4.7 Cranial Nerve VII: Facial Nerve

The facial nerve (CN VII) provides innervation to the facial muscles, platysma, and taste sensation to the anterior tongue. Motor function of CN VII to the face is tested by testing the platysma, smiling, pursing the lips, closing the eyes, and raising the eyebrows. Distinction of whether unilateral facial weakness is forehead sparing is pertinent to localization of the lesion. The cortex supplies innervation to the frontalis muscle bilaterally, and a stroke or mass lesion of the primary motor cortex will lead to a forehead-sparing paralysis on the contralateral side. Destruction of the facial nucleus or nerve will lead to complete paralysis of the ipsilateral side. Sensation of the facial nerve is assessed by taste to the anterior two-thirds of the tongue.

1.4.8 Cranial Nerve VIII: Vestibulocochlear Nerve

The vestibulocochlear nerve (CN VIII) provides sensation for sound and balance. Testing these nerves in an awake patient requires detailed assessment of each testable division of each nerve.

Oculocephalic Reflex: Doll's Eye Reflex

The oculocephalic reflex is important for the stabilization of images on the retina as the body and head move through space. As the semicircular canals change in orientation, signals are sent to the vestibular nuclei and through the medial longitudinal fasciculus to stabilize the eyes. Movement of the head in a patient with a functional reflex will cause the eyes to move to the contralateral side. Absence of this will result in no reflexive movement of the eyes. The absence of movement of the eyes is referred to as the doll's eye reflex because, at the time when the reflex was discovered, the eyes of dolls were painted on and would hence not move with movement of the head.

Vestibulo-ocular Reflex

The vestibulo-ocular reflex is tested by instilling approximately 30 to 100 mL of ice water into the external auditory canal (with an intact tympanic membrane) with the head of the bed at approximately 30 degrees. Patients with intact function will have a slow, tonic gaze toward the side of stimulation. Those without this reflex continue to stare ahead. This test evokes severe nausea and vomiting in an awake patient. This is most often performed on deeply comatose patients or those with suspected brain death.

1.4.9 Cranial Nerve IX: Glossopharyngeal Nerve

Gag Reflex

Glossopharyngeal (CN IX) and vagus (CN X) nerve function can be assessed with the gag reflex. This may be performed in an awake patient by stimulating the posterior pharynx with a tongue blade. The afferent sensory limb of the reflex stems from the glossopharyngeal nerve, and the motor limb from the vagus nerve.

1.4.10 Cranial Nerve X: Vagus Nerve

Cough Reflex

This reflex involves deep bronchial suctioning of an intubated patient. Sensory nerves within the bronchi respond to mechanical stimulation, sending afferents along the superior laryngeal nerve to the medulla. The efferents travel back along the vagus nerve to initiate a cough.

1.4.11 Cranial Nerve XI: Accessory Nerve

The accessory nerve is responsible for innervation of the sternocleidomastoid and trapezius muscles. The sternocleidomastoid can be tested by having patients rotate their head against the examiner's hand. The trapezius can be tested by having patients shrug their shoulders against resistance.

1.4.12 Cranial Nerve XII: Hypoglossal Nerve

The hypoglossal nerve innervates the muscles of the tongue and can be tested by having a patient stick the tongue out. Injury to this nerve can be visualized when a patient's tongue deviates to the ipsilateral side of injury. Caution should be exerted in a patient with facial paralysis because it can give the illusion of tongue deviation. To avoid this, the physician can ask the patient to touch the tongue to the nose.

1.5 Cortical Examination

1.5.1 Broca's Aphasia

Broca's aphasia results from damage to the dominant hemisphere's pars opercularis and pars triangularis. It is an expressive aphasia in which patients can comprehend what is said and they know what they would like to say in return, but they are unable to form the words. Patients are often able to use simple words, such as *yes* or *um*, or their name. Patients are often visibly frustrated. Patients with this aphasia are said to not have fluent speech.

1.5.2 Wernicke's Aphasia

Wernicke's aphasia results from damage to the dominant hemisphere's superior frontal gyrus. In this aphasia, patients are unable to comprehend what is heard and are unable to respond appropriately. They are unaware of their deficit and produce speech that either is inappropriate to the question or is composed of nonsensical words. This is considered an aphasia with fluent speech.

1.5.3 Conduction Aphasia

Conduction aphasia results from damage to the arcuate fasciculus, which is involved in direct transfer of information from the Wernicke's to the Broca's area. Patients with conduction aphasia are able to comprehend speech and string together novel sentences but are unable to repeat a phrase given to them. A way to test this would be to ask a patient to repeat "no ifs, ands, or buts."

1.5.4 Gaze Deviation

Prévost's Sign

Also known as Vulpian's sign, this refers to the acute and transient gaze palsy in a frontal lesion (e.g., infarct), which is toward the side of the lesion and away from the concurrent hemiparesis. The eyes can be brought to the other side with the oculocephalic maneuver or caloric testing. In contrast, thalamic and basal ganglia hemorrhages produce forced deviation of the eyes to the side contralateral to the lesion (wrong-way eyes).

Setting Sun Sign

The setting sun sign is defined as tonic downward deviation of the eyes and may include downbeating nystagmus. This results from midbrain compression of the interstitial nucleus of Cajal. It may exist with a constellation of other symptoms in Perinaud's syndrome. Perinaud's syndrome results from significant midbrain compression and presents with the setting sun sign, loss of pupillary light reflex, loss of convergence, and upper eyelid retraction.

1.5.5 Visual Fields

In order to understand deficits to the visual fields and how to localize the lesion within the brain, knowledge of the anatomy is crucial. The retina can be divided into the nasal hemiretina and the temporal hemiretina. Once light impacts the retina, impulses travel down the optic nerve where nerve fibers from the nasal hemiretina decussate at the optic chiasm to become the optic tract. Nerves of the optic tract synapse at the lateral geniculate ganglion. Nerve impulses then travel via the optic radiations to the primary visual cortex. Nerve fibers pertaining to the contralateral superior quadrant travel to the visual cortex via Meyer's loop, which travels in the temporal lobe.

The visual fields can be tested by either kinetic or static perimetry at an ophthalmologist's office or at the bedside by a confrontational field exam. A bedside confrontational examination is difficult to perform and must be carried out in a specific way, and in experienced hands it is capable of detecting only approximately 40% of lesions.[9] First a patient must cover one eye, then the physician will place a number of fingers in the right and left superior fields. A patient can then either state the number of fingers seen or note which ones appear blurrier or dimmer. The physician then can move to the inferior visual fields for testing. This is repeated for the contralateral eye and then without either eye being covered.

Monocular Blindness

Monocular blindness occurs from damage to the visual pathway anterior to the optic chiasm, which includes damage to the retina or the optic nerve. This typically occurs as a result of an embolic phenomenon from atherosclerotic disease. Temporary loss of vision as a result of embolic disease is termed amaurosis fugax.

Bitemporal Hemianopsia

Bitemporal hemianopsia results from damage to the central portion of the optic chiasm. This leads to bilateral loss of the temporal visual fields. The classic cause of this is a sellar mass, typically a pituitary adenoma.

Homonymous Hemianopsia

Homonymous hemianopsia results from damage to the visual pathway posterior to the optic chiasm. A complete lesion to the pathway leads to complete loss of vision of the contralateral visual fields. Typical causes include hemorrhagic stroke, ischemic stroke, or a mass lesion.

1.5.6 Hemineglect

Tactile Extinction

Tactile extinction is tested by applying a tactile stimulation bilaterally at the same time and asking the patient which side the stimulus occurred on. This can detect even subtle neglect at times. This can localize the lesion to the contralateral hemisphere.

Visual Extinction

Visual extinction is tested by asking a patient to add up the number of fingers simultaneously displayed bilaterally. The number of fingers on the side of neglect will often not be counted or recognized as present. This can localize the lesion to the contralateral hemisphere.

Hippus

This exam finding is characterized by irregular rhythmic dilation and contraction of the pupillary sphincter muscles. Hippus is often a normal phenomenon and may be seen in recovery from oculomotor nerve injury. It has been suggested by studies as an indication of underlying nonconvulsive status epilepticus.[10,11,12]

1.6 Cerebellar Examination

1.6.1 Dysdiadochokinesia

Dysdiadochokinesia represents a patient's difficulty with performing rapid alternating movements. This can be assessed by either rapid pronation/supination of the arms or hands, or by having patients tap their foot on the floor as fast as possible. This can localize the lesion to the ipsilateral cerebellar hemisphere.

1.6.2 Dysmetria

Dysmetria is also referred to as past-pointing sign. Patients are asked to touch their index finger to the examiner's finger, which is placed at the far end of the patient's reach. Patients with dysmetria will reach for a point that exists past the examiner's finger. This can localize the lesion to the ipsilateral cerebellar hemisphere.

1.6.3 Heel to Shin

This maneuver is performed by asking a patient to run the heel up and down the contralateral shin. Jerky performance or poor coordination can localize the lesion to the ipsilateral cerebellar hemisphere.

1.7 Spinal Cord Examination

Patients presenting to the emergency room or trauma bay with a spinal cord injury require special consideration in their initial management. This initial management and the potential need for immediate versus delayed surgical management will depend on the neurological findings on presentation and subsequent examinations during the patient's hospital stay.

The first indication that a patient may have a spinal cord injury occurs during the primary survey with the assessment of the ABCs. A patient presenting with hypotension and bradycardia may be the first indication of spinal cord injury and is suggestive of the patient being in either spinal shock or neurogenic shock.

Spinal shock must be differentiated from neurogenic shock during the initial evaluation to guide further management. Neurogenic shock results from a disruption of the autonomic pathways of the spinal cord above the level of T6[13] and can last from 24 hours to 6 weeks. Neurogenic shock presents as a distributive shock with warm extremities, hypotension, and often bradycardia. Spinal shock is a complete loss of all spinal cord functions, reflexes, and autonomic support. Therefore all patients with spinal shock are also in neurogenic shock. The end of spinal shock is heralded by the return of spinal cord reflexes, with the deep plantar response typically being the first to return, followed by the bulbocavernosus reflex, the cremasteric reflex, the ankle jerk, Babinski's reflex, and finally the knee jerk.[14]

The degree of injury is classified using the American Spinal Injury Association (ASIA) grading system. Ten muscle groups (the deltoid or biceps, wrist extensors, triceps, flexor digitorum profundus, hand intrinsics, iliopsoas, quadriceps, tibialis anterior, extensor hallucis longus, and gastrocnemius) are tested individually and graded on a scale of 0 to 5, and a detailed sensory exam with a pin must be conducted to define the sensory level of the patient.

Injuries that lead to spinal cord injury typically require significant forces and high mechanisms of injury. As such it is not uncommon to have patients with concurrent brain injury who may be unresponsive or unable to participate in an examination. In such patients, as long as they are not in spinal shock, localization of the level of injury by physical exam will rely heavily on the spinal reflex portion of the exam because this will be unaffected by level of consciousness.

1.7.1 Strength Exam

Muscle strength is graded using the Royal Medical Research Council of Great Britain Scale. It is scored on a range from 0 to 5 (▶ Table 1.4), and muscle groups that are unable to be assessed secondary to casting or other immobilization must be recorded as not testable.

A knowledge of which nerves innervate a muscle or at which level they leave the spinal canal is also necessary for localization of a lesion and can be seen in ▶ Table 1.5.

Table 1.4 Muscle strength grading

The most caudal segment of the spinal cord with *normal* sensory and motor function on both sides of the body denotes the intact level.	
Motor level is the caudal key muscle with at least grade 3 provided the key muscles above that level are judged to be normal	
0	Total paralysis
1	Palpable or visible contraction
2	Active movement, gravity eliminated
3	Active movement against gravity
4−	Active movement against less resistance
4	Active movement against some resistance
4+	Active movement against more resistance
5	Active movement against full resistance
NT	Not testable

Table 1.5 Muscle innervation

Dermatome	Nerve	Action	Muscle	Reflex
XI	Spinal accessory	Shoulder shrug	Trapezius	
C2–C4		Neck flexion	Sternocleidomas-toid	
C3–C4	Spinal accessory	Fixes scapula	Trapezius	
C3–C5	Phrenic	Inspiration, tV, FEV1	Diaphragm	
C4–C5	Dorsal scapular	Hand behind back and palm resistance	Rhomboids	
C5	Suprascapular	Lateral rotate arm at shoulder	Infraspinatus	
C5	Suprascapula	Arm abduction 0–15 degrees	Supraspinatus	
C5	Axillary	Arm abduction > 90 degrees	Deltoid	
C5	Musculocutane-ous	Flex supinated elbow	Biceps, brachialis	Biceps C5
C5–C6	Subscapular	Medial rotate arm at shoulder	Subscapularis	
C6–C7	Posterior interosseus	Supination	Supinator	
C5–C7	Long thoracic	Push at wall, scapula and back	Serratus anterior	

Table 1.5 continued

Dermatome	Nerve	Action	Muscle	Reflex
C6	Radial	Flex 1/2 supinated elbow	Brachioradialis	Brachioradialis C6
C6	Radial	Wrist extension 2–3	Extensor carpi radialis brevis/longus	
C5–T1	Anterior thoracic	Adduct arm	Pectoralis major	Pectoral
C6–C7	Median	Pronation	Pronator teres	
C6–C7	Median	Flex palm at wrist and hold 2–3 digit	Flexor carpi radialis	
C5–C7	Subscapular	Adduct horizontal arm	Teres major	
C7	Thoracodorsal	Adduct horizontal arm cough scapula > contract	Latissimus dorsi	
C7	Radial	Extend forearm	Triceps	Triceps C7
C7	Interosseous	Thumb away 1st digit in plane of palm	Abductor pollicis longus	
C7	Posterior interosseous	Finger extension at MP joint	Extensor digitorum	
C7	Posterior interosseous	Extend thumb	Extensor pollicis	
C7–C8	Ulnar	Flex palm at wrist and hold 4–5 digit	Flexor carpi ulnaris	
C8	Median	Flex fingers at DIP, 2–3 digit	Flexor digitorum profundus	
C8	Ulnar	Flex fingers at DIP, 3–4 digit	Flexor digitorum profundus	
C8	Median	Flex fingers at MP	Flexor digitorum superficial	
T1	Median	Extend fingers at PIP	Lumbricals	
T1	Median	Thumb at little finger	Opponens pollicis	
T1	Median	Thumb away (MC) from index plane palm	Abductor pollicis brevis	

(continued)

Table 1.5 continued

Dermatome	Nerve	Action	Muscle	Reflex
T1	Median	Flex first phalanx thumb	Flexor pollicis brevis	
C8–T1	Ulnar	Thumb at palm	First interossei	
C8–T1	Anterior inter-osseus	Flex distal pha-lanx thumb	Flexor pollicis longus	
T1	Ulnar	Fingers apart	Palmar interossei	
T1	Ulnar	Fingers together	Dorsal interossei	
T1	Ulnar	Thumb at index, in plane palm	Adductor pollicis	
T1	Ulnar	Abduct and flex 5 digit	Hypothenar (ab-ductor digiti quinti)	
T5–L2	Intercostal	Lift trunk umbil-icus deviation	Rectus abdomi-nis, I/E oblique	Abdominal cutaneous
L2	Femoral	Hip flexion	Iliopsoas	Cremasteric
L2–L3	Obturator	Adduct thigh	Adductor mag-nus, brevis/longus	
L3–L4	Femoral	Knee extension	Quadratus femoris	Patella L3–L4
L4	Deep peroneal	Dorsiflexion	Tibialis anterior	
L4–L5	Tibial/peroneal	Foot inversion	Tibialis anterior/ posterior	Medial ham-string
L4–L5	Superior gluteal	Abduct thigh medial rotation leg	Gluteus medius	
L4–L5	Superior gluteal	Flex thigh	Tensor fasciae latae	
L4–S3	Sciatic	Adducts thigh	Adductor magnus	Gluteal
L5	Deep peroneal	Great toe exten-sion	Extensor hallucis longus	
L5–S2	Inferior gluteal	Hip extension	Gluteus maximus	
S1	Sciatic	Knee flexion	Hamstrings bi-cep/ semitendi-nosus, semimem-branosus and biceps femoris	
L5–S1	Superficial peroneal	Foot eversion	Peroneus longus/ brevis	
L5	Deep peroneal	Toe 2–5 exten-sion	Extensor digito-rum longus/brevis	

Table 1.5 continued

Dermatome	Nerve	Action	Muscle	Reflex
S1–S2	Tibial	Plantar flex foot	Gastrocnemius/soleus	Achilles S1–S2
S1–S2	Tibial	Plantar flex toes	Flexor hallucis longus	
S2–S4		Clamp during rectal	Bladder, bowel, sphincter	Bulbocaver-nosus

Abbreviations: DIP, distal interphalangeal joints; I/E, internal/external; FEV1, forced expiratory volume in 1 second; MC, metacarpal; MP, metacarpophalangeal joints; PIP, proximal interphalangeal joint; tV, tidal volume.

Table 1.6 Reflex grading scale

Score	Description
0	Absent reflex
1+	Trace, or seen only with reinforcement
2+	Normal
3+	Brisk
4+	Nonsustained clonus (i.e., repetitive vibratory movements)
5+	Sustained clonus

1.7.2 Reflex Exam

Reflexes are graded as well on a scale of 0 to 5 as described in ▶ Table 1.6. During the exam it is important to note not only abnormal reflexes but also asymmetry between reflexes because this too will help in localization of a lesion. In the setting of spinal cord injury, reflexes will be normal above the level of injury, absent or hypoactive at the level of injury, and hyperactive below the lesion. In cases of malingering, when there is a question of an acute spinal cord injury, normal and symmetrical reflexes throughout would lead to questioning the validity of no movement and no response to painful stimuli in the awake patient.

1.7.3 Sensory Exam

Pinprick

Sensory examination using pinprick is the best way to localize a lesion—better than a motor or reflex exam. The assessment of fine touch checks for integrity of the posterior column–medial lemniscus pathway that transmits the sense of touch to the ipsilateral spinal cord's posterior column, decussates in the medulla, synapses in the thalamus, and ends in the postcentral gyrus. The sensory examination should be carried out by checking each dermatomal distribution in sequence (▶ Fig. 1.1). The subjective feeling of one dermatome should be compared to the contralateral side to detect subtle differences. Examination can be initiated with light touch but must be performed with pinprick to determine the specific dermatome.

Proprioception

The assessment of proprioception also checks for integrity of the posterior column–medial lemniscus pathway. It can be checked by movement of a patient's digits either upward or downward and asking the patient to identify the direction. Impaired proprioception is also suggested by a positive Romberg's sign.

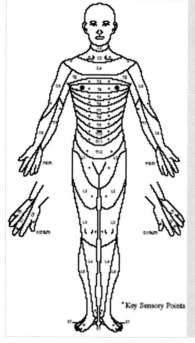

Fig. 1.1 Dermatomal and sensory nerve distribution. (Reproduced with permission from the American Spinal Injury Association.)

Temperature

The sensation of temperature first enters the spinal cord, where it immediately decussates before ascending in the anterolateral spinothalamic tract and synapses in the contralateral thalamus before traveling to the postcentral gyrus. It can be assessed by running an alcohol swab or cold utensil submerged in ice water over the dermatome of interest.

Hoffmann's Sign

This maneuver is performed by flicking the distal phalanx of the middle finger with reflexive flexion of either the index finger or the thumb. The presence of this finding is suggestive of a pyramidal tract lesion about the level of C5–C6. This sign should be interpreted with caution because it may be a normal finding in patients with hyperreflexivity, anxiety, or hyperthyroidism. Studies vary in terms of its accuracy, with sensitivity ranging from 58 to 94% and specificity ranging from 74 to 78%.[15,16,17]

Clonus Maneuver

The clonus maneuver is performed by rapid dorsiflexion of the foot with maintenance of the foot in the dorsiflexed position. The number of beats elicited from this maneuver is counted and is considered pathological if five or more beats are present. The presence of this exam finding is highly suggestive of pyramidal tract dysfunction.[18]

Babinski Maneuver

The Babinski maneuver is performed by scratching the lateral plantar surface with continuation to the transverse arch, lasting 5 to 6 seconds. Initial *extension* of the great toe with subsequent downward fanning of the other toes is the classic abnormal extensor response. The presence of this exam finding indicates pyramidal tract dysfunction. While Babinski's sign has a low sensitivity (~ 50%), it has a specificity for pyramidal tract dysfunction of 99%.[19]

Priapism

Priapism is sustained, unintended penile erection. In the context of spinal cord injury it is an ominous sign and is strongly associated with complete ASIA classification A (ASIA A) spinal cord injury. It is also associated with spinal shock. Priapism occurs immediately after injury and will not occur in a delayed fashion.

1.7.4 Rectal Exam

During the rectal examination of a patient five things should be noted in regard to spinal cord injury and can be recorded as present or absent. Pinprick sensation, active and passive rectal tone, anal wink reflex, and bulbocavernosus reflex (BCR). The BCR is a test of integrity of the S2, S3, and S4 nerve roots and involves contraction of the anal sphincter in response to squeezing of the glans penis or clitoris; it is the first reflex to return as spinal shock starts to recede, and as such is critical to determining the validity of the neurological exam after spinal cord injury. In a patient with a Foley catheter, this can be stimulated by gentle tugging on the catheter. The anal wink reflex tests the integrity of the S4, S5 nerve roots and is elicited by scratch or pinprick to the perianal region with reflexive contraction of the external sphincter ani muscle.

1.8 Malingering

Defined by the *Diagnostic and Statistical Manual of Mental Disorders, 4th edition* (DSM-IV) as "the intentional production of false or grossly exaggerated physical or psychological symptoms motivated by external incentives such as avoiding military duty, avoiding work, obtaining financial compensation, evading criminal prosecution, or obtaining drugs."[20] DSM-IV also recommends suspicion of malingering for patients who present with two or more of the following: medicolegal issues, disagreement between objective and subjective stress, noncompliance with evaluation or treatment, or antisocial personality disorder. Testing reflexes will help confirm malingering. An acute spinal cord injury will not have equal and symmetric reflexes; if this occurs additional methods must be used to confirm malingering. There are many physical exam tests to help support the diagnosis; however, evidence supporting it is lacking and is class C at best.

For the Hoover test, the physician places a hand under the thigh of the "paralyzed" leg and asks the patient to flex the contralateral thigh. A patient with true paralysis will not exert a downward force with the affected leg; however, patients with a nonorganic cause of paralysis should exert a downward force. One study tested a group of normal controls, patients with true hemiparesis, and patients suspected of feigning paralysis. A strain gauge was used under the affected leg to detect the downward force. The results of the study accurately distinguished between each group. However, in the study the strain gauge results were not compared to results of a physician-performed Hoover exam.[21]

Case Management

The mere presence of a spontaneous CN III palsy, especially one involving a large pupil unilaterally, should be considered an expanding or ruptured posterior communicating artery aneurysm until proven otherwise. The transient history of severe headache in this patient is suspicious for a sentinel bleed from a posterior communicating artery aneurysm. This patient needs a workup for subarachnoid hemorrhage, and at the minimum a computed tomographic angiogram to rule out an aneurysm. Should the patient turn out to have a ruptured aneurysm, or even an enlarging nonruptured aneurysm, she should be admitted to the NICU, with planned surgical or endovascular treatment of the aneurysm, because she has a high risk of catastrophic bleed.

References

[1] De Renzi E, Barbieri C. The incidence of the grasp reflex following hemispheric lesion and its relation to frontal damage. Brain. 1992; 115(Pt 1):293–313

[2] Lam BL, Thompson HS, Corbett JJ. The prevalence of simple anisocoria. Am J Ophthalmol. 1987; 104(1):69–73

[3] Ettinger ER, Wyatt HJ, London R. Anisocoria. Variation and clinical observation with different conditions of illumination and accommodation. Invest Ophthalmol Vis Sci. 1991; 32(3):501–509

[4] Tuite GF, Chong WK, Evanson J, et al. The effectiveness of papilledema as an indicator of raised intracranial pressure in children with craniosynostosis. Neurosurgery. 1996; 38(2):272–278

[5] Trobe JD. Managing oculomotor nerve palsy. Arch Ophthalmol. 1998; 116(6):798

[6] Yasumoto Y, Abe Y, Tsutsumi S, Kondo A, Nonaka S, Ito M. Rare complication of anterior spinal surgery: Horner syndrome [in Japanese]. No Shinkei Geka. 2008; 36(10):911–914

[7] Fountas KN, Kapsalaki EZ, Nikolakakos LG, et al. Anterior cervical discectomy and fusion associated complications. Spine. 2007; 32(21):2310–2317

[8] Keane JR, Baloh RW. Posttraumatic cranial neuropathies. Neurol Clin. 1992; 10(4):849–867

[9] Trobe JD, Acosta PC, Krischer JP, Trick GL. Confrontation visual field techniques in the detection of anterior visual pathway lesions. Ann Neurol. 1981; 10(1):28–34

[10] Jirsch J, Hirsch LJ. Nonconvulsive seizures: developing a rational approach to the diagnosis and management in the critically ill population. Clin Neurophysiol. 2007; 118(8):1660–1670

[11] Husain AM, Horn GJ, Jacobson MP. Non-convulsive status epilepticus: usefulness of clinical features in selecting patients for urgent EEG. J Neurol Neurosurg Psychiatry. 2003; 74(2):189–191

[12] Centeno M, Feldmann M, Harrison NA, et al. Epilepsy causing pupillary hippus: an unusual semiology. Epilepsia. 2011; 52(8):e93–e96

[13] Guly HR, Bouamra O, Lecky FE, Trauma Audit and Research Network. The incidence of neurogenic shock in patients with isolated spinal cord injury in the emergency department. Resuscitation. 2008; 76(1):57–62

[14] Ko HY, Ditunno JF, Jr, Graziani V, Little JW. The pattern of reflex recovery during spinal shock. Spinal Cord. 1999; 37(6):402–409

[15] Sung RD, Wang JC. Correlation between a positive Hoffmann's reflex and cervical pathology in asymptomatic individuals. Spine. 2001; 26(1):67–70

[16] Wong TM, Leung HB, Wong WC. Correlation between magnetic resonance imaging and radio-graphic measurement of cervical spine in cervical myelopathic patients. J Orthop Surg (Hong Kong). 2004; 12(2):239–242

[17] Glaser JA, Curé JK, Bailey KL, Morrow DL. Cervical spinal cord compression and the Hoffmann sign. Iowa Orthop J. 2001; 21:49–52

[18] Adams SE, Hoffman AF. Multi-beat clonus in a patient without an upper motor neuron lesion. A case report. J Am Podiatr Med Assoc. 1989; 79(4):194–196

[19] Isaza Jaramillo SP, Uribe Uribe CS, García Jimenez FA, Cornejo-Ochoa W, Alvarez Restrepo JF, Román GC. Accuracy of the Babinski sign in the identification of pyramidal tract dysfunction. J Neurol Sci. 2014; 343(1–2):66–68

[20] American Psychiatric Association. Diagnostic and Statistical Manual of Mental Disorders: DSM-IV. 4th ed. Washington, DC: American Psychiatric Association; 1994

[21] Ziv I, Djaldetti R, Zoldan Y, Avraham M, Melamed E. Diagnosis of "non-organic" limb paresis by a novel objective motor assessment: the quantitative Hoover's test. J Neurol. 1998; 245(12):797–802

2 Altered Mental Status and Coma: Pathophysiology and Management

Jason Duong, Shokry Lawandy, Jeffery M. Jones, Dan E. Miulli, and Javed Siddiqi

Abstract
Coma is not a lack of function but should be considered a derangement of function and possibly a disruption in neuroanatomy. When there is a change in the mental status usually there are lateralizing signs, but the brain's environment can be effected by seizures, metabolic changes, and other pathologies; it is the physician's responsibility to evaluate these processes.

Keywords: altered mental status, coma, consciousness, delirium, dementia, lateralizing signs, nonconvulsive status epilepticus, sundowning

---

Case Presentation

A 57-year-old woman was brought to the emergency room after being found on the kitchen floor in their home after the husband returned from the store. She was lethargic and confused, and this lasted about 5 hours in the emergency room. Her deficits included some slurred speech and mild left-sided weakness, but these symptoms seemed to resolve within the hour. She was in good health and took no medication other than hormone replacement for postmenopausal symptoms. The patient reported worsening early morning mild headaches over the last 2.5 years. Upon further workup, a computed tomographic (CT) scan demonstrated a 4 cm homogeneously enhancing left frontal-parietal mass with edema and 4 mm of midline shift.

See end of chapter for Case Management.

2.1 Altered Mental Status

2.1.1 Introduction

Before discussing the causes, categories, workup, or treatment of altered mental status (AMS), it is necessary to give a brief description of the term *consciousness*. Although this subject has philosophical, religious, and ethical connotations, simply stated, consciousness is the awareness of one's self and of one's environment, which includes people, places, and things. Consciousness also includes a multitude of higher mental functions, such as concept formation and the ability to manipulate these concepts. It is the physician's responsibility to evaluate these mental processes and compare them within the context of the patient's age, medical condition, baseline level of mental functioning, and numerous other factors, including comparison to the average mental functioning of the general population. This chapter discusses the evaluation process, differential diagnosis, and initial management of these patients in the neurosurgical intensive care unit (NICU).

2.1.2 Definitions

There are three major categories of AMS that should be defined: delirium, dementia, and coma. Dementia is a progressive and persistent loss of cognitive function, where both short- and long-term memory are impaired. These are typically associated with disorders such as aphasia, apraxia, and agnosia, and impairments of personality, planning, and critical and cognitive thinking.[1] It is critical to understand that dementia is a diagnosis of exclusion when other behavioral manifestations, such as delirium and other psychiatric diseases, have been ruled out.

Delirium, by definition of the American Psychiatric Association's *Diagnostic and Statistical Manual of Mental Disorders (DSM) 5th Edition*, consists of four key features[2]:

1. Disturbance in attention (i.e., reduced ability to direct, focus, sustain, and shift attention) and orientation to the environment.
2. Disturbance develops over a short period of time (usually hours to a few days) and represents an acute change from baseline that is not solely attributable to another neurocognitive disorder and tends to fluctuate in severity during the course of a day.
3. A change in an additional cognitive domain, such as memory deficit, disorientation, or language disturbance, or perceptual disturbance that is not better accounted for by a preexisting, established, or evolving other neurocognitive disorder.
4. Disturbances in numbers 1 and 3 must not occur in the context of a severely reduced level of arousal, such as coma.

The distinction between dementia and delirium is based on etiology and the time course of the disease process. Delirium is generally due to more acute, reversible processes, whereas dementia tends to be due to chronic, irreversible diseases. The following table summarizes and provides an overview of the characteristics of each (▶ Table 2.1).[3] Coma is a more severe depressed state, which will be further discussed later in this chapter.

Table 2.1 Comparison of altered states of consciousness[3]

Consciousness state	Definition	Pathophysiology	Time course	Disposition
Delirium	Acute confusional state, with impaired attention, perception, thinking, and memory	Always has an organic cause -Primary intracranial disease -Systemic disease -Exogenous toxins -Drug withdrawal	Acute	Often reversible when underlying etiology is addressed
Dementia	Implies a loss of mental capacity, short-term memory is particularly affected as well as cognitive abilities	Most are idiopathic (e.g., Alzheimer's, Parkinson's, vascular dementia)	Usually chronic and progressive	Usually not reversible, but can be treated symptomatically to a limited extent; only 10–20% have a reversible condition
Coma	Reduced state of alertness and responsiveness in which the patient cannot be aroused	Complex with many different sources (see below)	Usually acute or subacute	May be reversible if source is rapidly identified. The more time a patient spends in a coma the less favorable the prognosis

2.1.3 Approach to the Patient with Altered Mental Status

History

Because the patient most often will not be able to provide an accurate history, when evaluating the AMS patient for the first time, most of the history can be obtained from interviewing relatives or caregivers. A thorough history may reveal a recent illness, a history of drug abuse or alcoholism, depression, or a current medication list. If preceded by a trauma, mechanisms of insult and on-scene reports may help guide differential diagnoses and general approach to the examination.

Physical Exam

Within the NICU, the most common method for evaluating the patient's altered level of consciousness and confusional states is the Glasgow Coma Scale (GCS) (▶ Table 2.2). It is the most widely accepted score among physicians secondary to its high level of interexaminer and intraexaminer reliability. If the patient is uncooperative or confused, we should focus on the patient's vital signs, fluid balance, and general appearance. One can suspect hepatic failure if the patient is jaundiced, possible recreational drug abuse if needle tracks are noted, or possible seizure in a postictal state if there are signs of a bitten tongue. Any change in the GCS score of 2 points or more should be taken seriously and not dismissed as artifact.

The neurological exam in the NICU can reveal lateralizing signs of possible intracranial pathologies. Careful attention should be given to visual fields, cranial nerves, and motor deficits. It is also prudent to notice any changes from the initial presentation. Please see Chapter 1 for an overview of the neurological exam. However, it is important to note that absence of any focal findings does not exclude the possibility of focal neurologic lesions as the cause of the patient's delirium. If the patient is awake and alert with stable vital signs and no focal neurologic deficit, an assessment of mental status should be performed. The Mini Mental Status Examination (▶ Table 2.3) evaluates the patient's overall appearance, attitude, disorders of thought or perception, mood, insight, and judgment, as well as sensorium and intelligence. Points are allotted, with scores greater than 27, between 19 and 24, between 10 and 18, and less than 9 indicating normal, mild, moderate, and severe cognitive impairment, respectively (▶ Table 2.2, ▶ Table 2.3, ▶ Table 2.4).[1,5,6]

Table 2.2 Glasgow Coma Scale (3–15 points, higher points better)[4]

Score	Best motor response	Best verbal response	Best eye response
1	No response	No response	No response
2	Decerebrate posturing (extensor)	Incomprehensible sound	Open eyes to pain
3	Decorticate posturing (flexor)	Inappropriate speech	Open eyes to voice
4	Withdraws to pain	Confused (not oriented)	Opens spontaneously
5	Localizes to pain	Oriented	
6	Follows commands		

Table 2.3 Mini Mental Status Exam (0–30 points, higher points better)[4]

Total points	Test
5	What is the date, month, year, day of the week and season of the year (1 point each)
5	What is the hospital name, city, county, state, country (1 point each)
3	Name three objects after examiner, eg, apple, envelope, pen, eyeglasses (1 point each)
3	Recall the names of the three objects at 5 minutes (1 point each)
5	Serial 7's: Count back from 100 in 7's (1 point each correct answer up to 5)
2	Name a pencil and a watch
1	Repeat the phrase "No ifs, ands, or buts"
3	Three-stage command: e.g., "Take the paper in your right hand, fold it in half, and put it on the floor"
1	On a piece of paper or screen, read and obey: "Close your eyes"
1	Write a sentence
1	Copy the diagram shown to the right

2.1.4 Causes of Altered Mental Status

Careful attention must be given to the time of onset and the course of cognitive decline. It is prudent always to entertain delirium as a part of the working diagnosis and to rule out medical etiologies. The causes of altered mentation in the NICU are often different than those in the emergency room. NICU patients have head trauma, strokes, intracranial surgery, or other known sources of intracranial insult that could lead to an altered level of consciousness. Many times the neurointensivist is faced with a patient that was previously alert and aware prior to deterioration. The challenge to the neurointensivist is to identify the cause of the altered level of consciousness and institute the appropriate intervention for life-threatening conditions if need be. Acute neurologic disorders can include delayed presentations of subdural or epidural hematomas or seizures with the postictal state. Other common causes include the following:

- Drug or alcohol toxicity, including withdrawal syndromes (e.g., chronic alcoholics)
- Metabolic disorders (e.g., hypoglycemia, thyrotoxicosis)
- Infections (e.g., urinary tract infections, respiratory tract infections)
- Fluid and electrolytes (e.g., hyponatremia, hypernatremia)
- Cardiovascular issues (e.g., heart failure, acute myocardial infarction)
- Postoperative states (more common in the elderly)

Altered Mental Status and Coma: Pathophysiology and Management

Table 2.4 National Institutes of Health Stroke Scale (0–67 points)[4]

Item (score)	Item (score)	Item (score)
1a. Level of consciousness • Alert (0) • Drowsy (1) • Stuporous (2) • Coma (3)	4. Facial Paresis • Normal (0) • Flat nasolabial fold (1) • Partial paralysis (2) • Complete paralysis (3)	7. Limb ataxia • No ataxia (0) • Present in one limb (1) • Present in two limbs (2)
1b. Month and patient age • Both correct (0) • One correct (1) • None correct (2)	5a. Motor right arm • Normal (extends to 90 degrees without drift × 10 s) (0) • Drift (1) • Some effort against gravity (2) • No effort against gravity (3) • No movement (4) • Not testable (9)	8. Sensory • Normal (0) • Mild to moderate decrease (1) • Severe to total decrease (2)
1c. Open and close eyes or Squeeze and let go • Both (0) • One (1) • None (2)	5b. Motor left arm • Normal (extends to 90 degrees without drift × 10 s) (0) • Drift (1) • Some effort against gravity (2) • No effort against gravity (3) • No movement (4) • Not testable (9)	9. Best language • Normal (0) • Mild to moderate aphasia (1) • Severe aphasia (2)
2. Best horizontal eye movement • Normal (0) • Partial gaze palsy (1) • Forced deviation (2)	6a. Motor right leg • Normal (leg to 30 degrees for 5 s) (0) • Drift (1) • Some effort against gravity (2) • No effort against gravity (3) • No movement (4) • Not testable (9)	10. Dysarthria • Normal articulation (0) • Mild to moderate slurring (1) • Near complete dysarthria (2) • Intubated/not testable (9)
3. Visual field testing • Normal (0) • Partial hemianopia (1) • Complete hemianopia (2) • Bilateral hemianopia (blind) (3)	6b. Motor left leg • Normal (leg to 30 degrees for 5 s) (0) • Drift (1) • Some effort against gravity (2) • No effort against gravity (3) • No movement (4) • Not testable (9)	11. Inattention or extinction • Normal (0) • Extinction to one sensory modality (1) • Severe hemi-neglect (2)

It is beyond the scope of this book to give an exhaustive list of the possible causes of AMS. ► Table 2.5 presents the categories of causes and some of the most common etiologies of AMS in each category.

Table 2.5 Common causes of altered level of consciousness

Drugs and toxins: Prescription medications; nonprescription medications; drugs of abuse; withdrawal states, including delirium tremens, medication side effects, poisons (e.g., carbon monoxide, cyanide)

Infections: Sepsis, systemic infections, pneumonia, urinary tract infections, fever-related delirium

Metabolic derangements: Electrolyte disturbances (e.g. sodium, calcium, magnesium, phosphate), endocrine disturbances, hypercarbia, hyperglycemia, hypoglycemia, hyperosmolar and hypo-osmolar states, hypoxemia, Wernicke's encephalopathy, vitamin B12 deficiency, folate deficiency, niacin deficiency

Intracranial disorders: Encephalitis, meningitis, brain abscesses, epidural abscesses, epileptic seizures, nonconvulsive epilepticus, traumatic brain injury, increased intracranial pressure, hydrocephalus, hypertensive encephalopathy, psychiatric disorders

Systemic organ failure: Cardiac failure, acute myocardial infarction, hematologic disorders (e.g., thrombocytosis, hypereosinophilia, leukemic blast cell crisis, polycythemia), pulmonary disorders, pulmonary embolisms, renal failure

Physical disorders: Burns, electrocution, hyperthermia, hypothermia, polytrauma

Sundowning

This is a frequent, though poorly understood, symptom complex that generally occurs in patients with dementia or cognitive impairment, and usually manifests around sunset. Sundown syndrome refers to the emergence of neuropsychiatric symptoms, such as agitation, confusion, anxiety, and aggressiveness in the evening or at night.[7] It is thought to be associated with impaired circadian rhythmicity, and it appears to be mediated by degeneration of the suprachiasmatic nucleus of the hypothalamus and decreased production of melatonin.[7] Studies have shown that patients wakened from sleep during darkness experienced agitation, with a trend indicating the apparent worsening of agitation during the winter. This may suggest involvement of the circadian timing system.[2,8]

The diagnosis is clinical. There have been no laboratory values or imaging studies associated in the literature review. Management of sundowning includes encouraging increased activity, having the patient ambulate out of bed to the chair, exposure to light therapy during the day, and keeping a quiet and a dark environment during the night. It has been shown that bright light therapy has helped with agitated patients and restlessness in the elderly and patients with dementia.[9,10,11]

Nonconvulsive Status Epilepticus

Nonconvulsive status epilepticus (NCSE) can be underrecognized and can be a fairly common cause of altered mental status in the NICU. Once structural, metabolic, and iatrogenic causes of coma have been excluded, and NCSE workup should be the next step. Some clinical signs that may suggest NCSE include prominent bilateral facial twitching, unexplained nystagmus in obtunded patients, and unexplained automatisms, such as lip smacking, chewing, swallowing movements, acute aphasia, or neglect without a structural lesion. Continuous electroencephalographic (EEG) monitoring is necessary for the diagnosis and management of NCSE.

2.1.5 Workup for Altered Mental Status

The workup for AMS is driven mainly by the clinician's suspicion for a certain etiology. For example, a patient that has sudden onset of AMS with tonico-clonic-type movements would lead the physician toward a workup and intervention for a seizure. In a patient who has a known small epidural hematoma with a GCS score of 15 upon admission and deteriorates to a GCS score of 12, a stat CT should be ordered to further evaluate for possible hematoma expansion and the possible need for surgical intervention. If a postoperative craniotomy patient has a decreasing level of consciousness and fever, the suspicion of a postop infection should be entertained and a CT scan with contrast and a lumbar puncture will likely need to be performed. The noncontrast CT scan is used in many situations as the initial study for AMS because it gives information quickly as to whether there is a need for immediate surgical intervention. Once an anatomical source is ruled out, further testing should be ordered to find an etiology for the AMS. ▶ Table 2.6 gives common interventions for each major category of disease process.[4,12,13,14,15,16]

Table 2.6 Testing for altered level of consciousness for patients in the neurosurgical intensive care unit[16]

Category	Most common diagnostic modalities
1. Trauma	CT without contrast, ICP monitoring, brain metabolic monitoring
2. Epileptic	EEG, continuous EEG, MRI
3. Cerebrovascular	CT without contrast, carotid duplex, MRA, four-vessel angiography
4. Infectious	CT/MRI with and without contrast if warranted, blood cultures, sputum cultures, urine cultures, immunocompromised workup if warranted
5. Toxic/drug	CT (rule out anatomical disease), drug screen, toxin screen, EtOH level

Table 2.6 continued

Category	Most common diagnostic modalities
6. Metabolic	CT (rule out anatomical disease), metabolic profile (serum electrolytes, creatinine, glucose, calcium, complete blood count, urinalysis, urine cultures), liver function, Schilling test, EEG, folate, B12, thyroid function
7. Cardiopulmonary	EKG, cardiac enzymes, ABG, spiral CT, CT (rule out anatomical disease) if warranted
8. Psychiatric	CT (rule out anatomical disease), psychiatric consult, review medications and side effects

Abbreviations: ABG, arterial blood gas; CT, computed tomography; EEG, electro-encephalography; EKG, electrocardiography; EtOH, ethanol; ICP, intracranial pressure; MRA, magnetic resonance angiography; MRI, magnetic resonance imaging.

2.1.6 Interventions for Altered Mental Status in the Neurosurgical Critical Care Unit

Any particular intervention for AMS will be dependent upon the disease process. Processes that cause anatomical derangement should be managed in an emergent fashion. Subdural hematomas, epidural hematomas, contusions, and the like, are all disease processes that, if severe enough, will require emergent surgical intervention. A seizure will require anticonvulsant therapy, and if prolonged, in the case of status epilepticus or multiple seizures, may require emergent benzodiazepines. Cerebrovascular accidents of the ischemic type may be treated with clot-busting drugs or other interventional techniques if the time period is within certain guidelines. A large middle cerebral artery territory ischemic stroke may require a lifesaving decompressive craniectomy. Hemorrhagic strokes may require surgical intervention for evacuation of clot if the patient meets certain criteria (see Chapter 7). ▶ Table 2.7 shows some of the common interventions in each category. Many of these treatments and their specific implementation are covered in more detail in Chapters 26 and 27 of this book.

Table 2.7 Intervention for altered level of consciousness[16]

Category	Most common treatment modalities
1. Trauma	Craniotomy for evacuation of hematoma, craniectomy for ICP control, CSF drainage, osmotic diuretics
2. Epileptic	Anticonvulsants; benzodiazepines for status epilepticus, future vagal nerve stimulation, future epilepsy surgery
3. Cerebrovascular	Clipping/coiling of aneurysms, clot lyses, Merci extractor, stenting, endarterectomy, hematoma evacuation, craniectomy for ICP control in MCA strokes

(continued)

Table 2.7 continued

Category	Most common treatment modalities
4. Infectious	IV antibiotics, surgical debridement of infected hardware or abscess, sepsis management
5. Toxic/drug	Symptomatic treatment of drug and EtOH withdrawal
6. Metabolic	Lactulose, glycemic control, electrolyte correction
7. Cardiopulmo-nary	Anticoagulation, cardiology consult
8. Psychiatric	Psychiatric consult, antipsychotics, review of medication and side effects

Abbreviations: CSF, cerebrospinal fluid; EtOH, ethanol; ICP, intracranial pressure; IV, intravenous; MCA, middle cerebral artery.

2.2 Coma

Plum and Posner defined the normal wakeful conscious state in humans as serially time-ordered, organized, restricted, and reflective awareness of self and the environment and an experience of graded complexity and quantity.[16] Coma is a more severe form of depressed consciousness in which the person is incapable of perceiving self or environment, and the brain is not able to receive stimuli from the environment without aggressive stimulation. The patient's interaction with the environment during coma is at best reflexive.

Brain function has been found to show that cerebral oxygen had declined to 20% below normal levels in hepatic encephalopathy, lethargy, and global confusion. Other studies have shown deficiency in cholinergic function and excess release of dopamine, norepinephrine, and glutamate. The cholinergic system has been shown to provide the main input relay and the reticular nuclei of the thalamus from the upper brainstem. In fact, some studies have related coma to sleep states, where both conditions are due ultimately to the lack of activity of the ascending arousal system and where both impaired states of consciousness and non–rapid eye movement sleep are characterized by EEG patterns that include high-voltage slow waves.[17]

The GCS is the most commonly used grading system of consciousness (or coma) within the trauma setting. Coma is usually defined as a person who has a GCS score of 8 or less. These patients, at best, may open their eyes to painful stimulation and will localize to pain. Anatomically, coma can be caused by diffuse cortical dysfunction or by a dysfunction of the reticular activating system located in the brainstem (midbrain) (▶ Table 2.8).[18] Comatose patients remain motionless in an eyes-closed state without spontaneous eye movement, with total absence of patterned behavioral arousal or EEG features of the normal sleep–wake cycle. By definition, coma implies the state has endured for at least

1 hour, while eventually progressing through functional stages of the vegetative state (VS) and minimally conscious state (MCS).

The VS was first discussed by Jennett and Plum in 1972 and was associated with alternating periods of eye opening and closing in patients who do not show any signs of awareness of their environment. The most common causes of the VS are traumatic brain injury and cardiac arrest. Postmortem autopsies of patients who had been in VS show a loss of thalamic neurons near the thalamic intralaminar nuclei. Although diffuse axonal injury and hypoxic brain injury can cause severe loss of thalamic neurons, significant brainstem damage is not commonly found, emphasizing that VS is primarily a disorder of the corticothalamic system.

A VS is labeled as persistent once it lasts more than a month. It is considered permanent after 3 or 12 months, depending on the nature of the initial injury.[20] MCS is the first level of behavior recovery beyond VS, characterized by evidence of bedside responses to environmental stimuli. Such behavior can be visual tracking or fixation. Autopsies of patients who have died while in the MCS show no significant evidence of thalamic cell loss or severe diffuse axonal injury but show overall reduced cerebral cell death. Giacino et al[21] have suggested demonstration of the following behaviors in order to make the diagnosis of MCS:

1. Following simple commands.
2. Gestural or verbal yes/no responses (regardless of accuracy).
3. Intelligible verbalization.
4. Purposeful behavior, such as the following:
   a) Appropriate emotional responses to the linguistic or visual but not to neutral topics or stimuli.
   b) Vocalizations or gestures that occur in direct response to the linguistic content of questions.

Table 2.8 Glasgow Coma Scale[19]

Score	Best motor response	Best verbal response	Best eye response
1	No response	No response	No response
2	Decerebrate posturing (extensor)	Incomprehensible sound	Opens eyes to pain
3	Decorticate posturing (flexor)	Inappropriate speech	Opens eyes to voice
4	Withdraws to pain	Confused (not oriented)	Opens spontaneously
5	Localizes to pain	Oriented	
6	Follows commands		

c) Reaching for objects, demonstrating a relationship between object location and direction of reach.

d) Touching or holding objects, accommodating the size and shape of the object.

e) Pursuit eye movement or sustained fixation that occurs in direct response to moving or salient stimuli.

2.2.1 Initial Care of the Comatose Patient

There are often three types of comatose and obtunded patients a neurosurgical consultant will encounter. The first type is a patient with overwhelming structural brain injury with a poor prognosis for persistent VS. The second type is a patient who initially shows an early recovery. The third type of patient has a mix of both structural brain injuries with diffuse metabolic alterations. Most neurosurgical services do not become involved in the initial evaluation of a patient presenting to the emergency room in a coma of unknown etiology; however, it is useful to review the proper initial management of a comatose patient who has not received any laboratory or radiographic workup (▶ Table 2.9).

Table 2.9 Initial management of comatose patient[18,19]

Ensure patent airway and adequate oxygenation	Start mechanical ventilation or O_2 by mask if patient breathing on own
Protect C-spine	Immobilize C-spine with cervical collar
Maintain MAP above 100	Use fluids and vasopressors as necessary
Treat possible metabolic issue after initial blood draw	Thiamine 100 mg IV then glucose 25 g IV (d50)
Treat increased ICP if there is strong suspicion	Mannitol 0.25–1 g/kg bolus
Treat seizures	Benzodiazepine IV (lorazepam 2 mg IV)
Restore acid–base balance	Judicious use of fluids (0.9% saline preferred)
Treat any suspected drug overdose	Naloxone 0.2 mg IV and repeat; physostigmine 1 mg IV; Flumazenil 0.2 mg IV
Rule out space-occupying lesion	Stat CT scan of head
Normalize body temperature	Warm fluids and warming blankets
Treat any suspected meningitis or systemic infection	Wide spectrum antibiotics
Specific therapy ASAP	

Abbreviations: ASAP, as soon as possible; CT, computed tomography; ICP, intracranial pressure; IV, intravenous; MAP, mean arterial pressure.

2.2.2 Examination of a Comatose Patient

The exam for a comatose patient is much simpler than that for the awake patient, similar to the general format previously in this chapter. An advantage is the short length of the exam that must be performed within an emergent situation to yield critical information for patient care. The following exam items will allow specific localizations in unresponsive patients:

1. Mental status: document the level of consciousness with details of the specific responses along with the GCS. The subtle examination findings may be interpreted differently in a comatose patient when the scale is vague. In addition, this will allow repeating exams to be followed in a more detailed manner.
2. Cranial nerve exam.
   a) Ophthalmoscopic exam (CN II).
   b) Vision (CN II): blink to threat.
   c) Pupillary responses (CN II, III) (see oculomotor responses).
   d) Extraocular movements and vestibulo-ocular reflexes (CN III, IV, VI, VIII)
      1. Spontaneous ocular movements, nystagmus, dysconjugate gaze, oculo-cephalic maneuvers, caloric testing (brainstem reflexes).
   e) Corneal reflex, facial asymmetry, grimace response (CN V, VII).
   f) Gag reflex (CN IX, X).
3. Sensory and motor exam.
   a) Spontaneous movements.
   b) Withdrawal form painful stimuli.
4. Reflexes.
   a) Deep tendon reflexes.
   b) Plantar response.
   c) Posturing reflexes.
   d) Special reflexes suspected spinal cord lesions.

2.2.3 Causes of Coma

Causes of coma can be broken down into four main categories: structural, metabolic, electrical, and self-induced or iatrogenic. Structural lesions cause coma by physically interfering with nervous system pathways, either by trauma, compression by tumor, or increased pressure. Structural brain dysfunction is due to anatomical derangement of pathways due to physical phenomena. Metabolic causes of coma result from chemical derangements leading to improper functioning of the nervous system or some of its components (▶ Table 2.10).[18] Irrespective of specific etiology, for coma to occur there are limited final common pathways of damage necessary, including the following:

1. Diffuse impairment of both cerebral hemispheres.

Table 2.10 Structural and metabolic causes of coma[16]

Structural coma	Metabolic coma	
Hematoma	Hypoglycemia	Hypo-/hyperthermia
Trauma	Adrenal failure	Hypo-/hyperosmolality
Tumor	Liver disease	Diabetic ketoacidosis
Hydrocephalus	Renal disease	Encephalopathy
Abscess	Pulmonary disease	Drugs
	Dialysis dysequilibrium	Toxins

2. Impairment of the midline and paramedian upper brainstem and basal forebrain regions containing nuclei associated with the ascending reticular activating system.

Structural lesions can cause coma through three general mechanisms: compression of the brainstem, direct damage to the brainstem, or diffuse dysfunction of bilateral cerebral hemispheres. Damage to the brainstem can occur through a primary effect on the brainstem, such as a tumor, hemorrhage, or infarct of the brainstem, or it can be due to external pressure on the brainstem by another part of the brain that contains the pathology. This can be due to pathology that causes transtentorial herniation of the diencephalon or medial temporal lobe, or it can be due to a posterior fossa lesion causing compression of the brainstem. On the other hand, unilateral hemispheric lesions or lesions of the brainstem at the level of the midpons or below, should not cause coma.[17]

Supratentorial pathology tends to lead to one of the herniation syndromes as listed here. The herniation syndromes, especially uncal and central herniation, pass through four general stages: the diencephalic stage, the mesencephalic–pontine stage, the pontomedullary stage, and the medullary stage. The relay of the thalamic nuclei provides the largest source of input to the cerebral cortex; therefore, thalamic lesions that are sufficiently large can produce the same result as bilateral hemispheric cortical injury. For example, the "tip of the basilar" syndrome can cause bilateral thalamic infarction. The tonsillar and cingulate herniation syndromes may be progressive, but their progression is less well defined. Posterior fossa lesions may also cause supratentorial type herniation by causing an obstructive hydrocephalus, which can also lead to herniation (▶ Table 2.11, ▶ Table 2.12, ▶ Table 2.13).[17,19]

Table 2.11 Supratentorial herniation syndromes[22]

	Central herniation	Uncal herniation	Tonsillar herniation	Cingulate herniation
Lesion location	Diffuse supratentorial increase in intracranial pressure with no pressure gradient from right to left	Usually unilateral lesions, especially those located in the temporal lobes	Posterior fossa space-occupying lesions	Usually unilateral lesions, especially those located above the temporal lobes
Structures involved	Diencephalic compression progressing to pressure on the reticular activating system	Ipsilateral cranial nerve III, ipsilateral posterior cerebral artery, contralateral cerebral peduncle	Medullary respiratory center	Anterior cerebral artery
Signs/symptoms	Altered level of consciousness	Ipsilateral pupil dilation, ipsilateral hemiparesis (Kernohan's notch phenomenon)	Respiratory arrest	Leg weakness

Table 2.12 Stages of herniation[22]

Central herniation	Diencephalic stage	Mesencephalic-pontine stage	Pontomedullary stage	Medullary stage
Consciousness	Agitation or drowsiness	Comatose	Comatose	Comatose
Respiration	Sighs and yawns	Cheyne–Stokes respiration or tachypnea	Regular or shallow and rapid	Slow, irregular rate and depth and possible hyperpnea with apneic periods
Systemic responses	Diabetes insipidus (DI)	Hypothalamic dysfunction (DI, poikilothermia)		Fluctuating pulse, drop in blood pressure
Pupils	Small (1–3 mm) reactive	Midposition (3–4 mm), fixed	Small-midposition and fixed	Dilated and fixed
Eye movements	Roving eye movements	Vestibulo-ocular reflex im-	No vestibulo-ocular reflex	No vestibulo-ocular reflex

(continued)

Table 2.12 continued

Central herniation	Diencephalic stage	Mesencephalic-pontine stage	Pontomedullary stage	Medullary stage
	Vestibulo-ocular reflex may be weak or brisk No caloric response No vertical eye movement	paired with possible dysconjugate response	No oculocephalic response	No oculocephalic response
Motor	Worsening of existing hemiplegia Decorticate posturing	Decerebrate posturing	Flaccid flexor response	Flaccid, no deep tendon reflexes

Table 2.13 Stages of uncal herniation[19]

	Early third nerve stage	Late third nerve stage
Consciousness	Agitated or drowsy	Obtunded
Respiration	Normal	Hyperventilation
Pupils	Relative dilation of ipsilateral pupil	Fully dilated pupil
Eye movements	Oculocephalic normal or dysconjugate	
Motor	Appropriate to pain (localizes), contralateral Babinski's sign	Possible ipsilateral hemiplegia (Kernohan's notch) decerebrate

Metabolic causes of coma can include respiratory changes leading to acid–base changes, hyperventilation, and metabolic encephalopathy.[17] Mechanisms that can cause irreversible anoxic-ischemic brain damage, disorders of glucose (including both hypoglycemia and hyperglycemia), diseases of the liver, kidneys, or pancreas, and adrenal disorders can cause changes in mental status and coma. Diabetes is the most common endocrine disorder presenting as undiagnosed stupor and coma where most diabetic patients are prone to nonketotic hyperglycemic hyperosmolar coma, ketoacidosis, lactic acidosis, hyponatremia, hypophosphatemia, uremia-hypertensive encephalopathy, hypotension, or even sepsis. Other endocrine disorders that one may see in the neurosurgical setting include thyrotoxicosis in an elderly patient, where the usual signs of hypermetabolism are masked with depression and apathy. ▶ Table 2.10 can be reviewed for common causes of coma.[18]

Electrical causes of coma include seizure disorder or nonconvulsive status epilepticus. In status epilepticus, generalized convulsions occur in intervals so closely spaced that consciousness is not regained between them. It is important to recognize status epileptics because the cumulative systemic and cerebral anoxia can produce irreversible brain damage or death. NCSE is especially difficult to diagnose because of the absence of visible seizure activity; thus the layperson's description of this entity as silent or invisible status epilepticus. NCSE is usually characterized by delirium, stupor, and coma with trace or no motor activity.[17] In one study of 236 comatose patients with no overt clinical seizure activity, EEG demonstrated 8% of patients meeting the criteria of no convulsive status epilepticus.[18] The patients at risk are usually noncompliant with anticonvulsant drugs, or during the neurological exam subtle twitching of the face and/or extremities can be seen. When the diagnosis is still suspected and not seen on EEG, a trial of intravenous anticonvulsant may be warranted where improvement in EEG or clinical state can also confirm the diagnosis. Instead of spot EEG testing in suspected NCSE patients, continuous EEG is recommended.

Self-induced or iatrogenic causes of coma include sedative and psychotropic drugs, ethanol intoxication, drugs of abuse, or any drugs that cause intoxication causing metabolic acidosis. Coma may be caused by amphetamines, cocaine, 3,4-methylenedioxymethamphetamine (MDMA), tricyclic antidepressants, lithium, benzodiazepines, methaqualone, barbiturates, alcohol, and opioids.[17]

2.2.4 Respiratory Patterns in Coma

The pattern of respiration can give some insight as to the source of coma and possibly indicate where in the brain the dysfunction lies. ▶ Table 2.14 summarizes the different types of respirations and their meaning. Both metabolic and structural lesions can give rise to abnormal respiratory patterns.[22,23]

Table 2.14 Abnormal respirations in coma[23,24]

Respiration type	Description	Anatomical structure	Causes
Cheyne–Stokes	Periodic breathing, tachypnea alternates regularly and gradually with apnea	Unknown	Prolonged circulation time, bilateral suprapontine neurologic injury
Hyperventilation	Rapid, regular breathing	Not associated with a particular lesion site	Metabolic and physiological disorders acidosis
Apneustic	Inspiration cramp; excessive inspiration relative to expiration	Structure responsible remains unclear Pontine transaction just rostral to the	Brainstem demyelinating lesions and cervicomedullary compression have

(continued)

Table 2.14 continued

Respiration type	Description	Anatomical structure	Causes
		trigeminal motor nuclei and to the nucleus parabrachiales (case reports)	been associated with this ventilatory pattern
Ataxic	Breathing varies irregularly in depth as well as in frequency	Pons and medulla	Medullary lesions are probably the only reliable predictor of lesion site

2.2.5 Ocular Findings in Coma

A patient's ocular findings are the most informative findings in a comatose patient, especially in those patients who do not have a motor response to noxious stimuli. Some generalizations can also be made, especially concerning the pupillary responses:

1. Normal pupillary responses strongly favor a metabolic process in a coma of unknown origin.
2. The size of the pupils can give a clue as to the type of metabolic process that may be involved (e.g., narcotic overdose, anticholinergic toxicity).
3. Pupillary responses can be the most useful information regarding metabolic versus structural lesions, short of imaging (▶ Table 2.15).[24]

Table 2.15 Ocular and periocular findings and their meaning[18,19]

Structure	Finding	Meaning
Eyelids	Widened palpebral fissure	Facial paralysis
	Absent corneal reflex	Dysfunction of 5th or 7th CN or their connection
Ocular movements	Ping-pong gaze	Bilateral cerebral dysfunction
	Horizontal gaze deviation	• Ipsilateral frontal eye field dysfunction • Contralateral seizure • Unilateral pons lesion gives ipsilateral gaze palsy
	Vertical gaze disturbance	Posterior diencephalic and midbrain dysfunction
	Ocular bobbing	Extensive structural pontine damage
	Dysconjugate ocular bobbing	Pontomesencephalic damage
	Reverse bobbing (fast phase upward)	Metabolic encephalopathy, most prominently in anoxia

2.2.6 Outcome and Prognosis

Although there is continued uncertainty regarding the outcome for any individual patient in coma, VS, or MCS, this section discusses some clinical pearls and the overall prognosis for these patients.[25] A general guide to developing a prognosis has already been discussed and is presented in ▶ Table 2.16. While understanding that coma, VS, and MCS are transitional states with unpredictable time frames, 40 to 50% of patients in a coma resulting from traumatic brain injury and 54 to 88% of patients in a coma resulting from cardiac arrest die. Generally, comatose patients post–traumatic brain injury have a higher likelihood of recovery than those post–cardiac arrest, and the younger the patients, the better the outcome.

Time frames for VS can vary, where posttraumatic VS are typically longer than those resulting from metabolic causes. It is generally accepted that a VS lasting 1 year will more likely be permanent. The prognosis in MCS is still being studied since it is relatively new. Luauté followed the course of 12 patients in VS and 39 in MCS for 5 years, and the data suggested the possibility of significant further recovery from MCS, albeit with severe disabilities, after 1 year follow-up.[25]

The prognosis for brain injury depends on the portion of the brain affected, the duration of the effect, and the quantity of the brain affected. Advances in recent years have led to 20% of those with GCS 3 surviving, with 10% having a functional survival. Those patients older than 60 years have the worst outcome. The complications of injury also affect outcome. If there is a single episode of hypotension or hypoxia, the morbidity and mortality increase. In patients with traumatic brain injury, traumatic subarachnoid hemorrhage and a midline shift greater than 0.5 to 1.5 cm predict a poor outcome. The brain part injured correlates directly with the amount of life alteration. Brain lesions in the dominant hemisphere are usually more devastating than nondominant hemisphere lesions. Injuries to the brain usually have short-term effects of depression, headaches, and changes in mood, judgment, memory, and behavior. The amount of change to normal lifestyle frequently depends on the degree of

Table 2.16 Level of consciousness and disability from National Traumatic Coma Data Bank

Duration of altered level of consciousness $N = 486$	Bad outcome (%)	Moderate disability (%)	Severe disability (%)
<7 days	12	2	0
7–14 days	25	8	0
15–28 days	28	18	3
>28 days	35	72	97

preinjury education, with those patients having higher education levels able to return to some productive lifestyle, whereas those with less formal education are often less able to meet the same expectations. In addition to education level portending prognosis, the length of loss of consciousness lends itself to disability prediction.

Case Management

The patient's condition had worsened despite the fact that her postoperative CT scan of the head showed a good surgical evacuation and correction of the midline shift. After ensuring the metabolic panel was normal, it was felt that obvious structural and metabolic causes of coma had been excluded, leaving the final possible cause of silent status epilepticus, a condition only diagnosable with EEG. A subsequent EEG scan confirmed the diagnosis of silent status epilepticus, which was then treated medically until resolution of the electrical abnormality on her EEG was realized. The patient awoke from her coma 2 days later, and ultimately was discharged from the hospital in good condition.

References

[1] Rummans TA, Evans JM, Krahn LE, Fleming KC. Delirium in elderly patients: evaluation and management. Mayo Clin Proc. 1995; 70(10):989–998

[2] Bliwise DL. What is sundowning? J Am Geriatr Soc. 1994; 42(9):1009–1011

[3] Giacino JT, Ashwal S, Childs N, et al. The minimally conscious state: definition and diagnostic criteria. Neurology. 2002; 58(3):349–353

[4] Greenberg M. Handbook of Neurosurgery. 4th ed. New York, NY: Thieme; 1996:553–563

[5] Folstein MF, Folstein SE, McHugh PR. "Mini-mental state". A practical method for grading the cognitive state of patients for the clinician. J Psychiatr Res. 1975; 12(3):189–198

[6] Fleming KC, Adams AC, Petersen RC. Dementia: diagnosis and evaluation. Mayo Clin Proc. 1995; 70(11):1093–1107

[7] Khachiyants N, Trinkle D, Son SJ, Kim KY. Sundown syndrome in persons with dementia: an update. Psychiatry Investig. 2011; 8(4):275–287

[8] Bliwise DL, Carroll JS, Lee KA, Nekich JC, Dement WC. Sleep and "sundowning" in nursing home patients with dementia. Psychiatry Res. 1993; 48(3):277–292

[9] Haffmans PM, Sival RC, Lucius SA, Cats Q, van Gelder L. Bright light therapy and melatonin in motor restless behaviour in dementia: a placebo-controlled study. Int J Geriatr Psychiatry. 2001; 16(1):106–110

[10] Lovell BB, Ancoli-Israel S, Gevirtz R. Effect of bright light treatment on agitated behavior in institutionalized elderly subjects. Psychiatry Res. 1995; 57(1):7–12

[11] Olde Rikkert MG, Rigaud AS. Melatonin in elderly patients with insomnia. A systematic review. Z Gerontol Geriatr. 2001; 34(6):491–497

[12] Siu AL. Screening for dementia and investigating its causes. Ann Intern Med. 1991; 115(2):122–132

[13] Lipowski ZJ. Delirium (acute confusional states). JAMA. 1987; 258(13):1789–1792

[14] Clarfield AM. The reversible dementias: do they reverse? Ann Intern Med. 1988; 109(6):476–486

[15] Consensus conference. Differential diagnosis of dementing diseases. JAMA. 1987; 258(23):3411–3416

[16] Plum F, Posner J. The Diagnosis of Stupor and Coma. Philadelphia, PA: FA Davis; 1980

[17] Posner JB, Saper C. Schiff N, Plum F. Plum and Posner's Diagnosis of Stupor and Coma. 4th ed. New York, NY: Oxford Press; 2007

[18] Towne AR, Waterhouse EJ, Boggs JG, et al. Prevalence of nonconvulsive status epilepticus in comatose patients. Neurology. 2000; 54(2):340–345

[19] Fisher CM. Brain herniation: a revision of classical concepts. Can J Neurol Sci. 1995; 22(2):83–91

[20] Fins JJ, Schiff ND. Shades of gray: new insights into the vegetative state. Hastings Cent Rep. 2006; 36(6):8

[21] Giacino JT, Ashwal S, Childs N, et al. The minimally conscious state: definition and diagnostic criteria. Neurology. 2002; 58(3):349–353

[22] Simon R. Respiratory manifestations of neurologic disease. In: Goetz C, Tanner C, Aminoff M, eds. Handbook of Clinical Neurology. Vol 19 (63). Elsevier Science Publishers, B.V.; 1993:477–501

[23] North JB, Jennett S. Abnormal breathing patterns associated with acute brain damage. Arch Neurol. 1974; 31(5):338–344

[24] Levy DE, Knill-Jones RP, Plum F. The vegetative state and its prognosis following nontraumatic coma. Ann N Y Acad Sci. 1978; 315:293–306

[25] Luauté J, Maucort-Boulch D, Tell L, et al. Long-term outcomes of chronic minimally conscious and vegetative states. Neurology. 2010; 75(3):246–252

3 Neuroimaging and the Neurosurgical Intensive Care Unit Patient

Christopher Elia, Blake Berman, and Dan E. Miulli

Abstract

Once the clinician has obtained a history and performed a detailed physical examination inclusive of a sophisticated neurologic exam, a differential diagnosis can be determined. For the patient in the neurosurgical intensive care unit, imaging is vital to confirm pathology to begin treatment when such treatment should be precise to gain the best outcome. All imaging modalities, whether X-ray, magnetic resonance imaging, or ultrasound, can add details for the clinician in an attempt to provide the best possible care.

Keywords: blood signal, CT scan, MRI, spine fracture, spine stability, subluxation, transcranial Doppler, X-rays

Case Presentation

A 14-year-old boy sustains a head injury during a head-on collision with a tree while snowboarding without a helmet. He is brought to the emergency room, still awake and alert, but with a 4-cm laceration over his right temple and obvious cerebrospinal fluid (CSF) leaking from the injury site. A computed tomographic (CT) scan of the head shows a right temporal region skull fracture under the laceration, with the inner table of the skull depressed 1.5 cm into the cranial cavity.

See end of chapter for Case Management.

3.1 Introduction

The patient must be stabilized according to the ABCDEs. Most important to determine neurologic injuries is the history and neurologic exam. After the initial evaluation, the secondary survey includes lateral cervical spine X-rays. Some institutions have supplemented lateral cervical X-rays with CT scans with reconstructed views to rule out obvious fractures and malalignments. The quality of the lateral reconstructed cervical spine views depends on the thickness of the base films and their overlap; the smaller the thickness the better the quality of reconstruction. Additional X-rays or films will be taken as needed.

3.2 X-rays of the Skull and Spine

Skull X-rays may show nontraumatic abnormalities, such as congenital skull defects, skull lesions, or even foreign bodies.[1]

Traumatic linear fractures must be differentiated from vessel grooves and suture lines. Vessel grooves are thicker, and they may curve and branch. Suture lines are wide, jagged, and follow the course to meet other sutures.[2] Traumatic linear fractures are often associated with an epidural hematoma (EDH) or a subdural hematoma (SDH).[3]

Traumatic depressed skull fractures are best evaluated by CT scan using bone windows. It is important to determine if there is trauma to underlying brain if depression is greater than the thickness of the skull (8–10 mm). Contrecoup injuries of the brain must also be assessed. Do not confuse this with a bone shadow from bony prominences of the skull.

The fracture may appear within the suture of the calvarium, called diastasis or widening of the suture line. On follow-up films the fracture may grow if associated with a dural tear. This is rarely seen in pediatric patients and less so in the adult population (▶ Table 3.1).

Skull X-rays also demonstrate foreign bodies, postoperative changes, and extracranial material, such as reservoirs, plates, or screws, and intracranial material, such as shunt tubing, coils, or clips.

Spine X-rays may show nontraumatic abnormalities, such as congenital defects, degenerative processes, or pathological fractures. They are also useful in determining normal bony alignment and confirming stability of a fracture with the patient in a spinal orthosis.

Table 3.1 Classification of types of factures[1]

Types of fractures	Characteristics
Linear	Differentiate from vessel grooves and suture lines, often associated with EDH or SDH
Depressed	Best evaluated by CT bone window, depression is greater than thickness of the skull (8–10 mm)
Diastatic	Widens the suture line
Growing fracture	Wide fracture associated with dural tear, confirm with repeat imaging, rarely seen in pediatric patients and less so in adult population
Ping-pong fracture	Most likely seen in newborn, nonsurgical except for cosmetic purposes

Abbreviations: CT, computed tomography; EDH, epidural hematoma; SDH, subdural hematoma.

Table 3.2 Plain film imaging views and their uses[1,2,3]

X-ray	
Lateral cervical	Contours of anterior and posterior marginal line, spinolaminar line, and posterior spinous line Fanning of the spinous processes Prevertebral soft tissue swelling Atlantodental interval of 2.5–3 mm in adults Normal lordotic curvature Loss of vertebral height, fracture lines, disk height
Anterior-posterior	Evidence of rotation and compression
Open mouth odontoid	Evaluation of odontoid fractures Occipitoatlantal joints Lateral masses overhang of C1 and C2 not more than 7 mm Atlantoaxial alignment
Oblique anteroposterior and lateral views	Neural foramina, lamina, pedicles Measure angulation caused from compression or burst fractures
Oblique	Pedicles, lamina, facet joint, and pars interarticularis Useful to rule out spondylolysis

Traumatic findings include fractures, dislocation, subluxation, or rotation. The completed cervical spine evaluation must see from the craniocervical junction through T1. If there is too much soft tissue shadow on lateral views, reorder the X-ray, obtaining the "swimmer's view" X-ray (vs. standard lateral C-spine X-ray). A consistent process must be adhered to every time a cervical spine X-ray is obtained. On a lateral X-ray look for smooth contours of the anterior and posterior marginal line, and the alignment of the spinolaminar line. The alignment of the posterior spinous line is an approximation. When reviewing the posterior elements attention should be paid to the fanning of the spinous processes. After the bone is inspected the soft tissue should be reviewed. Prevertebral soft tissue swelling may indicate pathology. Approximations of normal width of the prevertebral tissue are 6 mm at C3 and 12 mm at C6.[2] The lateral cervical spine X-ray should include measurement of the atlantodental interval as an indicator of atlantoaxial subluxation; it should be 2.5–3 mm in adults. Other areas of concern are the normal cervical lordotic curvature and loss of vertebral height, or fracture lines, or a change in disk height. The same areas should be reviewed in the thoracic and lumbar spine. If there is a mechanism of injury that leads to cervical spine radiographs then it is usually a good idea to X-ray the thoracic and lumbar spines (▶ Table 3.2).

X-rays in the neurosurgical intensive care unit may be done after the application of a halo or tongs for traction to evaluate reduction after each addition of weights or manipulation of the device. X-rays will look for postoperative instrumentation placement. Dynamic films or flexion and extension films evaluate motion. These are most often used for cervical spine clearance but are also used to evaluate subluxation with spondylolisthesis and compression fractures. For cervical-spine clearance the patient must be alert and cooperative; the cervical spine cannot be cleared if there is more than 3.5 mm subluxation seen on the lateral film or if the patient has neurologic deficits.

3.3 CT Scans

3.3.1 Brain CT Scan

A CT scan is the best imaging tool for studying bone, hemorrhage, or other calcified structures. It is based on attenuation of the electron density of the material in the path of the X-ray beam. It is good for the initial assessment of head injury and neurologic deficits and patients who cannot have a magnetic resonance imaging (MRI) scan. However, a CT scan is prone to artifact from the densest material and cannot differentiate between soft tissues of similar densities and therefore is less advantageous for posterior fossa evaluation. It is contraindicated with contrast enhancement if the patient is in renal failure and blood urea nitrogen (BUN) is > 2.0 or there is a first-trimester pregnancy. CT scans can be completed with or without contrast. If suspecting a hemorrhage, obtain a noncontrasted CT head initially. Noncontrast CT scans can also be used to evaluate hardware placement and function with deep brain stimulators, intracranial pressure monitors and drains, external ventricular drains, and subdural catheters and as follow-up for residual or reaccumulation of hemorrhage. Contrasted CT scans are helpful when evaluating residual tumor or abscess when MRI is not accessible or tolerated by the patient.

The CT scan measures exposures in Hounsfield units from −1000 to 4000 progressing from dark (hypodense) to light (hyperdense):

Air → fat → water → CSF → brain tissue → subacute blood → liquid blood → clotted blood → bone → contrast → metals[4]

CT scans can demonstrate deleterious changes for the neurologic patient. This is useful when the neurologic exam is compromised by sedation or overmedication. The following are some CT scan signs of increased intracranial pressure[4]:

- Loss of sulci.
- Compressed ventricles, loss of fourth ventricle.
- Loss of cisterns.
- Midline shift.

Table 3.3 Types of herniation[3,4,5,6]

Subfalcine	Cingulated gyrus shifts under the falx
Central transtentorial	Diencephalon is forced through the incisura, obliteration of the quadrigeminal and perimesencephalic cisterns
Uncal	Uncus and hippocampal gyrus forced over the edge of the tentorium, decrease in suprasellar cistern followed by parasellar and interpeduncular cisterns
Upward	Cerebellar vermis ascends above tentorium, may cause hydrocephalus by compression of aqueduct of Sylvius and quadrigeminal cistern
Tonsillar	Cerebellar tonsils descend through foramen magnum (more likely seen on sagittal section of magnetic resonance imaging scan)

As the condition worsens the patient may progress to herniation (▶ Table 3.3).

Brain CT scans are useful for the evaluation of neurologic deficits, both new-onset and progressive, for following the progression of known pathology, such as hydrocephalus, infarction, edema, and intra-axial and extra-axial hemorrhage. Contrasted CT scans evaluate neurologic deficits when there is a suspected mass or infection.

The following are characteristic CT scan findings for bleeds[6]:

• Epidural hematoma (EDH): Biconvex or lentiform appearance, often underlying fractures, located between the skull and dura, may be limited by suture lines, usually seen in the acute phase when the lesion is hyperdense, areas of hypodensity indicate active bleeding.
• Subdural hematoma (SDH): Crescent shaped, between the brain and dura, may be acute (hyperdense), subacute (nearly isodense), or chronic (hypodense); areas of hypodensity indicate active bleeding in an acute SDH; areas of calcification may be seen in chronic SDH.
• Subarachnoid hemorrhage (SAH): Seen within the cisterns and sulci.
• Intracerebral hemorrhage (ICH): Seen in the putamen, caudate, cerebellum, and brainstem where hypertensive hemorrhages are likely to occur spontaneously.

EDHs are seen less frequently than SDHs and are usually the result of bleeding from a lacerated middle meningeal artery or dural venous sinus. If there is a loss of sulcal and gyral patterns on axial views near the vertex, order coronal and sagittal views to assess for a vertex EDH. These can be associated with fractures that extend midline and may be associated with damage to the superior sagittal sinus.

SDH is usually the result of bleeding from bridging cortical veins. SDHs conform to the contours of the brain and usually do not cross the midline but may cross suture lines. It is important to correlate the SDH width with the midline shift and edema. When patients present with what may seem like a small chronic SDH on imaging with edema and midline shift out of proportion to the SDH size, one must consider other possibilities, such as intracranial hypotension, subdural empyema, or even metastatic disease.

SAH should be suspected before or after an accident or in association with the worst headache of the patient's life. Most CT scans should be repeated in 12 to 24 hours. ICHs tend to recur after 6 to 12 hours. These patients can present posttrauma, and a careful history must be obtained to decipher if the patient ruptured an aneurysm, which led to a fall or motor vehicle collision, or if the fall/collision caused the SAH.

3.3.2 Spine CT Scan

CT scans of the cervical, thoracic, and lumbar spine in the acute setting are useful in the trauma patient when fractures or dislocations are suspected. The most important use of the CT scan when evaluating spine fractures is to identify unstable fractures.

For the mid and lower cervical spine, there are many criteria to identify unstable fractures. Sagittal plane displacement > 3.5 mm or 20% and/or sagittal plane angulation > 11 degrees on neutral films can be described as an unstable fracture. Flexion/extension films can also be assessed for > 3.5 mm or 20% displacement on the sagittal plane and/or > 20-degree rotation on the sagittal plane.[7,8] These patients will need an MRI scan of the cervical spine.

CT is useful for evaluating the bone and its alignment, such as when considering canal stenosis, degeneration, spontaneous hemorrhage, bony lesions, pathological fractures, traumatic fractures, or subluxation, or when planning for surgical approach and instrumentation. When suspecting a fracture obtain sagittal and coronal reconstructions for maximum benefit. There are also three-dimensional (3D) reconstructions that assist even further with fracture and malalignment identification. Although its use to evaluate soft tissue is limited, when used after myelography it becomes extremely helpful, such as when instrumentation obscures the view with MRI, the patient cannot tolerate MRI, or the patient has a history of multiple back surgeries. However, when concerned about changes within the spinal canal other than stenosis consider using MRI as the first advanced test. Contrasted CT scans can help identify osteomyelitis and tumor.

3.4 Establishing Cervical Spine Stability with the Use of Neuroimaging

Although a heavily debated topic, the use of neuroimaging is oftentimes required to establish stability in a cervical spine, such as in the awake/symptomatic patient, or even with the more controversial obtunded patient with a cervical collar. Some authors advocate for the use of MRI as the gold standard and for being superior to flexion-extension plain films, which they describe as being significantly less sensitive.[9] However, other studies attribute the inadequacy of flexion-extension plain films to poor study quality and stress that MRI should be reserved for the cases in which adequate flexion-extension films cannot be obtained.[10] "Adequate" flexion-extension plain films can identify underlying injury.[10] With the growing dependency on MRI as the most sensitive for detecting ligamentous injury and instability, the risk of overuse becomes an issue. A prospective study published in 2005 ($N = 2854$) identified 93 symptomatic patients with normal motor exams at the time of admission and found none of the MRI scans to be positive for occult injury. They concluded that MRI is not necessary in the awake/alert, symptomatic patient with a negative CT scan and a normal motor exam.[11]

Atlanto-occipital dislocation (AOD) is oftentimes missed on the initial survey of the CT C-spine. This injury should be suspected in all major trauma patients because it is highly unstable and needs emergent stabilization. MRI is not necessary to diagnose this condition. Type I odontoid fractures are very rare and are often associated with other underlying injury, such as AOD. Although individual measurements, such as atlanto-occipital interval (AOI), basion–axial interval (BAI), basion–dental interval (BDI), and Powers ratio are useful in diagnosing AOD, these values may be normal in patients with AOD. The subaxial cervical spine injury classification system (SLICS) is helpful in evaluating cervical spine injuries.[12] Please see Chapter 6 on spinal cord injury for further information.

3.5 Thoracolumbar Spine Stability

The thoracolumbar spine is commonly evaluated with CT scans, and MRI is useful for assessing ligamentous integrity, tumors, infections, and spinal cord injury. The three-column model is useful in identifying instability.[13] The thoracolumbar injury classification and severity (TLICS) score is helpful in evaluating thoracolumbar spine injuries.[14] (Please see Chapter 6 for further information.) Sagittal balance should be assessed on patients prior to surgical instrumentation to achieve normal curvature and avoid failed back syndrome.

Overall, with the growing accessibility of MRI and the advances in MRI technology, this modality has been used more frequently to assess for cervical spine stability. However, one must also be aware that other reasonable modalities exist for the clearance of a cervical spine and that MRI, although very sensitive, is not the only option available, especially in the awake and alert patient, regardless of whether the patient is with or without symptoms.

3.6 CT Scan Reformatted

CT scan information can be formatted in newer ways that have proven to be extremely beneficial, such as CT angiography (CTA). CTA provides a less invasive test than conventional angiography, with comparable results for many clinical situations. It aids with the diagnosis of arterial dissections, acute stroke, and aneurysms.

3.7 MRI

MRI is based on the relaxation characteristics of protons in differing chemical states. For the optimal scan the patient must not contain any ferromagnetic material in the area of interest. The MRI scan is quite different from the CT scan in that different information can be sought based on the different radiofrequency pulsations and magnetic gradients programmed prior to scanning. MRI does not use ionizing radiation, unlike CT. In the past the MRI scan has been more expensive because it was newer technology. Now the costs of MRI and CT are comparable so the initial advanced test after the history and physical should be an MRI scan when appropriate. It is not cost-effective to use CT first.

3.7.1 MRI Protocols

- T1-weighted image (T1WI):
  - Echo time (TE) < 50 ms, repetition time (TR) < 1000 ms.
  - Measured in intensity hypointense, isointense, hyperintense (from dark to bright): bone–calcium–CSF–gray matter–white matter–fat/melanin/blood > 48 h old.[5]
  - Most pathology is dark (hypointense = low signal).
  - Good for detecting gadolinium contrast enhancement.
- T2-weighted image (T2WI):
  - TE > 80, TR > 2000.
  - Dark to bright: fat–bone–white matter–gray matter–CSF–edema/water.
  - Notice that fat becomes dark on T2WI, whereas it is bright on T1WI.
  - Most pathology is light.
  - Gadolinium contrast enhancement does not cause much change in intensity of the signal.
  - Good for detecting pathological areas with edema, inflammation, or water (▶ Table 3.4, ▶ Table 3.5).
- Diffusion-weighted images (DWIs):
  - Based on movement of water in tissues.

Table 3.4 Characteristics of T1- and T2-weighted MRI[1,2,3]

	TR (ms)	TE (ms)	Bright to dark	Pathology
T1-weighted image	< 50	< 1000	Fat/melanin/ blood > 48 h White matter Gray matter Calcium CSF Bone	Dark
T2-weighted image	> 80	> 2000	Edema/water CSF Gray matter White matter Bone/Fat	Light

Abbreviations: CSF, cerebrospinal fluid; MRI, magnetic resonance imaging; TE, echo time; TR repetition time.

Table 3.5 Hemorrhage on MRI

Hemorrhage	T1-weighted image	T2-weighted image
Acute	Isointense (Gray)	Hypointense (Black)
Subacute	Hyperintense (White)	Hyperintense (White)
Chronic	Hypointense (Black)	Hypointense (Black)

- ○ Freely diffusing water (CSF) appears dark, whereas restricted diffusion seen with intracellular-edema-associated cell swelling from infarction appears bright.
- ○ Acute infarction appears bright within minutes.
- Perfusion-weighted images (PWIs):
  - ○ Use a bolus of gadolinium.
  - ○ Provide information on microcirculation and further insight into tissue infarction.
  - ○ Used in combination with DWIs to define the area of ischemic penumbra (tissue near the infarction zone that may be salvageable by thrombolytic therapy).

Other MRI protocols include fast spin echo, gradient echo, fluid-attenuated inversion recovery (FLAIR), short T1 inversion recovery (STIR), and proton density.

3.7.2 MRI and Brain Clinical Conditions

In general MRI is good for evaluation of soft tissue, posterior fossa lesions, small lesions, and seizure workup when quantifying the amount of specific tissue present, such as the size of the hippocampus. MRI is still not the most accepted study when evaluating acute bleeding in the brain or for bone evaluation. An MRI scan is much slower than a CT scan, the former being 20 to 40 minutes and the latter being seconds. It should not be used when patients have active pacemakers, known life-sustaining ferromagnetic implants, or any ferromagnetic implants directly in the area to be examined. Gunshot is not ferromagnetic unless a steel jacketed bullet is used, such as in the military.

MRI of the brain should be the first advanced scan in numerous conditions:

- Plain MRI.
  - Demyelinating disease.
  - Degenerative disease.
  - Edema.
  - Infarct to distinguish between old and new strokes.
  - Diffuse axonal injury—caused by shearing from rotation or deceleration/ acceleration, seen at the gray–white junction, corpus callosum, dorsolateral aspect of the upper brainstem, in order of frequency.
  - Midbrain and pontine injury.
  - Orbital compartment syndrome.
- Contrasted MRI.
  - Tumor.
  - Infection.
  - Inflammation of nerves.
  - Tumor residual.

3.7.3 MRI and Spine Clinical Conditions

MRI is also very useful in the spine, especially when soft tissue evaluation is essential. It is the evaluation of choice after the history and physical for a herniated disk and nerve root impingement, congenital abnormalities, stroke, hemorrhage, ligamentous injury, spinal cord injury, and spinal cord hemorrhage. In the spine MRI contrast and noncontrasted films are the imaging modalities of choice for tumors, including drop metastases; infection, including paravertebral lesion fistulas; extent of tumor removal; and postoperative infection.[6]

In facilities with a neurocritical care unit an MRI scanner must be available at all times, 24 hours a day. It is used emergently in patients with incomplete spinal cord injury, worsening neurologic deficit, or clinical evidence without radiographic proof of spinal cord injury.[4]

3.7.4 MRI and Other Clinical Conditions

It is used without contrast for peripheral nerve injury. Just as CT angiography provides detailed anatomy of the vessels in the brain or the large vessels of the spine, magnetic resonance angiography (MRA) demonstrates normal and pathological vascular anatomy, such as carotid-cavernous fistulas and vascular malformations, including aneurysms and arteriovenous malformations (AVMs). The venous phase of the circulation can also be specifically probed when one is looking for venous sinus thrombosis. MRI has been used in neuroscience for decades. It was once called nuclear magnetic resonance (NMR) but was changed because of the connotation with *nuclear*. However, NMR peered into tissue samples to examine their characteristic molecules. MR spectroscopy does the same thing on a much larger scale; it produces a graph based on chemical shift and is used primarily in the brain to help distinguish tumor from infection.[2]

3.8 Additional Imaging in the Neurosurgical Intensive Care Unit

Angiography is an invasive test having a 0.5 to 2% risk of major morbidity or mortality.[3] It also carries the risk of ionizing radiation. Although still the gold standard in many vascular cases it has been replaced in some large universities with CTA or MRA. In the community neurosurgical setting it remains the procedure of choice to investigate cerebral AVM, aneurysm, and carotid-cavernous fistula; evaluate tumor blood supply and embolization of arterial feeders and vasculitis; administer injection for vasospasm; and evaluate blunt cerebral vascular injuries, vessel injury in penetrating injuries like gunshot wounds, and pseudoaneurysm development. In the spine the angiogram can evaluate spinal AVM and dural fistula. However, recent studies investigating the use of 64-channel CTA demonstrates higher sensitivity rates than the previously reported 32-channel CTA and suggest that the 64-channel CTA may replace digital subtraction angiography as the primary screening tool for blunt cerebrovascular injury (BCVI).[15]

Nuclear medicine scans, such as bone scans, tagged white blood scans, and others, evaluate osteoblastic activity seen in infection, tumor, and abnormal metabolism. They can be used to differentiate between old and new fractures.

Transcranial Doppler has become an extremely useful tool in both trauma and cerebral vascular disease. It is performed at bedside to determine if there are vasospasms in the intracranial circulation as well as to assess the efficacy of thrombolysis in acute stroke and assist with the determination of brain death.

CT perfusion is performed using iodinated contrast with focus on different designated areas and vascular territories. Scans through the areas of interest are repeated every few seconds to assess perfusion.

Cerebral radionuclide angiography may be used as an adjunct for determining brain death, especially if an apnea test cannot be performed (e.g., in patients with chronic obstructive pulmonary disease or congestive heart failure). It is obtained by injecting 99mTc-labeled albumin and then obtaining serial anteroposterior images to assess uptake into the brain tissue.

Ultrasound has become critical to evaluating extracranial circulation, both carotid and vertebral, for the degree of stenosis as well as to evaluate the neonatal brain.

3.9 Radiology in the Neurocritical Care Unit

The brain and spinal cord cannot be directly visualized in the intact patient. The most important information for determining the disease process and treatment modalities in the neurocritical patient is acquired through the history and physical. After obtaining those details the disease and treatment should be highly suspected, and an opinion must be formed. Only after the opinion is formed may a radiographic examination be performed to confirm the clinical theorems. As such, good clinical skills will always surpass radiographic information.

Case Management

The patient has an open depressed skull fracture. In light of the CSF leakage from the laceration over the fracture, almost certainly this patient has an associated dural tear. Despite the good clinical condition of the patient, this is a serious condition with high infection risk, requiring early irrigation and debridement, elevation of the skull fracture, and repair of the dural laceration. The patient was taken to the operating room soon after arrival in the emergency room.

References

[1] Novelline RA. Squire's Fundamentals of Radiology. 5th ed. Cambridge, MA: Harvard University Press; 1997

[2] Osborn AG. Diagnostic Neuroradiology. St. Louis, MO: Mosby; 1994

[3] Greenberg M. Handbook of Neurosurgery. 7th ed. New York, NY: Thieme; 2010

[4] Layon AJ, Gabrielli A, Friedman W. Textbook of Neurointensive Care. Philadelphia, PA: Saunders; 2004

[5] Flaherty A. The Massachusetts General Hospital Handbook of Neurology. Philadelphia, PA: Lippincott Williams & Wilkins; 2000

[6] Winn HR. Youmans Neurological Surgery. 6th ed. Philadelphia, PA: Saunders; 2011

[7] White AA, III, Panjabi MM. The problem of clinical instability in the human spine: A systematic approach. In: White AA, Panjabi MM. Clinical Biomechanics of the Spine. 2nd ed. Philadelphia, PA: Lippincott Williams & Wilkins; 1990:277–378

[8] Panjabi MM. Clinical spinal instability and low back pain. J Electromyogr Kinesiol. 2003; 13 (4):371–379

[9] Duane TM, Cross J, Scarcella N, et al. Flexion-extension cervical spine plain films compared with MRI in the diagnosis of ligamentous injury. Am Surg. 2010; 76(6):595–598

[10] Insko EK, Gracias VH, Gupta R, Goettler CE, Gaieski DF, Dalinka MK. Utility of flexion and extension radiographs of the cervical spine in the acute evaluation of blunt trauma. J Trauma. 2002; 53 (3):426–429

[11] Schuster R, Waxman K, Sanchez B, et al. Magnetic resonance imaging is not needed to clear cervical spines in blunt trauma patients with normal computed tomographic results and no motor deficits. Arch Surg. 2005; 140(8):762–766

[12] Vaccaro AR, Hulbert RJ, Patel AA, et al. Spine Trauma Study Group. The subaxial cervical spine injury classification system: a novel approach to recognize the importance of morphology, neurology, and integrity of the disco-ligamentous complex. Spine. 2007; 32(21):2365–2374

[13] Denis F. The three column spine and its significance in the classification of acute thoracolumbar spinal injuries. Spine. 1983; 8(8):817–831

[14] Vaccaro AR, Lehman RA, Jr, Hurlbert RJ, et al. A new classification of thoracolumbar injuries: the importance of injury morphology, the integrity of the posterior ligamentous complex, and neurologic status. Spine. 2005; 30(20):2325–2333

[15] Paulus EM, Fabian TC, Savage SA, et al. Blunt cerebrovascular injury screening with 64-channel multidetector computed tomography: more slices finally cut it. J Trauma Acute Care Surg. 2014; 76(2):279–283, discussion 284–285

4 Diagnostic Laboratory Studies in the ICU Patient: What, When, and How Often?

John Ogunlade, Dan E. Miulli, and Jon Taveau

Abstract

Diagnostic laboratory studies assist in excluding or confirming a diagnosis when combined with a thorough history and physical examination so that a treatment plan can ultimately be formulated and performed in a precise manner. Laboratory studies are not meant to be ordered indiscriminately but strictly and critically to unmask the underlying pathological process.

Keywords: ASA Classification, blood dyscrasias, coagulopathy, electrolyte abnormalities, fluid disorder, metabolic disorders, preoperative testing, tumor markers

---

Case Presentation

An 18-year-old woman presents with acute onset of the worst headache of her life and decreased consciousness.

See end of chapter for Case Management.

4.1 Introduction

Diagnostic laboratory studies are tools used to enhance the overall clinical picture. They assist in excluding or confirming a diagnosis when combined with a thorough history and physical examination so that a treatment plan can ultimately be formulated and performed. Reassessing the patient and repeating diagnostic studies continue to confirm the diagnosis is accurate. This circular assessment sequence is the foundation of clinical medicine. It should be repeated as often as necessary.

In the intensive care unit (ICU) patient, every laboratory test order is critical to unmasking the underlying process, and proper use of every bit of information is imperative. Ordering multiple studies indiscriminately, the so-called shotgun approach, adds much confusion to the assessment as well as a terrible cost burden. By using a strict, sequenced, clinical approach to diagnosis, costs, mistakes, and misdiagnoses are lessened. ▶ Table 4.1 and ▶ Table 4.2 list common laboratory panels and normal laboratory values, respectively. This chapter serves to help streamline decision making in laboratory test selections and to better interpret the information provided by these tests.

Table 4.1 Common laboratory panels[1,2,3,4,5,6,7]

Adrenal function
Cortisol
Dexamethasone suppression test (DST)
Cosyntropin
Metyrapone test and corticotropin (ACTH)–releasing hormone (CRH)
Stimulation
Dehydroepiandrosterone sulfate (DHEA-S)
17-ketosteroids
17-hydroxycorticosteroids

Blood products
Type and cross: blood group (ABO), type (Rh type), Rh cross-match
Antibody
Coombs's antiglobulin (direct and indirect)
HLA analysis
Leukoagglutinin
Platelet antibody

Cardiac markers
CK
CK-MB
Troponin (I, t)
Homocysteine (Hcy)
Myoglobin

Coagulation
PT
INR
Partial thromboplastin time, activated (aPTT)
Bleeding time
Platelet count

Comprehensive metabolic panel (CMP)
Sodium
Potassium
Chloride
Carbon dioxide
BUN
Creatinine
Glucose
Calcium
Magnesium
Phosphorus
Total protein
Albumin
Alkaline phosphatase
ALT
AST
Bilirubin, total

CSF analysis (routine)
Color and clarity
Gram stain C&S
Cell count with differential (tubes 2 and 4)
Protein
Glucose

CSF analysis (selective for infection)
LDH
Lactate
Protein
Immunoglobulin
IgG–albumin index
IgG, IgA, and IgM against *Borrelia*, parasites, and viruses
Gram and Ziehl–Neelsen stain, touch prep
Bacterial, fungal, viral, and mycobacterial culture
DNA amplification (PCR) for tuberculosis and viral pathogens
Syphilis (VDRL and FTA)
Lyme disease
Candida albicans

CSF analysis (selective for cerebrovascular disease)
Cystatin C
Disseminated intravascular coagulopathy (DIC)
PT
INR
Partial thromboplastin time, activated (aPTT)
Bleeding time
Platelet count
D dimer
Thrombin time (TT), thrombin clotting time
Fibrin split products
Protein C&S
Antithrombin III
Fibrinogen antithrombin (I)
Coagulation factors
Encephalopathy
Folic acid
Vitamin B_{12}
TSH, T4 ammonia
Creatinine
Glutamine (CSF)

Hemogram with differential (CBC)
Hemoglobin
Hematocrit
Platelet count
RBC count
Red blood cell indices (MCV, MCH, MCHC)
WBC count
Absolute neutrophils, eosinophils, basophils, lymphocytes, and monocytes

(continued)

61

Hypercoagulable states
Protein C
Protein S
Antithrombin III
Factor V Leiden (activated protein C)
Homocysteine
Anticardiolipin antibodies
Lupus anticoagulant

Inflammation
ESR
CRP
ANA
Rheumatoid factor
Uric acid

Liver function
Total protein
Albumin
Alkaline phosphatase
ALT
AST
Bilirubin, total
Ammonia (NH_3)
γ-glutamyltransferase (GGT)
Prothrombin time (PT)
Platelet count
Serum protein electrophoresis

Renal function
CBC
CMP
24-hour urine creatinine
24-hour urine protein
Creatinine clearance

Toxicology screen
Acetaminophen
Carbon monoxide
Barbiturate
Ethanol
Ethylene glycol
Cocaine
Cyanide
Benzodiazepines
Tricyclic antidepressants
Methanol
Insulin

Abbreviations: ACTH, adrenocorticotropic hormone; ALT, alanine aminotransferase; ANA, antinuclear antibody; AST, aspartate aminotransferase; BUN, blood urea nitrogen; CBC, complete blood count; CK, creatine kinase; CK-MB, creatine kinase–MB mass; CMP, cytidine monophosphate; CRP, C-reactive protein; CSF, cerebrospinal fluid; DNA, deoxyribonucleic acid; ESR, erythrocyte sedimentation rate; FTA, fluorescent treponemal antibody; HLA, human leukocyte antigen; Ig, immunoglobulin; INR, international normalized ratio; LDH, lactate dehydrogenase; MCH, mean corpuscular hemoglobin; MCHC, mean corpuscular hemoglobin concentration; MCV, mean corpuscular volume; PCR, polymerase chain reaction; PT, prothrombin time; RBC, red blood cell; TSH, thyroid-stimulating hormone; VDRL, Venereal Disease Research Laboratory; WBC, white blood cell.

Table 4.2
Normal laboratory values [1,2,3,4,5,6,7]

Test	Specimen	Method	Normal range conventional units	SI units
Acetylcholine receptor antibody	Serum	Immunoassay	<0.5 nmol/L	<0.5 nmol/L
Acetylcholinesterase	RBC	Enzymatic colorimetry	11,000–15,000 U/L	11–15 kU/L
Adrenocorticotropic hormone (ACTH)	Plasma	Immunoassay	<70 pg/mL	<15pmol/L
Alanine aminotransferase (ALT)	Serum	Enzymatic colorimetry	<48 U/L	<0.80 mkat/L
Albumin	Serum	Colorimetry	3.5–5.0 g/dL	35–50 g/L
Aldolase	Serum	Enzymatic colorimetry	<8.1 U/L	<135 nkat/L
Aldosterone	Serum	Immunoassay	Supine: <16 ng/dL Upright: 4–31 ng/dL	Supine: <444 pmol/L Upright: 111–860 pmol/L
Alkaline phosphatase Isoenzymes	Serum	Electrophoresis	Intestinal: <18% of total activity Bone: 23–62% of total activity Liver: 38–72% of total activity	Intestinal: <0.18 of total activity Bone: 0.23–0.62 of total activity Liver: 0.38–0.72 of total activity
Total	Serum	Enzymatic colorimetry	20–125 U/L	0.33–2.08 mkat/L
Ammonia	Plasma	Enzymatic colorimetry	0.17–0.80 mg/mL	10–47 µmol/L
Amylase	Serum	Enzymatic colorimetry	30–170 U/L	0.50–2.83 mkat/ L
Androstenedione	Serum	Immunoassay	65–270 ng/dL Postmenopausal: <180 ng/dL	2.3–9.4 nmol/L Postmenopausal: <6.3 nmol/L

(continued)

Table 4.2 continued

Test	Speci-men	Method	Normal range conventional units	SI units
Angiotensin-con-verting enzyme (ACE)	Serum	Enzymatic color-imetry	8–52 U/L	133–867 nkat/L
Antidiuretic hor-mone (ADH)	Plasma	Extraction/immu-noassay	< 2.2 pg/mL (serum Osm < 285 mOsm/kg)	2.2–8.5 pg/mL (serum Osm > 290 mOsm/kg)
			< 2.2 ng/L (serum Osm < 285 mOsm/kg)	2.2–8.5 ng/L (serum Osm > 290 mOsm/kg)
Anti-DNA anti-body (double-stranded)	Serum	Immunoassay	< 30 U/mL	< 30 kU/ L
Antimicrosomal antibody (thyroid)	Serum	Immunoassay	< 0.3 U/mL	< 300 U/L
Antimitochondrial antibody	Serum	Immunofluores-cence	Negative (< 1:20)	
Antineutrophil cytoplasmic anti-body (ANCA)	Serum	Immunofluores-cence	Negative (< 1:20)	
Antinuclear anti-body (ANA)	Serum	Immunofluores-cence	Negative (< 1:40)	
Antithrombin III activity	Plasma	Nephelometry	85–130% of normal activity	0.85–1.3 of nor-mal activity
Antithrombin III antigen	Plasma	Enzymatic color-imetry	25–33 mg/dL	250–330 mg/L
Antithyroglobulin antibody	Serum	Immunoassay	< 1 U/mL	< 1 kU/L
α1-antitrypsin	Serum	Nephelometry	80–200 mg/dL	0.8–2.0 g/L
Apolipoprotein A-I	Serum	Nephelometry	Male: 94–176 mg/dL	Male: 0.94–1.76 g/L
			Female: 101–198 mg/dL	Female: 1.01–1.98 g/L
Apolipoprotein B	Serum	Nephelometry	Male: 52–109 mg/dL	Male: 0.52–1.09 g/L
			Female: 49–103 mg/dL	Female: 0.49–1.03 g/L

Table 4.2 continued

Test	Specimen	Method	Normal range conventional units	SI units
Apolipoprotein E	Serum	Nephelometry		
Apolipoprotein E4	Serum	Nephelometry		
Arsenic	Urine	ICP-MS	< 50 mg/d	< 0.65 mmol/day
Aspartate aminotransferase (AST)	Serum	Enzymatic colorimetry	< 42 U/L	< 0.7 mkat/L
Bilirubin				
Direct	Serum	Colorimetry	< 0.4 mg/dL	< 7 mmol/L
Indirect	Serum	Colorimetry	< 1.3 mg/dL	< 22 mmol/L
Total	Serum	Colorimetry	< 1.3 mg/dL	< 22 mmol/L
Bleeding time, template	Not applicable	Template method	2.5–9.5 minutes	
Cancer antigen (CA) 15.3	Serum	ABBOTT AXSYM	< 32 U/mL	< 32 kU/L
		CA15–3MEIA		
CA 19.9	Serum	CIS ELSA-CA 19–9 IRMA	< 33 U/mL	< 33 kU/L
CA 27.29	Serum	BIOMIRA TRUQANT	< 38 U/mL	< 38kU/L
		BR RIA		
CA 125	Serum	CENTOCOR-CA125IIRIA	< 35 U/mL	< 35 kU/L
Calcitonin	Serum	Immunoassay	Male: < 13.8 pg/mL	Male: < 13.8 ng/L
Calcitonin	Serum	Immunoassay	Female: < 6.4 pg/mL	Female: < 6.4 ng/L
Calcium	Serum	Colorimetry	8.5–10.3 mg/dL	2.12–2.57 mmol/L
	Urine	Colorimetry	Male: < 300 mg/d	Male: < 7.5 mmol/day
			Female: < 250 mg/d	Female: < 6.2 mmol/d
Carbon dioxide	Serum	Colorimetry	20–32 mmol/L	20–32 mmol/L
Carboxyhemoglobin	Blood	Spectrophotometry	< 2% of total Hb (nonsmoker)	< 0.02

(continued)

65

Table 4.2 continued

Test	Specimen	Method	Normal range conventional units	SI units
Carcinoembryonic antigen (CEA)	Serum	CHIRON ACS: 180 ICMA	< 2.5 ng/mL (nonsmoker)	< 2.5 mg/L (nonsmoker)
Catecholamines Fractionated	Plasma	HPLC	Dopamine	Dopamine
			Supine: < 90 pg/mL	Supine: < 588 pmol/L
			Standing: < 90 pg/mL	Standing: < 588 pmol/L
			Epinephrine	Epinephrine
			Supine: < 50 pg/mL	Supine: < 273 pmol/L
			Standing: < 90 pg/mL	Standing: < 491 pmol/L
			Norepinephrine	Norepinephrine
			Supine: 110–410 pg/mL	Supine: 650–2423 pmol/L
			Standing: 125–700 pg/mL	Standing: 739–4137 pmol/L
Total	Plasma	HPLC	Supine: 120–450 pg/mL	Supine: 709–2660 pmol/L
			Standing: 150–750 pg/mL	Standing: 887–4433 pmol/L
Ceruloplasmin	Serum	Nephelometry	25–63 mg/dL	250–630 mg/L
Chloride	Serum	ISE	95–108 mmol/L	95–108 mmol/L
Cholesterol, total	Serum	Colorimetry	Desirable: < 200 mg/dL	Desirable: < 5.17 mmol/L
			Borderline-high: 200–239 mg/dL	Borderline-high: 5.17–6.18 mmol/L
			High: > 240 mg/dL	High: > 6.21 mmol/L
Complement				
C3	Serum	Nephelometry	75–161 mg/dL	0.75–1.61 g/L
C4	Serum	Nephelometry	16–47 mg/dL	0.16–0.47 g/L
Total (CH 50)	Serum	Liposome lysis	31–66 U/mL	31–66 kU/L

Table 4.2 continued

Test	Speci-men	Method	Normal range conventional units	SI units
Complete blood count (CBC)	Blood	Automated analyzer		
Hemoglobin (Hb)			Male: 13.8–17.2 g/dL	Male: 138–172 g/L
			Female: 12.0–15.6 g/dL	Female: 120–156 g/L
Hematocrit (Hct)			Male: 41–50%	Male: 0.41–0.50
			Female: 35–46%	Female: 0.35–0.46
RBC count			Male: 4.4–5.8×10^6/mL	Male: 4.4–5.8×10^{12}/L
			Female: 3.9–5.2×10^6/mL	Female: 3.9–5.2×10^{12}/L
RBC indices			Mean corpuscular volume: 78-102 fL	Mean corpuscular volume: 78-102 fL
			Mean corpuscular Hb: 27–33 pg	Mean corpuscular Hb: 27–33 pg
			Mean corpuscular Hb concentration: 32–36 g/dL	Mean corpuscular Hb concentration: 320–360 g/L
			RBC distribution width: < 15%	RBC distribution width: < 0.15
WBC count			$3.8–10.8 \times 10^3$/µL	$3.8–10.8 \times 10^9$/L
WBC differential			Absolute neutrophils: 1,500–7,800 cells/mL	Absolute neutrophils: 1.5–7.8×10^9/L
			Absolute eosinophils: 50–550 cells/mL	Absolute eosinophils: 0.05–0.55×10^9/L
			Absolute basophils: 0–200 cells/mL	Absolute basophils: 0–0.2×10^9/L
			Absolute lymphocytes: 850–4100 cells/mL	Absolute lymphocytes: 0.85–4.10×10^9/L
			Absolute monocytes: 200–1100 cells/mL	Absolute monocytes: 0.2–1.10^9/L

(continued)

Table 4.2 continued

Test	Specimen	Method	Normal range conventional units	SI units
Platelet count			130–400 × 103/mL	130–400 × 10⁹/L
Cortisol, free	Urine	Immunoassay	20–90 mg/d	55–248 nmol/d
Cortisol	Serum	Immunoassay	4–22 mg/dL (morning specimen)	110–607 nmol/L (morning specimen)
			3–17 mg/dL (afternoon specimen)	83–469 nmol/L (afternoon specimen)
C-peptide	Serum	Immunoassay	0.8–4.0 ng/mL	0.26–1.32 nmol/L
C-reactive protein (CRP), creatine kinase (CK)	Serum	Nephelometry	< 0.8 mg/dL	< 8 mg/L
Isoenzymes	Serum	Electrophoresis	CK-MM: 97–100% of total	CK-MM: 0.97–1.00 of total
			CK-MB: < 3% of total	CK-MB: < 0.03 of total
			CK-BB: 0% of total	CK-BB: 0 of total
Total	Serum	Enzymatic colorimetry	Male: < 235 U/L	Male: < 3.92 mkat/L
			Female: < 190 U/L	Female: < 3.17 mkat/L
Creatinine	Serum	Enzymatic colorimetry	< 1.2 mg/dL	< 106 mmol/L
	Urine	Enzymatic colorimetry	Male: 0.8–2.4 g/d	Male: 7.1–21.2 mmol/day
			Female: 0.6–1.8 g/d	Female: 5.3–15.9 mmol/d
Creatinine clearance	Serum, urine	Calculation:	Male: 82–125 mL/min	Male: 1.37–2.08 mL/s
			Female: 75–115 mL/min	Female: 1.25–1.92 mL/s
Cyanide	Blood	Colorimetry	< 0.1 mg/L	< 3.8 mmol/L
D-dimer	Plasma	Slide latex agglutination	< 250 mg/L	< 250 mg/L
Dehydroepiandrosterone (DHEA), unconjugated	Serum	Immunoassay	130–1200 ng/dL	4.5–41.6 nmol/L

Table 4.2 continued

Test	Speci-men	Method	Normal range conventional units	SI units
Dehydroepian-drosterone sul-fate (DHEA-S)	Serum	Immunoassay	Male (age): 29 years 1.4–7.9 mg/mL	Male (age): 29 years 3.8–21.4 mmol/L
			30–39 years 1.0–7.0 mg/mL	30–39 years 2.7–19.0 mmol/L
			40–49 years 0.9–5.7 mg/mL	40–49 years 2.4–15.5 mmol/L
			50–59 years 0.6–4.1 mg/mL	50–59 years 1.6–11.1 mmol/L
			60–69 years 0.4–3.2 mg/mL	60–69 years 1.1–8.7 mmol/L
			70–79 years 0.3–2.6 mg/mL	70–79 years 0.8–7.1 mmol/L
			Female (age):	Female (age):
			29 years 0.7–4.5 mg/mL	29 years 1.9–12.2 mmol/L
			30–39 years 0.5–4.1 mg/mL	30–39 years 1.4–11.1 mmol/L
			40–49 years 0.4–3.5 mg/mL	40–49 years 1.1–9.5 mmol/L
			50–59 years 0.3–2.7 mg/mL	50–59 years 0.8–7.3 mmol/L
			60–69 years 0.2–1.8 mg/mL	60–69 years 0.5–4.9 mmol/L
			70–79 years 0.1-0.9 mg/mL	70–79 years 0.3–2.4 mmol/L
11-deoxycortisol	Serum	Immunoassay	<0.8 µg/dL	<23 nmol/L
Erythrocyte sedimentation rate (ESR)	Blood	Modified Westergren	Male: <20 mm/h	Male: <20 mm/h
			Female: <30 mm/h	Female: <30 mm/h
Erythropoietin	Serum	Immunoassay	<25 U/L	<25 U/L
Estradiol	Serum	Immunoassay	Male: <50 pg/mL	Male: <184 pmol/L
			Female:	Female:
			Follicular phase 10–200 pg/mL	Follicular phase 37–734 pmol/L

(continued)

Table 4.2 continued

Test	Speci-men	Method	Normal range conventional units	SI units
			Midcycle 100–400 pg/mL	Midcycle 367–1468 pmol/L
			Luteal phase 15–250 pg/mL	Luteal phase 55–954 pmol/L
			Postmenopaus-al < 50 pg/mL	Postmenopaus-al < 184 pmol/L
Estrone	Serum	Immunoassay	Male: 29–81 pg/mL	Male: 107–300 pmol/L
			Female:	Female:
			Follicular phase 37–152 pg/mL	Follicular phase 137–562 pmol/L
			Midcycle 72–200 pg/mL	Midcycle 266–740 pmol/L
			Luteal phase 49–114 pg/mL	Luteal phase 181–422 pmol/L
			Postmenopaus-al < 65 pg/mL (without HRT)	Postmenopaus-al < 240 pmol/L (without HRT)
Fatty acids, free	Plasma	Enzymatic color-imetry	0.19–0.90 mEq/L	0.19–0.90 mmol/L
Ferritin	Serum	Immunoassay	Male: 18–350 ng/mL	Male: 18–350 mg/L
			Female (age):	Female (age):
			15–49 years 12–156 ng/mL	15–49 years 12–156 mg/L
			> 49 years 18–204 ng/mL	> 49 years 18–204 mg/L
Fibrinogen	Plasma	Photo-optical clot detection	200–400 mg/dL	2–4 g/L
Folic acid	RBC	Immunoassay	> 95 ng/mL	> 215 nmol/L
	Serum	Immunoassay	> 1.9 ng/mL	> 4.3 nmol/L
Follicle-stimulat-ing hormone (FSH)	Serum	Immunoassay	Male (age): 20–70 years: 0.9–15.0 U/L	Male (age): 20–70 years: 0.9–15.0 U/L
			> 70 years: 2.8–55.5 U/L	> 70 years: 2.8–55.5 U/L
			Female: follicular phase 1.1–9.6 U/L	Female: Follicular phase 1.1–9.6 U/L

Table 4.2 continued

Test	Specimen	Method	Normal range conventional units	SI units
			Midcycle 2.3–20.9 U/L	Midcycle 2.3–20.9 U/L
			Luteal phase 0.8–7.5 U/L	Luteal phase 0.8–7.5 U/L
			Pregnancy < 0.9 U/L	Pregnancy < 0.9 U/L
			Postmenopausal 34.4–95.8 U/L	Postmenopausal 34.4–95.8 U/L
Free erythrocyte protoporphyrin (FEP)	Blood	Fluorometry	< 35 mg/dL RBGs	< 0.62 mmol/L RBGs
Fructosamine	Serum	Colorimetry	1.6–2.6 mmol/L	1.6–2.6 mmol/L
Gastrin	Serum	Immunoassay	< 200 pg/mL (nonfasting)	< 200 ng/L (nonfasting)
			< 100 pg/mL (fasting)	< 100 ng/L (fasting)
Glucagon	Plasma	Immunoassay	50–200 pg/mL	50–200 ng/L
Glucose				
Fasting	Plasma	Enzymatic colorimetry	< 110 mg/dL	< 6.1 mmol/L
Random	Serum	Enzymatic colorimetry	70–125 mg/dL	3.9–6.9 mmol/L
Glucose-6-phosphate dehydrogenase (G6PD)	Blood	Enzymatic colorimetry	5–13 U/g Hb	5–13 U/gHb
γ–glutamyl transferase (GGT)	Serum	Enzymatic colorimetry	Male: < 65 U/L	Male: < 1.08 mkat/L
			Female: < 45 U/L	Female: < 0.75 mkat/L
Growth hormone (GH)	Serum	Immunoassay	< 8 ng/mL	< 8 mg/L
Haptoglobin	Serum	Nephelometry	43–212 mg/dL	0.43–2.12 g/L
Hematocrit (Hct)	Blood	Automated analyzer	Male: 41–50%	Male: 0.41–0.50
			Female: 35–46%	Female: 0.35–0.46
Hemoglobin (Hb) A1c	Blood	Automated analyzer	Male: 13.8–17.2 g/dL	Male: 138–172 g/L

(continued)

Table 4.2 continued

Test	Specimen	Method	Normal range conventional units	SI units
			Female: 12.0–15.6 g/dL	Female: 120–156 g/L
	Blood	HPLC	< 6.0% of total Hb	< 0.06 of total Hb
Electrophoresis	Blood	Electrophoresis	Hb A1: < 96.0%	Hb A1: < 0.96
			Hb A2: 1.5–3.5%	Hb A2: 0.015–0.035
			Hb C: 0%	Hb C: 0
			Hb F: < 2.0%	Hb F: < 0.02
			Hb S: 0%	Hb S: 0
High-density lipoprotein (HDL) cholesterol	Serum	Precipitation/colorimetry	> 35 mg/dL	> 0.9 mmol/L
			"Negative" risk factor: > 60 mg/dL	"Negative" risk factor: > 1.55 mmol/L
Homocysteine	Plasma	HPLC	6.1–17.0 mmol/L	6.1–17.0 mmol/L
Homovanillic acid	Urine	HPLC	< 10 mg/d	< 55 mmol/d
Human chorionic gonadotropin (hCG)				
Qualitative	Urine	Immunoassay	Nonpregnant: negative	
			Pregnant: positive	
Quantitative (intact and free b)	Serum	Immunoassay	Male: < 2 U/L	Male: < 2 U/L
			Female:	Female:
			Premenopausal: < 5 U/L	Premenopausal: < 5 U/L
			Postmenopausal: < 10 U/L	Postmenopausal: < 10 U/L
			Pregnancy:	Pregnancy:
			0–2 wk < 500 U/L	0–2 wk < 500 U/L
			2–3 wk 100–5,000 U/L	2–3 wk 100–5000 U/L
			3–4 wk 500–10,000 U/L	3–4 wk 500–10,000 U/L

Table 4.2 continued

Test	Speci-men	Method	Normal range conventional units	SI units
			1–2 months 1,000–200,000 U/L	1–2 months 1000–200,000 U/L
			2–3 months	2–3 months
			10,000–100,000 U/L	10,000–100,000 U/L
17-hydroxycorti-costeroids	Urine	Enzymatic color-imetry	Male: 3–15 mg/d	Male: 8.3–41.4 mmol/d
			Female: 2–12 mg/d	Female: 5.5–33.1 mmol/d
5-hydroxyindole-acetic acid (5-HIAA)	Urine	HPLC	0.5–9.0 mg/d	3–47 mmol/d
Immunoglobulin				
IgA	Serum	Nephelometry	81–463 mg/dL	0.81–4.63 g/L
IgD	Serum	Radial immuno-diffusion	<14 mg/dL	<0.14 g/L
IgE	Serum	Immunoassay	<180 U/mL	<432 mg/L
IgG, subclasses	Serum	Nephelometry	Subclass IgG 1:450–900 mg/dL	Subclass IgG 1:4.5–9.0 g/L
			Subclass IgG 2: 180–530 mg/dL	Subclass IgG 2:1.8–5.3 g/L
			Subclass IgG 3:1380 mg/dL	Subclass IgG 3: 0.13–0.80 g/L
			Subclass IgG 4: 8–100 mg/dL	Subclass IgG 4: 0.08–1.00 g/L
IgC, total	Serum	Nephelometry	723–1685 mg/dL	7.23–16.85 g/L
IgM	Serum	Nephelometry	48–271 mg/dL	0.48–2.71 g/L
Insulin	Serum	Immunoassay	5–25 mU/mL	36–179 pmol/L
Iron	Serum	Colorimetry	25–170 mg/dL	4–30 mmol/L
Iron-binding capacity	Serum	Colorimetry	200–450 mg/dL	36–81 mmol/L
			% saturation: 12–57%	% saturation: 0.12–0.57
17-ketogenic ste-roids	Urine	Colorimetry	Male: 5–23 mg/d	Male: 17–80 mmol/d

(continued)

Table 4.2 continued

Test	Speci-men	Method	Normal range conventional units	SI units
17-ketosteroids, total			Female: 3–15 mg/d	Female: 10–52 mmol/d
	Urine	Colorimetry	Male: 9–22 mg/d	Male: 31–76 mmol/d
Lactate dehydro-genase (LD)			Female: 5–15 mg/d	Female: 17–52 mmol/d
Isoenzymes	Serum	Electrophoresis	LD1: 20–36% of total	LD1: 0.20–0.36 of total
			LD2: 32–50% of total	LD2: 0.32–0.50 of total
			LD3: 15–25% of total	LD3: 0.15–0.25 of total
			LD4: 2–10% of total	LD4: 0.02–0.10 of total
			LD5: 3–13% of total	LD5: 0.03–0.13 of total
Total	Serum	Enzymatic colorimetry	<270 U/L	<4.5 mkat/L
Lactic acid	Plasma (ve-nous)	Enzymatic colorimetry	9–16 mg/dL	1.0–1.8 mmol/L
Lead	Blood	Atomic spectroscopy	<25 mg/dL	<1.21 mmol/L
Lipase	Serum	Enzymatic colorimetry	7–60 U/L	0.12–1.00 mkat/L
Low-density lipo-protein (LDL) cholesterol, direct	Serum	Immunosepara-tion	Desirable: <130 mg/dL	Desirable: <3.36 mmol/L
		Colorimetry	Borderline–high: 130–159 mg/dL	Borderline–high: 3.36–4.11 mmol/L
			High: >160 mg/dL	High: >4.14 mmol/L
Luteinizing hor-mone (LH)	Serum	Immunoassay	Male (age): 20–70 years	Male (age): 20–70
			1.3–12.9 U/L	years 1.3–12.9 U/L
			>70 years 11.3–56.4 U/L	>70 years 11.3–56.4 U/L

Table 4.2 continued

Test	Speci-men	Method	Normal range conventional units	SI units
			Female:	Female:
			Follicular phase 0.8–25.8 U/L	Follicular phase 0.8–25.8 U/L
			Midcycle 25.0–57.3 U/L	Midcycle 25.0–57.3 U/L
			Luteal phase 0.8–27.1 U/L	Luteal phase 0.8–27.1 U/L
			Pregnancy < 1.4 U/L	Pregnancy < 1.4 U/L
Lymphocyte surface markers (T cell)			Postmenopausal 5.0–52.3 U/L	Postmenopausal 5.0–52.3 U/L
CD3	Blood	Flow cytometry	Absolute: 840–3060 cells/mL	Absolute: 0.84–3.06 × 109 cells/L
			Percentage: 57–85%	Percentage: 0.57–0.85 (57–85%)
CD4	Blood	Flow cytometry	Absolute: 490–1740 cells/mL	Absolute: 0.49–1.74 × 109 cells/L
			Percentage: 30–61%	Percentage: 0.30–0.61 (30–61%)
CD8	Blood	Flow cytometry	Absolute: 180–1170 cells/mL	Absolute: 0.18–1.17 × 109 cells/L
			Percentage: 12–42%	Percentage: 0.12–0.42 (12–42%)
Helper/suppressor (CD4/CD8) ratio	Blood	Flow cytometry	0.86–5.00	0.86–5.00
Magnesium	Serum	Colorimetry	0.6–1.0 mmol/L	0.6–1.0 mmol/L
Mercury metanephrines	Blood	Atomic spectroscopy	< 1 mg/dL	< 50 nmol/L
Fractionated	Urine	HPLC	Metanephrine: < 0.4 mg/d	Metanephrine: < 2.2 mmol/d
			Normetanephrine: < 0.9 mg/d	Normetanephrine: < 4.9 mmol/d
Total	Urine	HPLC	< 1.3 mg/d	< 7.1 mmol/d

(continued)

Table 4.2 continued

Test	Speci-men	Method	Normal range conventional units	SI units
Methemoglobin	Blood	Spectrophotome-try	<2% of total Hb	<0. 02 of total Hb
β2–microglobulin	Serum	Immunoassay	<3 mg/L	<3 mg/L
Muramidase (ly-sozyme)	Serum	Turbidimetry	2.8–8. 0 mg/L	0.20–0. 56 mmol/L
Myelin basic pro-tein	CSF	Immunoassay	<4 ng/mL	<4 mg/L
Myoglobin	Serum	Immunoassay	<55 ng/mL	<55 mg/L
Nitrogen, total	Feces	Acid digestion/ titrimetry	<2 g/d	<143 mmol/d
Osmolality	Serum	Freezing point depression	278–305 mOsm/ kg	278–305 mmol/ kg
	Urine	Freezing point depression	50–1200 mOsm/ kg	50–1,200 mmol/ kg
Oxalate	Urine	Colorimetry	<40 mg/d	<456 mmol/d
Parathyroid hor-mone (PTH), in-tact	Serum	Immunoassay	11–54 pg/mL	1.2–5.8 pmol/L
Partial thrombo-plastin time, acti-vated (aPTT)	Plasma	Photo-optical clot detection	20–36 s	20–36 s
Phosphorus	Serum	Colorimetry	2.5–4.5 mg/dL	0.81– 1.45 mmol/L
Platelet count	Blood	Automated analyzer	130–400 × 103/ mL	130–400 × 109/L
Porphobilinogen	Urine	Column chroma-tography/ spec-trophotometry	<2 mg/d	<8.8 mmol/d
Porphyrins, frac-tionated (proto-porphyrin)	Feces	HPLC	Dicarboxypor-phyrin <1,830 mg/d	Dicarboxypor-phyrin <3.26 mmol/d
			(protoporphyrin)	
			Heptacarboxy-porphyrin <20 mg/d	
			Octacarboxypor-phyrin <80 mg/d	Octacarboxypor-phyrin <96 nmol/d
			(uroporphyrin)	(uroporphyrin)

Table 4.2 continued

Test	Specimen	Method	Normal range conventional units	SI units
			Tetracarboxyporphyrin	Tetracarboxyporphyrin
			<640 mg/d	<977 nmol/d
			(coproporphyrin)	(coproporphyrin)
Potassium	Serum	ISE	3.5–5.3 mmol/L	3.5–5.3 mmol/L
Prealbumin	Serum	Nephelometry	18–45 mg/dL	180–450 mg/L
Progesterone	Serum	Immunoassay	Male: <1.2 ng/mL	Male: <3.8 nmol/L
			Female:	Female:
			Follicular phase <1.4 ng/mL	Follicular phase <4.5 nmol/L
			Luteal phase 2.5–28.0 ng/mL	Luteal phase 8.0–89.0 nmol/L
			Pregnancy	Pregnancy
			1st trimester	1st trimester
			9.0–47.0 ng/mL	28.6–149.5 nmol/L
			2nd trimester	2nd trimester
			17.0–146.0 ng/mL	54.1–464.3 nmol/L
			3rd trimester	3rd trimester
			55.0–255.0 ng/mL	174.9–810.9 nmol/L
			Postmenopausal <0.7 ng/mL	Postmenopausal <2.2 nmol/L
Prolactin	Serum	Immunoassay	Male: 2–18 ng/mL	Male: 2–18 mg/mL
			Female:	Female:
			Nonpregnant 3–30 ng/mL	Nonpregnant 3–30 mg/L
			Pregnant 10–209 ng/mL	Pregnant 10–209 mg/L
			Postmenopausal 2–20 ng/mL	Postmenopausal 2–20 mg/L
Prostate-specific antigen (PSA)	Serum	Immunoassay	<4 ng/mL (male)	<4 mg/L (male)
Protein, total	Serum	Colorimetry	6.0–8.5 g/dL	60–85 g/L
	Urine	Colorimetry	<150 mg/d	<150 mg/d

(continued)

Table 4.2 continued

Test	Specimen	Method	Normal range conventional units	SI units
Protein C activity	Plasma	Photo-optical clot detection	70–140% of normal	0.7–1.4 of normal
Protein C antigen	Plasma	Immunoassay	70–140% of normal	0.7–1.4 of normal
Protein electrophoresis	Serum	Electrophoresis	Albumin: 3.5–5.5 g/dL	Albumin: 35–55 g/L
			α_1-globulins: 0.1–0. 3 g/dL	α_1-globulins: 1–3 g/L
			α_2-globulins: 0.2–1.1 g/dL	α_2-globulins: 2–11 g/L
			β-globulins: 0.5–1.2 g/dL	β-globulins: 5–12 g/L
			γ-globulins: 0.5–1.5 g/dL	γ-globulins: 5–15 g/L
Protein S activity	Plasma	Photo-optical clot detection	Male: 70–150% of normal	Male: 0.7–1.5 of normal
			Female: 58–130% of normal	Female: 0.58–1.30 of normal
Protein S antigen	Plasma	Immunoassay	Male: 70–140% of normal	Male: 0.7–1.4 of normal
			Female: 70–140% of normal	Female: 0.7–1.4 of normal
Prothrombin time (PT)	Plasma	Photo-optical clot detection international normalized ratio (INR): 0.9–1.1 (patients not on anticoagulant therapy)	10.0–12.5 s	10. 0–12. 5 s
Protoporphyrin				
Free erythrocyte	Blood	Fluorometry	<35 mg/dL RBCs	<0.62 mmol/L RBCs
Zinc	Blood	Fluorometry	<70 mg/dL	<700 mg/L
Pyruvate	Blood	Enzymatic colorimetry	0.3–0.9 mg/dL	34–102 mmol/L
Pyruvate kinase	Blood	Fluorometry	Enzyme activity detected	
RBC count	Blood	Automated analyzer	Male: 4.4–5.8 × 10^6/mL	Male: 4. 4–5. 8 × 10^{12}/L

Table 4.2 continued

Test	Specimen	Method	Normal range conventional units	SI units
			Female: 3.9–5.2 × 10^6/mL	Female: 3.9–5.2 × 10^{12}/L
RBC indices	Blood	Automated analyzer	Mean corpuscular volume: 78–102 fL	Mean corpuscular volume: 78–102 fL
			Mean corpuscular Hb: 27–33 pg	Mean corpuscular Hb: 27–33 pg
			Mean corpuscular Hb	Mean corpuscular Hb
			concentration: 32–36 g/dL	concentration: 320–360 g/L
			RBC distribution width: < 15%	RBC distribution width: < 0.15
Renin activity	Plasma	Immunoassay	1.3–4.0 ng/mL/h (upright)	1.00–3. 07 nmol/L/h (upright)
			(Normal sodium intake: 100–200 mEq/d)	(Normal sodium intake: 100–200 mmol/d)
Reticulocyte count	Blood	Automated analyzer	0.5–2.3% of RBCs	0.005–0.023 of RBCs
Rheumatoid factor	Serum	Nephelometry	< 40 U/mL	< 40 kU/L
Schilling test	Urine	Radio-isotopic measurement	> 7% of administered dose in 24-hour urine	> 0.07 of administered dose in 24-hour urine
Scleroderma antibody (Scl-70)	-70) Serum	Immunoassay	Negative	
Serotonin	Blood	HPLC	46–319 ng/mL	0.26–1.81 mmol/L
Sodium	Serum	ISE	135–146 mmol/L	135–146 mmol/L
Somatomedin-C	Serum	Immunoassay	Male: 90–318 ng/mL	Male: 90–318 mg/L
			Female: 116–270 ng/mL	Female: 116–270 mg/L
T3 (triiodothyronine) Free	Serum	Immunoassay	230–420 pg/dL	3.5–6.5 pmol/L
Reverse	Serum	Immunoassay	2.6–18.9 ng/dL	0.04–0. 29 nmol/L

(continued)

79

Table 4.2 continued

Test	Specimen	Method	Normal range conventional units	SI units
Total T4 (thyroxine)	Serum	Immunoassay	60–181 ng/dL	0.9–2. 8 nmol/L
Free	Serum	Immunoassay	0.8–1.8 ng/dL	10–23 pmol/L
Total	Serum	Immunoassay	4.5–12.5 mg/dL	58–161 nmol/L
Testosterone, total	Serum	Immunoassay	Male: 194–833 ng/dL	Male: 6.7–28.9 nmol/L
			Female: 62 ng/dL	Female: < 2.1 nmol/L
Thrombin time	Plasma	Photo-optical clot detection	10.0–13.5 s	10.0–13.5 s
Thyroglobulin	Serum	Immunoassay	< 60 ng/mL	< 60 mg/L
Thyroid-stimulating hormone (TSH), ultrasensitive (third generation)	Serum	Immunoassay	0.50–4.70 mU/mL	0.50–4.70 mU/L
Thyroxine-binding globulin (TBG)	Serum	Immunoassay	16–34 mg/L	16–34 mg/L
Transferrin	Serum	Nephelometry	188–341 mg/dL	1.88–3.41 g/L
Triglycerides	Serum	Enzymatic colorimetry	< 200 mg/dL	< 2.26 mmol/L
Urea nitrogen, blood (BUN)	Serum	Colorimetry	7–30 mg/dL	2.5–10.7 mmol urea/L
Uric acid	Serum	Enzymatic colorimetry	Male: 4.0–8.5 mg/dL	Male: 238–506 mmol/L
			Female: 2.5–7.5 mg/dL	Female: 149–446 mmol/L
	Urine	Enzymatic colorimetry	200–750 mg/d	1.2–4.5 mmol/d
Urinalysis, complete	Urine	Reagent-impregnated strips	Appearance: clear, yellow	
		Microscopy	Specific gravity: 1.001–1.035	
			pH: 4.6–8.0	
			Protein: negative	
			Glucose: negative	

Table 4.2 continued

Test	Specimen	Method	Normal range conventional units	SI units
			Reducing substances: negative	
			Ketones: negative	
			Bilirubin: negative	
			Occult blood: negative	
			WBC esterase: negative	
			Nitrite: negative	
			WBC: < 5/high-power field	
			RBC: < 3/high-power field	
			Renal epithelial cells: < 3/high-power field	
			Squamous epithelial cells: none or few/high-power field	
			Casts: none	
			Bacteria: none	
			Yeast: none	
Vanillylmandelic acid (VMA)	Urine	HPLC	< 10 mg/d	< 50 mmol/d
Viscosity	Serum	Viscometer	1.5–1.9 viscosity units (relative to water)	
Vitamin A	Serum	HPLC	30–95 mg/dL	1.05–3.32 mmol/L
Vitamin B$_6$	Plasma	HPLC	5–24 ng/mL	30–144 nmol/L
Vitamin B$_{12}$	Serum	Immunoassay	200–800 pg/mL	> 150–590 pmol/L
Vitamin C	Plasma	Colorimetry	0.2–2.0 mg/dL	11–114 mmol/L
1,25-dihydroxy-vitamin D	Serum	Chromatography	24–65 pg/mL	58–156 pmol/L

(continued)

Table 4.2 continued

Test	Speci-men	Method	Normal range conventional units	SI units
25-hydroxy-vita-min D	Serum	Acetonitrile extraction/ immunoassay	10–55 ng/mL	25–137 nmol/L
Vitamin E	Serum	Fluorometry	5–20 mg/mL	12–46 mmol/L
WBC count	Blood	Automated analyzer	$3.8–10.8 \times 10^3$/mL	$3.8–10.8 \times 10^9$/L
WBC differential	Blood	Automated analyzer	Absolute neutro-phils: 1,500–7,800 cells/mL	Absolute neutro-phils: 1.5–7.8×10^9/L
			Absolute eosino-phils: 50–550 cells/mL	Absolute eosino-phils: 0.05–0.55×10^9/L
			Absolute baso-phils: 0–200 cells/mL	Absolute baso-phils: 0–0.2×10^9/L
			Absolute lym-phocytes: 850–4100 cells/mL	Absolute lym-phocytes: 0.85–4.10×10^9/L
			Absolute mono-cytes: 200–1100 cells/mL	Absolute mono-cytes: 0.2–$1.1 0^9$/L
Zinc	Plasma	Atomic spectroscopy	60–130 mg/dL	9.2–19.9 mmol/L

Abbreviations: CSF, cerebrospinal fluid; DNA, deoxyribonucleic acid; HPLC, high-performance liquid chromatography; HRT, hormone replacement therapy; ICMA, immuno-chemiluminometric assay; ICP-MS, inductively coupled mass spectroscopy; IRMA, immunoradiometric assay; ISE, ion-selective electrode; MEIA, microparticle enzyme immunoassay; RBC, red blood (cell) count; RIA, radioimmunoassay; SI, International System of Units; WBC, white blood (cell) count.

4.2 Preoperative Testing

Routine preoperative laboratory tests should include a complete blood count (CBC) with differential (white blood cell [WBC], hemoglobin, hematocrit, and platelets), an electrolyte panel (CHEM-7: sodium, potassium, chloride, carbon dioxide, blood urea nitrogen [BUN], creatinine, and serum glucose), and coagulation studies (prothrombin time [PT], international normalized ratio [INR], and partial thromboplastin time [PTT]). Depending on age and clinical suspicion, electrocardiography (EKG) and chest X-ray may be appropriate. For all intracranial procedures and extensive spine procedures, blood should be typed and crossed. For other neurosurgical procedures, blood should at least be typed and screened. The American Society of Anesthesiologists (ASA) Practice Advisory for Pre-Anesthesia Evaluation is a set of guidelines, most recently updated in 2012, to include scientific evaluation of the proposed guidelines from 2002. The 2012 ASA guidelines may be summarized as follows:

1. No laboratory study may clear a patient for surgery, there is insufficient evidence to identify explicit decision parameters or rules for ordering preoperative testing. A thorough history and physical is the most important factor in determining if a patient is medically fit for surgery. Medical risk stratification should be obtained for patients with multiple comorbidities.
2. Evaluation must occur prior to the day of surgery.
3. Preoperative laboratory testing should be carried out on a selective basis, with great consideration of the patient's medical history, physical, and type of procedure planned and its invasiveness.
4. Pregnancy testing should be routine for women of childbearing age 11 to 55 irrespective of the patient's belief that "there is no way" that she could be pregnant.

On the whole, not much benefit appears to result from unindicated routine laboratory testing. There is little evidence to suggest that patients classified as ASA I or II benefit from laboratory testing. Furthermore, in the absence of laboratory tests ASA I patients' medical care is not shown to be adversely affected.[1,8,9]

4.3 Infection

A patient with suspected infection, sustained fever of 100.4°F or more, without any obvious source, requires proper investigation for the cause. Fever workup should include, but is not limited to, CBC + differential, Chem 10, urinalysis, blood culture, sputum culture, urine culture, and chest X-ray. Often ordered in high suspicion of infection is C-reactive protein (CRP). CRP is an inflammatory marker produced by the liver that is often used as a nonspecific sign of infection and/or value to trend so as to measure treatment efficacy. More recent studies support the use of procalcitonin as a more reliable marker for infection.

Procalcitonin is normally synthesized by thyroid C cells; however, during severe infection (e.g., sepsis), procalcitonin originates outside the thyroid. Procalcitonin may be elevated in as little as 4 hours following a nonseptic systemic inflammatory response syndrome (SIRS) or immediately after surgery or trauma, without any obvious infection. Procalcitonin is best established as a diagnostic marker of bacterial meningitis in children and sepsis in critically ill adults, but studies continue to suggest an expanded use of procalcitonin as a marker of infection, often indicating that it is a superior marker to CRP.[10]

4.4 Tumors

4.4.1 Postoperative Markers for Tumors

Radiological studies and surgical biopsy are the primary methods used to diagnose central nervous system (CNS) tumors; however, in the ICU setting, diagnostic laboratory studies may assist with diagnosis and therapeutic monitoring following surgical intervention.

A variety of CNS tumors can arise from hormone-producing cells and are thus called neuroendocrine tumors. They often cause an abnormal increase in hormones, which can manifest as an array of symptoms. Checking for these specific hormones and other markers can aid in the diagnosis of the tumor prior to surgical resection and can be used to monitor the effectiveness of treatment. Pituitary tumors are a common example of neuroendocrine tumors, which often produce endocrine abnormalities that are measured in serum. Most commonly prolactinomas cause high levels of prolactin and can sometimes result in panhypopituitarism (decrease in all other pituitary hormones). A general rule of thumb is that the percent chance of a pituitary mass being a prolactinoma is calculated by dividing the serum level of prolactin by 2.

Some parasellar and pineal region embryonal tumors secrete hormones and proteins: alpha-fetoprotein (AFP), beta subunit of human chorionic gonadotropin (β-hCG), and placental alkaline phosphatase (PLAP). Cerebrospinal fluid (CSF) cytology may be used to diagnose tumor type. CSF analysis may reveal polyamines that localize tumors to ventricles or subarachnoid space, or pleocytosis may increase suspicion for lymphoma. Hemangioblastomas rarely causes polycythemia.[11] Polycythemia occurs in the setting of hemangioblastomas due to tumor cell production of erythropoietin. With the exception of pituitary tumors, following the removal of these primary CNS tumors the abnormal levels of these multiple tumor markers should normalize.

4.4.2 Tumors of the Sellar Region

Pituitary tumors present clinically by symptoms of pituitary hypersecretion (70% of cases), symptoms of pituitary hyposecretion, or neurologic symptoms of compression of the pituitary or other adjacent sellar structures. Diagnostic laboratory studies are very sensitive indicators of endocrine dysfunction and are focused on measuring pituitary and/or target-organ hormones in basal and provoked states to discriminate between various pituitary adenoma subtypes.

Screening tests include the following:

1. *Adrenal axis:* AM cortisol, 24-hour urine free cortisol, dexamethasone suppression test, cosyntropin stimulation test, insulin tolerance test.
2. *Thyroid axis:* thyroid-stimulating hormone (TSH), thyroxin (T_4), thyrotropin-releasing hormone (TRH) stimulation test.

3. *Gonadal axis:* serum luteinizing hormone/follicle-stimulating hormone (LH/FSH).
4. *Prolactin levels:* PRL.
5. *Growth hormone:* somatomedin-C (IGF-I), growth hormone–releasing hormone (GH-RH) stimulation test, glucose suppression test.
6. *Neurohypophysis:* water deprivation test, serum antidiuretic hormone (ADH).

Craniopharyngiomas produce effects seen using endocrine studies. They may reflect arrested pituitary function in children (growth failure, diabetes insipidus, and primary amenorrhea) and some degree of hypopituitarism in adults.

Hypersecretory syndromes include acromegaly, Cushing's disease, amenorrhea–galactorrhea syndrome, and secondary hyperthyroidism from hypersecretion of growth hormone (GH), adrenocorticotropic hormone (ACTH), PRL, and TSH, respectively.

Hypopituitarism results in fatigue, weakness, hypogonadism, regression of secondary sexual characteristics, and hypothyroidism. Pituitary insufficiency also occurs acutely in pituitary apoplexy.

Chronic progressive compression of the pituitary is accompanied by decline in functional reserve of secretory elements: gonadotrophs are most vulnerable and are affected first, next thyrotrophs, somatotrophs, and finally corticotrophs (the most resilient among pituitary hormones).

Acute processes produce the opposite effect. Panhypopituitarism results in compromise of all of the pituitary hormones, but hypocortisolism from ACTH deficit produces life-threatening adrenal insufficiency. Large adenomas may result in compression of the hypothalamus or in obstruction of CSF outflow and subsequent noncommunicating hydrocephalus. Also inhibition of dopamine transport from the hypothalamus via the portal vessels to the anterior lobe of the pituitary results in loss of suppression of PRL output (the "stalk section effect"). This phenomenon may result in PRL levels elevating to 150 ng/mL or greater (normal levels are < 25 ng/mL).

4.5 Trauma

Following trauma several delayed conditions may present. Diagnostic laboratory studies may be implemented to diagnose and/or prevent delayed hemorrhage, posttraumatic diffuse cerebral edema, seizures, metabolic abnormalities, and meningitis.

4.5.1 Intracranial Hematoma

Initial or delayed hemorrhage may be anticipated in 75% of patients with traumatic brain injury. Epidural hematoma (EDH), subdural hematoma (SDH), and traumatic intracerebral hemorrhage (TICH) may be present in either initial or delayed fashions.

Following initial management (intubation, sedation, elevation of the head of the bed, and management of hypertension, etc.), the focus is turned toward correction of coagulopathy if present, administration of anti-epileptic drugs (AEDs), and monitoring of electrolytes and osmolarity anticipating the onset of syndrome of inappropriate antidiuretic hormone (SIADH).

Coagulopathy is identified using PT, INR, PTT, bleeding time, and platelet count. Coagulopathy is treated with fresh frozen plasma (FFP), Aquamephyton (Phytonadione, a synthetic Vitamin K, Merck), and Kcentra (CSL Behring) (prothrombin complex concentrate) and is carefully monitored using coagulation studies every 4 hours until it is corrected.

Phenytoin is the first-line antiseizure medication and levels are observed as per the above protocol.

Serum and urine electrolytes, serum and urine osmolarity, and urine specific gravity are ordered every 6 hours to screen for SIADH. Serum uric acid may also be a helpful study to rule in the presence of SIADH (serum uric acid is decreased in SIADH).[4,5,6,12]

4.5.2 Diffuse Cerebral Edema

Increased cerebral blood volume may result from loss of cerebral vascular autoregulation. It occurs in children more frequently than in adults and carries a rate of mortality close to 100%. Diagnostic studies should be geared toward monitoring serum electrolytes and glucose, BUN, creatinine, and serum osmolarity. Also, hemoglobin and hematocrit should be measured to allow for optimization of volume status and oxygenation.[4,5,6] High tonicity (> 320 mOsm/L) and hypovolemia ("running dry") have little advantage to prevent cerebral edema and may result in renal dysfunction. Prevention of hypoglycemia is also important because it aggravates cerebral edema.

4.5.3 Posttraumatic Seizure

Posttraumatic seizures may occur early (< 7 days) or late (> 7 days) following head trauma and may precipitate adverse events as the result of elevation of intracranial pressure, alterations in systolic blood pressure, changes in oxygenation, and excessive neurotransmitter release. Anticonvulsants may be used to prevent *early* posttraumatic seizures in patients that meet high-risk criteria: (1) presence of SDH, EDH, ICH, TICH, or delayed traumatic intracerebral hematoma (DTICH); (2) open-depressed skull fracture with parenchymal injury; (3) penetrating brain injury; (4) seizure within the first 24 hours following trauma; (5) Glasgow Coma Scale score < 10, or 6); or history of substance abuse.

Patients meeting criteria should be started on phenytoin, carbamazepine, valproic acid, or phenobarbital for 1 week. Diagnostic laboratory studies to monitor AED levels are per specific agent:

Phenytoin: Peak serum drug concentrations are achieved between 3 and 12 hours after administration of an oral dose. Therapeutic drug concentrations can be obtained in 1 to 2 hours when the drug is administered intravenously. Time to steady state is highly variable, ranging from 1 to 5 weeks. The therapeutic range is 10–20 µg/mL.

Carbamazepine: Single oral dose, the carbamazepine tablets or chewable form, yield peak plasma concentrations of unchanged carbamazepine within 4 to 24 hours. Carbamazepine suspension is absorbed faster than the tablet; peak plasma levels are reached within 2 hours. Time to steady state is up to 10 days. The therapeutic range is 6 and 12 µg/mL.

Valproic acid: Peak serum drug concentrations are achieved between 1 and 4 hours with oral dosing. Time to steady state is between 2 and 4 days. Therapeutic range is 50–100 µg/mL.

Phenobarbital: Peak serum drug concentrations are achieved between 1 and 6 hours after oral or intramuscular dosing. Time to steady state is 16 to 30 days. Therapeutic range is 15–30 µg/mL.[4,5,6]

4.5.4 Metabolic Disorders

Several metabolic disorders may result from trauma (directly or indirectly) that affect the CNS: hypoxia, hyponatremia, hypoglycemia, renal failure, adrenal insufficiency, and hepatic encephalopathy.

Acute Renal Failure

Acute renal failure (ARF) is categorized as prerenal, postrenal, and intrinsic renal. Prerenal and postrenal causes are potentially reversible if diagnosed and treated early. Prerenal azotemia (50–80% of ARF) results from inadequate renal perfusion caused by extracellular fluid volume depletion or cardiovascular disease. Patients will be oliguric (not making much urine), have an elevated creatine (Cr > 1), a BUN to creatine ratio greater than 20, and a fractional excretion of sodium (FeNa) less than 1%. The patient's volume status will help determine the appropriate treatment.

Patients who are volume overloaded will need diuresis. These patents can be in congestive heart failure or can be cirrhotic and therefore third spacing. The patients who are in congestive heart failure are volume overloaded in the intravascular space, causing the heart to have an increased preload, thus decreasing cardiac output. These patients have pitting edema and audible abnormal heart sounds. Treatment for these patients is adequate diuresis.

Cirrhotic patients are clinically third spacing and are intravascularly "dry." They may have ascites, appear puffy or edematous, and may have wet lungs identified by auscultation and percussion or visible on chest X-ray. Treatment for these patients is to increase the intravascular solute concentration with albumin (or other substitutes).

Patients who are volume depleted will need fluids. These patients clinically look dehydrated, have dry mucosa, and have poor capillary refill and poor skin turgor.

Postrenal azotemia (5–10% of ARF) results from various types of obstruction in the voiding and collecting systems. This diagnosis should be considered for patients who have been first ruled out for prerenal disease, are oliguric (or anuric), and have an elevated creatine level. These patients should be screened for obstruction with an ultrasound of the kidney, ureters, and bladder. Hydro-ureter and or hydronephrosis indicates obstruction, and a consult to urology is warranted once a Foley catheter is successfully placed but has no urine return, or if the catheter is unable to be passed.

Intrinsic renal causes of ARF are the result of prolonged renal ischemia (hem-orrhage, surgery) or a nephrotoxin. This diagnosis should be considered once prerenal and postrenal causes of renal failure have been successfully ruled out.

Adrenal Insufficiency

Secondary adrenal insufficiency may occur in panhypopituitarism, in isolated failure of ACTH production, in patients receiving corticosteroids, or after dis-continuance of corticosteroid therapy.

Panhypopituitarism occurs in a trauma setting resulting directly from destruction of pituitary tissue or secondarily from infection. Also, patients receiving corticosteroids for > 4 weeks or who have discontinued their use after a period of weeks to months may have insufficient ACTH secretion during met-abolic stress to stimulate the adrenals to produce adequate quantities of corti-costeroids, or they may have atrophic adrenals that are unresponsive to ACTH.

Patients with secondary adrenal insufficiency are not hyperpigmented, as are those with Addison's disease. They have relatively normal electrolyte levels. Hyperkalemia and elevated BUN are not present because of the near-normal secretion of aldosterone. Hyponatremia may occur on a dilutional basis. Patients with panhypopituitarism have depressed thyroid and gonadal func-tion and hypoglycemia; coma may result when symptomatic secondary adre-nal insufficiency occurs.

Function of the hypothalamic–pituitary–adrenal axis during long-term ste-roid treatment can be determined by the cosyntropin-stimulation test:

intravenous injection of 5 to 250 mg cosyntropin results in plasma cortisol level > 20 mg/dL 30 minutes following the injection. Also, AM cortisol, 24-hour urine free cortisol, dexamethasone suppression test, and insulin tolerance test may be used to test adrenal function.[4,5,7]

Hepatic Encephalopathy

Hepatic encephalopathy may result from hepatic failure resulting from trauma. The liver metabolizes and detoxifies digestive products brought from the intestine by the portal vein. In hepatic failure these products escape into the systemic circulation if portal blood bypasses parenchymal cells or if the function of these cells is severely impaired. The resulting toxic effect on the brain produces the clinical syndrome.

Personality changes (e.g., inappropriate behavior, altered mood, impaired judgment) are common early manifestations. Psychomotor testing can detect such abnormalities not suspected clinically. Usually, impaired consciousness occurs. Initially, subtle sleep pattern changes or sluggish movement and speech may be present. Drowsiness, confusion, stupor, and frank coma indicate increasingly advanced encephalopathy. Constructional apraxia, in which the patient cannot reproduce simple designs (e.g., a star), is a characteristic early sign. A musty sweet odor of the breath, fetor hepaticus, occurs. A peculiar, characteristic flapping tremor, asterixis, is elicited when the patient holds his arms outstretched with the wrists dorsiflexed; as coma progresses, this sign disappears and hyperreflexia and the Babinski response may occur. Agitation or mania may occur. Seizures and localizing neurologic signs may also occur.

Diagnostic laboratory studies for hepatic function include serum total protein, albumin, alkaline phosphatase, alanine aminotransferase (ALT), aspartate aminotransferase (AST), total bilirubin, ammonia (NH_3), γ-glutamyltransferase (GGT), PT, platelet count, and serum protein electrophoresis.

The diagnosis of hepatic encephalopathy is clinical. There is no correlation with liver function tests. Blood ammonia levels are elevated, but values correlate poorly with clinical status. The CSF is unremarkable except for mild protein elevation.

An electroencephalogram usually shows diffuse slow-wave activity, even in mild cases, and may be useful in questionable early encephalopathy.[4,7]

4.5.5 Posttraumatic Meningitis

Posttraumatic meningitis occurs in up to 20% of patients with moderate to severe head injuries. Most cases occur within 2 weeks of trauma, 75% of which have demonstrable basal skull fracture and 50% have obvious CSF rhinorrhea.

Antibiotic coverage should be broad spectrum, targeting both gram-positive and gram-negative organisms. They should be continued for 1 week following CSF sterilization.

Routine CSF analysis should include Gram stain, culture and sensitivity, protein, glucose, cell count with differential, color, and clarity. Pathogens frequently cultured following basal skull fracture include gram-positive cocci (*Staphylococcus hemolyticus, Staphylococcus warneri, Staphylococcus cohnii, Staphylococcus epidermidis*, and *Streptococcus pneumoniae*) and gram-negative bacilli (*Escherichia coli, Klebsiella pneumoniae, Acinetobacter anitratus*). Elevations of protein and WBCs polymorphonuclear leukocytes (PMNs), low glucose, and cloudy/turbid CSF suggest bacterial infection. CSF should be collected for CSF analysis weekly until sterilization is achieved.[4,5,6]

4.6 Cerebrovascular Disease

4.6.1 Cerebrovascular Accident

Cerebrovascular accidents (CVAs) can be divided into ischemic and hemorrhagic. Approximately 85% of CVAs are ischemic, 15% are hemorrhagic.

Ischemic infarction: Of patients presenting with focal deficit, 5% of cases are seizure, tumor, or psychogenic in etiology, and 95% are vascular. Eighty-five percent of CVAs are attributed to ischemic infarct, whereas only 15% are from hemorrhage. With the mainstream use of thrombolytic therapy in the management of ischemic infarction it is important to be familiar with the exclusion criteria used to make decisions regarding their administration. The use of anticoagulants (heparin or coumadin), and extreme values of serum glucose may exclude a patient from receiving thrombolytic agents. Initial laboratory tests should include a fasting lipid panel, random blood glucose, hemoglobin A1C, and a coagulation panel (PT/PTT/INR).[13]

Computed tomography (CT) of the head will rule out hemorrhagic stroke and should be the first imaging modality completed. Once the patient is stable, further workup for the etiology can be pursued with magnetic resonance imaging/magnetic resonance angiography, carotid Doppler, and transesophageal echocardiography.

If the history and imaging fail to provide a clear etiology, then the patient should receive a hypercoagulable panel that includes a test for antiphospholipid antibodies (anti-cardiolipin antibodies), lupus anticoagulant, factor V Leiden and prothrombin gene mutation, protein C and S activity, heparin-induced thrombocytopenia HIT antibodies and in rare cases a genetic investigation for inherited thrombophilia or hyperhomocysteinemia.

Intracerebral hemorrhage: Intracerebral hemorrhage (ICH) accounts for 10% of strokes. Etiologies of ICH include amyloid angiopathy, trauma, hemorrhagic transformation of an ischemic infarct, tumors, cerebrovascular malformations (cerebral aneurysms, arteriovenous malformations [AVMs], venous malformations, cavernomas, capillary telangiectasias). Several risk factors are associated with ICH: age, gender, race, prior CVA, alcohol consumption and substance abuse, cigarette smoking, and liver dysfunction. Diagnostic laboratory studies may be used in both diagnosis and management.

Factors complicating or leading to ICH are coagulopathy, seizure, inflammatory disease, and SIADH.

Coagulopathy is identified using PT, INR, PTT, bleeding time, and platelet count. Coagulopathy is treated with FFP and Aquamephyton and is carefully monitored using coagulation studies every 4 hours until it is corrected.

Inflammatory disease is initially identified using erythrocyte sedimentation rate (ESR) or CRP.

Phenytoin is the first-line antiseizure medication, and levels are observed as per the preceding protocol.

Serum and urine electrolytes, serum and urine osmolarity, and urine specific gravity are ordered every 6 hours to screen for SIADH. Serum uric acid may also be a helpful study to rule in the presence of SIADH (serum uric acid is decreased in SIADH).

Toxicology screening may be ordered if there is suspicion for substance abuse.[4,5,12]

4.6.2 Subarachnoid Hemorrhage

Many etiologies for subarachnoid hemorrhage (SAH) exist: rupture of intracranial aneurysms (80%), cerebral AVM (5%), spinal AVM, arterial dissection or rupture, vasculitides, tumors, coagulation disorders, dural sinus thrombosis, drugs, sickle cell disease, and pituitary apoplexy. Risk factors include hypertension, use of oral contraceptives, substance abuse, tobacco abuse, alcohol abuse, pregnancy, lumbar puncture, and advanced age. Along with radiological studies, diagnostic laboratory studies may assist with diagnosis and are essential for management of SAH. These include coagulopathy and the causes of coagulopathy, as well as inflammatory disease. A simple ESR and CRP should be ordered prior to more specific tests for inflammation.

Patients having high suspicion for SAH will have noncontrast CT performed. If CT is negative, lumbar puncture may be performed. Lumbar puncture is the most sensitive test for SAH, albeit false-positives may occur as the result of a traumatic tap. Elevations of opening pressure and xanthochromia of CSF present during the lumbar puncture are consistent with SAH. CSF analysis will reveal nonclotting bloody fluid that does not clear with sequential tubes. Xanthochromia results from hemoglobin breakdown into bilirubin, leaving a yellow discoloration to CSF. In general, it takes 12 to 48 hours for xanthochromia to develop after an SAH, but it may be seen early on. Xanthochromia is tested by having the CSF spun down in a centrifuge to have the supernatant evaluated via spectrophotometry. The cell count reveals > 100,000 red blood cells (RBCs)/ mm^3, and when the first and last tubes are compared there should not be a significant drop in counts. Protein elevations are from blood breakdown products. Glucose may be normal or reduced.

Once the diagnosis of SAH has been made, initial management is directed toward preventing rebleeding, detection and treatment of hydrocephalus and vasospasm, monitoring for hyponatremia, deep vein thrombosis (DVT) prophylaxis, seizure prevention, and determining a source of bleeding. Arterial blood gas (ABG), electrolytes, CBC, and PT/INR/PTT should be ordered on admission.

Coagulopathy is expeditiously corrected and anticoagulants, to include aspirin or other nonsteroidal anti-inflammatory drugs, enoxaparin or other low-molecular weight heparin products, and coumadin are discontinued. Therefore, DVT prophylaxis is by mechanical means: application of knee-high T.E.D. (thromboembolic deterrent) hose (Covidien) and pneumatic compression boots. Coagulation panels should be monitored every 4 hours until coagulopathy is corrected, and then daily.

Blood rheology should be optimized using hemodilution; hemoglobin and hematocrit of 10 mg/dL and 30–35%, respectively, enhances perfusion when vasospasm is present.

SIADH and cerebral salt wasting may be detected by following serum and urine electrolytes, serum and urine osmolarity, and urine specific gravity.

AEDs are administered, phenytoin is preferred.[4,5,12,14]

4.7 Brain Death

Prior to the determination of brain death the patient should have a normal blood glucose level. The patient should have no abnormal labs that would confound the neurologic examination or suppress brainstem reflexes and muscle function.

Case Management

The patient has a high suspicion for SAH and therefore will have noncontrast CT performed. If CT is negative, lumbar puncture may be performed. There should be elevations of opening pressure and xanthochromia of CSF. There should be nonclotting bloody fluid that does not clear with sequential tubes. Xanthochromia, or yellow discoloration, may take 48 hours to develop but may be seen early on. This may be subtle and will require fluid to be spun down to have supernatant evaluated via spectrophotometry (visual inspection is less accurate). The cell count should reveal > 100,000 RBCs/mm^3, and when the first and last tubes are compared there should not be a significant drop in counts. Protein elevations are from blood breakdown products. Glucose may be normal or reduced; RBCs present within CSF may metabolize glucose.

Once the diagnosis of SAH has been made, initial management is directed toward preventing rebleeding, detection and treatment of hydrocephalus and vasospasm, monitoring for hyponatremia, DVT prophylaxis, seizure prevention, and determining a source of bleeding. ABG, electrolytes, CBC, and PT/INR/PTT should be ordered on admission.

Blood rheology should be optimized using hemodilution; hemoglobin and hematocrit of 10 mg/dL and 30–35%, respectively, enhances perfusion when vasospasm is present.

SIADH and cerebral salt wasting may be detected by following serum and urine electrolytes, serum and urine osmolarity, and urine specific gravity.

AEDs are administered; phenytoin is preferred.

References

[1]   Miller RD. Miller's Anesthesia. 7th ed. Philadelphia, PA: Elsevier; 2010
[2]   Lawrence W, Lenhard RE, Murphy GP. American Cancer Society Textbook of Clinical Oncology. Atlanta, GA: American Cancer Society; 1995
[3]   DeVita VT, Hellman S, Rosenberg SA. Cancer: Principles and Practice of Oncology. 10th ed. Philadelphia, PA: Lippincott Williams & Wilkins; 2014
[4]   Greenberg MS. Handbook of Neurosurgery. 8th ed. New York, NY: Thieme; 2016
[5]   Youmans JR, ed. Neurological Surgery. 6th ed. Philadelphia, PA: WB Saunders; 2011
[6]   Narayan RK, Wilberger JE, Povlishock JT. Neurotrauma. New York, NY: McGraw-Hill; 1998
[7]   Fauci A, Kasper D, Hauser S, Longo D, Jameson J, Losxalzo J. Harrison's Principles of Internal Medicine. 16th ed. New York, NY: McGraw-Hill; 2015
[8]   Anderson R. Clinical and laboratory diagnosis of acute renal failure. Best Pract Res Clin Anaesthesiol. 2004; 18(1):1–20
[9]   Apfelbaum JL, Connis RT, Nickinovich DG, et al. , . Practice advisory for preanesthesia evaluation: an updated report by the American Society of Anesthesiologists Task Force on Preanesthesia Evaluation. Anesthesiology. 2012; 116(3):522–538
[10] Uzzan B, Cohen R, Nicolas P, Cucherat M, Perret GY. Procalcitonin as a diagnostic test for sepsis in critically ill adults and after surgery or trauma: a systematic review and meta-analysis. Crit Care Med. 2006; 34(7):1996–2003
[11] So C-C, Ho LC. Polycythemia secondary to cerebellar hemangioblastoma. Am J Hematol. 2002; 71 (4):346–347
[12] Singh S, Bohn D, Carlotti AP, Cusimano M, Rutka JT, Halperin ML. Cerebral salt wasting: truths, fallacies, theories, and challenges. Crit Care Med. 2002; 30(11):2575–2579
[13] Varona JF. Diagnostic Work-Up and Etiology in Ischemic Stroke in Young Adults: Before and Now. J Neurol Neurophysiol. 2012; 3:133
[14] McGirt MJ, Blessing R, Nimjee SM, et al. Correlation of serum brain natriuretic peptide with hyponatremia and delayed ischemic neurological deficits after subarachnoid hemorrhage. Neurosurgery. 2004; 54(6):1369–1373, discussion 1373–1374

5 Team Management of the Multisystem-Injured Neurosurgical Intensive Care Unit Patient

Mark Krel, Javed Siddiqi, Silvio Hoshek, Rosalinda Menoni, Vladimir Adriano Cortez, Jeff W. Chen, and David T. Wong

Abstract

The practice of neurocritical care medicine is vast, comprehensive, and detailed. In order to accomplish the task with the best patient outcome and experience, the neurointensivist needs to both rely on another pair of eyes and perform as part of a team. Because the body is an integration of the neuro, muscular, skeletal, and vascular systems, each working to support the whole, the heath care team should work together, each performing a vital function and relating that function to the entire care of the patient.

Keywords: hypotension, hypoxia, multisystem injury

Case Presentation

A 23-year-old man is involved in a motorcycle collision against a pole. On primary survey, the patient's blood pressure is 90/palpable with a heart rate of 120. His pupils are 4 mm symmetrical and sluggish. His only motor response is localization to noxious stimulation. His lung sounds are diminished on the right, and there is a flailed segment on the same side. He has multiple deformities to his extremity.

See end of chapter for Case Management.

5.1 Introduction

The management of a multisystem-injured patient requires the concerted effort of a nonhierarchical though rigorously structured and coordinated prehospital and hospital care team from multiple specialties and is best handled at a designated trauma center that is staffed, equipped, and prepared for such critically injured patients. There are approximately 150,000 trauma deaths annually, three times the number of Vietnam conflict deaths. Of these, approximately 50% are avoidable with the institution of well-organized and meticulously maintained trauma response systems. These systems must include both the field/prehospital teams as well as the in-hospital immediate and

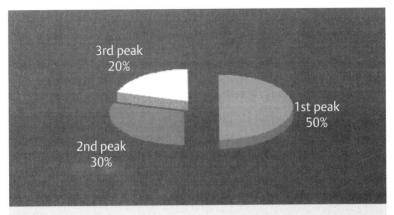

Fig. 5.1 Trauma mortality.

longer-term care teams. It is important to understand that there is actually a trimodal distribution of trauma-related death in the postinjury period. The first peak arises due to catastrophic and untreatable injuries that cause immediate posttraumatic death. The second and third peaks, the early posttraumatic mortality period, including secondary respiratory failure and systemic complications, such as overwhelming rhabdomyolysis, and the late posttraumatic mortality period, including hypercoagulable states and cerebral edema, respectively, are relatively preventable causes of death with implementation of efficacious trauma response systems (▶ Fig. 5.1). The first trauma mortality peak is due to catastrophic injury and untreatable injuries, the second and third peaks in trauma mortality can be reduced by trauma systems that include prehospital, emergency room, operative, and critical care.

Most traumatic injuries are time critical. The "golden hour" beginning from the time of injury to definitive treatment refers to the period during which an interdisciplinary trauma service can have a significant impact on the survival of the patient (▶ Fig. 5.2).[1] For example, the shorter the time to operative treatment for increased intracranial pressure, or, likewise, intra-abdominal hemorrhage, the better the chances for survival.

5.2 The "Safer Place"

Another important concept in trauma care involves improving the environment of the injured patient. The patient should be removed from the initial hostile, unpredictable, or otherwise inhospitable trauma scene as rapidly as is both safe and feasible and secured in a controlled environment. Typically, this initially involves the ambulance or medical evacuation helicopter followed by

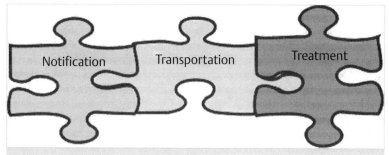

Fig. 5.2 Time Components to the golden hour.

Table 5.1 Environment, monitoring and treatment for the trauma patient

The injury site	Paramedics to the ER	Operating room or ICU
Unstable environment	More stable environment	Ultimate environmental control
No monitoring	Monitoring	Advance monitoring
No treatment	Stabilizing treatment	Definitive treatment
Abbreviations: ER, emergency room; ICU, intensive care unit.		

the emergency or trauma room and, ultimately, the operating room or intensive care unit. Hostile factors include not only the immediate proximal causes of the injury but environmental and situational factors, such as temperature, noise, and medical resource scarcity, all of which can adversely affect outcome. In point of fact, even the hospital environment can be hostile if the receiving physician is unable to control factors such as room temperature to prevent hypothermia or noise from poor crowd control, especially in the trauma bay, that can detrimentally affect communication and movement, and rapid utilization of studies and definitive treatment (e.g., decompressive craniotomy) (▶ Table 5.1).

Taking the patient to a safer place typically involves transportation to an environment such as the intensive care unit or the operating room, where environmental and treatment factors are predictable and controllable.

5.3 Prioritizing Care by the Trauma Team

5.3.1 Primary Assessment and Treatment

The primary assessment or the initial Advanced Trauma Life Support (ATLS) approach to an acutely injured patient requires the prioritized assessment and treatment of vital systems that are required for the support of all vital organs.

These systems are defined by the mnemonic ABC (airway, breathing, and circulation). The efficiency of assessment and treatment involves a team of trained professionals: trauma team captain, primary assessor, airway assessor, and trauma nurses. The trauma captain oversees the flow of the patient's overall care while the primary assessor carries out the majority of the physical examination and treatment. The care team member positioned at the head of the bed manages the airway and is usually an anesthesiologist or another emergency or trauma physician trained in airway management. In concert with the ATLS assessment, trauma nurses perform initial vital signs and placement of monitoring devices. They also start intravenous lines and administer the appropriate medications.

Airway

The loss of airway resulting in inadequate delivery of oxygenated blood to the brain and other vital organs is one of the earliest causes of death in the injured. This systematic approach includes immobilization of the cervical spine because, at this point in the trauma survey, there cannot have been time to fully clear the cervical spine; thus, out of an abundance of caution, it must be assumed that there is traumatic injury to the cervical spine. In the initial trauma survey, there are several indications for placement of an advanced airway to secure the respiratory pathway; some of these include decreased mentation (due to shock or true brain injury), severe maxillofacial injury, aspiration risk (from bleeding or vomiting), obstruction, and inadequacy of respiratory effort (▶ Fig. 5.3).

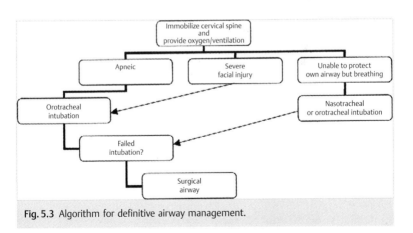

Fig. 5.3 Algorithm for definitive airway management.

Breathing

Hypoxia and anoxia are major contributors to brain injury mortality and to date are still found in 60% of head-injured patients at autopsy.[2] Life-threatening injuries, such as tension pneumothorax, hemothorax, flailed chest, and misplaced endotracheal intubation, must be identified and treated immediately. Inspection of the neck will help identify direct injury or tracheal deviation secondary to large hemothorax or tension pneumothorax (evidenced by deviation to the contralateral side). Auscultation of the chest bilaterally is important to confirm correct placement of the endotracheal tube as well as identification of hemo- or pneumothorax.

Circulation

A single incidence of hypotension increases the odds of mortality in brain-injured patients by 150%.[3,4] Recognition of shock as well as identification of exsanguinating hemorrhage requires an accurate history of the mechanism of injury as well as a thorough physical examination. Hypotension is rarely directly attributable to brain injury, and other sources for the hypotension must be investigated. Direct pressure to stop external hemorrhage controls both arterial and venous bleeding. In addition to external bleeding, internal bleeding and prehospital blood loss must also be recognized and addressed appropriately. For example, patients (particularly pediatric patients) can exsanguinate from a scalp laceration in the field, but on arrival, the bleeding may have stopped. Inaccurate history or poor recognition of this can be fatal due to delay in appropriate and adequate resuscitation. Other important steps in trauma resuscitation include securing two large-bore intravenous lines and early rewarming measures to prevent hypothermia-induced coagulopathies. ▶ Table 5.2 shows the correlation of vital signs and mental status changes to the degree of shock.

The so-called 3-for-1 rule is derived from the empirical observation that most patients in hemorrhagic shock require as much as 300 mL of crystalloid solution for each 100 mL of blood loss. In the trauma setting, patients who fail to restore vital signs after 2 liters of crystalloid bolus (nb: normal saline must be used in the brain-injured patient to prevent hyper- or hypo-osmotic states that may contribute to brain injury) may be in class III shock, and initiation of blood transfusion by massive transfusion protocol should be considered. Failure to recognize the severity of shock can result in excessive crystalloid resuscitation, itself a serious problem, as this may result in decreased perfusion and thereby diminished oxygen delivery to vital organs. The patient's response to resuscitation will help to guide trauma critical care management, summarized in ▶ Table 5.3.

Table 5.2 Estimated fluid and blood losses based on initial presentation[1,2]

	Class I	Class II	Class III	Class IV
Blood loss (mL)	Up to 750	750–1500	1500–2000	>2000
Blood loss (% blood volume)	Up to 15%	15–30%	30–40%	>40%
Pulse rate	<100	>100	>120	>140
Blood pressure	Normal	Normal	Decreased	Decreased
Pulse pressure (mm Hg)	Normal or increased	Decreased	Decreased	Decreased
Respiratory rate	14–20	20–30	30–40	>35
Urine output (mL/h)	>30	20–30	5–15	Negligible
Central nervous system/mental status	Slightly anxious	Mildly anxious	Anxious, confused	Confused, lethargic
Fluid replacement (3:1 rule)	Crystalloid	Crystalloid	Crystalloid and blood	Crystalloid and blood

Table 5.3 Responses to initial fluid resuscitation[a1,2]

	Rapid response	Transient response	No response
Vital signs	Return to normal	Transient improvement; recurrence of ↓ BP and ↑ HR	Remain abnormal
Estimated blood loss	Minimal (10–20%)	Moderate and ongoing (20–40%)	Severe (>40%)
Need for more crystalloid	Low	High	High
Need for blood	Low	Moderate to high	Immediate
Blood preparation	Type and cross-match	Type-specific	Emergent release (not crossed or type specific, usually O negative)
Need for operative intervention	Possibly	Likely	Highly likely
Early presence of surgeon	Yes	Yes	Yes

Abbreviations: BP, blood pressure; HR, heart rate.

[a]2 liters in adults, 20 mL/kg in children.

Disability

In the immediate trauma stabilization setting, prior to the arrival of the neuro-intensivist and/or neurosurgeon, as appropriate, a brief neurologic examination is performed by noting Glasgow Coma Scale on presentation, pupil size, equality, and reaction, and whether the patient spontaneously moves all extremities. It is important to note here that, while there is the tendency to treat brain and spinal injury as supreme to all else, it is vital to remember that the initial trauma stabilization must be allowed to proceed as necessary for the immediate survival of the patient and hemodynamic stabilization prior to any neurologic intervention.

5.3.2 Adjunct Tests/Treatments to the Primary Survey and Resuscitation

- Arterial blood gas.
- Electrocardiographic monitoring.
- Urinary for monitoring of hourly output.
- Gastric catheters (oral placement is preferred if brain injury or facial trauma is suggestive of a basal skull fracture in an intubated patient).
- Anterior-posterior chest, pelvic, lateral cervical spine X-ray if needed.
- CT scan of the abdomen or focused assessment with sonography in trauma (FAST) if there is suspicion of an abdominal injury.[5]
- Diagnostic peritoneal lavage if a FAST or CT exam cannot be done to evaluate the abdomen.[5]

If treatment is required during any part of the ABCs, the patient's airway, breathing, and circulation must be reassessed to assure that a fatal injury has not been missed.

5.3.3 Secondary Assessment

At the conclusion of the primary assessment, the trauma team must perform a thorough secondary assessment. The secondary assessment is a complete history and a more careful head-to-toe physical examination of the injured patient. Adjuncts to the secondary assessment, if warranted, include computerized axial tomographic (CAT) scans of the head, chest, abdomen, and pelvis and angiography. Consultation if warranted to specialized services, such as neurosurgery, orthopaedics, oromaxillofacial surgery, and/or cardiothoracic surgery must be obtained in a timely manner; however, as mentioned previously, the trauma service must be allowed to stabilize the patient prior to specialized intervention to ensure the viability and hemodynamic stability of the patient.

5.4 Conclusion

Traumatically induced injury, particularly brain injury, is a critically time-sensitive pathology. The rapid assessment and stabilization of the trauma patient require a well-coordinated prehospital as well as in-hospital nonhierarchical multidisciplinary system. The initial assessment, which is necessarily performed in minutes, must be detailed, thorough, and sufficiently accurate to recognize and correct life-threatening problems to the airway, breathing, and circulatory system. In the face of traumatic brain injury, the ultimate outcome is not solely affected by the transition to definitive care but is also fundamentally affected by the secondary insults of hypoxia and hypotension.[6,7]

Case Management

During prehospital care, the patient's airway was secured by oral intubation and cervical spine stabilization. Needle thoracostomy was performed on the right chest second intercostal space with a rush of air. Bilateral antecubital large-bore intravenous access was obtained with normal saline infused. After this fluid resuscitation, the blood pressure increased to 110/60 and the heart rate dropped to 98.

On arrival to the emergency room, the patient's airway was confirmed by direct laryngoscopy. Breath sounds continued to be diminished on the right, where a chest tube was placed, with 200 mL of blood released on initial entry. The patient's arterial saturation improved from 80 to 98% on 100% inspired oxygen. Blood pressure and heart rate remained unchanged. Body temperature was 94°F. Glasgow Coma Scale score was 6 T (E1 V1 T M4). Chest and pelvic X-rays were obtained that revealed wide mediastinum, pulmonary contusion, and pelvic fractures. The patient was then taken for head/chest/abdomen/pelvis CAT scans, which showed evidence of cerebral edema with no shift, bilateral pulmonary contusions, and a grade II liver laceration. The patient was transported to intensive care with continued resuscitation and warming measures. Intracranial pressure monitoring was placed via external ventricular drain with mechanical and pharmacological treatment of cerebral edema. The patient was also considered for advanced multimodal brain monitoring.[8] Pulmonary protective ventilation strategies were initiated.

References

[1] American College of Surgeons. Advanced Trauma Life Support–ATLS. 9th ed. Chicago, IL: American College of Surgeons; 2012

[2] US Dept of Transportation, Federal Highway Administration. ITS Benefits: Continuing Successes and Operational Test Results. Pub No. FHWA-JPO-98–002,12/97(1.5M)EW 10/97, p14. ntl.bts.gov/lib/jpodocs/repts_te/4003.pdf

[3] Graham DI, Ford I, Adams JH, et al. Ischaemic brain damage is still common in fatal non-missile head injury. J Neurol Neurosurg Psychiatry. 1989; 52(3):346–350

[4] Chesnut RM, Marshall LF, Klauber MR, et al. The role of secondary brain injury in determining outcome from severe head injury. J Trauma. 1993; 34(2):216–222

[5] Stengel D, Rademacher G, Ekkernkamp A, Güthoff C, Mutze S. Emergency ultrasound-based algorithms for diagnosing blunt abdominal trauma. Cochrane Database Syst Rev. 2015; 9(9): CD004446

[6] Wang HC, Sun CF, Chen H, et al. Where are we in the modelling of traumatic brain injury? Models complicated by secondary brain insults. Brain Inj. 2014; 28(12):1491–1503

[7] Algattas H, Huang JH. Traumatic Brain Injury pathophysiology and treatments: early, intermediate, and late phases post-injury. Int J Mol Sci. 2013; 15(1):309–341

[8] Citerio G, Oddo M, Taccone FS. Recommendations for the use of multimodal monitoring in the neurointensive care unit. Curr Opin Crit Care. 2015; 21(2):113–119

6 The Spinal Cord Injury Patient

Christopher Elia, Blake Berman, Jeffery M. Jones, Shokry Lawandy, Yancey Beamer, and Dan E. Miulli

Abstract

The management of spinal cord injuries is essentially no different than management of brain injuries. The goal of treatment is to prevent ischemia by decompressing the central nervous system, stabilizing the structures that support the spinal cord, and restoring blood flow. The examination of the spinal cord requires the same precision as the examination of the brain. The astute clinician should be able to distinguish a complete from an incomplete spinal cord injury as well as the conditions that make such a determination clouded.

Keywords: ASIA scale, autonomic dysfunction, bulbocavernosus reflex, complete spinal cord injury, incomplete spinal cord injury, neurogenic shock, spinal cord injury, spinal shock

Case Study

A 77-year-old woman is seen in the emergency department 5 hours after a mechanical fall down three steps. The patient's Glasgow Coma Scale score is 15 per the emergency department. She is also noted to have suffered a right midshaft femur fracture and multiple cuts and bruises on her knees and elbows. Physical examination reveals an awake and alert patient with stable vital signs. Focused neurologic exam reveals the pertinent positive findings to be 3/5 strength of her bilateral deltoid, biceps, and brachioradialis muscles; however, the remaining distal musculature is flaccid. She has preserved pinprick sensation only from the lateral elbow and up, and spinal reflexes are absent, including abdominocutaneous, cremasteric, anocutaneous, and bulbocavernosus reflexes. While the patient is being interviewed she begins to display signs of respiratory distress, including decreased pulmonary excursion and difficulty answering questions. The patient's blood pressure suddenly drops to 65 systolic and SPO$_2$ (saturation of peripheral oxygen) declines to 78. Neuroimaging reveals a flexion-distraction-type fracture at C6.

See end of chapter for Case Management.

6.1 Introduction

When encountering a patient with spinal cord injury (SCI), special consideration is paid to the basic principles of trauma in order to optimize the patient's outcome and survival, while also addressing the specific issues that are related to the spinal cord itself. Principles of treatment of spinal cord injury (SCI) patients include the following:

1. Preservation of life and prevention of complications.
2. Preservation of neurologic function.
3. Restoration of spinal stability and treatment of deformity.
4. Optimizing the potential for neurologic recovery and rehabilitation.

SCI may be emergently life threatening. SCI may acutely and adversely affect cardiopulmonary stability due to traumatic disruption of autonomic pathways in the spinal cord. Strict adherence to Advanced Trauma Life Support/Advanced Cardiovascular Life Support (ATLS/ACLS) protocols must be observed. Although radiographic findings and the neurologic exam are important in assessing SCI and spinal trauma, emergency measures are considered first. Emergent intubation, correction of blood pressure and volume, and similar emergency resuscitative measures may be indicated. A complete understanding of autonomic function and preservation of such is critical. Additionally, the physiology and consequences of cardiopulmonary events in SCI patients must be completely understood.

6.1.1 Effects of Spinal Cord Injury on Autonomic Function

Overview of the Autonomic Nervous System: Autonomic anatomy and physiology are complex and are only reviewed in brief detail here. The autonomic nervous system (ANS) is unique in that it requires a sequential two-neuron efferent pathway; the preganglionic neuron must first synapse onto a postganglionic neuron before innervating the target organ. The preganglionic, or first, neuron will begin at the "outflow" and will synapse at the postganglionic, or second, neuron's cell body. The postganglionic neuron will then synapse at the target organ. The two divisions of the ANS are the sympathetic and the parasympathetic divisions. The sympathetic nervous system outflow is from the thoracolumbar region (T1–L2/3) of the spinal cord. The parasympathetic nervous system outflow is from craniosacral neurons that begin at cranial nerves III, VII, IX, and X, and from the S2–S4 sacral nerve roots.

In spinal cord injury, a phenomenon known as traumatic sympathectomy, leading to *deafferentation*, may occur. This phenomenon is essentially a traumatic disconnection of sympathetic outflow, which is responsible for the maintenance of blood pressure and therefore blood flow and oxygen delivery to tissues. Traumatic sympathectomy leads to uninhibited parasympathetic outflow leading to vasodilation, decreased heart rate, and decreased cardiac contractility. This phenomenon may rapidly lead to *neurogenic shock*, which must be clinically distinguished from *spinal shock*,[1] a distinct entity.

6.2 Neurogenic Shock

Neurogenic shock results from excessive vasodilation and impaired distribution of blood flow; it typically presents with hypotension and bradycardia (vs. hypotension and tachycardia in hypovolemic/hemorrhagic shock). Decreased systemic vascular resistance results in pooling of blood within the extremities. Hypotension can cause secondary damage to an already injured spinal cord, while also dramatically worsening outcomes for any associated closed head injury. Neurogenic shock can be a potentially devastating complication, leading to organ dysfunction and death, if not promptly recognized and treated.

6.2.1 Treatment of Neurogenic Shock

Volume resuscitation and hemodynamic stability are the mainstays of treatment of neurogenic shock. Because patients with SCI frequently have multisystem injury, it is critical to rule out hemorrhagic shock in these patients, though that is typically associated with hypotension and tachycardia versus neurogenic shock, which is typically associated with hypotension and bradycardia or eucardia. Volume resuscitation for patients with neurogenic shock can be done with fluids and/or blood and blood products (cryoprecipitate, fresh frozen plasma, and platelets). Inotropic and vasopressor agents are also used—it makes intuitive sense to use sympathomimetics in the face of "traumatic sympathectomy." Sympathomimetics, such as epinephrine, noradrenaline hydrotartrate (norepinephrine), phenylephrine, dobutamine, and dopamine can be used. Most recommendations concerning vasopressor choice are based on class III evidence, and there are no prospective, randomized, placebo-controlled trials at this time. Most authors advocate the use of norepinephrine or dopamine. Dopamine is the precursor of norepinephrine, both of which act on alpha-1 and beta-1 receptors. In some studies dobutamine was used with good results. Vasopressin is not used because of the antidiuretic effects, which can lead to water retention and hyponatremia. Phenylephrine acts only on alpha-1 receptors and can theoretically cause worsened hypotension by a reflexive bradycardia, especially when not used in conjunction with another beta agonist.

The goal for mean arterial pressure (MAP) is generally regarded to be 85 mm Hg, although several studies have shown no mortality difference between a MAP of < 85 mm Hg and a MAP of < 90 mm Hg. The objective of higher MAPs than found in other forms of shock is to increase spinal perfusion.

6.3 Spinal Shock

Spinal shock is defined as the complete loss of all neurologic function, including reflexes and rectal tone, below the specific level of the SCI, which may also be associated with autonomic dysfunction. This kind of shock is a state of transient *physiological*, as opposed to *anatomical*, reflex depression of spinal cord function below the level of injury, with associated loss of all sensorimotor functions.[2] Spinal shock results in the release of catecholamines, causing an initial increase in blood pressure often followed by hypotension; flaccid paralysis, including of the bowel and bladder, and oftentimes sustained priapism are observed. Symptoms of spinal shock can last several hours to days until the reflex arcs below the level of the injury begin to function again; however, spinal shock typically starts to recede within 24 hours. The most reliable indicator of the return of spinal reflex arc function is the bulbocavernosus reflex (BCR), which is the first reflex to return as spinal shock begins to recede.[2] The last residue of spinal shock disappears weeks to months after an SCI as flaccid paralysis is replaced by muscle spasticity.

> **Key Clinical Point:** Until there is return of the bulbocavernosus reflex (BCR), the physical examination is unreliable and the patient may still be in spinal shock (▶ Table 6.1).

Table 6.1 Important reflexes

Abdominal cutaneous reflex	T8–T12	• A cortical reflex that is elicited by stroking one quadrant of the abdomen, which causes contraction of the underlying musculature, which causes the umbilicus to migrate toward that quadrant.
Bulbocavernosus reflex	S2–S4	• Bulbocavernosus reflex is used to determine the absence of spinal shock.[1] • First reflex to return. Absence of this reflex documents continuation of spinal shock or spinal injury at the level of the reflex arc itself. • The reflex is elicited by genital stimulation and produces anal contraction. • No injury may be considered a complete injury until spinal shock has resolved.
Cremasteric reflex	L1–L2	• Superficial reflex that consists of scrotal shrinkage following stroking of the inner thigh.

Table 6.1 continued

Anal cutaneous	S2–S4	• Known as anal wink. • Contraction of the anal sphincter following stimulation of the skin surrounding the anus.
Reverse radial reflex	UMN	• Indicates upper motor neuron dysfunction.
Hoffmann's reflex	UMN	• Indicates upper motor neuron dysfunction.
Priapism		• Indicates loss of sympathetic tone following cord injury and a predominance of parasympathetic tone.

6.4 Primary versus Secondary Spinal Cord Injury

SCI does not stop at the time of the ictus, or accident; it is a dynamic process in which the injury starts at the outset ("primary" SCI), and can progress with subsequent sequelae ("secondary" SCI). The key point is that, for SCI, the full extent of injury may not be initially apparent. Incomplete cord lesions may evolve into more complete lesions. Commonly, the level of injury may rise one or two spinal cord levels during the hours to days after the initial event, leading to devastating consequences. A complex cascade of pathophysiological events related to free radicals, vasogenic edema, and altered blood flow accounts for the clinical phenomena of secondary SCI. Normal oxygenation, blood perfusion, and acid–base balance are required to minimize secondary SCI.

Primary SCI arises from acute mechanical disruption, transection, or distraction of neural elements. It is usually, but not always, associated with fracture and/or dislocation of the spine. It may be caused by penetrating injuries from bullets, projectiles, stabbings, and the like, or it may be caused by displaced bony fragments. Primary SCI may be caused by extradural pathology due to direct cord compression (includes epidural hematomas, disk ruptures, bone fragments, and foreign bodies). Longitudinal distraction, with or without flexion and/or extension of the vertebral column, may result in primary SCI without spinal fracture or dislocation since the spinal cord is tethered more securely than the vertebral column. These injuries may not be apparent radiographically, resulting in the condition known as spinal cord injury without radiological abnormality (SCIWORA).

Secondary SCI occurs after the primary ictus, which serves as the nidus from which additional secondary mechanisms of injury extend. Secondary SCI mechanisms include, but are not limited to, ischemia, hemorrhage, thrombosis, edema, inflammation, free radical–induced cell injury and death, glutamate excitotoxicity, cytoskeletal degradation and induction of apoptosis,[3] fluid/electrolyte disturbances, mitochondrial dysfunction, immunologic injury, and

107

other miscellaneous processes.[4] Anoxic or hypoxic effects compound the extent of SCI. Neurocritical care goals are to minimize secondary SCI, largely by assuring spinal cord perfusion and oxygenation.

6.5 Complete Spinal Cord versus Incomplete Spinal Cord Injury

Complete SCI is characterized clinically as complete loss of motor and sensory function below the level of the traumatic lesion; incomplete SCI is characterized by variable neurologic findings with partial loss of sensory and/or motor function below the level of injury. The American Spinal Injury Association (ASIA) grading system is useful in describing the severity of SCI, complete versus incomplete (▶ Table 6.2). Incomplete SCIs are summarized in ▶ Table 6.3. All these patients end up in the neurosurgical critical care unit.

Table 6.2 American Spinal Injury Association (ASIA) Impairment Scale[5]

A	Complete	No motor or sensory function is preserved in the sacral segments S4–S5.
B	Incomplete	Sensory but not motor function is preserved below the neurologic level and extends through the sacral segments S4–S5.
C	Incomplete	Motor function is preserved below the neurologic level, and the majority of key muscles below the neurologic level have a muscle grade < 3.
D	Incomplete	Motor function is preserved below the neurologic level, and the majority of key muscles below the neurologic level have a muscle grade ≥ 3.
E	Normal	Motor and sensory function is normal.

Table 6.3 Incomplete spinal cord syndromes[6,7]

Syndrome	Mechanism	Motor loss	Sensory loss	Recovery
Brown–Séquard[8,9]	Hemisection of the spinal cord is usually caused by penetrating objects. Tumors or hematomas can also be a source.	Ipsilateral loss of motor below level of lesion.	Contralateral loss of pain and temperature below level of lesion. Ipsilateral loss of light touch, proprioception, vibration.	Most promising of the incomplete syndromes in terms of recovery. ~ 90% will regain independent ambulation, anal and urinary sphincter control.

Table 6.3 continued

Syndrome	Mechanism	Motor loss	Sensory loss	Recovery
Central cord[10, 11]	Accidents or minor falls resulting in neck extension are common causes.	Motor loss is greater in upper than lower extremities. UE recovery is variable. Fine motor of UEs usually does not recover so well.	Majority have intact bowel and bladder because of the peripheral arrangement of sacral fibers in the cord.	Will usually ambulate but commonly with spasticity.
Anterior cord[12]	Usually flexion-compression mechanism, diving accidents. Ischemic injury from compression of anterior spinal artery.	Loss of all motor function below lesion.	Loss of pain and temperature sensation below the lesion, in face of preservation of posterior column sensation; bowel/bladder also affected.	The poorest prognosis for any recovery of motor function of all the incomplete syndromes; only 10–20% may regain motor function.
Posterior cord		Preservation of motor function.	Preservation of pain and temperature function with loss of posterior column function (proprioception, two-point tactile discrimination, vibration modalities).	Patients can walk but rely on visual input for spatial orientation. Prognosis is unknown because it is so rare.
Conus medullaris	Injury to the terminal spinal cord usually just posterior to the bodies from T12 to L1. Trauma, tumor, infection.	Produces loss of bowel and bladder control, poor rectal muscle tone. No motor signs in legs (if pure). If motor loss, it is symmetrical and ankle jerk is absent (S1).	Loss of perirectal sensation. Saddle distribution of sensory loss.	Prognosis is poor for significant return of bowel and bladder.

Patients with incomplete SCI have a lot to lose, and they are at risk of progression to complete SCI. Various incomplete SCI syndromes need to be recognized, so appropriate management and prognosis can be considered. Incomplete SCI syndromes include anterior cord syndrome, Brown–Séquard syndrome, central cord syndrome, posterior cord syndrome, and cauda equina syndrome:

- Anterior cord syndrome: Involves a lesion causing variable loss of motor function and loss of pain and/or temperature sensation, with preservation of proprioception.

- Brown–Séquard syndrome: Is often associated with spinal cord hemisection and involves a relatively greater ipsilateral loss of proprioception and motor function, with contralateral loss of pain and temperature sensation.

- Central cord syndrome: Usually involves a cervical lesion and is associated with greater motor weakness in the upper extremities than in the lower extremities, with sacral sensory sparing. The pattern of motor weakness shows greater distal involvement in the affected extremity than proximally. Sensory loss is variable, and the patient is more likely to lose pain and/or temperature sensation than proprioception and/or vibration. Dysesthesias, especially those in the upper extremities, are common (e.g., sensation of burning in the hands or arms, allodynia, is not uncommon).

- Posterior cord syndrome: Involves damage to the dorsal columns of the spinal cord, thus the main deficit is poor coordination, whereas motor function and pain sensation are intact.

- Conus medullaris syndrome: Involves injury to the distal tip, or conus medullaris, of the spinal cord, usually located at the L1/L2 disk level. The most common symptoms include excruciating back pain, bowel and bladder dysfunction, sexual dysfunction, and variable motor and sensory disturbance of the lower extremities; Achilles reflex is typically suppressed or absent.

- Cauda equina syndrome: Although not strictly a "spinal cord" syndrome because the cauda equina is *anatomically distal* to the spinal cord and so a peripheral nerve injury, it is lumped together with neurologic injury associated with spinal fractures and disk herniations, and has a clinical presentation that is similar to that of conus medullaris syndrome. Cauda equina syndrome is characterized by injury to multiple lumbar nerve roots emerging from the conus medullaris, usually below the L1/L2 disk level. This syndrome can lead to unilateral, but usually bilateral, saddle sensory loss, bladder and bowel dysfunction, and variable lower extremity weakness and sensory problems; the patellar and Achilles reflexes are typically absent, and impotence is less common than in conus medullaris syndrome.

6.6 Spine Precautions: Immobilization

For the neurosurgical intensive care unit (NICU) patient with SCI, it is always safe to assume the spine is unstable until proven otherwise. Particular attention is paid to the unconscious or obtunded patient who may lack protective mechanisms. It is safest to maintain the entire spine in continuous "in-line" immobilization during any resuscitative maneuvers or during movement or transport of any kind. Rigid cervical collars, use of spine boards, and the "log roll" maneuver should be routine in the NICU. When intubation is necessary, maintain the cervical spine in constant in-line immobilization. Tracheal intubation may be required if emergent, or the use of fiberoptic laryngoscopy and topical anesthetics under titrated intravenous sedation may be needed. Since spinal immobilization has been the standard of care, it alone has had a dramatic impact resulting in a decline in percentage of complete SCIs from 55% in the 1970s to 39% in the 1980s.

6.7 Steroid Use in Spinal Cord Injury

Multiple studies have been done to explore the effect of low-, or high-dose, steroids in SCI. The three iterations of the North American Spinal Cord Injury Study (NASCIS I, II, and III) are summarized in ▶ Table 6.4. In brief, although initial results from NASCIS led to use of high-dose methylprednisolone looked promising, later findings showed adverse side effects, including the following potential adverse effects of high-dose steroid administration in trauma patients:

- Increased incidence of infectious and septic complications.
- Increased incidence and severity of respiratory complication.
- Increased incidence of pulmonary embolism.
- Worsening of head injury outcome.
- Increased incidence of gastrointestinal hemorrhage.
- Increased incidence of pancreatitis.
- Possibility of missed hollow viscus injury due to "masking" of abdominal signs.

In all three NASCIS studies and other, smaller studies, the incidence of sepsis and pneumonia was higher in the high-dose methylprednisolone groups than in the placebo or other treatment groups. In light of these serious side effects, the authors do not initiate high-dose steroid use for SCI at their trauma centers in Southern California.

Table 6.4 North American Spinal Cord Injury Study[13,14,15,16,17,18,19,20,21,22,23,24]

Study	Study type	Format	Results	Conclusion
NASCIS I	Multicenter randomized, double-blinded clinical trial 1979, reported in 1984	Compared MP 100 mg bolus and then MPS 100 mg/d × 10 d *versus* 1000 mg bolus and then 1000 mg/d × 10 d	There was no difference in neurologic recovery between the groups but there was no control.	MP at the tested levels did not significantly change outcome. Was the level of MPS to low?
NASCIS II	Multicenter reported in 1990	Standard dosage-30 mg/kg bolus then 5.4 mg/kg/h infusion for 23 hours was used compared to patients receiving naloxone at 5.4 mg/kg bolus then 4 mg/kg/h for 23 h or placebo Randomized within 12 hours	MP administered within 8 hours was associated with a significant improvement in motor score, sensation at 6-month follow-up. The authors also reported statistically significant improvement of motor scores at 1 year.	Post hoc analyses detected a small gain in the total motor and sensory score in a subgroup of patients who had received the drug within 8 hours after their injury.
NASCIS III	Double-blinded, multicenter study No placebo	Compared a 48-hour infusion of MP with a 24-hour infusion started within 8 hours after injury and found no benefit from extending the infusion beyond 24 hours	48-hour MP group showed improved motor score at 6 weeks and improved motor score and functional score at 6 months compared to MP 24 and 24 TM, especially if given between 3 and 8 hours	Found no benefit from extending the infusion beyond 24 hours
Cochrane review	Meta-analysis	Based on the controversial subgroup post hoc analyses in NASCIS II and III and the data from a Japanese study		Concluded that a 24-hour high-dose MP infusion within 8 hours after injury is efficacious

Abbreviations: MP, methylprednisolone; NASCIS, North American Spinal Cord Injury Study; TM, tirilazad mesylate.

Case Management

Preservation of life and prevention of complications: The patient was maintained with in-line cervical traction and emergently intubated for airway protection and optimization of cardiopulmonary function, oxygenation, and prevention of metabolic abnormalities. She was placed on intravenous (IV) norepinephrine 0.5 µg/kg/min, which was titrated to maintain a mean arterial pressure (MAP) of 85 mm Hg. She was placed on 100% FIO_2 (fraction of inspired oxygen) to maintain PaO_2 115 mm Hg. This would be temporary and to be titrated down. An arterial line was placed to properly monitor arterial pressure, and a triple lumen central venous catheter was placed for good venous access and for administration of medications, IV fluids, and/or blood or blood products. A 0.9% NaCl IV fluid bolus was given, and the patient's MAP was restored to 85–90 mm Hg. An arterial blood gas volume was obtained and was "normal," with the exception of a PaO_2 of 115 mm Hg.

Preservation of neurologic function: With the above completed, the patient is already on track to accomplish this goal. At this time, the examination is unreliable because the BCR has not yet returned. Serial neurologic examinations will be performed to confirm return of the BCR, and to obtain a fully reliable exam. Based on the results of the NASCIS trials, high-dose methylprednisolone treatment was not initialized. Radiographically, there was a flexion-distraction type injury and loss of normal physiological alignment. The patient was considered appropriate for placement of a halo ring, and weighted traction was initiated. After approximately 12 hours, the BCR returned, and follow-up radiographs showed markedly improved cervical alignment.

Restoration of spinal stability and treatment of deformity: On post-trauma day 4, the patient's neurologic exam was confirmed as a "complete" C6-level SCI. She was now off ventilator support and maintaining a MAP of 85 mm Hg. She was also determined to be clinically stable for surgery. Because magnetic resonance imaging revealed complete posterior ligamentous complex disruption, findings consistent with transection of the cervical spinal cord, she was taken to the operating room for surgical correction,[25] which was performed without incident.

Optimizing the potential for neurologic recovery and rehabilitation: On post-trauma day 20, she was transferred to acute inpatient rehabilitation.

References

[1] Atkinson PP, Atkinson JLD. Spinal shock. Mayo Clin Proc. 1996; 71(4):384–389

[2] Chin LS. Spinal cord injuries. http://emedicine.medscape.com/article/793582-overview#aw2aab6b2b3aa

[3] Trump BF, Berezesky I. Calcium-mediated cell injury and cell death. http://www.fasebj.org/content/9/2/219.short2001.pdf

[4] Acute spinal cord injury. Part I: Pathophysiologic mechanisms. In: Dumont RJ, et al, eds. Clinical Neuropharmacology. Vol. 24, no. 5. Philadelphia, PA: Lippincott Williams & Wilkins; 2001:254–264

[5] American Spinal Injury Association. Standards for the Neurologic Classification of Spinal Injury Patients. Chicago, IL: ASIA; 1982

[6] Schneider RC, Crosby EC, Russo RH, Gosch HH. Chapter 32. Traumatic spinal cord syndromes and their management. Clin Neurosurg. 1973; 20:424–492

[7] American Spinal Injury Association. Guidelines for Facility Categorization and Standards of Care: Spinal Cord Injury. Chicago, IL: ASIA; 1981

[8] Lim E, Wong YS, Lo YL, Lim SH. Traumatic atypical Brown-Sequard syndrome: case report and literature review. Clin Neurol Neurosurg. 2003; 105(2):143–145

[9] Rumana CS, Baskin DS. Brown-Sequard syndrome produced by cervical disc herniation: case report and literature review. Surg Neurol. 1996; 45(4):359–361

[10] Maroon JC, Abla AA, Wilberger JI, Bailes JE, Sternau LL. Central cord syndrome. Clin Neurosurg. 1991; 37:612–621

[11] Massaro F, Lanotte M, Faccani G. Acute traumatic central cord syndrome. Acta Neurol (Napoli). 1993; 15(2):97–105

[12] Schneider RC. The syndrome of acute anterior spinal cord injury. J Neurosurg. 1955; 12(2):95–122

[13] Bracken MB, Collins WF, Freeman DF, et al. Efficacy of methylprednisolone in acute spinal cord injury. JAMA. 1984; 251(1):45–52

[14] Bracken MB, Shepard MJ, Hellenbrand KG, et al. Methylprednisolone and neurological function 1 year after spinal cord injury. Results of the National Acute Spinal Cord Injury Study. J Neurosurg. 1985; 63(5):704–713

[15] Bracken MB, Shepard MJ, Collins WF, et al. A randomized, controlled trial of methylprednisolone or naloxone in the treatment of acute spinal-cord injury. Results of the Second National Acute Spinal Cord Injury Study. N Engl J Med. 1990; 322(20):1405–1411

[16] Bracken MB, Shepard MJ, Collins WF, Jr, et al. Methylprednisolone or naloxone treatment after acute spinal cord injury: 1-year follow-up data. Results of the second National Acute Spinal Cord Injury Study. J Neurosurg. 1992; 76(1):23–31

[17] Bracken MB, Shepard MJ, Holford TR, et al. Administration of methylprednisolone for 24 or 48 hours or tirilazad mesylate for 48 hours in the treatment of acute spinal cord injury. Results of the Third National Acute Spinal Cord Injury Randomized Controlled Trial. National Acute Spinal Cord Injury Study. JAMA. 1997; 277(20):1597–1604

[18] Bracken MB, Shepard MJ, Holford TR, et al. Methylprednisolone or tirilazad mesylate administration after acute spinal cord injury: 1-year follow up. Results of the third National Acute Spinal Cord Injury randomized controlled trial. J Neurosurg. 1998; 89(5):699–706

[19] Bracken MB. Pharmacological interventions for acute spinal cord injury. Cochrane Database Syst Rev. 2000;(2):CD001046. Review. Update in: Cochrane Database Sys Rev 2002;(3):CD001046

[20] Matsumoto T, Tamaki T, Kawakami M, Yoshida M, Ando M, Yamada H. Early complications of high-dose methylprednisolone sodium succinate treatment in the follow-up of acute cervical spinal cord injury. Spine. 2001; 26(4):426–430

[21] Galandiuk S, Raque G, Appel S, Polk HC, Jr. The two-edged sword of large-dose steroids for spinal cord trauma. Ann Surg. 1993; 218(4):419–425, discussion 425–427

[22] Gerndt SJ, Rodriguez JL, Pawlik JW, et al. Consequences of high-dose steroid therapy for acute spinal cord injury. J Trauma. 1997; 42(2):279–284

[23] Nesathurai S. Steroids and spinal cord injury: revisiting the NASCIS 2 and NASCIS 3 trials. J Trauma. 1998; 45(6):1088–1093

[24] Steroids for spinal cord injury. http://www.trauma.org/archive/spine/steroids.html

[25] Fehlings MG, Vaccaro A, Wilson JR, et al. Early versus delayed decompression for traumatic cervical spinal cord injury: results of the Surgical Timing in Acute Spinal Cord Injury Study (STASCIS). PLoS ONE. 2012; 7(2):e32037

7 Delayed Intracerebral Hemorrhage

Tyler Carson, Marc Billings, Todd M. Goldenberg, Vladimir Adriano Cortez, and Dan E. Miulli

Abstract

As much as 50% of the morbidity and mortality associated with head injury and possibly stroke comes from secondary injury. The secondary injury has been decreased due to dedicated intensive care unit awareness and management by the physician and the nursing and ancillary staff. Once the brain has been decompressed of its extravasated blood, the tamponing effect of that same condition is lost and allows a possible hyperemic condition in the setting of a broken blood–brain barrier. It is incumbent upon the clinician to recognize when and how the central nervous system should be decompressed in order to restore blood flow to prevent and reverse ischemia. The neuroscientist should also understand the possible results of the decompression, especially if the blood pressure is not controlled.

Keywords: anticoagulation, DTICH, epidural hematoma, evacuation ICH, intracerebral hemorrhage, intraventricular hemorrhage, rtPA, SBP < 140, subdural hematoma

Case Presentation

A 35-year-old man fell from a 6-foot ladder. His family describes a brief 2- to 3-minute loss of consciousness with significant confusion after the event. He was transported by emergency medical services to the hospital. On initial evaluation by paramedics, the patient was noted to have a Glasgow Coma Scale score (GCS) of 13 and continued as such at the hospital. He had no focal neurologic deficits at that time. A noncontrasted head computed tomographic (CT) scan obtained upon arrival at the hospital showed a 6 mm right frontoparietal subdural hematoma (► Fig. 7.1).

The radiologist reported no additional intracranial lesions or skull fractures. The patient was admitted for observation. After ~ 3 hours, the patient developed a fixed and dilated left pupil and a GCS score of 9. The patient received an emergent repeat CT scan that showed a 3 cm left frontoparietal epidural hematoma with a 1 cm midline shift (► Fig. 7.2).

See end of chapter for Case Management.

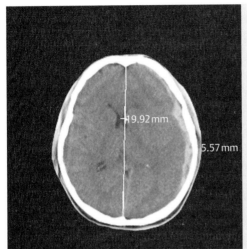

Fig. 7.1 Subdural hematoma.

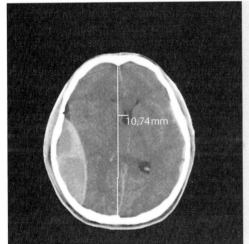

Fig. 7.2 Epidural hematoma.

7.1 Intracerebral Hemorrhages

Intracerebral hemorrhage (ICH) has been a topic of significant research in the past several decades and includes multiple etiologies, including uncontrolled hypertension, amyloid angiopathy, anticoagulant use, cerebrovascular disease, tumors, migraines, and invasive procedures. Bleeding is usually short lived and is tamponaded by anatomical and physiological means; however, it is associated with a 30-day morbidity and mortality of 60% and 30%, respectively.[1] Elevated blood pressure, defined as a systolic blood pressure (SBP) greater than 140 mm Hg, is seen in 75% of patients with acute ICH, and strict control of blood pressure is paramount in prevention of delayed rebleeding.[2]

The ICH score described by Hemphil in 2001 offers a good predictive factor for the 30-day mortality (▶ Table 7.1).[3] Any delayed rebleeding may result in increased clot size and increased ICH score and, as a result, in a significant increase in estimated mortality.

To decrease the risk of delayed nontraumatic intracranial hemorrhage from head injury during the first hour to 24 hours, large spikes in SBP or any blood pressure greater than 140 mm Hg systolic must be prevented. Helping to prevent delayed nontraumatic intracranial hemorrhage would also include avoiding the use of hypotonic fluid and preventing hyperthermia.

Table 7.1 Intracerebral hemorrhage scoring

Components	Finding	Points
Glasgow Coma Scale score	3–4	2
	5–12	1
	13–15	0
Volume	> 30 mL	1
	< 30 mL	0
Intraventricular	Yes	1
	No	0
Infratentorial origin	Yes	1
	No	1
Age	≥ 80 years	1
	< 80 years	0
Points	**Estimated 30-day mortality (%)**	
1	0	
2	13	
3	72	
4	97	
5	100	
6	100	

7.2 Treatment Guidelines for Spontaneous ICH

Many attempts to classify surgical indications for evacuation of ICH have been and continue to be studied.[4] The International Surgical Trial in Intracerebral Hematoma (STICH) looked at the outcome of 1,033 patients (from 83 centers in 27 countries) treated with early surgery (open craniotomy) versus initial conservative treatment.[5] Ultimately, the STICH trial showed no significant difference between early surgical treatment and nonsurgical treatment groups as a whole. However, there was a subset of the early surgical group that seemed to have a better outcome than conservatively treated patients. These patients had supratentoral ICH that came within 1 cm of the surface. Therefore, the STICH II trail was performed, which looked at early surgery (within 48 hours) versus initial conservative treatment, specifically for patients with ICH with a volume of 10–100 mL, within 1 cm of surface, without intraventricular hemorrhage (IVH) and a GCS motor score of 5–6 and a GCS eye-opening score of ≥ 2.[6] The results showed there was no increase in death or disability at 6 months between groups, and there was a small benefit in overall survival.

Clearly there is a subset of patients that benefit from evacuation of hematoma. To that end the MISTIE and MISTIE-II trials (Minimally Invasive Surgery Plus Recombinant Tissue Type Plasminogen Activator for Intracerebral Hemorrhage) looked to employ a minimally invasive approach to clot evacuation in hopes to decrease the clot size and perihematomal edema (PHE) more effectively than medical treatment alone.[7,8] Currently the MISTIE III trial is under way and has completed enrollment. MISTIE III will determine if the reduction in PHE and clot size results in improved neurologic outcome.

IVH, often accompanying ICH, is associated with increased 30-day mortality based on ICH score.[3] IVH can result in obstructive hydrocephalus and depressed mental status and often requires placement of an external ventricular drain (EVD) for cerebrospinal fluid (CSF) diversion. The tedious task of ensuring continued drainage of sanguineous CSF requires continued flushing, a replacement of EVD. Additionally, drainage of CSF with normalized ICH doesn't reverse the neurologic deficits likely due to toxicity of blood product.[9,10] The CLEAR IVH trial published in 2011 established that administration of intrathecal recombinant tissue plasminogen activator (rtPA) has an acceptable safety profile and has a dose-dependent response, with improved resolution of IVH compared to placebo.[11] CLEAR III study results came out in February 2016. Injecting low-dose tPA into ventricles after intraventricular hemorrhage did not significantly improve the primary endpoint of a good functional outcome. However, the treatment was associated with a 10% reduction in mortality without increasing the number of patients left in a vegetative state or requiring nursing home care. From subgroup analysis, it was also evident that the intervention had the best results in patients who had the most blood evacuated. In those who had bigger clots with more than 20 mL of blood evacuated, there was a significant 10% increase in the number of patients achieving a good functional outcome.

At our institution we have developed a standardized protocol for patients presenting with ICH to both prevent delayed interval increase in ICH and support maximal recovery of neurologic function (▶ Fig. 7.3).

The treatment for acute ICH after neurological evaluation is as follows:

- Immediate blood pressure reduction to SBP < 140 mm Hg (unless elevated creatinine/blood urea nitrogen [Cr/BUN] after control to indicate renal hypoperfusion).
- Immediate reversal of coagulopathy.
- Keep oxygenation in non-chronic obstructive pulmonary disease [COPD] patient ≥ 98%.

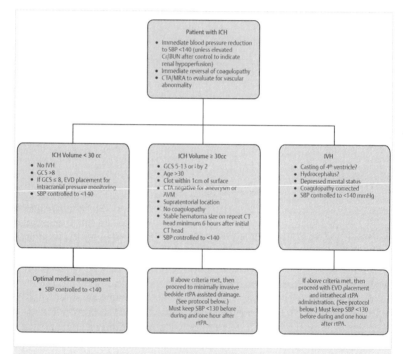

Fig. 7.3 Standardized protocol for patients presenting with intracerebral hemorrhage (ICH) at the authors' institution. AVM, arteriovenous malformation; BUN, blood urea nitrogen; Cr, creatinine; CT, computed tomography; CTA, computed tomographic angiography; EVD, external ventricular drain; GCS, Glasgow Coma Scale; IVH intraventricular hemorrhage; MRA, magnetic resonance angiography; rtPA, recombinant tissue plasminogen activator; SBP, systolic blood pressure.

- Start normal saline intravenous fluid.
- Elevate the head to 30–45 degrees (if trauma suspected then reverse Trendelenburg).
- Computed tomographic angiography/magnetic resonance angiography (CTA/MRA) to evaluate for vascular abnormality if the patient is less than 65 years old, or region of bleed is suspicious for aneurysm or arteriovenous malformation (AVM) bleed.
- If the GCS score is ≤ 8, use EVD placement for intracranial pressure monitoring.

The general guidelines for evacuation of an ICH are as follows:
- GCS score 5 to 13 or deterioration of 2 GCS points.
- Volume greater than 30 mL.
- No brainstem involvement, no active myocardial infarction (MI).

7.3 Protocol for Bedside Drainage of Intracerebral Hemorrhage

The criteria in ▶ Fig. 7.3 should be met before proceeding with bedside intra-clot drain placement.

The following supplies are needed:
- Cranial access kit.
- Trauma-style ventricular catheter.
- 10 or 12 Fr Frazier suction tip and suction tubing.
- Sterile gown/gloves/drape.
- Local anesthetic.

7.3.1 Procedure

After 6 hours post-ICH begin by using the bony anatomy to localize the entry point for trajectory of the drain placement. The entry site for the drain should be at a point where the clot comes closest to the cortical surface and 3 cm from the sylvian fissure, midline, or venous sinuses and avoids eloquent brain tissue, such as the motor strip. The hair should be clipped and sterile preparation of surgical site performed. After local anesthetic and appropriate conscious sedation is administered proceed with a 3 cm incision carried down to the cranium. Using the twist drill, create two holes in the same incision ~ 2 cm apart, with one hole directed toward the center of the ICH. Open the dura at both holes. Insert the brain needle with a stylet into the clot, keeping in mind the trajectory and depth at which the clot will be encountered based on CT imaging. Once the clot has been accessed, slowly dilate the tract by rotating the needle in a progressively wider circular motion. Insert Frazier suction with a stylet in into the tract, then remove the stylet and hook up the wall suction. Aspirate no more than 50% of the clot and do not aspirate to yield < 15 mL remaining. Stop suction and remove the Frazier sucker. Place a trauma EVD into the center of the hematoma along the previous tract, tunnel > 5 cm from the insertion site. Secure the drain to the skin and close the incision. Attach a three-way stopcock to the end of the catheter with bulb suction connected to one side of the stopcock; do not attach to sunction. Obtain a CT head scan immediately after the procedure. Make sure the EVD is in the center of the hematoma cavity. Then, if there is no active bleeding and SBP < 130 mm Hg, give 2 mg rtPA through a trauma-style EVD immediately upon return to the ICU, clamp the stopcock for 1 hour, then open to subdural bulb suction. Keep the SBP < 140 mm Hg during the interim. Repeat the CT head scan in 12 hours, and if there is no increase in the size of the hematoma, proceed with administration of 2 mg rtPA per EVD every 12 hours, clamping for 1 hour after each administration. Maintain a strict SBP goal of < 130 mm Hg before, during, and 1 hour after clamping. Continue administration of rtPA until the output is minimal or a CT head scan shows the clot volume to be < 15 mL. Check with a CT head scan at least after the first and eighth dose.

7.4 Protocol for Intrathecal rtPA Administration for Intraventricular Hemorrhage

Place the EVD using the standard method. Prior to administering intrathecal rtPA ensure the CTA is negative for aneurysm or AVM. Ensure that SBP is kept strictly < 130 mm Hg before, during, and after clamping. If blood pressure is labile, use nicardipine or an equivalent during and after clamping to keep SBP < 140 mm Hg. First remove 3 mL of CSF from the EVD and administer 2 mg of intrathecal rtPA mixed in 3 mL of sterile saline or water via EVD. Keep EVD clamped for 1 hour or as long as the patient can tolerate without sustained elevated intracranial pressures. Open the EVD and place level at 6 mm Hg above the external auditory canal. Obtain a repeat CT head scan within 12 hours of administration of the first dose of rtPA. If the scan is negative for new hemorrhage proceed with administration of rtPA every 12 hours using the same protocol as for the initial administration. Continue with rtPA administration until there is CT evidence of resolution of the IVH, especially within the fourth ventricle and CSF output becomes blood tinged to clear. Check the CT head scan at least after the first and eighth dose.

Case Example

A 48-year-old woman was found in her automobile in status epilepticus with generalized tonicoclonic seizures and a history of traveling cross-country for 1 month. Her past medical history and family medical history were negative except for a 6-week fast for religious reasons. She was intubated and sedated; seizure control was achieved via benzodiazepines. Initially, she had a GCS score of 7 T with mild (4/5) left-sided hemiparesis. A CT scan of the brain demonstrated a 1.3 cm intraparenchymal hematoma in the right parietal lobe with edematous changes associated with an infarct in the left parietal convexity (▶ Fig. 7.4).

A thrombus was directly visualized on CT in the superior sagittal sinus and the right transverse sinus and later confirmed on magnetic resonance imaging (MRI). The patient was diagnosed with venous sinus thrombosis secondary to severe dehydration with an associated intracranial hemorrhage and infarction. Aggressive rehydration and anticoagulation therapy with heparin were initiated. On reexamination of the patient 4 hours after beginning the heparin protocol, the patient had improved and was observed to have a GCS score of 11 T with residual left hemiparesis but moving all extremities. The patient was weaned to extubation and continued to become more alert. Thirty-six hours status postheparinization, the patient was noted to have a flaccid left side, although with a GCS score of 15. An emergent CT scan of the brain demonstrated a rebleed into the original intraparenchymal hemorrhage in the right parietal convexity, now measuring 3 cm, with worsening edema bilaterally (▶ Fig. 7.5). The heparin protocol was halted, and aggressive rehydration continued as the primary treatment. The patient's left hemiplegia gradually improved over the course of her hospital stay into a hemiparesis, and she was discharged to a rehabilitation center.

7.5 Delayed Traumatic Intracerebral Hemorrhage

Delayed hemorrhages previously discovered via angiography were considered relatively rare, yet with the advent of CT scanning, the ease of diagnosis and follow-up has increased, as well as the incidence. Etiologies are both posttraumatic and nontraumatic. The following section reviews the pathogenesis, diagnosis, management, and outcome of these lesions using three case examples. In most cases delayed hemorrhages can be prevented by following the same criteria for ICH:

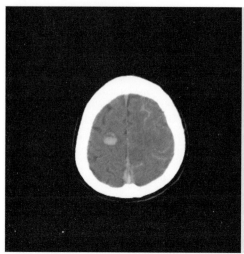

Fig. 7.4 A 1.3 cm intraparenchymal hematoma in the right parietal lobe with edematous changes associated with an infarct in the left parietal convexity.

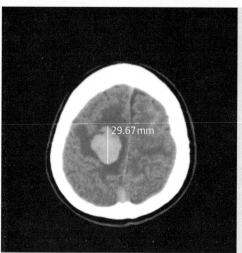

29.67 mm

Fig. 7.5 Rebleed into the original intraparenchymal hemorrhage in the right parietal convexity, now measuring 3 cm, with worsening edema bilaterally.

- Immediate blood pressure reduction to SBP < 140 mm Hg (unless elevated Cr/BUN after control to indicate renal hypoperfusion).
- Immediate reversal of coagulopathy.
- Keep oxygenation in non-COPD patients ≥ 98%.
- Start normal saline intravenous fluid.
- Elevate the head to 30–45 degrees (if trauma suspected then reverse Trendelenburg).

- CTA/MRA to evaluate for vascular abnormality if the patient is less than 65 years old or the hematoma is suspicious for an aneurysm or AVM-associated bleed.
- If the GCS score is ≤ 8, use EVD placement for intracranial pressure monitoring.

In 1891 Bollinger described delayed traumatic intracranial hemorrhages (DTICHs) as *traumatische Spät-Apoplexie* ("traumatic apoplectic event") events using three criteria[12]:
1. An apoplectic event preceded by a traumatic history.
2. A relatively symptom-free period followed by a neurologic decline.
3. The lack of preexisting vascular pathology.

Duret and other researchers expanded on Bollinger's work by delineating the stages of DTICH.[13,14] In the early 1900s, continued research led to theories of pathogenesis for DTICH, which we will discuss. Today, improved imaging has increased detection and diagnosis of DTICH, which was previously limited to operative and autopsy findings and has enhanced our understanding of the disease. DTICH can be divided into epidural, subdural, and intracerebral hemorrhages.

7.6 Delayed Traumatic Epidural Hematoma

A delayed traumatic epidural hematoma (DTEH) exists when there is evidence of an epidural collection of blood on follow-up CT scan that is not apparent on the initial CT scan. This may occur with or without an underlying skull fracture. It has classically been described as "talk and deteriorate." The symptoms vary according to the size and location of the hematoma and range from mild headache to focal neurologic deficits to deep comatose states. The delayed decline can occur anywhere from minutes to weeks after the initial traumatic event, most frequently between 6 and 48 hours after the trauma.[14,15]

The incidence of posttraumatic epidural hematoma in the pre-CT era occurred in less than 10% of all traumatic head injuries.[16,17] The recent widespread use of CT scans reveals an incidence as high as 30%.[18,19,20] DTEH specifically is estimated to occur in 2 to 10% of traumatic head injuries and as such has a predilection in males. It is more frequent in younger adults (average age 27) relative to the elderly.[21] One possible explanation for the accumulation is lifestyle differences; another is that, in advanced age, the dura mater can frequently adhere to the skull, preventing fluid accumulation.[14]

DTEH occurs most commonly in the temporal area (possibly secondary to thinner bone and the fragility of the middle meningeal artery) and with equal frequency in the frontal, parietal, and occipital areas.[22,23]

7.6.1 Pathogenesis

Delayed elevation of intracranial pressure, which may be caused by arterial bleeding or progressive edema, is a likely cause of the rapid deterioration these patients experience. Damaged vessels, initially in vasospasm, would allow increased blood flow and hematoma formation once the vasospasm has resolved.[16,24,25,26,27] Hematomas also occur secondary to damage to superficial veins running along the arteries in the bony grooves, or damage to venous sinuses. Venous bleeding is slower and could account for the delayed detection of these bleeds. Patients initially in shock would be resuscitated, and efforts reversing the hypovolemic state would encourage bleeding from a damaged vessel. Measures taken to treat and relieve elevated intracranial pressure, including surgical and medical techniques, decompress the brain and create new space for subsequent bleeding as the tamponade effect is reversed.[16,17,26] Piepmeier and Wagner[28] showed that 10% of patients with an evacuated traumatic extra-axial hematoma developed a second surgical hematoma at an alternate site within 24 hours of the original surgery. Skull fractures could act as a decompressive device for acute epidural hematoma, allowing blood to seep into the subgaleal space and delaying intracranial symptoms, leading physicians to incorrectly believe the diagnosis to be delayed epidural hematoma.

7.6.2 Treatment

The primary treatment is to prevent DTEH by immediate blood pressure reduction to SBP < 140 mm Hg (unless elevated Cr/BUN after control to indicate renal hypoperfusion) but keep cerebral perfusion pressure > 50 mm Hg in the trauma patient that has an external ventricular drain, begin immediate reversal of coagulopathy, keep oxygenation in non-COPD patients ≥ 98%, start normal saline intravenous fluid, elevate the head to 30–45 degrees (if trauma is suspected then use reverse Trendelenburg), if the GCS score ≤ 8, use EVD placement for intracranial pressure monitoring. The gold standard is craniotomy for the removal of the hematoma. The patients described by Ashkenazi et al[27] recovered completely after evacuation of the bleed with a craniotomy. They were discharged in excellent condition, and follow-up scans showed no reaccumulation. Smaller bleeds can be observed.

7.6.3 Outcome

Outcome is dependent on the initial presentation, the size and location of the bleed, and the aggressive treatment by the physician. Unsuccessful treatment of elevated intracranial pressure with an initial negative CT occurs in as many as 60% of cases of DTEH and is often used as an indication for follow-up scanning.[17] Overall mortality approaches 12%, yet 91% of initially noncomatose patients and 35% of initially comatose patients taken to the operating room have a good recovery.[21]

7.7 Delayed Traumatic Subdural Hematoma

Delayed subdural hematomas have been difficult to diagnose because of the frequently subacute and chronic presentation of this entity. A delayed traumatic subdural hematoma (DTSH) is an acute subdural hemorrhage, not apparent on initial imaging, appearing on follow-up CT scans within 30 days of a traumatic event. It usually presents as a decline in mental status, but significant neurologic deficit, though rarely seen, is a late finding of DTSH. The majority of cases are identified incidentally on follow-up scans or while being evaluated for new-onset headaches and mental status changes.

7.7.1 Incidence

Of completely evacuated acute subdural hemorrhages, 0.5% will develop subsequent delayed recurrence.[14] DTSH is most commonly associated with other intracerebral hemorrhages, mass lesions, and brain edema. As with acute subdural hematoma, DTSH is frequently attributed to the tearing of bridging veins.

7.7.2 Pathogenesis

The detection of subdural hemorrhages is often delayed because initial resuscitation efforts reverse low flow secondary to systemic hypotension or shock from other traumatic injuries.

The tamponade effect caused by elevated intracranial pressure would delay frank bleeding. Generalized traumatic edema and other intracranial lesions (e. g., hemorrhagic or mass effect) would cause just this type of tamponade. The evacuation or reversal of the offending agent, via medication, procedures (e.g., ventriculostomy), or surgery would allow expansion of the subdural hemorrhage appearing as a DTSH. Vascular malformations may also be traumatically induced and have been identified as causes of DTSH.[29]

7.7.3 Treatment

Treatment of DTSH depends on the size, location, overall mass effect, and neurologic status of the patient.

The primary treatment is to prevent DTSH by immediate blood pressure reduction to SBP < 140 mm Hg (unless elevated Cr/BUN after control to indicate renal hypoperfusion) but keep cerebral perfusion pressure > 50 mm Hg in the trauma patient that has an external ventricular drain, begin immediate reversal of coagulopathy, keep oxygenation in non-COPD patients ≥ 98%, start normal saline intravenous fluid, elevate the head to 30–45 degrees (if trauma is suspected then use reverse Trendelenburg), if the GCS score is ≤ 8, use EVD placement for intracranial pressure monitoring. Further guidelines for DTSH are similar to those for acute subdural hematoma. Symptomatic lesions, lesions over 1 cm thick, and lesions with more than 0.5 cm midline shift should be evacuated. Depending on the age of the hematoma and the presence of membrane formation on CT scan, burr hole drainage or bedside drain placement drainage may be an acceptable alternative to a full craniotomy.

7.7.4 Outcome

The outcome for DTSH is highly variable and very case specific, as most studies incorporate patients with different etiologies, hematoma subtypes, symptoms, and presentations.[30]

7.8 Delayed Traumatic Intracerebral Hematoma

As previously discussed, the ambiguity and multitude of classification systems surrounding a diagnosis of a "delayed" nature, as well as the varied courses of cases and the wide range of possible intracerebral locations, make a clear definition of delayed traumatic intracerebral hematoma (DTIH) difficult. Studies are under way to investigate the practicality of using contrasted CT scans and/ or MRI to detect future sites of DTIH.

Lipper et al's suggested definition of DTIH[31] mandates an initial CT scan with lesions smaller than 1 cm (including completely negative CT scans) and subsequent identification of a high-density intraparenchymal lesion on follow-up imaging.

Fukamachi et al[32] divided traumatic intracerebral hemorrhages into four subtypes:

- *Type 1:* Hematomas visible on initial CT without changes on further CT scans.
- *Type 2:* Hematomas that progressively enlarge.
- *Type 3:* Delayed hematoma, which developed in different areas from the original intracerebral hematoma on initial CT scan.
- *Type 4:* Hematomas that developed in areas with previous contusions but no intracerebral hemorrhage.

The clinical presentation of patients with DTIH can be classified into four groups:

- *Group I:* Patients with a GCS score of 8 to 15, mild to moderate head injuries, develop DTIH as identified on routine follow-up CT scans.

- *Group II:* Patients are asymptomatic for hours to weeks after a traumatic event, with subsequent later neurologic decline; DTIH is diagnosed on CT scan or at autopsy.
- *Group III:* Patients have an initial GCS score of less than 8 and no evidence of further neurologic decline; the initial CT scan shows no intracerebral hemorrhage, but follow-up imaging shows DTIH.
- *Group IV:* Patients have a GCS score of less than 8 and progressive neurologic decline and/or medically uncontrollable intracranial pressure.

7.8.1 Incidence

The detection of DTIH has increased significantly with improved imaging techniques. The incidence is highly dependent on patient selection and project inclusion criteria, as well as the timing, availability, and quality of imaging. Delayed posttraumatic intracerebral hemorrhage is the fourth most common cause of all intracerebral hemorrhages after hypertension, vascular malformations, and alcoholism, in that order.[24] As many as 50% of posttraumatic intraparenchymal enhancing lesions will develop into a hematoma.[14] The enhancing lesion may be due to a breakdown of the blood–brain barrier in this large percentage of patients. Since the advent of CT scanners, the overall incidence of delayed posttraumatic intracerebral hemorrhage is noted in 1.7 to 7.4% of all closed head injuries. It is generally accepted that ~ 10 to 20% of patients presenting with a GCS score of less than 8 will continue to develop DTIH (group III and IV).[33,34] There are few reliable data on the incidence of DTIH associated with group I and II patients.

7.8.2 Pathogenesis

Although the severity and extent of trauma sustained are variable, head motion at the time of impact is significant for the development of DTIH.[22,35] Bollinger initially hypothesized that necrotic brain softening around traumatized blood vessels led to DTIH.[12] Microscopically damaged blood vessels, including traumatic aneurysms, may develop into DTIH. Posttraumatic dysregulation of cerebral blood flow leading to vasodilatation, caused by focal hypoxia and hypotension, and subsequent increased intravascular pressure due to resuscitative efforts, leads to elevated intracranial pressure and possible hemorrhage.[36,37,38] In either case, there is disruption of the blood–brain barrier allowing changes in pressure whether blood pressure, hydrostatic pressure, or other causes of increased intracranial pressure to further push blood through the disruption in the blood vessels and small capillaries. Coagulopathy will cause poor hemostasis and clotting and can develop into a DTIH in 70 to 80% of patients.[38,39] Locally damaged brain will release thromboplastic substances, which will produce intravascular coagulation. Such coagulation will lead to small areas of infarct, injuring the brain and restarting the cycle. The small infarction also creates additional space for possible expansion of the hematoma or future hemorrhagic conversion.

7.8.3 Treatment

Treatment is not significantly different from that for other traumatic intracranial hemorrhages. To decrease the risk of DTIH up to the first 12 to 24 hours after head trauma, any spike in SBP over 140 mm Hg must be prevented, as well as hyperthermia, oxygenation less than 98% in non-COPD patients, and the use of hypotonic fluid. There must be immediate correction of coagulation factors. Blood pressure regulation must take into account cerebral perfusion pressure avoiding pressure less than 50 mm Hg as well as the other extreme, greater than 80 mm Hg. After the initial insult, after stabilization during 12 to 24 hours, during greatly elevated ICP greater than 25 mm Hg, there may be a need to increase mean arterial pressure as one possible mechanism to treat refractory intracranial pressure. However, this should not be the initial treatment. Intracranial pressure monitoring is indicated for all groups because rapid deterioration may be preventable with close monitoring and treatment of intracranial pressure. Any coagulopathies or other medical problems should be managed concurrently. Treatment is based on the clinical presentation, as follows[14]:

- *Group I:* Patients are generally observed and treated medically unless progression occurs.
- *Group II:* Patients are categorized as such because of their neurologic decline and should be operatively treated unless otherwise contraindicated because of location or comorbidity factors.
- *Group III:* Patients who have not progressed to group IV criteria warrant close observation and aggressive medical management of intracranial pressure.
- *Group IV:* Patients necessitate immediate operative intervention with aggressive intracranial pressure management.

7.8.4 Outcome

Prolonged low cerebral perfusion pressure directly correlates with poor outcome. Mortality rates as high as 75% are noted with group III and IV patients. Poor quality of life and vegetative states are not uncommon. The degree of secondary insult caused by the natural cascade of brain injury only adds to the underlying damage done by the hematoma itself and the associated mass effect. Coagulopathy needs to be corrected as soon as possible to decrease morbidity and mortality.[38,39,40] Prompt intervention where appropriate is our only current tool to counteract the natural progression of DTIH.

7.9 Anticoagulation and Intracerebral Hemorrhages

Anticoagulation in itself does not predispose patients to intracerebral hemorrhage; however, it does produce complications if a hemorrhage occurs.[41,42] Intracerebral hemorrhages associated with anticoagulation yield higher morbidity and mortality (67%) than those hemorrhages without anticoagulation treatment (55%). There is also documentation that the volume of hematoma is larger in those patients receiving anticoagulation treatment, although the volume itself is unrelated to the degree of anticoagulation.[4,2,43] Emergency reversal of anticoagulation after intracerebral hemorrhage detection is critical to preventing further bleeding. Fredriksson et al[44] suggested that treatment with prothrombin complex concentrate reverses anticoagulation more rapidly than fresh frozen plasma, and therefore is indicated with suspected intracerebral hemorrhage.

7.10 Rebleeding of Subarachnoid Hemorrhages

The incidence of subarachnoid hemorrhage varies significantly according to underlying pathology. When considering aneurysm rupture, the incidence of rebleeding is as high as 4% in the first 24 hours, then 1.5% per day for the first 2 weeks. A total of 50% will rebleed in the first 6 months. The higher the Hunt and Hess score,[45] the higher the risk of rebleed.[46] Nonaneurysmal subarachnoid hemorrhage has a lower incidence of recurrent hemorrhage, at ~ 1% each year.[45] Theories suggest the decreased rate of rebleed in these patients is secondary to the initial hemorrhagic rupture eradicating the offending pathology. No known prophylactic treatment options currently exist to prevent rebleeding.

7.11 Delayed Intracerebral Hemorrhage Secondary to Underlying Medical Pathology

7.11.1 Cerebrovascular Infarction

The frequency of hemorrhagic transformation of cerebrovascular accidents is still under debate, with multiple studies under way. The incidence increases as a function of the frequency at which follow-up neuroimaging studies are performed. A study of 200 patients determined that 68.6% underwent hemorrhagic conversion, most without further clinical deterioration.[47] Hemorrhagic transformation of ischemic strokes in the carotid artery distribution has an incidence of 43%.[48] Higher blood pressures may account for the repeat bleeding regardless of the presence or absence of arterial reopening.

7.11.2 Hypertension

Hypertensive hemorrhages account for 10 to 30% of all strokes. Studies of recurrent intracerebral hemorrhage without other identifiable etiology and a history of hypertension show a relatively infrequent incidence of 2.7%.[49,50,51,52] The recurrence rate is theorized to be low due to the lipohyalinosis and transmural necrosis affecting the vessels, leading to hemorrhage. The hemorrhage ultimately destroys the vessels and leads to thrombosis at the time of the event, thereby preventing a future repeat episode. Over 90% of recurrent hypertensive hemorrhages are in a different location from the original bleeding; however, the distribution of locations is similar, with most recurrent hypertensive bleeds occurring in the basal ganglia.

7.11.3 Tumors

Underlying tumors account for 1 to 2% of intracerebral hemorrhage cases, as determined in an autopsy series; however, they can range to as high as 10% in clinic-radiological series. The majority of hemorrhages into tumor beds occur in malignant tumors or metastatic tumors, rarely meningiomas or oligodendrogliomas.[53] Rebleeding itself is a rare entity, as the primary tumor is itself treated or the patient clinically deteriorates and follow-up studies are forgone. However, in an extensive study of postoperative hematomas, 56% of patients had a primary diagnosis of intracranial tumor that then bled into the resection site. Meningiomas are the most common tumor to hemorrhage after resection, at 40%.[54,55]

7.11.4 Migraines

Migraines have also been documented to be associated with recurrent hemorrhages, albeit rarely. Most cases arise from symptomatic grade IIA migraines or grade IIB migraine mimics. Reported cases are most frequently associated with a preexisting arteriovenous malformation, where hemorrhage occurs into the bed during a migraine attack. Also, lobar hemorrhages can occur after a migraine attack associated with sudden hypertensive episodes.[56]

7.11.5 Cerebral Amyloid Angiopathy

Beta amyloid protein depositions can accumulate in the media of small cerebral vessels with or without accumulation in other systemic vessels. Cerebral amyloid angiopathy (CAA) is present in 50% of those patients over 70 years old, accounts for 10% of all first-time intracerebral hemorrhages, and is the leading cause of angiographically negative recurrent hemorrhages in this age group.[57] Frequently, but not exclusively, apolipoprotein e4 allele is associated with CAA. Presentation is similar to hypertensive hemorrhages with location-specific findings and often an associated history of transient ischemic attacks.[58] Unlike hypertensive hemorrhages, CAA is more likely to be lobar than ganglionic, and recurrent hemorrhage is common. Confirmatory diagnosis is only possible via evaluation of brain tissue. No treatment is known.

Case Example

A 39-year-old woman presented with new-onset focal seizures of her right arm and no neurologic deficit. A CT scan of her head was performed and revealed a left parietal mass measuring 3 × 2 cm. MRI confirmed the lesion and showed minimal enhancement on contrasted study, little to no edema, and a 6 mm necrotic center. A stereotactic biopsy was scheduled and revealed a grade III astrocytoma. Postoperatively, the patient had elevated blood pressure with increased incision drainage. A repeat CT scan showed a 3 × 3 cm intracerebral hematoma at the end of the biopsy site. The patient was returned to the operating room for evacuation of the intracerebral hematoma. Upon recovery, the patient continues to have no neurologic deficit and is undergoing medical treatment of the tumor.

7.12 Postprocedural Intracerebral Hemorrhage

Factors contributing to delayed postprocedural hemorrhages include multiple passes through the brain, specifics of the clotting status of the patient, and the type of procedure performed. Bleeding often contributes to erosion of surface veins or disruption of superficial blood vessels during the procedure. Routine postprocedural imaging is the best source of detection of hemorrhaging. This entity is frequently underdiagnosed because of the lack of routine repeat imaging and because small hemorrhages tend not to cause any additional symptoms or deficits. After stereotactic biopsy, 0.8 to 59.2% of patients will have a postoperative hemorrhage, the wide range depending on the postprocedural scanning schedule.[43,59,60] Only 10% of those with hemorrhage will have suspicious symptoms or deficits. A review of the literature reveals the incidence of postventriculoperitoneal shunt placement hemorrhages to be 0.4 to 4.0%.[61] Even major surgeries have the possibility of rebleeding. A study of 230 patients revealed an incidence of rebleeding after aneurysm clipping to be as high as 2.6%.[62]

Case Management

The blood pressure *was not decreased* due to herniation (blown pupil) and the need to maintain perfusion. The patient was taken immediately to the operating room for evacuation of the hematoma, arriving within 5 minutes of the CT scan. The patient was intubated within 5 minutes of the CT scan. Coagulation studies were obtained. A delay in travel to the operating room could have been mitigated with immediate intubation, elevation of the head of bed using reverse Trendelenburg, and the use of 20 mL of IV 23.4% saline. After craniotomy the brain remained swollen 1 cm outside the outer table of the skull and the bone was not replaced during this surgery. An external ventricular drain was placed during surgery. After surgery the patient had a GCS score of 8 and the pupil returned to normal reactive size. He improved over 2 weeks after surgery and was eventually discharged to an acute rehabilitation facility with a helmet. The bone flap was replaced in 4 months when the contours of the brain were within the inner table of the skull.

References

[1] Gioia LC, Kate M, Dowlatshahi D, Hill MD, Butcher K. Blood pressure management in acute intracerebral hemorrhage: current evidence and ongoing controversies. Curr Opin Crit Care. 2015; 21 (2):99–106

[2] Qureshi AI, Ezzeddine MA, Nasar A, et al. Prevalence of elevated blood pressure in 563,704 adult patients with stroke presenting to the ED in the United States. Am J Emerg Med. 2007; 25(1):32–38

[3] Hemphill JC, III, Bonovich DC, Besmertis L, Manley GT, Johnston SC. The ICH score: a simple, reliable grading scale for intracerebral hemorrhage. Stroke. 2001; 32(4):891–897

[4] Morgenstern LB, Hemphill JC, III, Anderson C, et al. American Heart Association Stroke Council and Council on Cardiovascular Nursing. Guidelines for the management of spontaneous intracerebral hemorrhage: a guideline for healthcare professionals from the American Heart Association/American Stroke Association. Stroke. 2010; 41(9):2108–2129

[5] Mendelow AD, Gregson BA, Fernandes HM, et al. STICH investigators. Early surgery versus initial conservative treatment in patients with spontaneous supratentorial intracerebral haematomas in the International Surgical Trial in Intracerebral Haemorrhage (STICH): a randomised trial. Lancet. 2005; 365(9457):387–397

[6] Mendelow AD, Gregson BA, Rowan EN, Murray GD, Gholkar A, Mitchell PM, STICH II Investigators. Early surgery versus initial conservative treatment in patients with spontaneous supratentorial lobar intracerebral haematomas (STICH II): a randomised trial. Lancet. 2013; 382(9890):397–408

[7] Mould WA, Carhuapoma JR, Muschelli J, et al. MISTIE Investigators. Minimally invasive surgery plus recombinant tissue-type plasminogen activator for intracerebral hemorrhage evacuation decreases perihematomal edema. Stroke. 2013; 44(3):627–634

[8] Morgan T, Zuccarello M, Narayan R, Keyl P, Lane K, Hanley D. Preliminary findings of the minimally-invasive surgery plus rtPA for intracerebral hemorrhage evacuation (MISTIE) clinical trial. Acta Neurochir Suppl (Wien). 2008; 105:147–151

[9] Adams RE, Diringer MN. Response to external ventricular drainage in spontaneous intracerebral hemorrhage with hydrocephalus. Neurology. 1998; 50(2):519–523

[10] Lee KR, Kawai N, Kim S, Sagher O, Hoff JT. Mechanisms of edema formation after intracerebral hemorrhage: effects of thrombin on cerebral blood flow, blood-brain barrier permeability, and cell survival in a rat model. J Neurosurg. 1997; 86(2):272–278

[11] Naff N, Williams MA, Keyl PM, et al. Low-dose recombinant tissue-type plasminogen activator enhances clot resolution in brain hemorrhage: the intraventricular hemorrhage thrombolysis trial. Stroke. 2011; 42(11):3009–3016

[12] von Bollinger O. Ueber traumatische spät-Apoplexie: ein Beitrag zur Lehre von der Hirnerschutterung. In: Internationale Beiträge zur wissenschaftlichen Medizin: Festschrift, Rudolf Virchow gewidmet zur vollendung seines 70. Vol 2. Berlin, Germany: Hirchwald; 1891:459–470

[13] Duret H. Traumatismes craniocérébraux: accidents primitifs, leurs grandes syndromes. Paris: Felix Alcan; 1922:833–851

[14] Cohen TI, Gudeman SK. Delayed traumatic intracranial hematoma. In: Narayan RK, Wilberger JE, Povlishock JT, eds. Neurotrauma. New York, NY: McGraw-Hill Health; 1996:689–702

[15] Rockswold GL, Leonard PR, Nagib MG. Analysis of management in thirty-three closed head injury patients who "talked and deteriorated". Neurosurgery. 1987; 21(1):51–55

[16] Bucci MN, Phillips TW, McGillicuddy JE. Delayed epidural hemorrhage in hypotensive multiple trauma patients. Neurosurgery. 1986; 19(1):65–68

[17] Borovich B, Braun J, Guilburd JN, et al. Delayed onset of traumatic extradural hematoma. J Neurosurg. 1985; 63(1):30–34

[18] Teasdale G, Galbraith S. Acute traumatic intracranial hematomas. In: Krayenbuhl H, Maspes PE, Sweet WH, eds. Progress in Neurosurgery. Vol 10. Basel, Switzerland: Karger; 1980:14–42

[19] Poon WS, Rehman SU, Poon CY, Li AK. Traumatic extradural hematoma of delayed onset is not a rarity. Neurosurgery. 1992; 30(5):681–686

[20] Youmans JR, ed. Diagnosis and treatment of moderate to severe head injury in adults. In: Neurological Surgery. Philadelphia, PA: WB Saunders; 1996:1618–1718

[21] Rivas JJ, Lobato RD, Sarabia R, Cordobés F, Cabrera A, Gomez P. Extradural hematoma: analysis of factors influencing the courses of 161 patients. Neurosurgery. 1988; 23(1):44–51

[22] Diaz FG, Yock DH, Jr, Larson D, Rockswold GL. Early diagnosis of delayed posttraumatic intracerebral hematomas. J Neurosurg. 1979; 50(2):217–223

[23] Young HA, Gleave JR, Schmidek HH, Gregory S. Delayed traumatic intracerebral hematoma: report of 15 cases operatively treated. Neurosurgery. 1984; 14(1):22–25

[24] Alvarez-Sabín J, Turon A, Lozano-Sánchez M, Vázquez J, Codina A. Delayed posttraumatic hemorrhage. "Spät-apoplexie". Stroke. 1995; 26(9):1531–1535

[25] Elsner H, Rigamonti D, Corradino G, Schlegel R, Jr, Joslyn J. Delayed traumatic intracerebral hematomas: "Spät-Apoplexie". Report of two cases. J Neurosurg. 1990; 72(5):813–815

[26] Mendelow AD, Teasdale GM, Russell T, Flood J, Patterson J, Murray GD. Effect of mannitol on cerebral blood flow and cerebral perfusion pressure in human head injury. J Neurosurg. 1985; 63(1):43–48

[27] Ashkenazi E, Constantini S, Pomerans S, Rivkind AI, Rappaport ZH. Delayed epidural hematoma without neurologic deficit. J Trauma. 1990; 30(5):613–615

[28] Piepmeier JM, Wagner FC, Jr. Delayed post-traumatic extracerebral hematomas. J Trauma. 1982; 22(6):455–460

[29] Aoki N, Sakai T, Kaneko M. Traumatic aneurysm of the middle meningeal artery presenting as delayed onset of acute subdural hematoma. Surg Neurol. 1992; 37(1):59–62

[30] Dowling JL, Brown AP, Dacey RG. Cerebrovascular complications in the head-injured patient. In: Narayan RK, Wilberger JE, Povlishock JT, eds. Neurotrauma. New York, NY: McGraw-Hill Health; 1996:655–672

[31] Lipper MH, Kishore PR, Girevendulis AK, Miller JD, Becker DP. Delayed intracranial hematoma in patients with severe head injury. Radiology. 1979; 133(3 Pt 1):645–649

[32] Fukamachi A, Nagaseki Y, Kohno K, Wakao T. The incidence and developmental process of delayed traumatic intracerebral haematomas. Acta Neurochir (Wien). 1985; 74(1–2):35–39

[33] Young HA, Gleave JR, Schmidek HH, Gregory S. Delayed traumatic intracerebral hematoma: report of 15 cases operatively treated. Neurosurgery. 1984; 14(1):22–25

[34] Huneidi AH, Afshar F. Delayed intracerebral haematomas in moderate to severe head injuries in young adults. Ann R Coll Surg Engl. 1992; 74(5):345–349, discussion 349–350

[35] Jaimovich R, Monges JA. Delayed posttraumatic intracranial lesions in children. Pediatr Neurosurg. 1991–1992; 17(1):25–29

[36] Gudeman SK, Kishore PR, Miller JD, Girevendulis AK, Lipper MH, Becker DP. The genesis and significance of delayed traumatic intracerebral hematoma. Neurosurgery. 1979; 5(3):309–313

[37] Riesgo P, Piquer J, Botella C, Orozco M, Navarro J, Cabanes J. Delayed extradural hematoma after mild head injury: report of three cases. Surg Neurol. 1997; 48(3):226–231

[38] Pretorius ME, Kaufman HH. Rapid onset of delayed traumatic intracerebral haematoma with diffuse intravascular coagulation and fibrinolysis. Acta Neurochir (Wien). 1982; 65(1–2):103–109

[39] Kaufman HH, Moake JL, Olson JD, et al. Delayed and recurrent intracranial hematomas related to disseminated intravascular clotting and fibrinolysis in head injury. Neurosurgery. 1980; 7 (5):445–449

[40] Juvela S, Heiskanen O, Poranen A, et al. The treatment of spontaneous intracerebral hemorrhage. A prospective randomized trial of surgical and conservative treatment. J Neurosurg. 1989; 70 (5):755–758

[41] Rådberg JA, Olsson JE, Rådberg CT. Prognostic parameters in spontaneous intracerebral hematomas with special reference to anticoagulant treatment. Stroke. 1991; 22(5):571–576

[42] Snyder M, Renaudin J. Intracranial hemorrhage associated with anticoagulation therapy. Surg Neurol. 1977; 7(1):31–34

[43] Franke CL, de Jonge J, van Swieten JC, Op de Coul AA, van Gijn J. Intracerebral hematomas during anticoagulant treatment. Stroke. 1990; 21(5):726–730

[44] Fredriksson K, Norrving B, Strömblad LG. Emergency reversal of anticoagulation after intracerebral hemorrhage. Stroke. 1992; 23(7):972–977

[45] Winn HR, Richardson AE, Jane JA. The long-term prognosis in untreated cerebral aneurysms: I. The incidence of late hemorrhage in cerebral aneurysm: a 10-year evaluation of 364 patients. Ann Neurol. 1977; 1(4):358–370

[46] Hunt WE, Hess RM. Surgical risk as related to time of intervention in the repair of intracranial aneurysms. J Neurosurg. 1968; 28(1):14–20

[47] Hornig CR, Bauer T, Simon C, Trittmacher S, Dorndorf W. Hemorrhagic transformation in cardioembolic cerebral infarction. Stroke. 1993; 24(3):465–468

[48] Garcia JH. Pathology. In: Barnett HJ, Mohr JP, eds. Stroke. New York, NY: Churchill Livingstone; 1992:125–135

[49] Lee KS, Bae HG, Yun IG. Recurrent intracerebral hemorrhage due to hypertension. Neurosurgery. 1990; 26(4):586–590

[50] Field M, Witham TF, Flickinger JC, Kondziolka D, Lunsford LD. Comprehensive assessment of hemorrhage risks and outcomes after stereotactic brain biopsy. J Neurosurg. 2001; 94(4):545–551

[51] Park YC. Clinical diagnosis of cerebrovascular accidents. J Korean Med Assoc. 1973; 28:303–308

[52] Herbstein DJ, Schaumberg HH. Hypertensive intracerebral hematoma. An investigation of the initial hemorrhage and rebleeding using chromium Cr 51-labeled erythrocytes. Arch Neurol. 1974; 30(5):412–414

[53] Kase CS. Intracerebral hemorrhage. In: Barnett HJ, Mohr JP, eds. Stroke. New York, NY: Churchill Livingstone; 1992:561–616

[54] Little JR, Dial B, Bélanger G, Carpenter S. Brain hemorrhage from intracranial tumor. Stroke. 1979; 10(3):283–288

[55] Kalfas IH, Little JR. Postoperative hemorrhage: a survey of 4992 intracranial procedures. Neurosurgery. 1988; 23(3):343–347

[56] Cole AJ, Aubé M. Migraine with vasospasm and delayed intracerebral hemorrhage. Arch Neurol. 1990; 47(1):53–56

[57] Gilbert JJ, Vinters HV. Cerebral amyloid angiopathy: incidence and complications in the aging brain. I. Cerebral hemorrhage. Stroke. 1983; 14(6):915–923

[58] Greenberg SM, Rebeck GW, Vonsattel JP, Gomez-Isla T, Hyman BT. Apolipoprotein E epsilon 4 and cerebral hemorrhage associated with amyloid angiopathy. Ann Neurol. 1995; 38(2):254–259

[59] Jane JA, Kassell NF. The natural history of aneurysms and arteriovenous malformations. J Neurosurg. 1985; 62:321–323

[60] Kulkarni AV, Guha A, Lozano A, Bernstein M. Incidence of silent hemorrhage and delayed deterioration after stereotactic brain biopsy. J Neurosurg. 1998; 89(1):31–35

[61] Savitz MH, Bobroff LM. Low incidence of delayed intracerebral hemorrhage secondary to ventriculoperitoneal shunt insertion. J Neurosurg. 1999; 91(1):32–34

[62] Proust F, Hannequin D. Causes of morbidity and mortality after ruptured aneurysm surgery in a series of 230 patients. The importance of control angiography. Stroke. 1995; 26(9):1553–1557

8 Sedation and Pain Management in the Neurosurgical Intensive Care Unit Patient

Gohar Majeed and Dan E. Miulli

Abstract

Pain is the fifth vital sign because if it is not recognized and treated it leads to disorders of the remaining vital signs and further tissue damage. Pain may be the result of ischemic tissue, dilated blood vessels, or tissue being compressed. Although tissue ischemia may be due to large forces the specific chemical nature of the action and response should be understood in order to effectively treat it. The treatment of pain is as detailed as the treatment of any disease; it cannot be left to the individual unfamiliar with the details of the nervous system for the type and duration of treatment or lack of treatment will affect the patient's neurologic outcome.

Keywords: A delta fibers, C fibers, ice, narcotics, NMDA, nociceptors, NSAIDs, pain scale

Case Presentation

A 47-year-old woman was involved in a rollover motor vehicle accident, with resultant severe closed head injury, consisting of mild cerebral edema, right pneumothorax, pulmonary contusion, and multiple rib fractures. The patient's pupils are 2 mm and reactive; she does not open her eyes, is intubated, and is unable to move any of her extremities, yielding a Glasgow Coma Scale (GCS) score of 3 T. The trauma team has placed a chest tube. The patient will remain on the ventilator while her GCS score is ≤ 8 and while the trauma team remains concerned about lung injuries. The vital signs demonstrate an increased heart rate and increased blood pressure anytime there is attempted movement of the patient; therefore, the patient is sedated and given pain medication.

See end of chapter for Case Management.

8.1 Introduction: What Is Pain?

Pain is "whatever the experiencing person says it is, existing whenever s/he says it does."[1] It is an unpleasant sensory and emotional experience associated with actual or potential tissue damage, or described in terms of such damage.[2] In biological terms, stimulus energy from any source is converted into nerve impulses and transferred from the site of transduction to the central nervous system (CNS) and brain, during which time the signal is modulated at multiple levels before being perceived at the highest centers of the brain.

Nociceptors are specific receptors that respond to tissue trauma or stimuli that may cause tissue trauma.[3] They are located in skin, connective tissue, muscle, tendon, muscle spindle, joint capsules, bone, and viscera, and around nerves and blood vessels. Thankfully, they are not located in the brain substance itself. The tissue changes from injury-released prostaglandins, substance P, bradykinins, cytokines, histamine, and serotonin. This is the first area where pain can be modulated. The impulses from the nociceptors responding to these substances or responding to simple mechanical deformation travel along slow-conducting unmyelinated C fibers or faster-conducting, small myelinated A delta fibers. Although both C fibers and large A delta fibers respond to pain, it is the ratio of response that determines the passage through the dorsal horns as pain; the response from C fibers must be greater than the response from A delta fibers. The impulses are mostly from the trunk and limbs, and therefore go to the dorsal horn of the spinal cord, usually activating N-methyl-D-aspartate (NMDA) receptors, the second site of pain modulation. NMDA receptor stimulation causes intraneuronal elevation of Ca^{2+}, which stimulates nitric oxide synthase (NOS) and the production of nitric oxide (NO).[4] Substances known to block NMDA receptors include d-methadone, dextromethorphan, ketamine, naloxone, and amantadine. It is at the NMDA receptors that inherent spinal cord nociceptor modulators, such as γ-aminobutyric acid (GABA), serotonin, glutamate, substance P, norepinephrine, and endogenous opioids are released by spinal interneurons in laminae I, II, IV, and V of the dorsal horn, which are controlled by brain cortex centers, periaqueductal gray, or concurrent spinal cord input. The modified signal crosses in the spinal cord and ascends in multiple tracts, such as the spinoreticular, spinothalamic, spinomesencephalic, and spinohypothalamic, to the reticular formation, thalamus, mesencephalon, and hypothalamus, respectively, the third area of modulation. Sensations reaching the thalamus undergo complex modulation to determine if the sensation will be processed to reach the brain. From these intermediates, the signal passes to the frontal cortex, insular cortex, limbic structures, and sensory cortex to label the pain as good or bad, the fourth area of possible modulation.

A functioning brain is needed for the perception of pain. Each area through neurochemical release, such as GABA, norepinephrine, substance P, serotonin, and opioids, influences the pain. These same areas respond to memories, social influences, environmental influences, experiences, depression, and culture. Repeated stimuli at any location further change the characteristics of the pain and the threshold (▶ Table 8.1).

Table 8.1 Results of undertreatment and overtreatment of pain[5]

Undertreatment of pain	Overtreatment of pain
Suffering, anxiety, fear, anger, depression	Inability to perform neurologic exam
Slow recovery	Prolonged intubation
Decreased ability to participate in activities of daily living	Prolonged intensive care unit stay
Patient's family anxiety	Pneumonia
Weight loss, fever, increased heart and respiratory rates, increased blood pressure, chest pain, myocardial infarction; atelectasis, constipation, infection	Deep venous thrombosis

Acute injury is mostly transmitted as nociceptive pain. This differs in treatment from neuropathic pain associated with chronic repeated stimuli and caused by aberrant signal processing in the peripheral or central nervous system. After repeated stimulation, the pathophysiological abnormalities of neuropathic pain become unrelated to the provocative event. This type of pain occurs infrequently in the intensive care unit (ICU) but may be seen in patients with multiple strokes, multiple fractures, or cancer pain.

8.2 General Principles of Pain Management

Pain must be treated. Neglecting pain treatment results in undue suffering, anxiety expressed by the patient and the family, fear, anger, depression, slow recovery, decreased ability to participate in activities of daily living, weight loss, fever, increased heart and respiratory rates, increased blood pressure, chest pain, myocardial infarction (MI), atelectasis, constipation, and infection.[6,7,8]

8.3 Assessment of Pain

The first step in pain management involves an appropriate assessment of the pain, most often recorded on a pain scale. Pain assessment in the awake cooperative patient requires obtaining a detailed history along with the examination. This allows the physician to adequately assess and address these issues. However, neurosurgical patients present a unique challenge when it comes to assessment of pain as a large number of our patient population are either intubated and sedated or just unable to accurately describe their pain due to a variety of reasons, such as altered mental status, increased agitation secondary to fearfulness or pain, and so forth.

The characteristics of the pain also play a role in the treatment, including but not limited to, its quality, location, intensity, duration, periodicity, exacerbating and relieving factors, present and past pain management, and associated signs and symptoms.

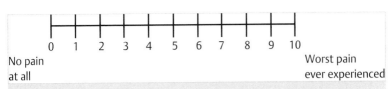

Fig. 8.1 Commonly used pain scale. Patient points to number on scale after health-care worker describes "0" as no pain at all and "10" as worst pain ever experienced.

Pain is an unpleasant sensory and emotional experience associated with actual or potential tissue damage. Therefore, assessment of pain requires an examination of the area of pain referral and any other diagnostic tests that will assist in determining the appropriate treatment.

Often only pain intensity is considered in the pain history; by itself, however, it may lead to unnecessary treatments. When there are difficulties in communication such as may occur in the very young, the very old, the mildly confused, and patients of different language, culture, or background, a pain assessment rating scale may be the only information available. Most widely used "pain scales" are based on 10 divisions. Because it is necessary to follow pain trends over time and with treatment, often between varying health care workers and health facilities, only a 10-division scale should be used until other scales become universal.[9,10]

A numeric rating scale asks the patient or the health care worker to rate the pain on a scale of 0 to 10, with 0 being no pain at all and 10 being the worst possible pain the patient or health care worker could imagine. Often patients will state that they have a high pain threshold, much higher than others. However, it must be emphasized to patients that the worst possible pain that they could imagine is a 10, and the current pain is in relation to that level, not based on others' perception. It may be appropriate at times to ask women who have had children by vaginal delivery, as ascertained in the history, to compare the current pain to the pain experienced during labor, which may have been a 10 (▶ Fig. 8.1).

The modified visual analog scale is a 10 cm line marked from 0 to 10, with 0 being no pain at all and 10 being the worst possible pain the patient could imagine. When teamed with the commonly used scales, such as the American Cancer Society Pain Scale, Facial Pain Scale, or Wong-Baker Faces Rating Scale for Children, all of which consist of multiple images of faces with varying expressions of pain, the modified Visual Analog Scale becomes the ultimate scale for the awake person (▶ Fig. 8.2).

Severely debilitated patients and those with severe head injuries are physically not able to use these scales to indicate their level of pain. In these cases, health care workers are responsible for acting in the best interest of the individual patient to relieve suffering without causing untoward side effects. A behavioral pain scale is useful when patients cannot communicate. One of the most widely accepted behavioral pain scales is the 10-point FLACC scale. The patient is assessed in five categories and given 0, 1, or 2 points depending on the behavior being demonstrated. The behaviors are *facial* expression, *leg* movement, general *activity*, *crying*, and ability to be *consoled* (▶ Table 8.2). The FLACC scale can also be used with children ages 6 months to 3 years.

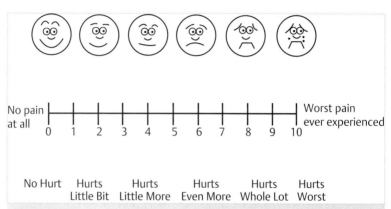

Fig. 8.2 Visual Analog Scale (VAS) and Wong-Baker Faces Scale allows additional clues for patients to adequately assess their pain. The health-care worker describes "0" as no pain at all and "10" as worst pain ever experienced. The faces help the patient decide how he or she currently feels.

Table 8.2 FLACC Behavioral Pain Scale[6,7]

	Score		
	0	1	2
Facial expression	Smiles or no particular expression	Occasional grimace, frown; withdrawn	Frequent to constant frown, clenched jaw, quivering chin
Leg movement	Relaxed or normal posture	Uneasy, restless, tense	Kicking or legs drawn up
General activity	Normal position; lying quietly, moves easily	Squirming, shifting back and forth, tense	Arched, rigid, or jerking
Crying	No crying while awake or asleep	Moans, whimpers; occasional complaints	Crying steadily; screams or sobs; frequent complaints
Ability to be consoled	Content, relaxed	Reassured by occasional touching, hugging, or talking; distractible	Difficult to console or comfort

8.4 Pain in the Neurosurgical Patient

Pain in the neurosurgery patient needs to be adequately controlled. In addition to the stressors in the ICU, neurosurgical patients can have physiological causes of pain, including postoperative pain, meningeal irritation due to subarachnoid hemorrhage (SAH) or meningitis, cranial nerve dysfunctions, invasive procedures, and neuropathy due to various conditions. Before the initiation of sedation, pain must be addressed adequately because it can cause significant anxiety, agitation, and deleterious neurological effects.

Overmedication results in the inability to perform a neurologic exam, which is the most important means of following a patient with neurologic disease or injuries. Overtreatment of pain and sedation leads to prolonged intubation, prolonged ICU stay, pneumonia, and deep venous thrombosis (▶ Table 8.1).[5]

In a severe head injury or comatose patient who is intubated, only subtle changes may foretell drastic intracranial changes and problems, such as contusions blossoming or other small abnormalities leading to midline shift and herniation. If the patient is overmedicated, a treatable lesion will be missed. Frequently, in patients with severe head injury or severe neurologic deficits, an intracranial pressure (ICP) monitor is inserted; however, the ICP, although rising and falling with movement, suctioning, and pain, will change exponentially as the brain has reached the ability to compensate. A gradual change in neurologic exam precedes large changes in ICP. Therefore, there must be a fine line that is maintained between pain and sedation, and under- and overmedication in the neurologic patient. A key principle in the use of analgesics and sedatives in the neurosurgical ICU (NICU) is *titration*: after proving the analgesic or sedative is actually effective for the given patient, dosing of the analgesic or sedative of choice should be titrated gradually to avoid side effects of overdosing.

Some of the most commonly used medications in neurocritical care are outlined here.

8.4.1 Nonsteroidal Anti-inflammatory Drugs

Once a patient's pain can be assessed using a pain scale, medication and other treatment can be quickly entertained. Pain that is rated as 4 or less can be managed with ice, acetaminophen, or nonsteroidal anti-inflammatory drugs (NSAIDs), with the last two inhibiting an isoform of the enzyme cyclo-oxygenase (COX 1–3) blocking prostaglandin synthesis.[11] The usual dose for acetaminophen (N-acetyl-*p*-aminophenol [APAP]) is 10 to 75 mg/kg/d in four to six divided doses. The maximum adult daily dose is 4,000 mg. It is now believed that an initial large dose of 50 mg/kg can be given, yielding relief comparable to that of some narcotics while maintaining a high safety profile. The side effects of acetaminophen are seen with elevated multiple doses, although they can occur with a single dose. They are acute hepatic necrosis, or liver toxicity

143

nephrotoxicity and, with chronic use, thrombocytopenia. Those with impaired liver function or regular alcohol use should take no more than 2 g daily. Anyone who takes more than three alcoholic drinks a day should be advised to avoid acetaminophen.

Analgesics, including aspirin (acetylsalicylic acid [ASA]) and APAP, inhibit cyclo-oxygenase, preventing the production of prostaglandins. COX receptors are found throughout the body, and a specific group's effect depends on which receptors are stimulated. COX-1 receptors are found in the CNS, kidneys, platelets, gastrointestinal (GI) system, skin, and other areas. COX-2 receptors are found in the brain and kidneys. COX-3 receptors are found in the CNS. Most NSAIDs are nonselective COX 1–3 receptor inhibitors. The location of the receptors in the CNS is the reason that APAP only lowers temperature and pain but does not inhibit platelet function or have any significant anti-inflammatory effect.

NSAIDs should be withheld for 4 to 10 days after mild bleeding and not given for at least 4 to 10 days after severe bleeding. NSAIDs inhibit platelet function only while at therapeutic dosage. They should be given with a stomach protectant and adequate hydration to help prevent side effects. The usual dose for ibuprofen is 50 mg/kg divided into 4 to 6 doses per day.

Ketorolac is another anti-inflammatory drug that can be given intravenously or orally. The usual dose for ketorolac is 30 to 60 mg per dose and can be given every 6 to 8 hours. Ketorolac can be given immediately after such neurosurgical procedures as lumbar diskectomy and lumbar spinal fusion when bleeding has been controlled. During these procedures, ketorolac 30 mg intravenous (IV) may be given initially, followed by 120 mg in 500 mL saline at 10 mL/h continuous drip until completed. This treatment modality, along with lidocaine patches or infusion, may greatly decrease or obviate the need for narcotics.

NSAIDs belong to multiple drug classes, with each class affecting individuals differently. Therefore, if one class of NSAID or even a drug in the same class does not work, consider treatment with another (▶ Table 8.3).

None of the drugs in this group should be given if there is a known sensitivity to an NSAID. Salicylates should not be given to children with viral infections. In general, the nonselective COX inhibitor NSAIDs have similar side effects, such as dyspepsia; ulcers; GI perforation and bleeding (antiplatelet activity lasts for 2–3 days while therapeutic); kidney and liver dysfunction; hypersensitivity reaction, such as urticaria-angioedema; respiratory, attention, and memory deficits; headache; and tinnitus. Rofecoxib, a COX-2 inhibitor, was recently shown to have cardiac side effects, such as MI and stroke, and has been voluntarily removed from the market. Celecoxib, another COX-2 inhibitor, has not been removed from the market. Celecoxib side effects are thought to be less problematic than those of other NSAIDs.

Table 8.3 Pain medication for pain rated as 4 or less on 0 to 10 pain scale[6,7,8,9,10,11,12]

Generic name	Average dose	Average frequency (hours)	Maximum daily dose	Class
Ice	Local area	Until it melts		
Acetaminophen	10–75 mg/kg/d	4–6	4,000 mg	p-aminophenol, COX-3 inhibitor
Aspirin	5–100 mg/kg/d	4–6	8,000 mg	Salicylate
Diflunisal	250–500 mg	8–12	1,500 mg	Salicylate
Choline, magnesium, trisalicylate	30–60 mg/kg/d	8–12	4,500 mg	Salicylate
Ibuprofen	5–50 mg/kg/d	4–6	3,200 mg	Propionic acid
Naproxen	250–500 mg	6–8	1,500 mg	Propionic acid
Ketoprofen	12.5–75.0 mg	6–8	300 mg	Propionic acid
Flubiprofen	50–100 mg	6–8	300 mg	Propionic acid
Oxaprozin	600–1200 mg	8–12	1,800 mg	Propionic acid
Indomethacin	25–75 mg	8	200 mg	Indoleacetic acid
Piroxicam	10–20 mg	24	20 mg	Benzothiazine
Meloxicam	7.5–15.0 mg	24	15 mg	Benzothiazine
Diclofenac	25–75 mg	6–8	200 mg	Pyrroleacetic acid
Ketorolac	30–60 mg	Intravenously, orally 6–8	150 mg	Pyrroleacetic acid
Celecoxib	200–400 mg	12–24	800 mg	COX-2 inhibitor

Abbreviation: COX, cyclo-oxygenase.

There is no significant difference between the GI effects of nonselective COX NSAIDs and a proton pump inhibitor and selective COX-2 NSAIDs. ASA inhibits platelet function irreversibly, whereas NSAIDs inhibit platelet function only while at therapeutic dosage.

8.4.2 Other Pain Treatment

There are numerous ways to administer effective pain treatment, and in the neurologic patient these routes must be tried unless there is a contraindication. Initially, local pain should be treated with ice. Icing works by stimulating large A delta fibers in the peripheral nervous system, increasing output above

145

C fibers, and inhibiting pain transmission. Longer-lasting pain, such as that caused by muscle spasm, may be treated with ice, heat, or both, depending on the response. If there is severe extremity or axial pain epidural at the approximate dermatome or caudal, anesthetics and analgesics may be delivered. The elevated pain from the disruption or destruction of large muscle areas may be treated appropriately with the local continuous infusion of long- or short-acting lidocaine derivatives. When the pain is of less severity, or to augment delivery of other pain medication, topical solutions can be used. Although used for chronic and neuropathic pain, they can be used for acute pain. Compounds such as a 5% lidocaine patch can significantly reduce pain and improve the quality of life. Lidocaine is believed to block sodium channels in the damaged nerve endings. It can be applied to the newly traumatized or operated tissue. The 5% lidocaine patch should not be applied directly to the open tissue or freshly sutured tissue. In those cases, it can be applied on both sides of the wound for 12 continuous hours per day (▶ Table 8.4).

Table 8.4 Initial pain medication and delivery[6,7,8,9,10,11,12]

Treatment	Dosage	Delivery	Injury
Ice	30 minutes on and off	Topical	Local soft tissue injury
Lidocaine 5% patch	12 hours on	Topical	Local soft tissue injury
EMLA cream (2.5% lidocaine, 2.5% prilocaine)	Apply every 2 hours	Topical	Local soft tissue injury
Capsaicin cream	Apply twice a day, three times a day	Topical	Neuropathic
NSAID cream (e.g., diclofenac, indomethacin)	Apply three times a day, four times a day	Topical	Nonacute tendon or ligament injury
Lidocaine intramuscular infusion	2 mg/min	Intratissue infusion	Local soft tissue injury
Bupivacaine epidural infusion	0.03–0.06%	Epidural	Soft tissue, bone
Bupivacaine epidural infusion with opioid	0.030–0.125% and 0.5–1.0 mg morphine or 1 µg fentanyl	Epidural	Soft tissue, bone

Abbreviations: EMLA, eutectic mixture of local anesthetics; NSAID, nonsteroidal anti-inflammatory drug.

8.4.3 Nonopioid Pain Treatment

For pain greater than 4 on a 0 to 10 pain scale, acetaminophen and NSAIDs, as well as other nonconventional, nonnarcotic complementary drugs, can be used (▶ Table 8.5). Each may be used with narcotics, potentiating the effects of a smaller narcotic dosage, resulting in less sedation and other deleterious side effects. The nonconventional medications can be beneficial, especially if the history can provide clues as to environmental, physiological, or psychological factors influencing the current pain. The nonconventional medications include antiepileptic drugs (AEDs), tricyclic antidepressants (TCAs), GABA, norepinephrine, α- and β-blockers, capsaicin, serotonin, benzodiazepines, caffeine, and barbiturates. These nonconventional medications are particularly beneficial in neuropathic and chronic pain.

Table 8.5 Nonopioid medication for pain rated as 4 or greater on the 0 to 10 pain scale[6,7,8,9,10,11,12]

Generic name	Average dosage	Average frequency (hours)	Major use	Maximum daily dose
Caffeine	65–325 mg	8	Stimulant	
Methysergide	2–8 mg	8–12	Headache	6–8 mg
Gabapentin	100–1,200 mg	8	Neuralgia	3,600 mg
Carbamazepine	5–35 mg/kg/d	6–12	Neuralgia	1,600 mg
Divalproex sodium	15–60 mg/kg/d	24	Migraine	4,000 mg
Phenytoin	4–8 mg/kg/d	6–8	Trigeminal neuralgia	600 mg
Amitriptyline	0.5–2.0 mg/kg/d	6–12	Depression	300 mg
Nortriptyline	20–150 mg	6–12	Depression	150 mg
Dexamethasone	0.0233–0.333 mg/kg/d	4–8	Inflammation	16 mg
Tramadol (opioid and SSRI)	50–100 mg	4–6	Pain	400 mg
Zolmitriptan	1.25–5 mg	2	Headache	10 mg
Propranolol	0.5–16 mg/kg/d		Migraine	640 mg
Baclofen	10–20 mg	6–8	Spasm	80 mg
Ketamine	5 µg/kg/min		Pain	
Benzodiazepines (e.g., alprazolam)	0.25–1.00 mg	8	Anxiety	10 mg
Calcium channel blocker	Multiple			

Abbreviation: SSRI, selective serotonin reuptake inhibitor.

Nonconventional pain medications work in multiple areas and by a variety of mechanisms, as listed here (▶ Table 8.6).

- *TCAs* inhibit neuronal discharge, decrease sensitivity of adrenergic receptors, block reuptake of norepinephrine and serotonin, and bind to histaminergic, cholinergic, and adrenergic receptors.
- *Selective serotonin reuptake inhibitors (SSRIs)* potentiate serotonin and norepinephrine pathways, inhibit cytochrome P-450, and assist in treating patients with depression and anxiety. Side effects include tremor, fever, diarrhea, delirium, and increased muscle tone.
- *AEDs* suppress abnormal neuronal discharges by blocking sodium channels, whereas others increase the inhibiting GABA transmission.
- *Benzodiazepines* potentiate inhibitory GABA transmission while also having antianxiety and antispasticity properties.
- *Alpha-adrenergic blockers* decrease hyperarousal symptoms by activating autoinhibitory presynaptic receptors of the locus cerulus.

Common potentiating adjuvant nonnarcotic pain medications are listed in ▶ Table 8.5. The medication should be carefully chosen and reflect the clinical situation associated with the drug's major use. For example, if depression exacerbates the pain, consider the addition of amitriptyline.

Table 8.6 Neurochemicals released and possible modulators of pain pathway areas[5,6,7,8]

Area in pain pathway	Neurochemical	Possible modulation
Nociceptor	Prostaglandins, substance P, bradykinins, cytokines, histamine, and serotonin	Local anesthetics, ASA, NSAIDs, opioids, acetaminophen, AEDs, and TCAs
Pain fiber C or A delta	Calcium and sodium channel	Channel blockers
Interneuron	NMDA, GABA, and endogenous opioids	Magnesium, PCP, GABA, and opioids
Reticular formation, thalamus, mesencephalon, and hypothalamus	GABA, norepinephrine, substance P, serotonin, and opioids	GABA, norepinephrine, β-blocker, capsaicin, serotonin, and opioids
Frontal cortex, insular cortex, limbic structures, and sensory cortex	GABA, norepinephrine, substance P, serotonin, and opioids	GABA, norepinephrine, β-blocker, capsaicin, serotonin, opioids, AEDs, TCAs, benzodiazepines, and barbiturates

Abbreviations: AEDs, antiepileptics; ASA, acetylsalicylic acid (aspirin); GABA, γ-aminobutyric acid; NMDA, N-methyl-D-aspartate; NSAIDs, nonsteroidal anti-inflammatory drugs; PCP, phencyclidine hydrochloride; TCAs, tricyclic antidepressants.

8.4.4 Opioids

Opioids are the most commonly used medication in the ICU. Opioids are mainly used to provide analgesia, but they also serve as sedatives/hypnotics in low doses. All opioids act by binding to opioid receptors in the central and peripheral nervous systems as agonists, partial agonists, or agonist-antagonists to produce the pharmacological effects like analgesia, decreased level of consciousness, respiratory depression, miosis, gastrointestinal hypo-motility, and vasodilatation. Fentanyl, remifentanil, and morphine are μ-receptor agonists most commonly used in the ICU. Opioids are generally well tolerated in the neurosurgical patients with minimal side effects. However, patients with traumatic brain injury (TBI) receiving some classes of opioids have had an increase in their intracranial pressures secondary to decreased respiratory drive, leading to vasodilation of cerebral blood vessels and an eventual increase in ICP. Miosis related to opioid use can also mask neurologic deterioration in a patient with TBI or preexisting increased ICP.[13]

High doses of morphine and fentanyl have been related to seizure-like activity in patients undergoing general anesthesia. This has been related to opioid-related muscle rigidity or myoclonus. Nonepileptic myoclonus has also been documented in patients receiving high-dose IV or intrathecal morphine. Other adverse reactions related to opioid use include somnolence, respiratory depression, chest wall and muscle rigidity (fentanyl and remifentanil), dysphoria or hallucinations (primarily with morphine), nausea and vomiting, histamine release causing urticaria, flushing and hypotension (most commonly related to morphine and meperidine). Fentanyl and remifentanil have shown to have little effect on blood pressure. Careful monitoring of vital signs, especially respiratory rate and pulse oximetry, is extremely important in patients receiving opioid therapy. The advantage of opioid analgesics is the ability to reverse their effect with the opioid antagonist naloxone.[13,14]

There are four classes of opioids, representing the particular receptor they stimulate: mu, kappa, delta, and the newest, nociceptin/orphanin FQ (N/OFQ).

Clinically, the effect of opioids is to raise the pain threshold, increasing the minimal intensity needed to feel pain. At the anatomical level, opioids act by inhibiting nociceptive transmission to the spinal cord, activating descending inhibitory pathways, and altering the higher-center activity of pain perception. The opiates may have a purely stimulatory effect on opiate receptors (agonists) or stimulate at low doses and block at higher concentrations (agonists/antagonists). At the cellular physiology level, all opioids decrease cyclic adenosine monophosphate (cAMP); increase K^+ efflux, especially mu and delta; decrease calcium entry into the neuron, especially kappa; cause cellular hyperpolarization; and decrease the release of neurotransmitters, providing a neuroprotective mechanism.

Kappa Opioid Receptor Stimulators

Opioid receptors are classified into four types: mu, delta, kappa, and N/OFQ. Among these types, the kappa receptor system has become most attractive. According to Ikeda and Matsumoto,[15] by targeting the kappa receptor, novel therapeutic agents beyond pain and its relief can potentially be developed. Endogenous opioid systems have been proposed as secondary or delayed brain injury factors, largely on the basis of the therapeutic efficacy of opioid receptor antagonists or agonists. Ikeda and Matsumoto[15] demonstrated that the novel kappa opioid agonist RU51599 has a neuroprotective effect on traumatic and ischemic brain edema, while also having an analgesic effect. Hudson et al[16] demonstrated the neuroprotective effects of the kappa opioid-related anticonvulsants U-50488 H and U-54494A in a neurotoxic model of NMDA-induced brain injury in the neonatal rat. Tortella and DeCoster[17] found that kappa receptor opioids, specifically the arylacetamide series of kappa opioid analgesics, are novel pharmacotherapeutic treatments for epilepsy, stroke, or trauma-related brain or spinal cord injury.[18,19] The kappa opioid shares common properties with all opioids, being neuroprotective but, unlike mu receptors, acting directly in the brain to reduce ICP by inhibiting antidiuretic hormone (arginine vasopressin [AVP]) secretion and promoting water excretion in humans.[20] AVP regulates brain water content and is elevated in the cerebrospinal fluid of patients with ischemia and TBIs. Ikeda et al[21] demonstrated the protective effect of RU51599, a selective kappa opioid agonist and AVP release inhibitor, thereby improving brain edema. Kappa receptor stimulation increases diuresis, reducing edema and increasing ICP, leading to increases in cerebral perfusion pressure. Kappa receptor stimulators cause respiratory depression but less than mu receptor stimulation. They also cause dysphoria, which can be problematic.

Nalbuphine is a potent kappa agonist and mu antagonist analgesic with a low side-effect profile and low abuse potential, possibly because it inhibits midbrain dopamine release. Because it is a mu antagonist, it should be used with caution in those individuals who are addicted to mu receptor stimulators, such as morphine, because it can cause a withdrawal problem.

Mu Opioid Receptor Stimulators

The prototypical mu receptor stimulator is morphine, which has many benefits. In neurologic disease, it is neuroprotective to the cell. Morphine may also be used for preoperative sedation and dyspnea associated with acute left ventricular failure and pulmonary edema. Camphorated tincture of opium, another mu receptor stimulator, can treat severe diarrhea and intestinal cramping, and codeine is helpful with severe persistent cough. At times when very mild hyperventilation may be used, such as after head injury, morphine blunts the reflex vasoconstriction caused by decreased PCO_2 and decreases peripheral vascular resistance.[12]

The potential adverse effects of ketamine in neurosurgical anesthesia have been well established. The side effects of this mu receptor stimulator are increased ICP and cerebral blood flow (CBF). De Nadal et al[22,23] demonstrated in human brain trauma subjects that when carbon dioxide reactivity was preserved, 56.7% of the patients showed impaired or abolished autoregulation to hypertensive challenge. In both groups after mu receptor stimulation with either morphine or fentanyl, there was a significant increase in ICP and a decrease in mean arterial blood pressure and cerebral perfusion pressure, but arterial-venous difference of oxygen ($AVDO_2$) estimated CBF remained unchanged. In patients with preserved carbon dioxide reactivity, the opioid-induced ICP increase was even greater. This demonstrated the vasodilating effects of fentanyl. In additional studies, de Nadal and others came to the conclusion that potent opioids cause greater increases of ICP due to methods other than activation of the vasodilator cascade. Sperry et al[24] showed that mu receptor stimulators are associated with a statistically significant ICP increase of 8.2 mm Hg for fentanyl, and an increase of 6.1 mm Hg for sufentanil. Both drugs caused statistically significant decreases in mean arterial blood pressure: fentanyl, 11.6 mm Hg; sufentanil, 10.5 mm Hg. No significant changes in heart rate occurred. Their results indicate that modest doses of potent opioids can significantly increase ICP in patients with severe head trauma.[24] Other investigators proved the same, that sufentanil, fentanyl, and alfentanil infusions cause a significant but transient increase in ICP accompanied by a significant decrease in mean arterial pressure.[25] Hydromorphone, a mu receptor agonist, also significantly increased regional CBF in the anterior cingulate cortex, both amygdalae, and the thalamus, all structures belonging to the limbic system.[26]

Not all mu receptor stimulators cause cerebral vasodilation.

Opioids and Their Side Effects

Just as NSAIDs belong to different groups, with considerable variability in efficacy, opioid groups vary in their ability to treat pain, even in the same individual. *If one opioid does not work, consider treatment with another one.* The first and most widely used opioid is the group that stimulates the mu receptor; these include morphine, meperidine (Demerol), hydromorphone (Dilaudid), and fentanyl. The side effects of this group share some commonality with most opioid receptor stimulators and, as expected, demonstrate unique risks. Mu receptor stimulators cause increased ICP, both directly and indirectly, by vasodilatory and nonvasodilatory ways[3,9,10,12,27]; respiratory depression; bronchoconstriction; chest wall rigidity; hypotension; increased edema by increasing antidiuretic hormone (ADH) release; stimulated dopamine release; constipation; reduced body temperature; sedation; nausea with or without vomiting;

itching; somnolence; confusion and disorientation; hallucinations; and seizures at high doses. The mu acting drug also stimulates dopamine release, leading to addiction.

Therefore, when prescribing a high-dose intravenous opioid or opioid infusion, vital signs must be closely monitored. There should be continuous pulse oximetry, and the physician should be notified for decreased oxygenation. Blood pressure and respirations should be recorded every 15 minutes for 2 hours, then every hour for 4 hours, then every 4 hours thereafter. With each increase in dosage, the vital sequence should restart. The medication should be stopped and the physician notified if the respiratory rate is less than 10 per minute or the systolic blood pressure (SBP) is less than 90 mm Hg. Antidotes for opioids must be immediately available. Naloxone 1 mg ampule should be on the patient's floor. If the respiratory rate is less than 8 per minute, give naloxone 0.2 mg intravenous push (IVP) and call the attending physician; the dose may be repeated in 5 minutes. For itching, have available diphenhydramine 25 mg IV/orally every 6 hours. For initial nausea and vomiting, which usually resolve with the second dose, have available an antiemetic, such as granisetron 10 μg/kg IV over 5 minutes every 4 hours, or a comparable agent. Furthermore, when discontinuing patient-controlled analgesia (PCA) if greater than 3 days of continuous infusion, wean the medication (▶ Table 8.7).

Table 8.7 Opioid receptors and side effects[6,7,8,9,10,11,12,15,16,20,21]

Receptor	Drug	Side effects	Contraindications or cautions
Mu	Morphine, fentanyl, hydromorphone, buprenorphine	Raises ICP, respiratory depression, bronchoconstriction, chest wall rigidity, hypotension; increases edema by increasing ADH release; stimulates dopamine release, pupil constriction (miosis); reduces body temperature; depresses cough reflex; constipation, sedation, and nausea with or without vomiting; itching; somnolence, confusion, and disorientation	Head injury, asthma, respiratory conditions, paralytic ileus
Kappa	Nalbuphine	Respiratory depression, euphoria, sedation, nausea, vomiting, sweating, headache vertigo, confusion, dry mouth	,
Delta	Experimental BW373U86, SB235863		

Abbreviations: ADH, antidiuretic hormone; ICP, intracranial pressure.

Opioid medication should be prescribed only after understanding the risks and benefits of the medication. Additional resources for prescribing dosage and administration should be checked before giving the medication. Following here are some of the commonly prescribed opiates with some general considerations. For each, the exact dose should be tailored to the patient and clinical circumstance.

- Ten percent of the population lacks the enzyme needed to activate codeine. As a desired treatment, codeine may cause nausea and constipation.
- Tramadol lowers the seizure threshold.
- Fentanyl transdermal takes 12 to 16 hours to produce a therapeutic effect and 48 hours to reach steady state.
- Seriously consider the use of meperidine in the NICU patient because of neurotoxic risks of anxiety, tremors, myoclonus, and seizures.
- Give a loading dose of the narcotic, then an hourly dose of approximately $1/6$ the loading dose.
- Most opiates are cleared by renal and hepatic means (▶ Table 8.8).

Table 8.8 Opioid pain medication for pain of 5 or 6 or greater on the 0 to 10 pain scale[6,7, 8,9,10,11,12,15,16,20,21]

Drug	Receptor agonist or antagonist	Route	Dosage	Frequency (hours)	Half-life (hours)
Morphine	Mu	IV	0.1 mg/kg	3–4	2.1–2.6
		IM	0.2 mg/kg	3–4	
		Oral	0.3 mg/kg	3–4	
Ketamine	Mu	IV	5 µg/kg/min	3–4	
Hydromorphone	Mu	IV, IM	0.015 mg/kg 0.5–1.0 mg/h	3–6	2.6–3.2
		Oral	0.06 mg/kg	3–6	
Fentanyl	Mu	IV	25–50 µg/h		3.7
		TC	25–100 µg/h 600–7200 µg	72-hour patch	3.7
Oxycodone	Mu	Oral	0.2 mg/kg	3–4	
Hydrocodone	Mu	Oral	0.2 mg/kg	3–4	
Meperidine	Mu	IV	0.75 mg/kg	2–3	3
		IM	75 mg		3
		Oral	Not given orally	Not given orally	3

(continued)

Table 8.8 continued

Drug	Receptor agonist or antagonist	Route	Dosage	Fre-quency (hours)	Half-life (hours)
Levorpha-nol	Mu	IM	0.02 mg/kg	6–8	11
		Oral	0.04 mg/kg	6–8	11
Buprenor-phine	Mu	IV	0.4 mg/kg	6–8	5
		SL	2–24 mg	6–8	5
Codeine	Mu	IV	1 mg/kg	6–8	3
		IM	1 mg/kg	6–8	3
		Oral	1 mg/kg	3–4	
Tramadol	Mu	Oral	50–100 mg	6	
Nalbu-phine	Kappa agonist, mu antagonist	IV	0.15–2.5 mg/kg	3–6	5
Butorpha-nol	Kappa agonist, mu agonist and antago-nist	IV, IM	2 mg 0.5–4.0 mg 0.25–32 mg/d max	3–4	3
		IN	1 mg spray, 1–4 mg/d	3–6	
Thyroid-releasing hormone		IV			
Naloxone	Binds mu receptor without stimulation; also binds kappa and delta	IV	0.4 mg every 2–3 min		1
Pentazo-cine	Kappa; mu agonist and antagonist	Oral	50 mg	4–6	4
Propoxy-phene HCl	Mu	Oral	65 mg	4–6	9

Abbreviations: HCl, hydrochloric; IM, intramuscularly; IN, intranasally; IV, intravenously; SL, sublingual; TC, transdermal transcutaneous.

8.5 General Considerations in Treating Pain

Treat pain early, when it begins; do not wait until pain is out of control. When pain becomes severe, it will require a much greater dosage. Consider providing medication around the clock when there is an initial injury, as opposed to giving medication only when asked for by the patient or only when the patient appears symptomatic. There will also be times when there is breakthrough pain. This pain is usually of moderate to severe intensity, occurs rapidly, usually in less than 3 minutes, is of relatively short duration, and occurs one to four times per day. Therefore, different medications should be prescribed for initial treatment and recurring pain. It is even beneficial to prescribe patient-controlled analgesia or continuous intravenous infusion of pain medication (▶ Table 8.9).

In addition to cautiously looking for reasons to decrease or discontinue the medication, NICU personnel must document the medication's efficacy. The attending physician must be notified if the pain remains greater than 4 on a 1–10 pain scale for 3 consecutive hours. If there is breakthrough pain, acetaminophen, 650 mg or more, can be given every 4 to 6 hours. Consider additional treatment should a pain pump or medication stop being available (▶ Table 8.10).

Table 8.9 Treatment of pain

Scale score	Treatment
0–4	Ice + APAP; possibly low-dose NSAIDs, possibly topical
5–9	Ice + APAP + ketorolac; possibly high-dose NSAIDs, low-dose opioids
10	Ice + APAP + ketorolac; possibly high-dose NSAIDs, high-dose opioids

Abbreviations: APAP, acetaminophen; NSAIDs, nonsteroidal anti-inflammatory drugs.

Table 8.10 Patient-controlled or continuous IV analgesia algorithm[6,7,8,9,10,11,12,15,16,20,21]

Document allergies:

Weight in kilograms:

Use continuous pulse oximeter; notify physician if less than____%.

Record blood pressure and respirations every 15 minutes for 2 hours, then every hour for 4 hours, then every 4 hours thereafter. With each increase in dosage, begin sequence of vital signs again. Stop infusion and notify attending physician if respiratory rate < 10/min or systolic blood pressure < 90 mm Hg. Keep pain < 4 on 1–10 VAS or 1–10 FLACC pain scale. Assess and record pain every hour while awake.

Choose one medication to use:

____morphine 1 mg/mL

____hydromorphone (Dilaudid) 0.5 mg/mL

____fentanyl 10 µg/mL

____butorphanol (Stadol) 0.1 mg/mL (for increased ICP)

____nalbuphine (Nubain) 1 mg/mL (for increased ICP)

Give initial bolus of the medication being used above:

____mg morphine sulfate (range: 1–5 mg)

____mg hydromorphone (Dilaudid) (range: 0.1–1.0 mg)

____mg fentanyl (range: 10–20 µg)

(continued)

____mg butorphanol (Stadol) (range: 0.5–2.0 mg)

____mg nalbuphine (Nubain) (range: 10–20 mg)

PCA pump settings of the medication chosen above (continuous basal rate):

____mg/h morphine sulfate (range: 1–4 mg)

____mg/h hydromorphone (Dilaudid) (range: 0.5–1.0 mg)

____μg/h fentanyl (range: 10–20 μg)

____mg/h butorphanol (Stadol) (range: 0.1–1.0 mg)

____mg/h nalbuphine (Nubain) (range: 5–10 mg)

PCA dose of the medication chosen above:

____mg morphine sulfate (range: 0.5–2.0 mg)

____mg hydromorphone (Dilaudid) (range: 0.1–0.2 mg)

____μg fentanyl (range: 10–20 μg)

____mg butorphanol (Stadol) (range: 0.1–0.5 mg)

____mg nalbuphine (Nubain) (range: 5–10 mg)

Lockout interval: ____5–30 minutes Maximum dose per 4 hours of the medication chosen above:

____mg morphine (range: 10–40 mg)

____mg hydromorphone (Dilaudid) (range: 2–6 mg)

____μg fentanyl (range: 100–300 μg)

____mg butorphanol (Stadol) (range: 2–4 mg)

____mg nalbuphine (Nubain) (range: 40 mg)

Notify attending physician if pain > 4 for more than 1 hour.

Have available on the floor naloxone (Narcan) 1 mg ampule. Give 0.2 mg IVP if respiratory rate is < 8/min and call physician; may repeat dose in 5 minutes. When discontinuing PCA if > 3 days of continuous infusion, wean:

____decrease morphine 1 mg/h until < 2 mg/h, then decrease 0.5 mg/h

____decrease hydromorphone (Dilaudid) 0.5 mg/h until < 1 mg/h, then decrease 0.2 mg/h

____decrease fentanyl 10 μg/h until < 20 μg/h, then decrease 5 μg/h

____decrease butorphanol (Stadol) 0.5 mg/h until less < 1 mg/h, then decrease 0.2 mg/h

____decrease nalbuphine (Nubain) 5 mg/h until < 10 mg/h, then decrease 1 mg/h

Primary IV line to run at a rate of at least____to be piggybacked into the PCA line.

Have available diphenhydramine (Benedryl) 25 mg IV/PO every 6 hours as needed for pruritus. Have available an antiemetic such as granisetron (Kytril) 10 μg/kg IV over 5 minutes every 4 hours as needed for nausea and vomiting.

For breakthrough pain, may give acetaminophen (Tylenol) 650 mg every 6 hours. If pump is interrupted for > 1 hour, not due to respiratory changes or blood pressure changes, may give hydrocodone 5 mg orally every 4 hours.

Abbreviations: IV, intravenously; IVP, intravenous push; PCA, patient-controlled analgesia; VAS, visual analog scale.

8.6 Sedation in Neurocritical Care

The indications for sedation that exist in the ICU population, such as cardiopulmonary stabilization, performing and maintaining endotracheal intubation, and reducing central hypoxemia, exist in neurocritical care as well. However, certain indications that are unique to this patient population include reducing ICP, maintaining adequate cerebral perfusion pressure, decreasing cerebral oxygen consumption, preventing central hyperventilation, refractory status epilepticus, and controlling agitation in patients with TBI or drug/alcohol withdrawal.[28] Neurosurgery patients are the most difficult ICU patients to manage as they require adequate sedation and analgesia with the need for frequent rapid reversal to obtain accurate neurologic exams.[13,14]

It must be remembered that sedation and paralytics have not been shown to increase positive outcome in patients with severe head injury. Sedation and paralytics, however, have been shown to increase the possibility of pneumonia, ventilator dependency, duration of delirium, and ICU length of stay.[5] Notwithstanding, sedation is sometimes required. During these times the initial agitation scale must be assessed, and the level of sedation required must also be recorded. Any sedation decreases the most sensitive and important means to assess neurologic injury: the neurologic exam. The favored assessment scale is the Ramsey or Modified Ramsey based on wakefulness (▶ Table 8.11).

Just like pain, sedation needs must also be appropriately assessed and scored prior to treatment. Based on this, an appropriate sedative is then chosen. The drug of choice should provide the clinician with an opportunity to examine the patient closely on a regular basis. It should also have a rapid onset of action, short half-life, and provide adequate sedation without significant side effects.

Majority of the sedatives used in neurocritical care cause dose-dependent respiratory depression. Thus it is vital for the patient to have a protected airway prior to the start of any sedation regimen. Careful monitoring of the hemodynamic and respiratory status of the patients should also be used throughout the process.[13]

Table 8.11 Modified Ramsey scale score[1,6,9,10,12]

Score	Description
1	Anxious, agitated
2	Cooperative, oriented, tranquil
3	Responds to commands
4	Responds to shaking
5	Responds to noxious stimuli only
6	Unresponsive

8.7 Common Sedative Agents Used in Neurocritical Care

8.7.1 Benzodiazepines

These are some of the most commonly used sedative agents in critical care. Some of the common agents include diazepam, midazolam, and lorazepam. They exert their clinical action by augmenting the action of GABA on the GABA$_A$ receptors and in turn affecting the movement of chloride ions. They have dose-dependent amnestic, sedative, muscle relaxant, anxiolytic, and anti-convulsive properties. Benzodiazepines have little or no analgesic properties. Thus appropriate analgesic supplementation should be added. Due to their anxiolytic and amnestic properties; benzodiazepines are of vital use in neuro-critical care, especially during painful procedures. They have little or no effect on blood pressure, heart rate, and respiratory status. Thus low-dose titrated infusions are generally well tolerated. However, high-dose benzodiazepine infusion can cause profound respiratory depression and significantly reduce blood pressure. This effect is augmented when other medications with a similar mechanism of action are used concomitantly. Thus careful hemodynamic monitoring and airway protection are highly recommended for any patients receiving continuous benzodiazepine infusion. No significant effect on ICPs has been noted.[13] However, hypercarbia secondary to respiratory depression can cause vasodilation of cerebral vasculature resulting in an increase in CBF and resultant increase in ICPs. Decrease in mean arterial pressure can lower cerebral perfusion pressure and cause negative outcomes in patients. This effect is profound in patients in whom the normal autoregulatory mechanism is disabled or altered secondary to TBI or some other pathological process.[14]

Benzodiazepines are extremely lipophilic in nature, and prolonged exposure can cause an extended effect, leading to a state of delirium. Compared to other benzodiazepines, lorazepam is the least lipophilic of all the benzodiazepines and leads to the least amount of redistribution affect, thus offering a longer duration of action. However, due to its propylene glycol dilutent it can be toxic if continuously infused. Anion gap metabolic acidosis, renal failure, and CNS toxicity are some of the markers of propylene glycol toxicity. An accurate estimation of renal function and serial arterial blood gas measurements should be obtained to evaluate for any renal or metabolic derangements.[13]

Midazolam is highly lipophilic and has a short onset and duration of action. It is primarily metabolized by the liver and excreted by the kidneys. Thus, in patients with concomitant liver disease, accumulation of active metabolites can cause prolonged sedation and a state of delirium even after cessation of therapy. Lorazepam and midazolam have also been used for the treatment of status epilepticus. However, this effect is diminished over time due to buildup of tolerance. Other common side effects include headache, nausea or vomiting, vertigo, confusion, somnolence, hypotonia, and muscular weakness.[13,14]

The effects of benzodiazepines can be reversed with Romazicon (flumazenil); 0.2 mg can be given IVP. Flumazenil's duration of action is ~ 30–60 minutes. Thus patients receiving longer-acting benzodiazepines can become resedated once it is metabolized.

8.7.2 Diprivan (Propofol)

Propofol is an ultra-short-acting alkylphenol. The exact mechanism of action still remains unclear. However, it is known to bind to the GABA$_A$ receptor, the primary inhibitory receptor of the CNS, thus causing hyperpolarization of the postsynaptic membrane resulting in inhibition of the postsynaptic neuron.

Propofol's sedative and hypnotic properties make it a popular agent for anesthesia induction, sedation in ventilated patients, and procedural sedation. Hailed by many as the sedative agent of choice in the neurosurgical patient, propofol's rapid onset of action coupled with its short duration makes it one of the most widely used agents in neurocritical care. Propofol can lead to a rapid decrease in ICP due to its sedative effects coupled with a dose-dependent decrease in cerebral metabolism. At high doses, propofol also exhibits antiepileptic properties and suppresses electroencephalographic activity in a similar fashion to barbiturates. However, due to its negative effects on blood pressure, propofol can lead to decreased cerebral perfusion pressure and worsening of neurologic dysfunction, especially in patients with TBI. Propofol requires close monitoring of the hemodynamic and respiratory status of patients. It has shown to cause a significant decrease in blood pressure due to its negative ionotropic and vasodilatory properties.[29] This effect is potentiated in patients with hypovolemia, reduced cardiac output, use of other cardiodepressant medications, and the elderly.[30]

Propofol causes dose-dependent respiratory depression and should be used in the setting of careful monitoring of pulse oximetry and respiratory rate. It is preferred that the patient has a protected airway while infusing continuous or bolus propofol dosing.

Propofol has no known analgesic properties and is most commonly used in combination with analgesic agents such as fentanyl or other opioid analgesics. Careful attention must be paid while dosing these agents in combination with propofol as they can further add to the hemodynamic and respiratory depressive properties of propofol.

One of the most serious side effects related to long-term use of high-dose propofol is development of "propofol related infusion syndrome" (PRIS). It is defined as acute onset of refractory bradycardia leading to asystole in the presence of one or more of the following: metabolic acidosis with base deficit > 10 mmol, rhabdomyolysis, hyperkalemia, and hyperlipidemia. PRIS is more commonly associated with infusion doses greater than 4 mg/kg for more than 48 hours, especially common in the pediatric population, patients with severe critical illness of the CNS or respiratory system, exogenous catecholamine or glucocorticoid administration, inadequate carbohydrate intake, and subclinical mitochondrial disease. The exact mechanism is unknown. However, it has been postulated that PRIS is due to the direct mitochondrial respiratory chain inhibition or impaired mitochondrial fatty acid metabolism mediated by propofol. Early signs of PRIS include cardiac instability with the development of acute-onset right bundle branch block with convex-curved ("coved type") ST elevation in the right precordial leads (V1 to V3) on electrocardiogram (EKG). Routine monitoring for electrolyte abnormalities, lactic acidosis, and increases in creatinine kinase and triglycerides is highly recommended, with immediate cessation of therapy if any of the aforementioned abnormalities are encountered.[30]

Propofol is insoluble in water and is normally suspended in an emulsified solution of soy, glycerol, and egg phospholipids. Careful attention must be paid in making sure the patients are not allergic to any of these products. Propofol's lipid suspension also provides 1.1 kcal/mL of caloric value. Thus nutritional requirements should be adjusted accordingly. Injection site pain is also a common complaint; this can be minimized by infusing propofol through a large-bore IV or central line.[13,14] The effects of propofol can also be reversed with Romazicon (flumazenil). If SBP becomes < 90 mm Hg or heart rate < 50, the attending physician should be notified.

8.7.3 Dexmedetomidine (Precedex)

Dexmedetomidine is a highly selective agonist at the alpha-2 adrenoreceptor. Its affinity for the alpha-2 receptors is considerably higher than its other counterparts, such as clonidine; thus leading to a stronger sedative, anxiolytic, anti-sympathetic, and analgesic effect. Its versatile properties make it a suitable drug when one is trying to avoid multiple agents. Some of the major side effects include hypotension and bradycardia due to decreased sympathetic outflow from postsynaptic alpha-2 receptors in the CNS.[13]

Precedex offers a dose-dependent decrease in vigilance and increase in sedation. The inability to provide anterograde amnesia coupled with maintenance of arousability even at deeper levels of sedation provide emergence from light sedation without disorientation and confusion and with increased levels of vigilance compared to some of its other sedative counterparts. Its ability to provide such "cooperative sedation" makes it ideal for conducting accurate neurologic exams.[31]

Precedex has been associated with decreased episodes of ICU delirium when compared to other sedatives. Its central mechanism of action is on the locus ceruleus; a nucleus located in the rostral pons that contains many noradrenergic neurons, and mediates arousal, vigilance, and the sleep–wake cycle. By decreasing transmission of the noradrenergic output, it produces anxiolysis and sedation. Opioid withdrawal, which can offer a major challenge to the neurointensivist, can be counteracted by Precedex's ability to decrease reflex noradrenergic release. This makes it a suitable agent for weaning off of high-dose opioid analgesics and counteracting agitation secondary to acute drug withdrawal.[31] Precedex has also shown not to cause respiratory depression. The respiratory pattern, even when on high doses of Precedex, mimics that of the natural sleep cycle. It has also been shown to facilitate weaning off from mechanical ventilation by decreasing agitation related to extubation and by decreasing dependence on opioids and benzodiazepines as stated previously.

The onset of action is within 15 minutes after bolus infusion, with peak concentration achieved within 1 hour. Initial infusion can cause transient hypotension and bradycardia. This is attenuated in patients with hypovolemia and preexisting cardiac conditions. These effects are treated with cessation of infusion or with medical management, either atropine, ephedrine, atipamezole, or volume infusion. Its half-life is around 6 minutes and its terminal elimination half-life is around 2 hours. The short half-life allows for easy titration. Precedex causes no change in ICP; however, it can cause a decrease in cerebral perfusion pressure due to a decrease in mean arterial pressure. In patients suffering from TBI this can be deleterious as decreased CBF can cause secondary brain injury; especially in the immediate postresuscitative period when the brain is most vulnerable to ischemic damage.

Currently, the use of Precedex is only approved for a maximum of 24 hours by the U.S. Food and Drug Administration secondary to risks of rebound hypertension and tachycardia upon discontinuation of therapy. However, randomized clinical trials evaluating this relationship are currently limited in number.[31]

8.8 Comparison of Different Sedative Agents

There have been a number of clinical trials evaluating the efficacy and reliability of the different sedative agents available. A variety of outcome measures have been assessed, including length of ICU stay, duration of mechanical ventilation, time to extubation, incidence of delirium, cardiovascular effects, and neurocognitive impairment.

The Maximizing Efficacy of Targeted Sedation and Reducing Neurological Dysfunction (MENDS) trial evaluated delirium- and coma-free days in patients receiving lorazepam versus Precedex. It showed that the use of Precedex was associated with decreased duration of delirium and coma as well as a more reliable level of sedation as compared to lorazepam. The MIDEX and PRODEX were large multicenter trials comparing the use of Precedex to midazolam and propofol, respectively. They showed that Precedex was not inferior to midazolam and propofol in maintaining the desired level of sedation in mechanically ventilated patients for prolonged periods of time. Precedex was also found to reduce the duration of mechanical ventilation compared to midazolam. Patients were also able to communicate their pain better while receiving treatment with Precedex versus midazolam or propofol.[32]

8.9 Barbiturate Therapy (Burst Suppression)

Barbiturates are centrally acting agents that exert their depressive effects on primarily the $GABA_A$ receptors and at higher concentrations directly activate these receptors.[13] They have dose-dependent sedative, hypnotic, anxiolytic, analgesic, anticonvulsant, and neuroprotective properties. The most commonly used barbiturates in neurocritical care are pentobarbital, phenobarbital, and sodium thiopental.

Barbiturates are primarily used in neurocritical care for the treatment of status epilepticus and controlling refractory intracranial hypertension. They exert their effect on intracranial pressure by causing a decrease in CBF and cerebral metabolic rate of oxygen ($CMRO_2$) and by having a neuroprotective effect at a cellular level. As per the most recent TBI guidelines, there is level II evidence that high-dose barbiturate therapy is effective in controlling intracranial hypertension refractive to maximal medical and surgical ICP-lowering strategies. Pentobarbital is the most widely used agent for controlling refractory ICPs in neurocritical care.[13,14]

The goal of therapy is to achieve a pentobarbital concentration between 3 and 5%. However, studies have shown poor correlation among serum concentrations of the drug and its therapeutic effects. On the other hand, the pattern of burst suppression on electroencephalography has been shown to more accurately represent a maximal decrease in CBF and cerebral metabolic demand and to prevent overmedication. When a burst suppression pattern is achieved on an electroencephalogram a patient is said to be in a pentobarbital coma. Listed here are some of the things that need to be taken into account and monitored before and during a pentobarbital or barbiturate coma.[33,34]

- All other medical and surgical options of decreasing intracranial pressures have been exhausted.
- No surgical lesion is present.
- Brain death is excluded.
- Serum sodium concentration is < 160 mEq/L and serum osmolality is less than 330 mOsm/Kg before initiating therapy.
- There is continuous electroencephalography and intracranial pressure/cerebral perfusion pressure monitoring.
- Airway protection and mechanical ventilation are provided.
- Avoid hypotension; keep SBP > 90 at all times. Consider invasive hemodynamic monitoring with pulmonary artery (PA) catheter or arterial line. Use ionotropic and vasopressive agents if needed.

- Monitor feeding intolerance. Consider early total parenteral nutrition if paralytic ileus is suspected.
- Daily complete blood count, comprehensive metabolic panel (CMP).
- Periodic liver function tests (LFT).
- Daily chest X-rays.
- Aggressive and early infectious/sepsis workup and treatment if suspected.

Pentobarbital burst suppression protocol is as follows:
1. Give pentobarbital 2.5 mg/kg every 15 minutes for four doses. *Follow blood pressure closely.*
2. Over the next 3 hours, give pentobarbital 10 mg/kg/h continuous infusion.
3. Then initiate maintenance pentobarbital 1.5 mg/kg/h infusion.
4. Maintain burst suppression 1–2 bursts/page.
5. Check daily levels; maintain pentobarbital level 5 mg% (a lab value, e.g., mg, µg/mL) or 50 µg/mL.
   a) Remember that this is not a pentobarbital level.
   b) Some people may not have burst suppression at higher levels.
   c) If ICP is controlled for > 48 hours, then start to wean off the drug.
   d) If ICP is not controlled in 24 hours, this procedure is unlikely to work.

Pentobarbital is primarily metabolized through a first-pass mechanism by the liver. It has an onset of action of approximately 15 minutes and a half-life of approximately 15 to 48 hours. It takes about 2 days for neurologic function to return after cessation of therapy.[35]

In conclusion, we recommend use of high-dose barbiturate therapy only in patients with refractory ICPs, with no surgical lesions and viable brain function. Prophylactic barbiturate therapy has not shown to improve outcome and should be avoided.[36] Patients should be closely monitored throughout the therapy (▶ Table 8.12).

Table 8.12 Patient sedation and analgesia intravenous schedule algorithm[6,7,8,9,10,11,12,15,16,20,21]

Initially, the patient is loaded with the appropriate analgesic and sedation. Further medication can be based on the following protocol being adjusted for patient characteristics.

Must fill out patient sedation schedule

Select single pain analgesia to be given:

____morphine sulfate 1 mg/mL

____hydromorphone (Dilaudid) 0.5 mg/mL

____fentanyl 10 µg/mL

____butorphanol (Stadol) 0.1 mg/mL (for increased ICP)

____nalbuphine (Nubain) 1 mg/mL (for increased ICP)

(continued)

Table 8.12 continued

For propofol (Diprivan) dose of 5–19 µg/kg/min, or midazolam (Versed) dose of 0.02–0.06 mg/kg/h, or lorazepam (Ativan) dose of 0.02–0.04 mg/h, administer:

morphine sulfate 1 mg/h by continuous IV infusion *or*

hydromorphone (Dilaudid) 0.2 mg/h by continuous IV infusion *or*

fentanyl 10 µg/h by continuous IV infusion *or*

butorphanol (Stadol) 0.2 mg/h by continuous IV infusion *or*

nalbuphine (Nubain) 5 mg/h by continuous IV infusion

For propofol (Diprivan) dose of 20 to 39 µg/kg/min, or midazolam (Versed) dose of 5 to 7 mg/h, or lorazepam (Ativan) dose of 3 mg/h, administer:

morphine sulfate 3 mg/h by continuous IV infusion *or*

hydromorphone (Dilaudid) 1 mg/h by continuous IV infusion *or*

fentanyl 40 µg/h by continuous IV infusion *or*

butorphanol (Stadol) 1 mg/h by continuous IV infusion *or*

nalbuphine (Nubain) 10 mg/h by continuous IV infusion

For propofol (Diprivan) dose above 40 µg/kg/min, or midazolam (Versed) dose above 7 mg/h, or lorazepam (Ativan) dose above 3 mg/h, administer:

morphine sulfate 5 mg/h to a maximum of____by continuous IV infusion *or*

hydromorphone (Dilaudid) 1.5 mg/h to a maximum of____by continuous IV infusion *or*

fentanyl 50 µg/h to a maximum of____by continuous IV infusion *or*

butorphanol (Stadol) 2 mg/h to a maximum of____by continuous IV infusion *or*

nalbuphine (Nubain) 15 mg/h to a maximum of____by continuous IV infusion

Naloxone 1 mg ampule must be available on the floor. Give 0.2 mg IVP, if SBP < 90 mm Hg, call physician. May repeat dose in 5 minutes.

When discontinuing the chosen analgesia if > 3 days of continuous infusion, wean:

____decrease morphine 1 mg/h until < 2 mg/h, then decrease 0.5 mg/h

____decrease hydromorphone (Dilaudid) 0.5 mg/h until < 1 mg/h, then decrease 0.2 mg/h

____decrease fentanyl 10 µg/h until < 20 µg/h, then decrease 5 µg/h

____decrease butorphanol (Stadol) 0.5 mg/h until < 1 mg/h, then decrease 0.2 mg/h

____decrease nalbuphine (Nubain) 5 mg/h until < 10 mg/h, then decrease 1 mg/h

Primary IV line to run at a rate of at least____to be piggybacked into the PCA line.

Have available diphenhydramine (Benedryl) 25 mg IV/orally every 6 hours as needed for pruritus.

Have available granisetron (Kytril) 10 µg/kg IV over 5 minutes every 4 hours prn nausea and vomiting.

If pain pump is interrupted for > 1 hour, not due to respiratory changes or blood pressure changes, may give hydrocodone 5 mg NG tube every 4 hours.

Abbreviations: ICP, intracranial pressure; IV, intravenously; NG, nasogastric; PCA, patient-controlled analgesia; SBP, systolic blood pressure.

Table 8.13 Medication for sedation per desired Ramsey score[1,6,9,10,12]

Medication	Desired sedation goal of burst suppression	Desired Ramsey score (4–6)	Desired Ramsey score (2–3)
Propofol (Diprivan)	15 µ/kg/min	10 µg/kg/min	5 µg/kg/min
Midazolam (Versed)	0.06 mg/kg/h	0.04 mg/kg/h	0.02 mg/kg/h
Lorazepam (Ativan)	0.06 mg/kg/h	0.04 mg/kg/h	0.02 mg/kg/h

It is often difficult to adequately sedate the patient while providing proper analgesia. However, the same delivery of analgesia and sedation according to predefined and measurable criteria is possible using the FLACC and Ramsey/Modified Ramsey scores, as stated earlier (▶ Table 8.11, ▶ Table 8.13).

8.9.1 Disclaimer

All medications and dosages listed in this chapter are taken from *AHFS Drug Information*[9] and *Drug Facts and Comparisons,* 2014 edition.[10] This information is intended as a supplement to, and not a substitute for, the actual information from the sources. It is not meant to substitute for the knowledge, expertise, skill, and judgment of physicians, pharmacists, or other health care professionals in patient care. The absence of a warning for any medication should not be interpreted to indicate that the medication is safe, appropriate, or effective in any given patient.

Case Management

The patient should be assessed initially using the FLACC scale and given an initial dose of intravenous morphine bolus, followed by incrementally titrated doses as necessary until a FLACC score < 4 is achieved. A dosage should be given every 3 to 6 hours based on the FLACC score at the time of assessment. The pain therapy should also be augmented with acetaminophen 10 to 75 mg/kg/d in four to six divided doses unless contraindications exist. Alternatives to this approach are discussed in the algorithm in ▶ Table 8.10.

References

[1] McCaffery M. Nursing Practice Theories Related to Cognition, Bodily Pain and Man-Environmental Interactions. Los Angeles: UCLA Student Store; 1968
[2] Merskey H, Bugduk N. Classification of Chronic Pain Syndromes and Definitions of Pain Terms. 2nd ed. Seattle, WA: IASP Press; 1994

[3] Brody TM, Larner J, Minneman KP. Human Pharmacology: Molecular to Clinical. 3rd ed. St. Louis, MO: Mosby; 1998

[4] Riedel W, Neeck G. Nociception, pain, and antinociception: current concepts. Z Rheumatol. 2001; 60(6):404–415

[5] Guidelines for the Management of Severe Head Injury. New York, NY: The Brain Trauma Foundation; 2000

[6] Joint Commission on Accreditation of Healthcare Organizations National Pharmaceutical Council, Inc. (JCAHO). Pain: Current Understanding of Assessment, Management, and Treatment. Oakbrook Terrace, IL: JCAHO; 2001

[7] Jacox AK, Carr DB, Chapman CR. Acute pain management: operative or medical procedures and trauma. Clinical Practice Guidelines No 1, AHCPR 92–0032. Rockville, MD: U.S. Department of Health and Human Services, Agency for Health Care Policy and Research; 1992

[8] Pasero C, Paice JA, McCaffery M. Basic mechanisms underlying the causes and effects of pain. In: McCaffery M, Pasero C, eds. Pain Clinical Manual. 2nd ed. St. Louis, MO: Mosby; 1999:15–34

[9] McEvoy GK, ed. AHFS Drug Information. Bethesda, MD: American Society of Health-System Pharmacists; 2004

[10] Drug Facts and Comparisons 2014. 68th ed. St. Louis, MO: Facts and Comparisons; 2014

[11] Chandrasekharan NV, Dai H, Roos KL, et al. COX-3, a cyclooxygenase-1 variant inhibited by acetaminophen and other analgesic/antipyretic drugs: cloning, structure, and expression. Proc Natl Acad Sci U S A. 2002; 99(21):13926–13931

[12] Hardmann JG, Limbird LE. Goodman and Gillman's The Pharmacological Basis of Therapeutics. 10th ed. New York: McGraw-Hill; 2001

[13] Paul BS, Paul G. Sedation in neurological intensive care unit. Ann Indian Acad Neurol. 2013; 16 (2):194–202

[14] Lewin J, Goodwin H, Mirski M. Sedation and Analgesia in Critically Ill Neurologic Patient. 2013 Neurocritical Care Society Practice Update

[15] Ikeda Y, Matsumoto K. Analgesic effect of kappa-opioid receptor agonist [in Japanese]. Nihon Rinsho. 2001; 59(9):1681–1687

[16] Hudson CJ, Von Voigtlander PF, Althaus JS, Scherch HM, Means ED. The kappa opioid-related anticonvulsants U-50488 H and U-54494A attenuate N-methyl-D-aspartate induced brain injury in the neonatal rat. Brain Res. 1991; 564(2):261–267

[17] Tortella FC, DeCoster MA. Kappa opioids: therapeutic considerations in epilepsy and CNS injury. Clin Neuropharmacol. 1994; 17(5):403–416

[18] McIntosh TK, Faden AI. Opiate antagonist in traumatic shock. Ann Emerg Med. 1986; 15 (12):1462–1465

[19] McIntosh TK, Fernyak S, Hayes RL, Faden AI. Beneficial effect of the nonselective opiate antagonist naloxone hydrochloride and the thyrotropin-releasing hormone (TRH) analog YM-14673 on long-term neurobehavioral outcome following experimental brain injury in the rat. J Neurotrauma. 1993; 10(4):373–384

[20] Bemana I, Nagao S. Effects of niravoline (RU 51599), a selective kappa-opioid receptor agonist on intracranial pressure in gradually expanding extradural mass lesion. J Neurotrauma. 1998; 15 (2):117–124

[21] Ikeda Y, Teramoto A, Nakagawa Y, Ishibashi Y, Yoshii T. Attenuation of cryogenic induced brain oedema by arginine vasopressin release inhibitor RU51599. Acta Neurochir (Wien). 1997; 139 (12):1173–1179, discussion 1179–1180

[22] de Nadal M, Munar F, Poca MA, Sahuquillo J, Garnacho A, Rosselló J. Cerebral hemodynamic effects of morphine and fentanyl in patients with severe head injury: absence of correlation to cerebral autoregulation. Anesthesiology. 2000; 92(1):11–19

[23] de Nadal M, Ausina A, Sahuquillo J, Pedraza S, Garnacho A, Gancedo VA. Effects on intracranial pressure of fentanyl in severe head injured patients. Acta Neurochir Suppl (Wien). 1998; 71:10–12

[24] Sperry RJ, Bailey PL, Reichman MV, Peterson JC, Petersen PB, Pace NL. Fentanyl and sufentanil increase intracranial pressure in head trauma patients. Anesthesiology. 1992; 77(3):416–420

[25] Albanèse J, Viviand X, Potie F, Rey M, Alliez B, Martin C. Sufentanil, fentanyl, and alfentanil in head trauma patients: a study on cerebral hemodynamics. Crit Care Med. 1999; 27(2):407–411

[26] Vink R, Portoghese PS, Faden AI. kappa-Opioid antagonist improves cellular bioenergetics and recovery after traumatic brain injury. Am J Physiol. 1991; 261(6 Pt 2):R1527–R1532

[27] Cottrell JE, Turndorf H. Anesthesia and Neurosurgery. 2nd ed. St. Louis, MO: Mosby; 1986

[28] Schwartz ML, Tator CH, Rowed DW, Reid SR, Meguro K, Andrews DF. The University of Toronto head injury treatment study: a prospective, randomized comparison of pentobarbital and mannitol. Can J Neurol Sci. 1984; 11(4):434–440

[29] Jones GM, Doepker BA, Erdman MJ, Kimmons LA, Elijovich L. Predictors of severe hypotension in neurocritical care patients sedated with propofol. Neurocrit Care. 2014; 20(2):270–276

[30] Erdman MJ, Doepker BA, Gerlach AT, Phillips GS, Elijovich L, Jones GM. A comparison of severe hemodynamic disturbances between dexmedetomidine and propofol for sedation in neurocritical care patients. Crit Care Med. 2014; 42(7):1696–1702

[31] Pandharipande PP, Pun BT, Herr DL, et al. Effect of sedation with dexmedetomidine vs lorazepam on acute brain dysfunction in mechanically ventilated patients: the MENDS randomized controlled trial. JAMA. 2007; 298(22):2644–2653

[32] Jakob SM, Ruokonen E, Grounds RM, et al. Dexmedetomidine for Long-Term Sedation Investigators. Dexmedetomidine vs midazolam or propofol for sedation during prolonged mechanical ventilation: two randomized controlled trials. JAMA. 2012; 307(11):1151–1160

[33] Majdan M, Mauritz W, Wilbacher I, Brazinova A, Rusnak M, Leitgeb J. Barbiturates use and its effects in patients with severe traumatic brain injury in five European countries. J Neurotrauma. 2013; 30(1):23–29

[34] Flower O, Hellings S. Sedation in traumatic brain injury. Emerg Med Int. 2012; 2012:637171

[35] Chen HI, Malhotra NR, Oddo M, Heuer GG, Levine JM, LeRoux PD. Barbiturate infusion for intractable intracranial hypertension and its effect on brain oxygenation. Neurosurgery. 2008; 63 (5):880–886, discussion 886–887

[36] Löscher W, Rogawski MA. How theories evolved concerning the mechanism of action of barbiturates. Epilepsia. 2012; 53 Suppl 8:12–25

9 Homeostatic Mechanisms in the Neurosurgical Intensive Care Unit Patient

Jerry Noel, Dan E. Miulli, Gayatri Sonti, and Javed Siddiqi

Abstract
Although the environment of the brain is within a closed box without the ability to infinitely expand, it is completely dependent on the response of other systems of the body to deliver substrate to optimally function and survive. The brain can regulate the flow and pressure of blood, the amount of cerebrospinal fluid, the edema, and the resultant substrate delivery. The changing delivery is in response to the ever changing brain milieu. If the brain's regulatory mechanisms cannot overcome the microscopic, tissue, or organ environment the neurointensivist should recognize the condition and assist the brain with its ability to heal without causing further damage.

Keywords: blood pressure, electrolyte balance, energy equilibrium, euvolemia, fluid balance, ICP, Monro–Kellie hypothesis, serum glucose

Case Presentation

A 28-year-old, right-handed, Caucasian man had a pituitary macroadenoma resection. Postoperatively, the patient's Glasgow Coma Scale (GCS) score decreased from 15 to 6. The patient started to have seizures. His temperature was 37.3°C (99.2°F), heart rate 80, respirations 16, and blood pressure 160/90. He was intubated and was transferred to the neurosurgical intensive care unit (NICU). An external ventricular drain was placed and demonstrated intracranial pressure (ICP) consistently above 30 mm Hg and cerebral perfusion pressure (CPP) 70–80 mm Hg. Arterial blood gas showed pH 7.53, pCO_2 20 mm Hg, and PaO_2 98%. Electrolytes showed serum sodium 129 mEq/L, potassium 3.2 mEq/L, chloride 105 mEq/L, bicarbonate 30 mEq/L, blood urea nitrogen (BUN) 5 mg/dL, creatinine 0.3 mg/dL, and serum osmolality 282 mosm/kg.
See end of chapter for Case Management.

9.1 Homeostasis of the Brain

The Monro–Kellie hypothesis[1] states the skull is a solid box within which the volume of all the components—the brain, cerebrospinal fluid (CSF), and blood—should remain constant. Alteration in pressure in one compartment of the skull

Table 9.1 Therapeutic targets for neurosurgical intensive care unit patients[1,2,4]

CPP	>70–95 or >60–95 if concerns about secondary injury from treatment
ICP	5–15 mm Hg
Hemoglobin	10
Hematocrit	30–35%
Core temperature	35–37.2°C, 95–99°F
PaO_2	>97%
PO_2	>115 mm Hg for 72 hours, then >100 mm Hg
Serum osmolality	<320 mOsm/L
PCO_2	35–40 mm Hg
Sodium	140–145 mmol/L
Glucose	80–110 mg/dL
PCWP	10–14 mm Hg
PAD	12–16 mm Hg
CVP	6–8 mm Hg

Abbreviations: CPP, cerebral perfusion pressure; CVP, central venous pressure; ICP, intracranial pressure; PAD, pulmonary artery diastolic pressure, PCWP; pulmonary capillary wedge pressure.

is compensated by volume changes in the other. The energy requirements of the brain are met through oxygenation of glucose. In addition, the autoregulation of the cerebral vasculature attempts to maintain adequate perfusion to the brain.[2,3] The homeostasis of the brain results from a balance of the foregoing mechanisms.

In the neurologically injured patient, this homeostasis is altered and must be understood because, if not treated, ischemia leading to infarction and death will occur. The treatment of patients in the NICU includes a thorough understanding of cerebral metabolism, intracranial pressure (ICP), cerebral perfusion pressure (CPP), management of fluids and electrolytes, and the correction of these parameters to achieve homeostasis after brain injury (▶ Table 9.1).

9.2 Cerebral Blood Flow and Perfusion

Cerebral blood flow (50–75 mL/100 g/min) is affected by regional cerebral metabolism, CPP, and oxygen and carbon dioxide tension.[5] Globally cerebral blood flow decreased to one-half normal after injury and reduced even further around contusions, in punctate hemorrhages. It is the lowest with subdural hematoma (SDH), diffuse axonal injury (DAI), and hypotension. There is 3–4% change CBF/mm Hg change PCO_2, increases 2–3 days after injury and if lower early worse outcome at 3 and 6 months. One of the main objectives of the neurointensivists is to prevent ischemia. Without blood flow, glucose and glycogen are depleted in 4 minutes. In the ischemic penumbra, also thought of as the "shadow of death" of the infarcted or dead core, there is an increased metabolism attempting to deliver more substrate that results in increased brain temperature.[6] If brain tissue oxygen drops below 20 mm Hg, there is anaerobic respiration, followed by glucose storage–dependent lactic acid accumulation, mitochondrial damage, decreased pH, vasodilation, failure of the Na–K adenosinetriphosphatase (ATPase) pump, and Na and Cl influx followed by water, all of which lead to cytotoxic edema.[2,3] Failure in the blood–brain barrier leads to vasogenic edema. Hydrogen ions accumulate and pH drops to 6.0 from 6.4, causing inhibition of mitochondrial respiration and failure to sequester calcium, and, in turn, leading to further cell activation in the face of no substrate, and in turn, the cell dies. Cerebral autoregulation attempts to maintain blood flow according to this or any other change in cerebral metabolism.

Cerebral perfusion is the blood pressure gradient across the cerebral vasculature and usually is equal to the mean arterial pressure minus the intracranial pressure (MAP – ICP). The ability to maintain cerebral autoregulation is affected by pathological conditions, such as hyperventilation, edema, and hypoxia. ICP is controlled through regulation of the intracranial constituents of CSF, blood, and brain volume. The pressure volume index is the ability of the brain to compensate for increased intracranial volume. ICP slowly rises to a point where a slight increase in intracranial volume causes a big change in ICP. When ICP is consistently increased to greater than 20 mm Hg, it may lead to ischemia and herniation, which eventually lead to brain death. The goal in the management of high ICP is to reduce the CSF, blood, and brain volume. This may be accomplished by CSF drainage, prevention of vasodilation, and surgery in the form of a decompressive craniectomy to allow more space for the brain to swell. ▶ Table 9.2 outlines the basic approach to managing elevated ICP and CPP.

Table 9.2 Management of elevated intracranial pressure and cerebral perfusion pressure[5]

Surgical evacuation of mass lesion
• Head of bed elevated to 30 degrees
• Mild hyperventilation to $PaCO_2$, of 32–35 mm Hg
• Diuretics (e.g., mannitol 0.25–1 g/kg) if signs of herniation
• Ventricular drainage if Glasgow Coma Scale score $\leq$ 8
• Vasopressors such as norepinephrine (0.2–0.4 µg/kg/min), low-dose dopamine (1.5–2.5 µg/kg/min), and phenylephrine (max 4 µg/kg/min)
• Sedation and paralytics using short-acting agent
• Pain control
Note: Initiate hypothermia and barbiturate coma if the above measures fail and if intracranial pressure is consistently above 25 mm Hg.

9.3 Control of Blood Pressure

CPP should be maintained > 70 mm Hg and < 80, as best as possible. If there is a concern about secondary injury from therapy, consider maintaining CPP above 50 mm Hg. Significant decreases in blood pressure are a direct effect of ICP treatments using sedation, paralytics, or diuretics. In these hypotensive situations, moderate intravenous (IV) fluids followed by vasopressors can elevate blood pressure. In brain injury, the autoregulation of cerebral blood flow is altered; if CPP increases above 95 to 125 mm Hg, there can be an increase in blood volume and an increase in ICP. The first-line antihypertensive medication should be beta blockers or angiotensin-converting enzyme (ACE) inhibitors. Other medications, such as nitrogen-containing compounds, act quickly, but because they cause a direct vasodilator effect, they increase ICP.[2]

Maintaining the appropriate control of blood pressure is essential in order to prevent severe hypotension that may lead to decreased blood flow and perfusion and ischemia. On the opposite end of the spectrum, uncontrolled hypertension may cause expansion of hematomas, cerebral edema (which may lead to cerebral ischemia), and ultimately deleterious sequelae. Every effort should be made to prevent secondary brain injury.

9.4 Control of Serum Glucose

Tight control of glucose concentration is essential in head injury patients.[7,8,9,10,11] Many authors express concern that even slightly elevated blood glucose levels can cause or exacerbate secondary brain injury. Investigators have conducted clinical trials to test the efficacy of "tight glucose control," or maintenance of blood glucose levels of less than 110–120 mg/dL by using continuous insulin infusions.

In a prospective study of 240 adult patients with severe traumatic brain injury (TBI), patients were randomly assigned either to a tight glucose control group (intensive insulin therapy) with glucose levels maintained at 80 mg/dL throughout their intensive care unit stay, or to a conventional glucose control group where insulin was not given unless serum glucose levels exceeded 200 mg/dL.[11] The groups were well matched according to several measures of severity of injury and age. Six-month mortality rates were similar for the two groups, though significantly more patients in the intensive insulin therapy group had good outcomes (i.e., a Glasgow Outcome Scale [GOS] score of 4 or 5) than did the conventional therapy patients. In addition, intensive insulin therapy was associated with a significantly lower infection rate and shorter intensive care unit stay.

Others advocate concern about the associated risk of hypoglycemic episodes and the further neuronal injury that can result from hypoglycemia.[7,9,10]

Episodes of hypoglycemia have been found to be associated with increased extracellular levels of glutamate, glycerol, and the lactate:pyruvate ratio, all measures of cellular distress.[8]

Hypoglycemia of 50 mg/dL causes neuronal injury by changing cerebral blood flow and cerebral metabolism. In addition, glucose levels > 110 to 150 mg/dL in nondiabetics and > 200 to 250 mg/dL in diabetics also have deleterious effects. Regular IV insulin infusion and frequent blood glucose checks are essential to maintain glucose levels between 80 and 110 mg/dL.[11]

In conclusion, the majority of currently available clinical and preclinical evidence does not support tight glucose control (maintenance of blood glucose levels below 110–120 mg/dL) during the acute care of patients with severe TBI without further injury. Therefore, it is recommended to maintain blood glucose below 150 mg/dL.

9.5 Fluids and Electrolyte Balance

The principles of homeostasis of body water are as follows: two-thirds of total fluid resides inside cells, and one-third of total fluid resides in the extracellular space. The extracellular space is composed of one-third plasma and two-thirds interstitial fluid. The osmotic forces created by solutes determine the movement of water across membranes. An estimate of serum osmolality is determined by the equation

$$2Na + BUN/2.8 + glucose/18,$$

where BUN is the blood urea nitrogen level.

Sodium is the main determinant of osmotic force because it does not easily cross the membrane. Therefore, an imbalance in sodium concentration and volume status results in disturbance in homeostasis.[5] The most common conditions seen are diabetes insipidus, syndrome of inappropriate antidiuretic hormone (SIADH), and cerebral salt wasting (CSW) (▶ Table 9.3).[2,3,5]

Table 9.3 Common conditions leading to sodium concentration imbalance[1,4]

Condition	Vascular volume	Serum sodium	Urine sodium	Urine osmolality
DI	Decrease	Increase	No change	Decrease
SIADH	Increase	Decrease	Increase	Increase
CSW	Decrease	Decrease	Increase	

Abbreviations: CSW, cerebral salt wasting; DI, diabetes insipidus; SIADH, syndrome of inappropriate antidiuretic hormone.

9.5.1 Hypernatremia

Hypernatremia is usually caused by hypovolemia due to free water loss. It is often related to defective antidiuretic hormone (ADH) release or due to osmotic diuresis. When sodium levels are > 160 mmol/L, decreased level of consciousness and confusion set in. Hypernatremia should be treated first with crystalloids, 0.45 or 0.9% NaCl; if needed, colloids such as 5% albumin can be used. Patients with diabetes insipidus should be carefully monitored for fluid balance, body weight, serum and urine sodium, and urine specific gravity. If urine output exceeds the input by 250 mL/h for 2 consecutive hours, hormonal replacement with IV 1-deamino-8-D-arginine vasopressin (DDAVP, or desmopressin) 0.5 to 2 µg may be administered with caution.[2,3,5,12]

Also, hypernatremia may intentionally be induced to combat cerebral edema due to a variety of conditions, for example, metabolic, infectious, neoplasia, cerebrovascular, and TBI disease states. Hyperosmolar therapy, such as hypertonic saline solution of different concentrations, may be used.

9.5.2 Hyponatremia

Hyponatremia is one of the most common electrolyte disorders encountered in clinical medicine.[12] Hyponatremia should further be investigated and treated when the serum sodium level is less than 131 mmol/L. Evaluation should include a combination of physical examination findings, basic laboratory studies, and invasive monitoring when available.[13]

In NICU patients, hyponatremia results primarily from SIADH and CSW. In SIADH, the extracellular volume is increased, and CSW is decreased. If sodium is less than 135 mmol/L, due to excessive water retention or sodium excretion, serum osmolality should be measured immediately. An increase in glucose concentration by 100 mg/dL also accounts for a fall in sodium by 1.6 mmol/L and a rise in serum osmolality by 2 mOsm/kg. Patients usually become symptomatic after a drop of sodium below 120 mOsm/L, although mentation changes can be seen with levels below 130 mmol/L in the acutely injured patient. Some of the common symptoms are headache, nausea, and vomiting. Patients may also become lethargic or develop tonicoclonic seizures at low levels. Hyponatremia should be corrected slowly to prevent central pontine myelinolysis—do not increase serum sodium more than 12 mEq/L in 24 hours or more than 1.3 mEq/L/h.[2,5]

Also, hypertonic saline solution may be used as a treatment modality.

The practitioner must distinguish the two disorders because the main treatment for SIADH is fluid restriction. Urea, diuretics, demeclocycline, and lithium may also be used. For CSW fluid and sodium chloride administration are the principal therapies. Fludrocortisone may be considered in subarachnoid hemorrhage patients at risk of vasospasm, and hydrocortisone may be used to prevent natriuresis.[13]

9.6 Hypothermia and Brain Injury

Hypothermia is a great neuroprotectant and has consistently shown benefit against a variety of brain injuries at the experimental level. It has recently been shown to improve neurological outcome in comatose survivors of cardiac arrest and neonatal hypoxia ischemia and is being increasingly used by many centers for these conditions. However, its use in clinical practice is not yet entirely clear and not widely accepted due to unique challenges. For instance, unlike patients cooled following cardiac arrest, most stroke patients are awake and not endotracheally intubated. Thus measures are needed to prevent shivering and other discomfort experienced by deliberate cooling. Return of circulation following cardiac arrest is also generally associated with return of cerebral perfusion. In the case of stroke, the affected vessel often remains occluded for days or indefinitely in the absence of reperfusion therapies.[6]

Brain temperature is higher than the core body temperature by 1°C. Several studies demonstrate that in head-injured patients, there are moderate to severe elevations in brain temperature. Hyperthermia is neurotoxic, and hypothermia attenuates these effects. Mild hypothermia is defined to range between 32 and 35°C, and moderate hypothermia, 30 and 33°C.[4,14] Although spontaneous hypothermia and hyperthermia result from damage to the hypothalamus, several studies demonstrate the neuroprotective effects of iatrogenically induced hypothermia.[6] Hypothermia can be induced by antipyretic medication, surface cooling using hypothermia blankets, gastric lavage with ice-cold water, or saline. However, the most efficient way is by an endovascular cooling device placed in the inferior vena cava via the femoral vein.[15] The duration, speed of cooling, and rate of rewarming are likely factors in determining whether hypothermia will be effective. ▶ Table 9.4 and ▶ Table 9.5 outline the advantages and disadvantages of hypothermia for brain-injured patients.[4,5,6,14,15,16]

Table 9.4 Advantages of hypothermia for brain-injured patients[4,6,14,15,16]

Attenuation of release of excitatory amino acids, such as glutamate, and other chemicals, such as pyruvate and glycerol
• Decrease in reperfusion injury
• Decrease in intracranial pressure
• Improvement in cerebral perfusion pressure
• High temperatures increase brain metabolism; the adverse effects can be reduced by induced hypothermia.

Table 9.5 Disadvantages of hypothermia for brain-injured patients[4,14,15,16]

Temperature below 35°C may impair brain tissue oxygenation
• Hypokalemia and hyperglycemia
• Infections

Case Management

The described patient had a seizure and was hyperventilating. He is subsequently postictal. The seizures should be treated and an emergent head CT is obtained to rule out a mass lesion, such as a newly acute hematoma. The patient is also hypervolemic as suggested by the low sodium, potassium, BUN, and creatinine values. The glucose is presumably high because the serum osmolality does not correlate with the sodium level. A rising glucose level is expected after falling sodium but can also occur with steroid administration after pituitary surgery. Although patients become lethargic or develop tonicoclonic seizures at sodium levels around 120 mmol/L, this can occur with higher levels of sodium when there is a rapid drop, such as > 0.5 mmol/h. When correcting hyponatremia, do not increase serum sodium more than 12 mEq/L in 24 hours or more than 1.3 mEq/L/h. The patient may benefit from furosemide intravenously to decrease fluid overload, and a fluid restriction to 1 liter per day.

References

[1] Mokri B. The Monro-Kellie hypothesis: applications in CSF volume depletion. Neurology. 2001; 56(12):1746–1748

[2] Broderick JP, Hacke W. Treatment of acute ischemic stroke: Part II: neuroprotection and medical management. Circulation. 2002; 106(13):1736–1740

[3] Layon AJ, Gabrielli A, Friedman WA. Textbook of Neurointensive Care. 2nd ed. Philadelphia, PA: Saunders; 2014

[4] Yasui N, Kawamura S, Suzuki A, Hadeishi H, Hatazawa J. Role of hypothermia in the management of severe cases of subarachnoid hemorrhage. Acta Neurochir Suppl (Wien). 2002; 82:93–98

[5] Bernard SA, Buist M. Induced hypothermia in critical care medicine: a review. Crit Care Med. 2003; 31(7):2041–2051

[6] Yenari MA, Hemmen TM. Therapeutic hypothermia for brain ischemia: where have we come and where do we go? Stroke. 2010; 41(10) Suppl:S72–S74

[7] Bruno A, Kent TA, Coull BM, et al. Treatment of hyperglycemia in ischemic stroke (THIS): a randomized pilot trial. Stroke. 2008; 39(2):384–389

[8] Schlenk F, Nagel A, Graetz D, Sarrafzadeh AS. Hyperglycemia and cerebral glucose in aneurysmal subarachnoid hemorrhage. Intensive Care Med. 2008; 34(7):1200–1207

[9] Vespa PM. Intensive glycemic control in traumatic brain injury: what is the ideal glucose range? Crit Care. 2008; 12(5):175

[10] Prakash A, Matta BF. Hyperglycaemia and neurological injury. Curr Opin Anaesthesiol. 2008; 21 (5):565–569

[11] Yang M, Guo Q, Zhang X, et al. Intensive insulin therapy on infection rate, days in NICU, in-hospital mortality and neurological outcome in severe traumatic brain injury patients: a randomized controlled trial. Int J Nurs Stud. 2009; 46(6):753–758

[12] Boscoe A, Paramore C, Verbalis JG. Cost of illness of hyponatremia in the United States. Cost Eff Resour Alloc. 2006; 4:10

[13] Rahman M, Friedman WA. Hyponatremia in neurosurgical patients: clinical guidelines development. Neurosurgery. 2009; 65(5):925–935, discussion 935–936

175

[14] Steinberg GK, Ogilvy CS, Shuer LM, et al. Comparison of endovascular and surface cooling during unruptured cerebral aneurysm repair. Neurosurgery. 2004; 55(2):307–314, discussion 314–315

[15] Soukup J, Zauner A, Doppenberg EM, et al. The importance of brain temperature in patients after severe head injury: relationship to intracranial pressure, cerebral perfusion pressure, cerebral blood flow, and outcome. J Neurotrauma. 2002; 19(5):559–571

[16] Schaller B, Graf R. Hypothermia and stroke: the pathophysiological background. Pathophysiology. 2003; 10(1):7–35

10 Neurophysiology in the Neurosurgical Intensive Care Unit: Options, Indications, and Interpretations

Tyler Carson, Dennis Cramer, and Dan E. Miulli

Abstract

The neurointensivist should at all cost prevent nervous tissue ischemia and infarction. The greatest decrease in nervous system blood flow is understandably when the brain or spinal cord is the most injured. When injury is extensive, function is minimal and therefore difficult to assess for minor changes that could lead to major injury. The neurointensivist fortunately has available at many, but not all, times, technology to assess changing physiological conditions that may lead to a change in neurosurgical intensive care unit management of the patient.

Keywords: brain tissue oxygenation, BAER, burst suppression, EEG, EMG, Lindegaard ratio, pentobarbital coma, SSEP, TCD

> **Case Presentation**
>
> A 70-year-old man, who works as a musician in an orchestra, is undergoing resection of a right cerebellopontine angle mass. Monitoring for the operation includes brainstem auditory evoked response (BAER) and somatosensory evoked potentials (SSEPs). During the resection there is an increase in SSEP latency by 50% in the left upper extremity and left lower extremity. BAER detects a prolonged III–V interpeak latency on the right.
> *See end of chapter for Case Management.*

10.1 Electroencephalogram

The electroencephalogram (EEG) records the sum of neuronal activity of approximately 10,000 neurons within the pyramidal layer of the cerebral cortex, which is 1 cm from the cortical surface.[1] It is not useful to detect the function of the midbrain or brainstem. The electrode system uses channels (two electrodes per channel) arranged in different combinations, termed montages. Each channel reflects the summation of both excitatory and inhibitory potentials produced by the cell membranes between the two electrodes. Neurosurgical intensive care unit (NICU) EEG monitoring can be acute or chronic using a

177

full montage to localize specific activity or four electrodes to determine the type of activity. EEG monitoring can be complicated by patient movement, head wrapping, transportation, need for computed tomographic (CT) scan or magnetic resonance imaging (MRI). Its role must be considered before or after other tests. Furthermore, with long-term use the scalp should be inspected for skin breakdown. EEG monitoring can be effectively used in the following[2]:

- Seizure monitoring and differentiation.
- Alterations in mentation due to clinically silent status epilepticus or metabolic dysfunction.
- Intracranial pressure (ICP) monitoring.
- Hydrocephalus.
- Postoperative monitoring and depth of anesthesia.
- Cerebral perfusion alterations.
- Vasospasms.
- Monitoring effectiveness of ischemia therapy.

The four basic frequency patterns generated by the brain are referred to as beta, alpha, theta, and delta. Beta is associated with acts of mental concentration, alpha can be found in relaxed patients who have their eyes closed, theta waveforms are often seen during general anesthesia and rapid eye movement (REM) sleep and head injury, and delta is most often pathological or representative of deep sleep (▶ Fig. 10.1).

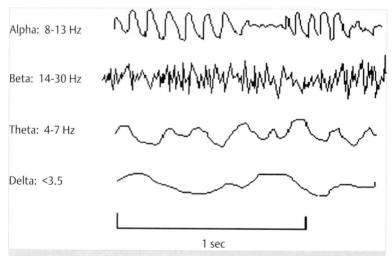

Alpha: 8-13 Hz

Beta: 14-30 Hz

Theta: 4-7 Hz

Delta: <3.5

1 sec

Fig. 10.1 The four basic frequency patterns generated by the brain, as seen in electroencephalogram readings.

The EEG electrodes are attached in a standardized fashion, termed the International 10–20 system (▶ Fig. 10.2, ▶ Fig. 10.3, ▶ Fig. 10.4). Even-numbered electrodes are on the patient's right, and odd-numbered electrodes are on the left, while electrodes with a z are midline. The letters used are P for parietal attachment, T for temporal, O for occipital, F for frontal, and A for auricular.

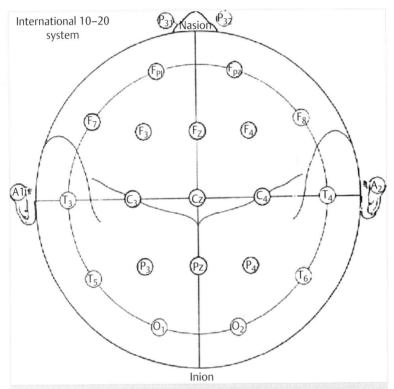

Fig. 10.2 The international 10–20 system of electrode attachment for an electro-encephalogram (EEG). The signal processing in an EEG machine converts the voltage versus time plot to one of frequency plus power versus time. An EEG can filter out extraneous electrical input (e.g., 60 Hz interference) but not physiological "noise" (e.g., cardiac activity). This should be taken into account during analysis. When examining an EEG tracing, the key considerations are the patient's degree of alertness during the recording and any increased or decreased waveform, particularly if localized to specific channels, which can then be correlated to specific cerebral locations. A normal adult tracing is shown in ▶ Fig. 10.3, and common pathological tracings are depicted in ▶ Fig. 10.4a–d.

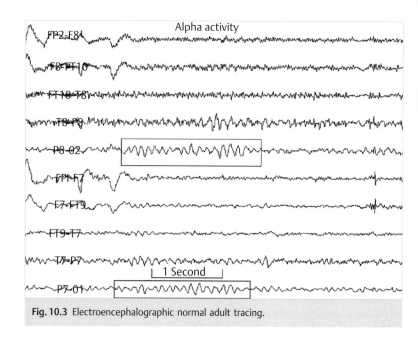

Fig. 10.3 Electroencephalographic normal adult tracing.

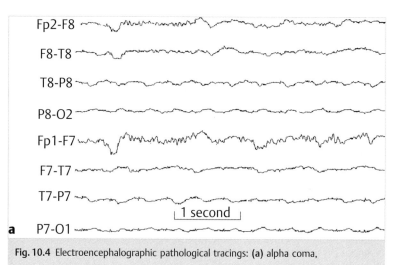

Fig. 10.4 Electroencephalographic pathological tracings: (a) alpha coma,

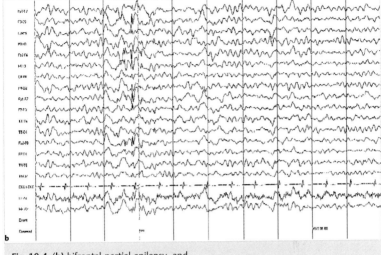

Fig. 10.4 (b) bifrontal partial epilepsy, and

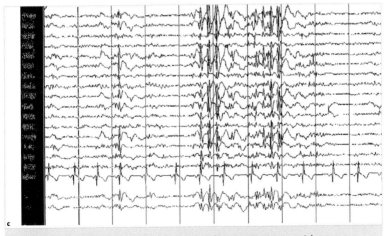

Fig. 10.4 (c) generalized tonicoclonic seizure with increasing intracranial pressure.

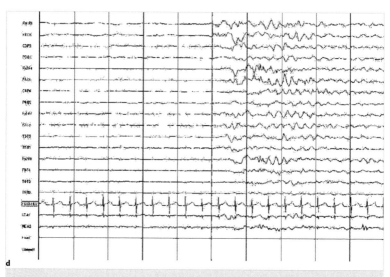

Fig. 10.4 (d) Closed head injury with increased intracranial pressure.

10.1.1 Burst Suppression

Burst suppression is an abnormal pattern characterized by bursts of higher-voltage sharp wave (8–12 Hz) and slow wave (1–4 Hz) activity appearing out of a background of relatively suppressed voltage. A flurry of activity is seen, followed by a period of electrical silence on the tracing. This can be seen during high-dose anesthesia administration. A common use of burst suppression monitoring is the titration of neuroprotective medications. The end point of titration is the induction of the burst suppression pattern on the EEG of one to two electrical bursts per page (► Fig. 10.5). Bursts occurring less often have not been shown to be more neuroprotective. Giving higher doses of medication to achieve fewer bursts can be associated with lower blood pressure and therefore decreased cerebral perfusion. Common burst suppression doses are listed here[3]:

- *Pentobarbital:* 10 mg/kg load, then 1 to 3 mg/kg/h.
- *Midazolam:* 200 µg/kg as a slow intravenous (IV) bolus, followed by 0.75 to 10.0 µg/kg/min.
- *Etomidate:* 0.4 to 0.5 mg/kg.
- *Propofol:* 1 mg/kg loading dose, titrate down rapidly starting at 20 mg/kg/h.

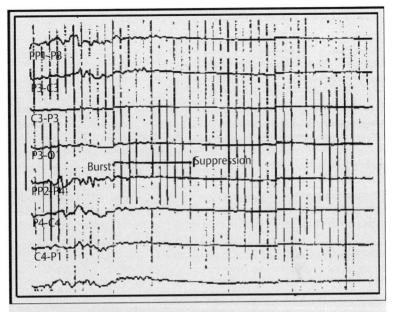

Fig. 10.5 Electroencephalographic burst suppression pattern.

10.1.2 Somatosensory Evoked Potentials

Somatosensory evoked potentials (SSEPs) allow for the monitoring of the spinal cord and peripheral nerves, as well as both cortical and subcortical structures. The evoked potential is generated when repetitive stimuli are applied to a peripheral nerve. Responses are then recorded centrally. Common nerves used are the median, ulnar, common peroneal, and posterior tibial. SSEPs are less affected by anesthesia than EEG and are more sensitive indicators of ischemia than EEG monitoring. SSEP waveforms move in parallel to regional blood flow and reflect changes when blood flow falls to near critical levels. It is notable to point out that SSEPs can be affected by medical equipment generating strong electrical fields (e.g., CT scanner is next door to the NICU). Any SSEP with amplitude reduction by more than 50% or latency increase by 1 millisecond should be further investigated.[4,5]

SSEPs have the following NICU applications[4]:

- Differentiating preganglionic versus postganglionic injury.
- Evaluating peripheral nerve trauma and postoperative progress.
- Evaluating postsurgical premotor and motor strip operations.
- Investigating postoperative paraplegia after posterior spinal fusion.
- Evaluating the comatose patient.

10.1.3 Limitations of SSEPs

SSEPs can be poor in predicting function in areas of the brain not involved with the somatosensory pathways.

10.1.4 Predictive Value of SSEPs

SSEPs have been used in evaluating the predicted prognosis of patients with spinal cord injury (SCI) in many studies. The tibial or common peroneal nerves are used, and the latency times are compared to those of normal subjects (▶ Fig. 10.6a). Further delineation between patients with ischemic and traumatic SCI allows for a more specifically tailored outcome. The outcome after rehabilitation can also be predicted using SSEPs (▶ Fig. 10.6b).[6]

▶ Fig. 10.7 shows a normal median nerve SSEP. The labels used stand for Erb's point (EP), a negative dorsal cervical spine potential (N13), a negative potential recorded from the contralateral scalp (N20), and a positive scalp potential (P22). The overlapping of tracings occurs as the previous tracing is retained while a new evoked potential is written over it for comparison. Each nerve has its own physiological limits on the SSEP. The criteria for an abnormal study are prolonged central conduction time,[1] abnormal internerve (right–left) central conduction time difference,[2] and absent EP, N13, N18, or N20 waves.[3] A typical value for the upper limit of normal for an EP–N20 is ~ 11 milliseconds.

10.2 Electromyogram

The electromyogram (EMG) captures electrical activity produced by the depolarization of muscle membrane. Most data regarding EMG usage are derived from the large number of studies that have been done on the facial nerve during acoustic neuroma removal. Spinal nerve EMG should not be attempted acutely but after 10–14 days. Prior to this time EMG may give a false-positive finding because the nerve would not have degenerated completely and the distal response may be recorded. EMGs may be used to monitor the following[7]:

• Cranial nerve functioning.
• Spinal nerve roots.

10.2.1 Interpretation of EMG Results

When a nerve is electrically excited using EMG, the signal is displayed visually, and the output can be coupled to a speaker for auditory feedback during a procedure. ▶ Fig. 10.8 shows the spectrum of EMG discharge types that are encountered during passive nerve monitoring.

No activity in an intact nerve is the best situation. The "popcorn" discharge is commonly caused by mechanical stimulation of the nerve. Sustained muscle activity indicates serious nerve irritation. The neurotonic discharge is

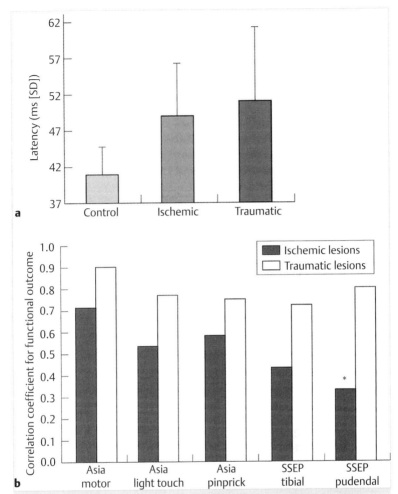

Fig. 10.6 Predictive value of somatosensory evoked potentials (SSEPs) from tibial or common peroneal nerve latency in groups of patients. **(a)** Comparison of SSEPs for normal (control) subjects with those from ischemic or traumatic spinal cord–injured (SCI) patients. **(b)** SSEPs can help predict outcomes for ischemic versus traumatic SCI patients.

indicative of serious nerve trauma. The amplitude of the EMG potentials shows how many nerve fibers are activated; accordingly, a reduction in amplitude indicates a conduction block. Anesthesia can induce spontaneous nerve discharge, which can mimic neurotonic discharge.[8]

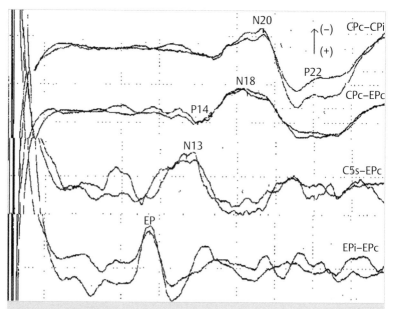

Fig. 10.7 Somatosensory evoked potential tracing of a normal median nerve. EP, Erb's point; N13, negative dorsal cervical spine potential; N20, negative potential recorded from the contralateral scalp; P22, positive scalp potential.

10.3 Transcranial Doppler Ultrasound

Transcranial Doppler ultrasound has been regarded as the earliest detector of impending damage because it detects blood flow abnormalities prior to ischemic injury. This noninvasive monitor is used in the early postoperative period to evaluate middle cerebral artery (MCA) flow for signs of velocity increases and pulsatile changes.[9] These early changes are predictive of an intracerebral hemorrhage (ICH) before the symptoms of headache or hypertension. Cerebral vasospasm can be assessed by comparing the ratio of blood flow in the MCA and the internal cerebral artery (ICA) (the Lindegaard ratio). This differentiates hyperemia from true vasospasm.

▶ Table 10.1 outlines the interpretation of values for the Lindegaard ratio.[4,10]
▶ Table 10.2 lists the clinical applications of transcranial Doppler ultrasound.[11]

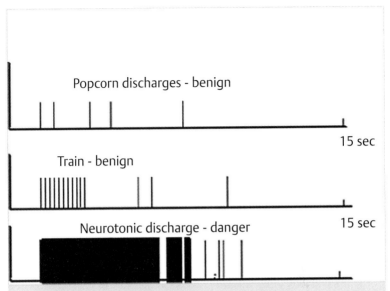

Fig. 10.8 Spectrum of electromyographic discharge types that are encountered during passive nerve monitoring.

Table 10.1 Lindegaard ratio interpretation[9,10,11]

0–3	Normal
3–6	Mild vasospasm
>6	Severe vasospasm

Table 10.2 Clinical applications of transcranial Doppler ultrasound[9,10,11]

		Evidence	
Applications	Rating	Quality	Strength
Sickle cell disease	Effective	Class I	Type A
Ischemic cerebrovascular disease	Established	Class II	Type B
Subarachnoid hemorrhage	Established	Class II	Type B
Arteriovenous malformations	Established	Class III	Type C
Cerebral circulatory arrest	Established	Class III	Type C
Perioperative monitoring	Possibly useful	Class III	Type C
Meningeal infection	Possibly useful	Class III	Type C
Periprocedural monitoring	Investigational	Class III	Type C
Migraine	Doubtful	Class II	Type D
Cerebral venous thrombosis	Doubtful	Class III	Type D

Recommendations for patients with subarachnoid hemorrhage (SAH) are as follows: if no vasospasm is detected by day 7–8 in patients with grade I SAH, transcranial Doppler ultrasound is usually discontinued. Transcranial Doppler ultrasound is performed every other day after days 8 through 10 in patients with higher SAH grades and no spasm.

10.4 Brainstem Auditory Evoked Response

The brainstem pathway for the auditory system includes the cochlea, spiral ganglion, eighth cranial nerve (CN VIII), cochlear nucleus (lower pons), superior olivary nucleus (lower three-fifths of pons), lateral lemniscus (upper pons), inferior colliculus (midbrain), and medial geniculate body (thalamus). Input from CN VIII ascends both ipsilateral and contralateral, and there are crossing fibers at each level.

Small ear inserts placed in the external auditory canal (EAC) apply a stimulus in which the patient hears a clicking noise or tone bursts. These bursts are recorded from electrodes placed on the scalp along the vertex and on each earlobe. The brainstem auditory evoked response (BAER; also known as the auditory brainstem response, evoked auditory potential, brainstem auditory evoked potential, and evoked response audiometry) consists of five waves (I, II, III, IV, and V). Waves I, III, and V are the most robust of the waveforms. The absolute and interpeak latencies, amplitude, and overall morphology of the waves are measured and evaluated. The auditory brainstem values have a normal range, which varies among patients and instruments used. It may be difficult to differentiate the origins of waves II to V because of the relatively small area of the auditory structures. The localization errors are ~ 1 cm at worst.[12]

10.4.1 Indications for BAER in the NICU

The following are indications for the use of BAER in the NICU:
- Lateralization of pathology.
- Hearing loss (including Meniere's disease).
- Neoplasms of the brainstem (including the cerebellopontine angle).
- Multiple sclerosis.
- Central pontine myelinolysis.
- Leukodystrophies and other degenerative diseases of the central nervous system.
- Infarctions and ischemia.
- Pontine hemorrhages.
- Screening for ototoxic drugs.
- Coma and brain death.

Abnormal auditory brainstem response findings may consist of delays in the absolute latency times of the individual waves, or an increased latency time between waves I to V, or waves I to III, or waves III to V. Poor wave morphology is also considered to be abnormal (▶ Table 10.3, ▶ Table 10.4, ▶ Table 10.5, ▶ Table 10.6; ▶ Fig. 10.9, ▶ Fig. 10.10).

Table 10.3 Anatomical correlations to brainstem auditory evoked response[12]

Wave	Location
I	Auditory nerve
II	Cochlear nucleus
III	Superior olive
IV	Lateral lemnisci
V	Inferior colliculus

Table 10.4 Brainstem auditory evoked response montage[12]

BAER channel	Recorded waveform location
Channel 1	Ai-CZ
Channel 2	Ac-CZ
Channel 3	Ai-Ac
Channel 4	Inion-CZ

Note: Ai and Ac refer to earlobe ipsilateral and earlobe contralateral, respectively, to the ear being stimulated; CZ refers to the center, midline, midplane between earlobes.

Table 10.5 Brainstem auditory evoked response reference values[12]

Wave	Mean latency (ms)	Range (ms)
Wave I	1.62	1.26–1.98
Wave II	2.80	2.23–3.37
Wave III	3.75	3.24–4.26
Wave IV	4.84	4.15–5.53
Wave IV/V	5.27	4.61–5.93
Wave V	5.62	4.93–6.31
	Female	**Male**
I–V (age < 60 years)	< 4.60	< 4.65
I–V (age > 60 years)	< 4.70	< 4.75
I–III	2.63	
I–IV/V	4.32	
III–V	2.31	

Table 10.6 Interpretation of brainstem auditory evoked response results[12]

Wave finding	Interpretation
Abnormal I–III IPL	This abnormality suggests the presence of a conduction defect in the brainstem auditory system between the CN VIII close to the cochlea and the lower pons.
Abnormal III–V IPL	This abnormality suggests the presence of a conduction defect in the brainstem auditory system between the lower pons and the midbrain.
I absent and III–V is normal	Wave I (CN VIII activation potential) could not be recorded. This is usually due to a peripheral hearing disorder. Because of this, the state of conduction in the brainstem auditory pathway between peripheral CN VIII and lower pons could not be determined. Lower pons to midbrain conduction was normal.
IV or V absent or of abnormally low amplitude	This abnormality suggests the presence of a conduction defect in the brainstem auditory system rostral to the lower pons.
Absent II, III, IV, and V with normal I	This abnormality indicates a significant lack of function in brainstem auditory tracts.

Abbreviations: CN, cranial nerve; IPL, interpeak latency.

Note: Normal adult auditory brainstem response waveform. I–V absolute latencies and interpeak intervals (I–III, III–V, I–V) are within normal limits bilaterally. Interaural differences for the I–V interpeak intervals (0.16 ms) and wave V absolute latencies (0.08 ms) are within normal limits.

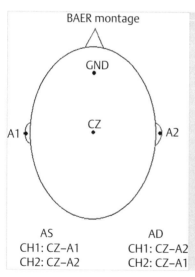

Fig. 10.9 Brainstem auditory evoked response (BAER) montage.

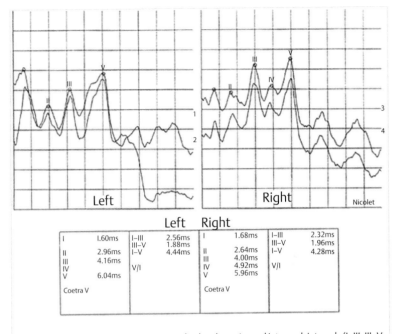

Left				Right			
I	I.60ms	I–III	2.56ms	I	1.68ms	I–III	2.32ms
		III–V	1.88ms			III–V	1.96ms
II	2.96ms	I–V	4.44ms	II	2.64ms	I–V	4.28ms
III	4.16ms			III	4.00ms		
IV		V/I		IV	4.92ms	V/I	
V	6.04ms			V	5.96ms		
Coetra V				Coetra V			

Normal adult ABR waveform response. I–V absolute latencies and interpeak intervals (I–III, III–V, I–V) are within normal limits bilaterally. Interaural differences for the I–V interpeak intervals (.16ms) and wave V absolute latencies (.08ms) are within normal limits.

Fig. 10.10 Normal adult auditory brainstem response (ABR) waveforms.

10.5 Brain Tissue Oxygenation

There is a direct way to measure cerebral cell oxygenation. Although the 0.5 mm sensor is stationary it can determine the partial pressure of oxygen from the area surrounding the probe. The probe is inserted in a similar manner to the external ventricular catheter and placed into functioning brain tissue, avoiding the hematoma. After sensor calibration and insertion the probe should be given time to reach equilibrium. Measurements before this time are not reliable. After equilibrium is reached, dependent upon brain temperature and blood flow, which can be minutes to hours, a partial pressure of oxygen below 6 mm Hg is not consistent with a return to functioning brain. This is also true of a reading less than 10 mm Hg for greater than 30 minutes. The partial pressure of oxygen should be maintained above 20 mm Hg for functional outcome and above 28 mm Hg for a good outcome. Controlling ICP and cerebral perfusion pressure (CPP) by itself does not prevent brain tissue hypoxia.

If the partial pressure of brain tissue oxygen decreases, which precedes changes in EEG, transcranial Doppler (TCD) and other monitoring equipment, measures must be taken to return the blood and nutrient flow to the brain. These include the following:

- Increase FiO_2—ventilator
- Increase mean arterial pressure—fluids.
- Increase perfusion—blood pressure.
- Improve blood cell deformability, optimize viscosity and O_2 carrying capacity —hemoglobin and hematocrit (H&H).
- Increase volume—fluids.
- Decrease hyperventilation.
- Decrease edema—mass, blood pressure, fluids.
- Decrease ICP—drainage.
- Decrease temperature.
- Decrease metabolism.
- Decrease vasospasm.

Case Management

In this patient, the change in BAER reflects an abnormality between the mid-brain and lower pons. The SSEP localizes the change to an area above the pyramidal decussation, possibly due to ischemia. Possible etiologies for the monitoring changes include vascular injury, increased edema from venous damage compression, retractor injury, increased iatrogenic compression, use of cold water irrigation, or decreased blood flow. First blood pressure and oxygenation should be addressed through the anesthesiologist; then the temperature of the irrigation must be checked. Ideally, the surgeon may need to stop until an explanation for the changes is available.

References

[1] Youman JR. Neurological Surgery: A Comprehensive Reference Guide to the Diagnosis and Management of Neurosurgical Problems. 4th ed. Philadelphia, PA: WB Sanders; 1996:402–430

[2] Vespa PM, Nenov V, Nuwer MR. Continuous EEG monitoring in the intensive care unit: early findings and clinical efficacy. J Clin Neurophysiol. 1999; 16(1):1–13

[3] Jordan KG. Continuous EEG monitoring in the neuroscience intensive care unit and emergency department. J Clin Neurophysiol. 1999; 16(1):14–39

[4] Greenberg MS. Handbook of Neurosurgery. 5th ed. New York, NY: Thieme; 2001:549–552

[5] Czosnyka M, Kirkpatrick PJ, Pickard JD. Multimodal monitoring and assessment of cerebral haemodynamic reserve after severe head injury. Cerebrovasc Brain Metab Rev. 1996; 8(4):273–295

[6] Iseli E, Cavigelli A, Dietz V, Curt A. Prognosis and recovery in ischaemic and traumatic spinal cord injury: clinical and electrophysiological evaluation. J Neurol Neurosurg Psychiatry. 1999; 67 (5):567–571

[7] Houlden DA, Schwartz ML, Klettke KA. Neurophysiologic diagnosis in uncooperative trauma patients: confounding factors. J Trauma. 1992; 33(2):244–251

[8] Murthy JM. Somatosensory evoked potentials by paraspinal stimulation in acute transverse myelitis. Neurol India. 1999; 47(2):108–111

[9] Wilterdink JL, Feldmann E, Furie KL, Bragoni M, Benavides JG. Transcranial Doppler ultrasound battery reliably identifies severe internal carotid artery stenosis. Stroke. 1997; 28(1):133–136

[10] Assessment: transcranial Doppler. Report of the American Academy of Neurology, Therapeutics and Technology Assessment Subcommittee. Neurology. 1990; 40:680–681

[11] Aaslid R, Huber P, Nornes H. Evaluation of cerebrovascular spasm with transcranial Doppler ultrasound. J Neurosurg. 1984; 60(1):37–41

[12] Chiappa KH. Evoked Potentials in Clinical Medicine. 3rd ed. Philadelphia, PA: Lippincott–Raven; 1997:199–268

11 Cerebral Perfusion

Deependra Mahato, Kevin Ray, Dan E. Miulli, and Javed Siddiqi

Abstract

Lack of blood flow and substrate delivery to the brain results in brain ischemia and, if not compensated, infarction. The brain should maintain cerebral blood flow, which is dependent upon many issues of resistance and supply. The brain tissue resists the flow when there is edema, or receives decreased flow from poor blood viscosity or vessel constriction. The supply of blood flow to the brain is dependent upon the perfusion pressure reaching it. The cerebral perfusion pressure is dependent upon the function of the cardiac system. Too low blood pressure leads to ischemia; even one episode of hypotension in severe head injury can double the morbidity and mortality. Likewise, too high blood pressure will push through a damaged blood–brain barrier and cause further edema and damage.

Keywords: blood–brain barrier, capillary membrane, CBF, CPP, cytotoxic edema, interstitial edema, MAP, vasogenic edema

Case Presentation

A 20-year-old man presents after a fall from a second-story window with obvious contusions to his chest, abdomen, and head. At the scene of the accident, he does not open his eyes or talk, and he exhibits extensor/decerebrate posturing. His pupils are equal and sluggishly reactive. There is no obvious distension or rigidity of the abdomen. His blood pressure is 90/50.

See end of chapter for Case Management.

11.1 Introduction

In light of any injury to the brain, whether it is due to a trauma, ischemic or hemorrhagic stroke, metabolic derangements, or neoplasm, it is imperative that hemodynamics be managed in a way that maintains adequate cerebral perfusion. Fortunately, the brain possesses some innate ability to respond to inadequate cerebral perfusion, though it is not a perfect system by far. To fully appreciate these mechanisms and gain insight into interventions that help us to maintain cerebral perfusion, it is first necessary to understand the underlying anatomy of the blood–brain barrier, circumventricular organs, and the mechanics of cerebral blood flow (CBF) and autoregulation.

11.2 Blood–Brain Barrier

The brain capillary varies from the systemic capillary by several unique features; these establish the blood–brain barrier. The brain capillary endothelial cells are the distinguishing elements of the blood–brain barrier. The brain capillary endothelial cells are not fenestrated, lack intracellular clefts, and are closed by intercellular tight gap junctions. The tight gap junctions of the brain capillary endothelial cells assist in keeping substances out of the brain interstitial space. The body systemic capillary endothelial cells are not in contact with one another; they do not make a circumferential ring barrier but instead have multiple fenestrations that allow fluid to pass freely (▶ Fig. 11.1).[1]

The circumferential ring of brain capillary endothelial cells regulates which substances reach the brain's interstitial space, the supporting astrocytes, and the neurons. In an intact blood–brain barrier, all substances pass through the capillary endothelial cell and the other regulator, the choroid plexus epithelial cell. The blood–brain barrier regulates the biochemical, immunological, and electrical passage of material into the brain. The tight gap junctions, the strong intercellular connections, have high electrical impedance, preventing ions from passing. The capillary endothelial cells exclude plasma proteins from the brain interstitial space because the endothelial cells have very little pinocytic vesicles to transport the proteins and contain unique cerebral enzymes, cellular channels, and transport systems (▶ Table 11.1). The brain capillary endothelial cells require large amounts of energy to serve as the complex regulatory interface between the brain and the blood circulation. The brain capillary endothelial cell energy-dependent transport organizations have three to five times the amount of mitochondria as the systemic capillary cells. Maintaining the blood–brain barrier's unique functions, the brain capillary membrane has a different structural surface, and its lack of permeability is assisted by pericytes and astrocytic foot processes.

The pericyte or perivascular cells are not unique to the brain; they are found partially wrapping systemic capillaries and venules in endothelial cells. The selective permissiveness into the brain interstitial space is not present in circumventricular organs, including the neural hypophysis, subfornical organ, median eminence, area postrema, and pineal gland (▶ Table 11.2).[1,2,3]

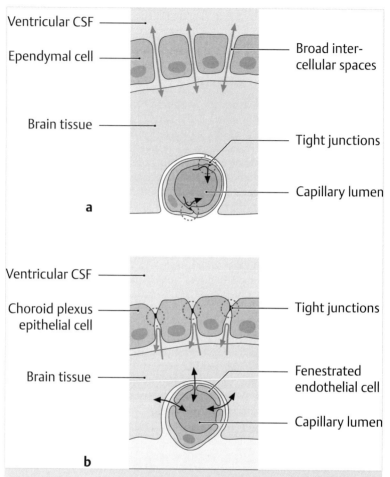

Fig. 11.1 Blood–brain barrier and blood-CSF barrier. (a) Normal brain tissue with an intact blood–brain barrier; (b) Blood-CSF barrier in the choroid plexus. (Reproduced with permission.[1])

Table 11.1 Blood–brain barrier characteristics: the brain capillary endothelial cell[2,3,4]

Tight gap junction	Different membrane structure
Basement membrane	Neuronal enzymes
Minimal pinocytic activity	Transport mechanisms
High mitochondrial content	Pericytes (also seen in systemic circulation)
High electrical impedance	Astrocytic foot processes

11.2.1 Circumventricular Organs

The circumventricular organs represent structures in the brain where the blood–brain barrier allows for communication between the central nervous system and peripheral blood flow. These structures are highly vascular and can be divided into sensory and secretory organs (▶ Fig. 11.2, ▶ Table 11.2)[1,2,3]

11.2.2 Brain Interstitial Circulation

In the normal state, for substances to pass from the blood to the brain interstitial space, they must pass through the capillary endothelial cell. The brain capillary endothelial cell allows certain compounds to pass with relative ease into the brain interstitial space via transcellular diffusion or ubiquitous transport mechanisms. These substances are lipid soluble, low molecular weight of ~ 500 daltons or less, nonpolarized, and not bound to proteins. Such substances include glucose, low-density lipoproteins, transferrin, bromide, morphine, and bile salts. These substances when not actively transported must still diffuse

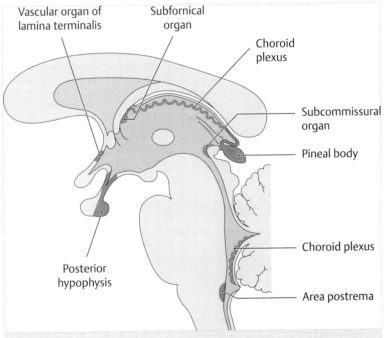

Fig. 11.2 Location of the circumventricular organs (midsagittal section, left lateral view). (Reproduced with permission.[1])

Table 11.2 Circumventricular organs[1]

Sensory organs	Function
• Area postrema	Zone associated with emetic reflex
• Vascular organ of the lamina terminalis	Sensitive to angiotensin II, secretes somatostatin, luliberin, motilin
• Subfornical organ	Sensitive to angiotensin II, secretes somatostatin, luliberin; plays active role in fluid balance regulation
Secretory organs	
• Subcommissural organ	Secretes subcommissural organ-spondin into third ventricle to create Reissner's fibers that maintain patency of sylvian aqueduct
• Posterior pituitary	Stores and secretes oxytocin and antidiuretic hormone
• Pineal body	Secretes melatonin, role in circadian rhythm

down a concentration gradient from blood to capillary endothelial cell to brain interstitial space. The blood–brain barrier is not permeable to ions and amino acids, and the exact type of permeability to water is controversial. Water does not enter through a lipid membrane but must pass through selective water channels regulated by aquaporins. The blood–brain barrier excludes water-soluble molecules with a molecular weight greater than 180 daltons. It is not permeable to vital dyes, epinephrine, curare, bile pigments, and fluorescein. Substances that enter the brain interstitial space fluid could alter nervous system function. These substances pass from the blood–brain capillary to the interstitial space, where they may be absorbed by neurons, glial cells, or others; they then pass through, but sometimes around, subependymal glial cells and ependymal gap junctions into the cerebrospinal fluid (CSF) of the ventricles, cisterns, and Virchow–Robin spaces, where they eventually circulate back into the blood via the arachnoid villi.[2,3,4]

11.2.3 Blood–Cerebrospinal Fluid Barrier

The choroid plexus epithelial circumferential junction actively secretes substances into the CSF. The blood–CSF barrier is similar to the blood–brain barrier of the capillary endothelial cell. Substances dissolved in the choroid capillary blood pass more easily through the choroid endothelium, are selectively passed by the connective tissue of the choroid plexus, and then are regulated by the choroid epithelium. The choroid epithelial cells contain circumferential junctions, which must secrete CSF into the ventricle. The CSF acts as a sink for the brain interstitial fluid, with a gradient of substances carrying components away from the interstitial space.

11.2.4 Blood–Brain Barrier Disruption

Diseases of the nervous system disrupt the blood–brain barrier, resulting in most of the devastation. The barrier is disrupted by hypertension, hypercapnia, hypocapnia, trauma, hyperthermia, chemicals such as intra-arterial lactated Ringer's solution, mannitol, leukotriene C_4, nitric oxide synthetase, arabinose, and lactamide, as well as in the center of tumors, but necessarily in the periphery. The disrupted blood–brain barrier leads to brain edema, accumulation of fluids and electrolytes, increased cerebral volume, increased intracranial pressure (ICP), cellular swelling, and cell death. There are many studies of brain edema in a variety of pathologies. However, there is a clinical situation that, when thoroughly understood, will clarify most questions about the blood–brain barrier and cerebral edema. That situation is head trauma.

11.2.5 Vasogenic Edema

At the moment of impact, the blood–brain barrier's tight gap junctions are stretched, which essentially turns the brain capillary for ~ 30 to 60 minutes into a sieve, leading to vasogenic edema. There is accumulation of serum, albumin, and proteins. The opening is also prolonged for an unknown duration by hypoxia and for a single time of 6 hours by a hypertension surge. The mechanical disruption traumatizes microvessels, cells, and cellular organelles, releasing calcium, ornithine decarboxylase, and free radicals. Sustained increases of free radicals meant to oxidize toxins will disrupt the cellular membrane. An increase in intracellular and extracellular stores of calcium will be sustained by hypoxia.

The activity of ornithine decarboxylase is increased 2,000% due to upregulation of its messenger ribonucleic acid (mRNA).[5] It acts to decarboxylate ornithine forming putrescine, which is then converted into spermidine, then finally into spermine. All three are released immediately after cellular injury because of the necessity for regeneration, development, cell growth, and neuronal survival. Putrescine accumulation induces shrinkage in cerebral microvessels after trauma, opening the blood–brain barrier and increasing vasogenic edema. Putrescine can be increased by isoflurane and decreased by ketamine.

Bradykinins are released, which, with other pathway products, increase calcium at the time of mechanical disruption. This calcium increases calcium-calmodulin and calcium protein kinase C and opens the blood–brain barrier.

The disrupted blood–brain barrier is stabilized by dexamethasone, copper, zinc, superoxide dismutase, serotonin antibodies, and progesterone.

11.2.6 Cytotoxic Edema

The most common type of edema after head injury, cytotoxic edema, occurs in the cell 30 to 60 minutes after insult as a response to the intracellular accumulation of the toxic levels of lactate, hydrogen-ion acidosis, potassium, oxygen free radicals, and glutamate, among others. The sodium potassium adenosine triphosphatase (ATPase) pump fails secondary to depletion of cellular energy, allowing sodium to build up intracellularly and drawing in water. Hydrogen accumulation is the most common reason for buffering the cell by increasing the water content. The cell osmotically swells, reacting to the increasing glycogen granules that are sequestered to provide more substrate to the tricarboxylic acid (TCA) cycle. The additional energy is required to supply cellular active transport mechanisms, including the following:

- Sodium potassium ATPase.
- Sodium potassium chloride cotransporter.
- Calcium-activated potassium channels.
- Sodium hydrogen antiporter.
- Chloride bicarbonate exchanger.
- Carrier-mediated transport of nutrients.
- Receptor-mediated transport of peptides.

As the cellular membrane starts to fail, glutamate is released, increasing cellular metabolism, which, under its current anaerobic conditions, leads to further lactate production and, without utilization, accumulation and then to failure of energy metabolism and cell death.[4]

11.2.7 Interstitial Edema

Interstitial fluid drains down the gradient into the CSF sink. That sink starts to become clogged with toxins and proteins. CSF production is increased to buffer the brain interstitial fluid acidosis runoff by upregulation of the chloride bicarbonate exchanger. One method to decrease interstitial edema and cytotoxic edema (the major contributor to traumatic brain injury) is by decreasing the sink into which brain fluid drains. Decreasing the CSF in the ventricles does this; decreasing the pressure of the intracranial contents does not.

There is no silver bullet to treat brain injury. Fortunately, the brain can adapt and recover from multiple insults. Brain injury occurs because several innate brain systems fail to compensate for the overwhelming insult. Currently, there are experimental chemicals that are available to ameliorate different types of edema (▶ Table 11.3).[6]

Table 11.3 Means to decrease brain edema[2,3,4,7]

Type of edema	Means to decrease
Cytotoxic (the most common type in head injury)	Alpha-difluoromethylornithine, alpha-trinositol, amiloride, THAM
Vasogenic	CuZn SOD, 5-HT1B receptor, progesterone, indomethacin, naloxone, dexamethasone, CSF drainage
Interstitial	CSF drainage, acetazolamide

Abbreviations: CSF, cerebrospinal fluid; CuZn SOD, copper-zinc superoxide dismutase; THAM, tris-(hydroxymethyl)-aminomethane.

The aim of aggressive early treatment is to prevent ischemia. Glucose and glycogen are depleted in 4 minutes; there is increased metabolism in the layer surrounding the ischemic penumbra, the brain temperature increases, metabolism increases, and brain tissue PO_2 drops to less than 20 mm Hg, favoring anaerobic respiration. Anaerobic respiration causes lactic acidosis and brings hydrogen into the cell. Lactate accumulation approximates glucose stores at the time of ischemia. The cell swells in response to increasing levels of hydrogen. Multiple neuromodulators stimulate cyclic adenosine monophosphate–dependent ion transport, bringing more hydrogen into the cell. The ischemia leads to the cellular pH dropping to 6.0 to 6.4, inhibiting mitochondrial respiration and the ability to sequester calcium. When the cell is deprived of energy and oxygen, calcium stores are released, stimulating phosphorylation of protein kinase C and further increasing intracellular hydrogen in a vicious cycle, leading to degradation of cell membranes. Therefore, increasing CBF in excess of edema is necessary to increase oxygen delivery.

11.3 Cerebral Blood Flow

CBF averages 45 to 65 mL/100 g/min (55 mL/100 g/min used by most references), being higher in gray matter (75–80 mL/100 g/min) and somewhat less in white matter (20–30 mL/100 g/min) (See ▶ Fig. 11.3). Changes occur sooner when the entire CBF is affected compared to changes in regional CBF. Protein synthesis declines at 40 to 50 mL/100 g/min, and anaerobic glycolysis at 35 mL/100 g/min. Drastic electroencephalographic (EEG) changes of absent activity are seen as early as 25 mL/100 g/min; however, brainstem auditory evoked responses (BAERs) occur at 12 mL/100 g/min, and loss of transcellular function begins at 10 to 20 mL/100 g/min and anoxic depolarization at 8 to 15 mL/100 g/min. Brain tissue tolerates slightly lower regional CBF changes before similar effects. Of course, the duration of decreased perfusion also differentiates ischemia from infarction.[7]

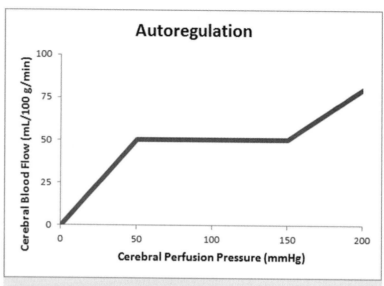

Fig. 11.3 Autoregulation. Average cerebral blood flow (CBF) is 55 mL/100 g/min and will remain relatively constant in the range of 50–150 mm Hg. CBF decreases when cerebral perfusion pressure (CPP) drops below 50 mm Hg and increases when CPP rises above 150 mm Hg.

11.3.1 Autoregulation

When compared to other organs of the body, brain tissue is more sensitive to changes in vascular perfusion due to its high metabolic demands. Autoregulation is the ability of the brain to maintain CBF and perfusion at a constant level despite changes in cerebral perfusion pressure (CPP). In normal individuals, ICP is relatively constant; therefore CPP is primarily influenced by changes in mean arterial pressure (MAP) and, by extension, systolic blood pressure (SBP). The normal threshold of CPP is between 50 and 150 mm Hg in adults (▶ Fig. 11.3), though it is usually in the range of 70–90 mm Hg. In order to maintain constant CBF, cerebral arteries constrict in response to rising CPP and dilate as CPP decreases. The mechanism by which this occurs is thought to be related to autonomically controlled changes in vascular smooth muscle tone in response to vasoactive substances released by vascular endothelium (myogenic hypothesis), and changes in transmural blood pressure detected by periadventitial nerves (neurogenic hypothesis). Under normal circumstances, autoregulatory changes occur within 15–30 seconds of detected changes in CPP or transmural pressure. There is some evidence to support metabolic feedback influencing autoregulation; however, the rapid time course over which the responses occur argue against metabolism playing a major role.[8]

11.3.2 Cerebral Vascular Resistance

The physiology of cerebral vascular resistance (CVR) differs from the systemic circulation. One-half of the systemic MAP is lost just distal to the cerebral arteries and arterioles. CVR is complex and neither always proportional nor linear to CPP. Therefore, knowing CPP does not allow direct calculation of CBF. CVR varies with edema, $PaCO_2$, and a host of other conditions. Under normal steady-state conditions, autoregulation occurs as CVR varies with CPP to maintain a constant CBF. However, during extremes of pathological states, or extremes of autoregulation, CVR cannot vary enough. Between a CPP of 50 and 125 mm Hg, the blood vessel dilates and constricts to maintain constant CBF. At CPP of 50 to 60 mm Hg, the blood vessel is maximally dilated, and further decrease in CPP only results in decreased CBF. Likewise, at a CPP of 125 mm Hg, the blood vessel is maximally constricted. Any further increase in CPP is similar to increasing the flow through a rigid tube. This will cause vasogenic edema as the tight gap junctions are split apart. The amount of autoregulation or the amount of CVR changes daily, hourly, and by the minute. During head trauma, unless secondary injury occurs, or hypotension, ischemia, or hyperventilation, autoregulation is maintained but shifted to the left.[9] To date there is no direct way to continuously measure CVR. Criteria are being developed utilizing transcranial Doppler ultrasound, its pulsatile index and resistance, in an attempt to quantify CVR and CBF, as given here:

$$CBF = CPP/CVR = MAP - ICP/CVR$$

11.3.3 Hypotension

After severe head injury around contusions, in punctate hemorrhages CBF cannot be maintained. CBF drops to less than 20 mL/100 g/min and remains less than 30 mL/100 g/min during the first 8 to 24 hours. It remains lowest under subdural hematomas and diffuse axonal injuries and, as expected, with hypotension. However, it is not only low around the area of injury; globally, it can be decreased to half the normal level after injury. A single episode of hypotension doubles the morbidity and mortality associated with severe head injury.[9] Hypotension leads to vasodilation 165% above baseline, increasing cerebral blood volume and ICP. Hypotension is not used initially to treat severe head injury. Although hypertension to maintain CPP in the normal range is beneficial,[10] if CPP exceeds the upper limit of autoregulation, whether artificially changed or not, it too will increase cerebral blood volume and ICP. The Brain

Trauma Foundation's *Guidelines for the Management of Severe Traumatic Brain Injury,* 3rd edition,[9] recommends the following:
- *Level II Recommendation*
  - Blood pressure should be monitored and SBP < 90 mm Hg avoided.[9]
- *Level III Recommendation*
  - Oxygenation should be monitored and hypoxia (apnea cyanosis in the field, PaO_2 < 60 mm Hg or O_2 saturation < 90%) avoided.[9]
- *Option*
  - Mean arterial pressures should be maintained above 90 mm Hg through the infusion of fluids throughout the patient's course to attempt to maintain cerebral perfusion pressure greater than 70 mm Hg.

SBP and MAP can be treated in the field. However, if there is severe head injury, the patient must be taken to a trauma center where a neurosurgeon is present. The neurosurgeon will insert an external ventricular drain and an ICP monitor.

11.3.4 Cerebral Perfusion Pressure

Older studies compared the CPP to mortality in the adult, mostly male, population and found that if the CPP was greater than 80 mm Hg the mortality at that time in history was only 35 to 40%. If the CPP was less than 80 mm Hg mortality increased for each 10 mm Hg decrease in CPP, yielding a mortality of 95% for a CPP less than 60 mm Hg. Other investigators also found that the single most important therapy was to keep the CPP greater than 60 mm Hg.[11] *Guidelines for the Management of Severe Traumatic Brain Injury,* 3rd edition, provides a Level III recommendation that a CPP < 50 mm Hg be avoided and that the target CPP lies within the range of 50–70 mm Hg, whereas patients with intact pressure autoregulation can tolerate higher CPP values.[9]

Several caveats exist. This is the recommendation for the average adult male, not for children and not for some adult females who have a normal SBP, let alone MAP lower than 90 mm Hg. A CPP greater than 70 mm Hg should not be maintained at the expense of causing other injuries, such as pulmonary edema and acute respiratory distress syndrome (ARDS). Hlatky et al[12] demonstrated that, for maximum CPP treatment in patients with difficult-to-manage ICP elevations, more fluids were used, more vasopressors were used, and there was a fivefold increase in ARDS. If secondary injury is becoming apparent, and that secondary injury may decrease outcome in the management of severe head injury, then CPP should be kept above a minimum of 60 mm Hg.

When attempting to manage the patient with severe head injury, orders must be written to maintain the CPP above a certain level. Clifton et al[13] state that a target for CPP threshold should be set to 10 mm Hg above what the critical threshold is determined to be for a particular patient in order to prevent the CPP from falling below the critical point. For instance, if the critical threshold is determined to be 50 mm Hg, orders should be written to maintain CPP > 60 mm Hg, as well as an order to maintain CPP below an upper limit, which typically varies from 90 to 120 mm Hg.

11.3.5 Blood Pressure Management in Infarction

There is considerable debate regarding the appropriate blood pressure to maintain in a patient who has suffered ischemia or who has suffered an intra-cerebral hemorrhage (ICH). Lowering blood pressure too aggressively during cerebral ischemia can lead to infarction. Blood pressure usually increases during the first few hours after ischemia in an attempt to correct the underlying physiological problem; but once the injury has equilibrated, the blood pressure decreases within 24 hours, returning to the patient's normal level in 4 to 7 days. The rise in blood pressure does not change CBF in areas of the brain where autoregulation is intact. However, elevated blood pressure is required in areas of ischemia to protect the penumbra, and even more important in areas with associated disturbances in autoregulation. Current guidelines from the American Heart Association (AHA) and American Stroke Association provide a Class I (Level of Evidence [LOE] B) recommendation stating that those patients diagnosed with an ischemic stroke that have significantly elevated blood pressure though are otherwise eligible for rtPA, should have their SBP lowered and stabilized below 185 mm Hg and diastolic blood pressure stabilized below 110 mm Hg prior to initiation of fibrinolytic therapy. Further, blood pressure must be maintained below 180/105 for at least 24 hours after intravenous recombinant tissue plasminogen activator (rtPA) is given.[14] The AHA provides another Class I recommendation (LOE C) for blood pressure management for patients with markedly elevated pressures that do not receive rtPA. While there are no explicitly defined parameters, the consensus is that antihypertensive medication should be withheld unless SBP exceeds 220 mm Hg, or diastolic exceeds 120 mm Hg. For those meeting this criteria, the goal is to lower blood pressure by 15% over the first 24 hours after onset of the stroke.[14]

Patients who have had a stroke and are hypertensive are at high risk for an additional stroke. Those patients should receive blood pressure treatment when elevated to 140/90 mm Hg or higher. However, the decision to treat blood pressure at these levels should be made 4 to 7 days after the return to baseline blood pressure was to be expected. Blood pressure should be gradually reduced to 120/80, the optimal level for reducing cardiovascular risk.[15]

11.3.6 Blood Pressure Management in Hemorrhage

There has been significant debate in the past concerning appropriate management of blood pressure in those suffering from ICH. Some have advocated lowering blood pressure to reduce the risk of bleeding, edema formation, and systemic hypertensive complications.[16,17,18,19] While the prevalence of elevated blood pressure in ICH is high, it is unclear whether it is the cause or an effect of the initial bleed. Additionally, pain, stress, increased ICP, and premorbid hypertensive conditions may also be contributing to persistent blood pressure elevations after acute ICH.[20] Complications arising from high SBP in the face of acute ICH include expansion of hematoma, rebleeding, worsening neurologic deficits, and death.[20,21,22,23]AHA 2015 guidelines for blood pressure management in acute hemorrhagic stroke are as follows:

- Class I (LOE A) Recommendation
  - For ICH patients presenting with SBP between 150 and 220 mm Hg and without contraindication to acute blood pressure treatment, acute lowering of SBP to 140 mm Hg is safe and can be effective for improving functional outcome.[20]
- Class II (LOE B) Recommendation
  - For ICH patients presenting with SBP > 220 mm Hg, it may be reasonable to consider aggressive reduction of blood pressure with a continuous intravenous infusion and frequent blood pressure monitoring.[20]

Concerning cerebral ischemia after ICH, Butcher et al[24] used CT perfusion in a randomized clinical trial to show there was no evidence of perihematomal reduction in CBF related to lowering the SBP below 140 mm Hg within several hours of onset in small and medium-sized ICH. The Antihypertensive Treatment of Acute Cerebral Hemorrhage (ATACH) trial as well as both phase 1 and phase 2 of the Intensive Blood Pressure Reduction in Acute Cerebral Hemorrhage (INTERACT1, INTERACT2)[20,25,26] trials showed that not only was rapid lowering of SBP to < 140 mm Hg safe but there was no increase in mortality or morbidity from early intensive antihypertensive therapy.[20,25,26] Further, the INTERACT2 trial showed a slight trend toward better functional outcomes, reduced incidence of death, and major disability.[26]

There remains some debate in treating patients with ICH on whether surgery improves perfusion and thus outcome. The Surgical Trial in Intracerebral Hemorrhage randomized 1,033 patients from 83 centers and reported that patients with spontaneous supratentorial ICH in neurosurgical units show no overall benefit from early surgery when compared to initial conservative treatment.[27]

There is new evidence that ICH progression can be minimized with recombinant activated factor VII (RFVII) and that morbidity and mortality can consequently be reduced after ICH.[28] One to three IV doses of 40, 80, or 160 μg/kg given within the first 3 to 4 hours after symptom onset, or in patients at risk of additional bleeding, such as those with coagulopathy, demonstrated a 3-month mortality of 18% when compared to the placebo group mortality of 29%.[29]

However, there still remain subsets of patients that may benefit from surgical evacuation of ICH. The risk for rebleed is highest in the first 3 to 6 hours and lowest after 12 hours. Waiting until the patient is herniating before surgical intervention is no better than medical management alone.

The following patients may benefit from surgery for ICH:

- Patients who are symptomatic from a cerebellar hemorrhage > 3 cm or > 30 mL.
- Patients who have a supratentorial ICH > 20 to 30 mL and who present with a Glasgow Coma Scale (GCS) score of 13–5 or a decrease of 2 GCS points (carefully weigh the decision to take the patient to surgery if the bleed is in the left deep gray matter).
- Patients with lobar ICH.

The goal of surgery is volume reduction to less than 20 mL. It should be noted that patients with amyloid ICH, on average, do not require surgery.

Finally, the question of elevated blood pressure in aneurysmal subarachnoid hemorrhage (SAH) must be addressed. There is concern that the patient may rebleed if blood pressure is high and/or pulse pressure is large. However, patients with a lower GCS score may require higher perfusion pressures to prevent infarction.

The following are recommended for hypertension treatment in acute SAH:

- If the patient has a GCS score of 3 to 6 (World Federation of Neurological Surgeons scale[30] grade 5) or has a history of hypertension, maintain SBP < 140 mm Hg.
- If the patient has a GCS score > 6 and no history of hypertension, maintain SBP < 120 mm Hg.

At times the patient's blood pressure or CPP is too low despite adequate fluid resuscitation. There is no consensus regarding which vasopressor to use. Small-dose intravenous vasopressin infusion may be beneficial in patients with acute brain injuries and with unstable hemodynamics who are refractory to fluid resuscitation and catecholamine vasopressors.[31] Biestro et al[32] commented that noradrenaline at a dose of 0.5 to 5.0 mg/h is effective and safe and might be considered the drug of choice, whereas dopamine was not as effective at a high dose of 10.0 to 42.5 µg/kg/min, and methoxamine given as a bolus controls sudden decreases in MAP. The use of vasoconstrictor drugs to increase CPP may impair oxygenation in the ischemic penumbra and to other tissues of the body, such as the intestinal mucosa and the kidneys. Several human and animal studies suggest that norepinephrine improves CBF better than dopamine at high doses (▶ Table 11.4).[33]

Table 11.4 Vasopressors used in hypertension treatment in subarachnoid hemorrhage[33]

Agent	Receptor stimulus	Dosage	Effects
Dopamine	B2	1–3 µg/kg/min, 5 µg/kg/min	Vasodilates, increases CO and SV
	B1	+10 µg/kg/min; titrate up to 20 µg/kg/min	Vasoconstricts
Dobutamine	A B1	5–20 µg/kg/min	Increases CO/HR/SV, vasodilates
Phenylephrine (Neosynephrine)	B2 A	2–180 µg/min	Vasoconstricts, increases SVR
Epinephrine	A high and B low	1–8 µg/min	Increases HR/CO/SVR
Norepinephrine (Levophed)	A mostly and B little	8–12 µg/min	Increases CO/HR/SVR
Isuprel (Isoproterinol)	B	1–4 µg/min	Vasodilates, increases HR/CO

Abbreviations: CO, cardiac output; HR, heart rate; SVR, systemic vascular resistance.

11.4 Cerebral Oxygenation

The brain cells need oxygen and need adenosine triphosphate (ATP). In an injured state, the brain does not respond well to blood pressure or volume that is excessively elevated. Blood pressure that is too high will cause cerebral edema, bleeding, and increased ICP. Therefore, a dilemma exists as to the exact titration of therapy; this dilemma has been answered with the introduction of technology that allows the monitoring of cerebral metabolism and brain oxygenation. The literature is replete with documentation that supernormal PaO_2 improves brain tissue oxygenation and outcome in hundreds of patients.[11,34,35,36,37,38,39,40,41,42,43,44,45,46,47] The hemoglobin molecule has the capacity to carry 17 to 21 mL O_2/100 mL blood when all four binding sites are saturated. PaO_2 reflects only free oxygen molecules dissolved in plasma and not those bound to hemoglobin. Neither PaO_2 nor SaO_2 reflects total oxygen in the blood. At 100% saturation, PO_2 can be as low as 80 mm Hg; at 75% saturation, PO_2 can be as low as 40 mm Hg; and at 50% saturation, PO_2 can be as low as 27 mm Hg. It must be remembered that blood cells plus plasma carry more oxygen than can be accounted for by the hemoglobin molecule. The red blood cells reach only 85% of the brain cells, with plasma supplying the remainder. Treating the patient must account for decreased affinity of hemoglobin from increased temperature, PCO_2, 2,3-diphosphoglycerate, and a decrease in pH. A rightward shift, by definition, causes a decrease in the affinity of hemoglobin for oxygen. This makes it harder for the hemoglobin to bind to oxygen (requiring a higher partial pressure to achieve the same oxygen saturation), but it makes it easier for the hemoglobin to release bound oxygen. Physiologically, increasing FIO_2 past the maximal saturation of hemoglobin only increases the dissolved O_2 in plasma by 2 to 3%. Furthermore, FIO_2 levels higher than 60% may be harmful when used for longer than 24 hours in adults.

Increasing PO_2 to higher levels than necessary to saturate hemoglobin drives O_2 into the oxygen-starved brain tissue. With supernormal PO_2, during the early period after severe head injury, the lactate levels in brain tissue are reduced, and outcome is improved. Brain-injured patients may benefit from 100% O_2 during the first 8 to 24 hours, $PaO_2 > 150$ mm Hg for 2 to 4 days during peak edema, and > 100% thereafter, each in an attempt to maintain brain tissue oxygenation around 40 mm Hg and not below 20 mm Hg. Cerebral tissue monitoring systems measure four areas of brain metabolism, as well as physiological information about the progression of secondary injury at the cellular level, which may indicate the onset of ischemic injury. Experiments have demonstrated good recovery with mean brain partial oxygen pressure at 39 ± 4 mm Hg, moderate to severe disability with mean brain partial oxygen pressure at 31 ± 5 mm Hg, and dead or vegetative disability with a mean brain partial oxygen pressure at 19 ± 8 mm Hg.[35,36,39,40,41,42,43,44,45,46,47]

Cerebral perfusion must be provided in a tightly regulated manner. The blood pressure must be maintained so that appropriate CPP and CBF continue without causing additional edema, increased ICP, or bleeding. Oxygen has to be supplied in supernormal levels to prevent the ischemic penumbra from infarcting.

Case Management

A 20-year-old man presents after a fall from a second-story window with obvious contusions to his chest, abdomen, and head. At the scene, he does not open his eyes or talk, and he exhibits extensor/decerebrate posturing. His pupils are equal and sluggishly reactive. There is no obvious distension or rigidity of the abdomen. His blood pressure is 90/50.

The patient has a GCS score of 4 and is hypotensive. The patient must first be resuscitated with fluids and his GCS reassessed. If he remains at GCS ≤ 8 or less, an ICP monitor and a cerebral metabolic monitor should be placed. FIO_2 and blood pressure should be adjusted to maintain a brain tissue oxygenation of 40 mm Hg. The CPP should be maintained > 70 and < 90 mm Hg. The patient should have augmentation of blood pressure with vasopressors such as norepinephrine or low-dose dopamine if CVP is in the desired range of 6 to 8 or pulmonary capillary wedge pressure is 10 to 14 mm Hg or pulmonary artery diastolic pressure is 12 to 16 mm Hg. The patient should be placed on 100% O_2 for 8 to 24 hours.

References

[1] Schuenke M, et al. Atlas of Anatomy—Head and Neuroanatomy - (corr.). New York, NY: Thieme; 2010:196–197

[2] Kandel E, Schwartz J, Jessel TH, eds. Principles of Neural Science. 3rd ed. New York, NY: Elsevier; 1991

[3] Joynt R, Griggs R. Clinical Neurology. Baltimore, MD: Lippincott-Raven; 1996

[4] Youmans JR, ed. Neurological Surgery. 5th ed. Philadelphia, PA: WB Saunders; 2004

[5] Henley CM, Muszynski C, Cherian L, Robertson CS. Activation of ornithine decarboxylase and accumulation of putrescine after traumatic brain injury. J Neurotrauma. 1996; 13(9):487–496

[6] Edvinsson L, Krause DN. Cerebral Blood Flow and Metabolism. 2nd ed. Philadelphia, PA: Lippincott Williams & Wilkins; 2002

[7] Narayan RK, Wilberger JE, Povlishock JT. Neurotrauma. New York, NY: McGraw-Hill; 1994

[8] Friedman JA, Khurana VG, Anderson RE, Meyer FB. Cerebral blood flow: physiology and measurement techniques. In: Moore AJ, Newell DW, eds. Neurosurgery Principles and Practice. New York, NY: Springer; 2005:301–314

[9] Guidelines for the Management of Severe Traumatic Brain Injury. 3rd ed. New York, NY: The Brain Trauma Foundation; 2007

[10] Bouma GJ, Muizelaar JP. Relationship between cardiac output and cerebral blood flow in patients with intact and with impaired autoregulation. J Neurosurg. 1990; 73(3):368–374

[11] Kiening KL, Härtl R, Unterberg AW, Schneider GH, Bardt T, Lanksch WR. Brain tissue pO2-monitoring in comatose patients: implications for therapy. Neurol Res. 1997; 19(3):233–240

[12] Hlatky R, Valadka AB, Robertson CS. Intracranial hypertension and cerebral ischemia after severe traumatic brain injury. Neurosurg Focus. 2003; 14(4):e2

[13] Clifton GL, Miller ER, Choi SC, Levin HS. Fluid thresholds and outcome from severe brain injury. Crit Care Med. 2002; 30(4):739–745

[14] AHA/ASA Guidelines for the Early Management of Patients with Acute Ischemic Stroke. https://www.aan.com/guidelines/home/getguidelinecontent/581. American Heart Association; 2013

[15] Cohen S. Management of Ischemic Stroke. New York, NY: McGraw-Hill; 2000

[16] Kanji S, Corman C, Douen AG. Blood pressure management in acute stroke: comparison of current guidelines with prescribing patterns. Can J Neurol Sci. 2002; 29(2):125–131

[17] Broderick JP, Adams HP, Jr, Barsan W, et al. Guidelines for the management of spontaneous intracerebral hemorrhage: A statement for healthcare professionals from a special writing group of the Stroke Council, American Heart Association. Stroke. 1999; 30(4):905–915

[18] Qureshi AI, Tuhrim S, Broderick JP, Batjer HH, Hondo H, Hanley DF. Spontaneous intracerebral hemorrhage. N Engl J Med. 2001; 344(19):1450–1460

[19] Ohwaki K, Yano E, Nagashima H, Hirata M, Nakagomi T, Tamura A. Blood pressure management in acute intracerebral hemorrhage: relationship between elevated blood pressure and hematoma enlargement. Stroke. 2004; 35(6):1364–1367

[20] Hemphill JC, III, Greenberg SM, Anderson CS, et al. Guidelines for the Management of Spontaneous Intracerebral Hemorrhage: A Guideline for Healthcare Professionals From the American Heart Association/American Stroke Association. Stroke. 2015; 46(7):2032–2060

[21] Zhang Y, Reilly KH, Tong W, et al. Blood pressure and clinical outcome among patients with acute stroke in Inner Mongolia, China. J Hypertens. 2008; 26(7):1446–1452

[22] Rodriguez-Luna D, Piñeiro S, Rubiera M, et al. Impact of blood pressure changes and course on hematoma growth in acute intracerebral hemorrhage. Eur J Neurol. 2013; 20(9):1277–1283

[23] Sakamoto Y, Koga M, Yamagami H, et al. SAMURAI Study Investigators. Systolic blood pressure after intravenous antihypertensive treatment and clinical outcomes in hyperacute intracerebral hemorrhage: the stroke acute management with urgent risk-factor assessment and improvement-intracerebral hemorrhage study. Stroke. 2013; 44(7):1846–1851

[24] Butcher KS, Jeerakathil T, Hill M, et al. ICH ADAPT Investigators. The Intracerebral Hemorrhage Acutely Decreasing Arterial Pressure Trial. Stroke. 2013; 44(3):620–626

[25] Anderson CS, Huang Y, Wang JG, et al. INTERACT Investigators. Intensive blood pressure reduction in acute cerebral haemorrhage trial (INTERACT): a randomised pilot trial. Lancet Neurol. 2008; 7 (5):391–399

[26] Anderson CS, Heeley E, Huang Y, et al. INTERACT2 Investigators. Rapid blood-pressure lowering in patients with acute intracerebral hemorrhage. N Engl J Med. 2013; 368(25):2355–2365

[27] Mendelow AD, Gregson BA, Fernandes HM, et al. STICH investigators. Early surgery versus initial conservative treatment in patients with spontaneous supratentorial intracerebral haematomas in the International Surgical Trial in Intracerebral Haemorrhage (STICH): a randomised trial. Lancet. 2005; 365(9457):387–397

[28] Grotta JC. Management of primary hypertensive hemorrhage of the brain. Curr Treat Options Neurol. 2004; 6(6):435–442

[29] Mayer SA, Brun NC, Begtrup K, et al. Recombinant Activated Factor VII Intracerebral Hemorrhage Trial Investigators. Recombinant activated factor VII for acute intracerebral hemorrhage. N Engl J Med. 2005; 352(8):777–785

[30] Drake CG. Report of World Federation of Neurological Surgeons Committee on a universal subarachnoid hemorrhage grading scale. J Neurosurg. 1988; 68(6):985–986

[31] Yeh CC, Wu CT, Lu CH, Yang CP, Wong CS. Early use of small-dose vasopressin for unstable hemodynamics in an acute brain injury patient refractory to catecholamine treatment: a case report. Anesth Analg. 2003; 97(2):577–579

[32] Biestro A, Barrios E, Baraibar J, et al. Use of vasopressors to raise cerebral perfusion pressure in head injured patients. Acta Neurochir Suppl (Wien). 1998; 71:5–9

[33] Kroppenstedt SN, Sakowitz OW, Thomale UW, Unterberg AW, Stover JF. Influence of norepinephrine and dopamine on cortical perfusion, EEG activity, extracellular glutamate, and brain edema in rats after controlled cortical impact injury. J Neurotrauma. 2002; 19(11):1421–1432

[34] Sheinberg M, Kanter MJ, Robertson CS, Contant CF, Narayan RK, Grossman RG. Continuous monitoring of jugular venous oxygen saturation in head-injured patients. J Neurosurg. 1992; 76 (2):212–217

[35] van Santbrink H, Maas AI, Avezaat CJ. Continuous monitoring of partial pressure of brain tissue oxygen in patients with severe head injury. Neurosurgery. 1996; 38(1):21–31

[36] Zauner A, Doppenberg EM, Woodward JJ, Choi SC, Young HF, Bullock R. Continuous monitoring of cerebral substrate delivery and clearance: initial experience in 24 patients with severe acute brain injuries. Neurosurgery. 1997; 41(5):1082–1091, discussion 1091–1093

[37] Kiening KL, Schneider GH, Bardt TF, Unterberg AW, Lanksch WR. Bifrontal measurements of brain tissue-PO2 in comatose patients. Acta Neurochir Suppl (Wien). 1998; 71:172–173

[38] Zauner A, Doppenberg E, Soukup J, Menzel M, Young HF, Bullock R. Extended neuromonitoring: new therapeutic opportunities? Neurol Res. 1998; 20 Suppl 1:S85–S90

[39] Menzel M, Doppenberg EM, Zauner A, Soukup J, Reinert MM, Bullock R. Increased inspired oxygen concentration as a factor in improved brain tissue oxygenation and tissue lactate levels after severe human head injury. J Neurosurg. 1999; 91(1):1–10

[40] Menzel M, Doppenberg EM, Zauner A, et al. Cerebral oxygenation in patients after severe head injury: monitoring and effects of arterial hyperoxia on cerebral blood flow, metabolism and intracranial pressure. J Neurosurg Anesthesiol. 1999; 11(4):240–251

[41] Manley GT, Pitts LH, Morabito D, et al. Brain tissue oxygenation during hemorrhagic shock, resuscitation, and alterations in ventilation. J Trauma. 1999; 46(2):261–267

[42] van den Brink WA, van Santbrink H, Steyerberg EW, et al. Brain oxygen tension in severe head injury. Neurosurgery. 2000; 46(4):868–876, discussion 876–878

[43] Rockswold SB, Rockswold GL, Vargo JM, et al. Effects of hyperbaric oxygenation therapy on cerebral metabolism and intracranial pressure in severely brain injured patients. J Neurosurg. 2001; 94(3):403–411

[44] Longhi L, Valeriani V, Rossi S, De Marchi M, Egidi M, Stocchetti N. Effects of hyperoxia on brain tissue oxygen tension in cerebral focal lesions. Acta Neurochir Suppl (Wien). 2002; 81:315–317

[45] Reinert M, Alessandri B, Seiler R, Bullock R. Influence of inspired oxygen on glucose-lactate dynamics after subdural hematoma in the rat. Neurol Res. 2002; 24(6):601–606

[46] Reinert M, Barth A, Rothen HU, Schaller B, Takala J, Seiler RW. Effects of cerebral perfusion pressure and increased fraction of inspired oxygen on brain tissue oxygen, lactate and glucose in patients with severe head injury. Acta Neurochir (Wien). 2003; 145(5):341–349, discussion 349–350

[47] Tolias CM, Reinert M, Seiler R, Gilman C, Scharf A, Bullock MR. Normobaric hyperoxia-induced improvement in cerebral metabolism and reduction in intracranial pressure in patients with severe head injury: a prospective historical cohort-matched study. J Neurosurg. 2004; 101 (3):435–444

12 Cerebrospinal Fluid Dynamics and Pathology

Deependra Mahato, Kevin Ray, John D. Cantando, Dan E. Miulli, and Javed Siddiqi

Abstract
The cerebrospinal fluid (CSF) is a vital fluid providing nutrients to brain tissue and removing products of metabolism and disease from the brain. The flow of CSF throughout the brain tissue is likewise as significant as the flow of blood through its vessels. CSF is so important that its rate of production and reabsorption is meticulously controlled. It is constantly made at roughly half a liter per day in the adult and removed at roughly the same rate. When the constituents of CSF, the flow of CSF, or the pressure of CSF is altered significantly there is disease, which can be recognized and treated.

Keywords: arachnoid granulations, beta2-transferrin, choroid plexus, CSF, CSF glucose, hydrocephalus, NPH, ring sign

Case Presentation

A 21-year-old woman was struck in the head by falling objects, resulting in a loss of consciousness. Her Glasgow Coma Scale (GCS) score was 7. A computed tomographic (CT) scan revealed a small amount of epidural intracranial air. There were multiple facial fractures, including fractures of the orbit and zygoma. An intraventricular drain and monitor were placed upon admission. During her hospital course the external ventricular drain was raised to 15 mm Hg after 5 days. She remained intubated. She developed fluid leakage from her nostrils.

See end of chapter for Case Management.

12.1 Introduction

Cerebrospinal fluid (CSF) is found within the four ventricles of the brain, the subarachnoid space, and the central canal of the spinal cord. It is also called liquor cerebrospinalis.[1] CSF circulates a variety of chemicals and nutrients necessary for normal brain function and metabolism; it also acts as a shock absorber, cushioning the brain from both day-to-day activity and traumatic events.

12.2 Cerebrospinal Fluid Identification

Grossly, CSF should be a colorless, odorless, serous fluid. There is an estimated 70 to 160 mL of fluid in the central nervous system at any given time (~ 50% intracranial, 50% spinal). Certain pathological conditions will change both the chemical and the gross appearance of CSF. In the majority of cases, it is simple to ascertain whether fluid is CSF or not by a simple halo test described later in this chapter. If the source was suspicious for CSF then it is more likely. However, at times, especially when contaminated with other fluids, it is necessary to analyze the fluid for its constituents to determine if an unknown fluid is CSF, contains CSF, or is another bodily fluid.[2,3,4,5,6,7,8] ▶ Table 12.1 compares the composition of CSF with plasma. The following tests can determine if a fluid is CSF:

- *Glucose analysis:* Analysis should be done immediately after collection to prevent fermentation. Nasal/lacrimal fluid or mucosal secretion will have < 5 mg/dL of glucose. A negative test is more reliable because, even with meningitis, the glucose level is usually 5 to 20 mg/dL and associated with other changes. However, there is a 45 to 75% chance of a false-positive[2,3,6,7,9,10]

- *Beta2-transferrin:* This test can be performed only by electrophoresis of at least 0.5 mL of sample. Beta2-transferrin is found only in CSF and vitreous humor. (Note: This test is not reliable in patients with liver disease or in newborns.[11,12])

- *Ring sign:* Also known as the halo, this sign is particularly useful for blood-tinged samples. A drop of suspected fluid is placed on linen; as the fluid feathers out into the surrounding area, blood and mucus will stay centrally placed, and the CSF (which is less viscous) will continue spreading, creating a clear ring around the central colored area.

Table 12.1 Chemical constituents of cerebrospinal fluid and plasma[2,3,4,5,6,7,8]

Constituent	Units	CSF	Plasma
Formation	mL/min	0.35	–
Osmolarity	mOsm/L	295	295
H_2O	%	99%	93%
Sodium	mEq/L	138–150	135–145
Potassium	mEq/L	2.2–3.3	4.1–4.5
Chloride	mEq/L	119–130	102–112
Calcium	mEq/L	2.1	4.8
Bicarbonate	mEq/L	22.0–23.3	24.0–26.8
Magnesium	mEq/L	2.3–2.7	1.7–1.9
Phosphorus	mg/dL	1.6	4.0
Ammonia	µg/dL	22–42	37–70

Table 12.1 continued

Constituent	Units	CSF	Plasma
PCO$_2$	mm Hg	43–47	38–41
pH		7.33–7.35	7.41
PO$_2$	mm Hg	43	104
Glucose	mg/dL	45–80	90–110
Lactate	mEq/L	0.8–2.8	0.5–1.7
	mg/dL	10–20	6–13
Pyruvate	mEq/L	0.08	0.11
lactate: pyruvate		26	17.6
Glutamine	mg/dL	<20	>23
	µmol/L	552	641
Glutamate	µmol/L	26.1	61.3
GABA	µmol/L	3.5	29.8
Total protein	mg/dL	5–45, 5–15 ventricular, 10–25 cisternal, 15–45 lumbar	7,000
Albumin	mg/L	155	36,600
Prealbumin	mg/L	17.3	238
Amino acids	% blood	30	3.6–7.2
	mEq/L	0.72–2.62	
IgG	mg/L	5–12	9870
RBCs	/mm^3	0	3.6–5.4 M
WBCs	/mm^3	<6/mm^3; in children, up to 20/mm^3	5,000–10,000
Oligoclonal bands		<2	0
GOT	U	7–49	5–40
LDH	U	15–71	200–680
CPK	U	0–3	0–12
BUN	mg/dL	5–25	6–28
Bilirubin	mg/dL	0	0.2–0.9
Iron	µg/dL	1.5	15

Abbreviations: BUN, blood urea nitrogen; CPK, creatine phosphokinase; CSF, cerebrospinal fluid; GABA, γ-aminobutyric acid; GOT, glutamic-oxaloacetic transaminase; IgG, immunoglobulin G; LDH, lactate dehydrogenase; RBC, red blood cell; WBC, white blood cell.

12.3 Chemical Regulators of Cerebrospinal Fluid

Constituents of CSF are affected by secretion and absorption rates of CSF, hormones, and chemicals. The secretion rates and effects of hormones and chemicals on CSF vary from the vascular to the ventricular side of the choroid plexus.[13,14,15] These are described in ▶ Table 12.2.

Table 12.2 Hormone and chemical secretions in cerebrospinal fluid[13,14,15]

Vascular side of choroid plexus
Nonadrenergic sympathetic innervation (near CP epithelial cells and blood vessels) decreases CSF flow by 30%.
Cholinergic input primarily near the third ventricle stimulates CSF production up to 100%.
Endothelin binding sites are found in CP of lateral and third ventricles. Endothelin decreases blood flow and subsequently CSF production.
Antidiuretic hormone (ADH) regulates norepinephrine, dopamine, and endorphin release within the ventricle. ADH has been shown to indirectly decrease plasma Na^+.

Ventricular side of choroid plexus
5-hydroxytryptamine (5HT) The CP contains 10 times the amount of 5HT receptors relative to other areas of the brain. It is released from the supraependymal nerve fibers into the CSF and interacts with the CP-5HT receptors. 5HT reduces the rate of CSF secretion.
Melatonin binding sites are located in the fourth ventricle and stimulate CSF secretion.
Carbonic anhydrase High concentrations within the CP increase CSF production by facilitating Na^+ transport.
L-dopa is the most abundant monoamine in the CSF. The CP has D_1 receptors but lacks direct dopaminergic innervation. Dopamine effects on the CP are via the CSF, similar to 5HT.
Norepinephrine is secreted by noradrenergic periventricular neurons in contact with the ventricles and decreases CSF production. It follows circadian variations similar to systemic circulation.
Arginine vasopressin (AVP) is released by vasopressinergic neurons into the CSF, which stimulates CSF production. AVP in the CSF follows circadian variations, whereas plasma levels do not. The CP has V_1 receptors for AVP. AVP has been shown to indirectly lower plasma Na^+.
Arial natriuretic peptide (ANP) reduces CSF production. It is elevated in hydrocephalus cases. Evidence supports ANP involvement in the regulation of water and electrolyte passage across the blood–brain barrier. ANP has a direct negative effect on CSF production as substantiated by increased levels of ANP circulating within the CSF in hydrocephalic patients (both normal and high pressure). Systemically, ANP stimulates renal inhibition of Na^+ and water absorption, leading to hyponatremia. Within the brain, ANP reduces the net flux of Na^+ from the circulation by inhibiting the $Na^+/K+/Cl$ cotransport system that is known to decrease CSF production.[8,9]

Abbreviations: CP, choroid plexus; CSF, cerebrospinal fluid.

12.4 Flow Pattern of Cerebrospinal Fluid

CSF from blood plasma is actively transported by the choroid plexus (80%), or invaginations of the pia mater, into the ventricles, with the remaining 10 to 20% produced by ventricular ependymal cells, brain parenchyma, and indirect cellular fluid shifts. The approximate CSF secretion is 450 mL per day, which corresponds to a rate of 0.3 (0.35–0.37) mL/min. The CSF is in constant flow in a continuous pattern. Starting from the choroid plexus in the lateral ventricles, CSF continues through the foramen of Monro into the third ventricle and passes into the cerebral aqueduct prior to the fourth ventricle. From the fourth ventricle, fluid escapes into the cisterns and subarachnoid space via the foramen of Luschka and the foramen of Magendie. Some enters the central canal of the spinal cord, although most spinal fluid then circulates through the subarachnoid space and is reabsorbed in the venous system via the arachnoid villi. To keep the total spinal fluid in circulation throughout the ventricular system and subarachnoid space at ~ 150 mL, the absorption into the venous system is relatively constant at 450 mL/d, matching the daily production. There should be at least 3 to 5 mm Hg pressure of CSF for absorption to take place. Pathological states can alter the production, secretion, and/or circulatory flow of CSF.

12.4.1 Monro–Kellie Doctrine

The brain is unique among other bodily organs in that it is fully encased within the skull, which provides a rigid covering for the brain, CSF, and blood. The Monro–Kellie doctrine states that, because each of these compartments is non-compressible, their volume within the skull remains constant. Expansion of any one compartment (e.g., hydrocephalus, a developing mass, or an expanding hematoma) will result in compression of the others and an eventual rise in intracranial pressure (ICP). There is some leeway due to the compressibility of the venous sinuses and caudal displacement of CSF into the spinal canal. However, once this buffering capacity is exhausted, ICP will begin to rise and lead to a decrease in cerebral perfusion pressure (CPP) (given that CPP = mean arterial pressure − ICP) and will possibly lead to a host of different herniation syndromes determined by the location of the source of compression; particularly if the ICP is greater than 30 mmHg.[16]

12.5 Pathology Involving Cerebrospinal Fluid

▶ Table 12.3 notes changes in the gross appearance and the chemical composition of CSF due to certain disease states.

Cerebrospinal Fluid Dynamics and Pathology

Table 12.3 Cerebrospinal fluid findings in pathological conditions

Constituent	Color	Clarity	Pressure	Glucose mg/dL	Lactate mg/dL	Protein mg/dL	Cells/mm³	Oligoclonal bands
SAH bleed	Xanthochromic in <6–12 hours	Bloody, no clots	↑	Normal	Normal	↑	RBC to 5 days, PMN, then lymphocytes	
Multiple sclerosis	Colorless	Normal	Normal	Normal	Normal	Minimum ↑ 25–50	Lymphocytes	≥2
Spinal obstruction	Colorless	Normal	Normal	Normal	Normal	>500	Normal	
Spinal tumor	Sl xanthochromic	Cloudy	↓	Normal	Normal	↑, Froin's syndrome	Lymphocytes	
Bacterial infection	White, yellow	Cloudy	↑	↑, ½ or less serum glucose	>35 mg/dL	↑ 80–500	PMN >500	
Viral infection	Colorless	Clear	Mild ↑	Normal	Normal	Normal-Sl ↑ 130–100	Lymphocytes <500	
TB meningitis	Colorless	Cloudy	↑	↓	>35 mg/dL	↑ 50–300	Lymphocytes 200–500	
Fungal meningitis	Colorless	Cloudy, varies	↑	↓, varies	↑	↑ 50–300	PMN/lymphocytes 50–150	
Aseptic meningitis	Colorless	Clear	Normal	Normal	Normal	Normal- Sl ↑	Lymphocytes	
Abscess	Colorless	Clear	↑	Normal	Normal, varies	↑ 20–120	PMN	
Infarction	Colorless	Clear	Sl ↑	Normal	Normal, varies	Sl ↑	Sl PMN <50	
Traumatic LP	Not xanthochromic	Bloody, does clot	Normal	Normal	Normal	4 mg/dL increase/5,000 RBCs	Same as peripheral	

Abbreviations: LP, lumbar puncture; PMN, polymorphonuclear neutrophil leukocytes; RBC, red blood (cell) count; SAH, subarachnoid hemorrhage; Sl, signal intensity; TB, tuberculosis.

Source: Adapted from Greenberg M. Handbook of Neurosurgery. 5th ed. New York, NY: Thieme, 2001, with permission.

12.5.1 Disorders of Volume and Pressure

Normal pressure hydrocephalus (NPH) is associated with a classic triad of symptoms: dementia, gait disturbance, and urinary incontinence. The etiology is usually idiopathic but can be secondary to other intracranial pathology, such as Alzheimer's disease, carcinomatosis, infectious meningitis, and subarachnoid hemorrhage.[17] Diagnosis is primarily clinical, with documented normal pressure via lumbar puncture and a full workup of other causes of dementia. Some clinicians augment clinical symptoms by performing a quantitative lumbar puncture or continual physiological drainage over 3 days. Usually a cognitive assessment, such as a neuropsychological test, precedes the lumbar puncture or continuous drainage. The lumbar puncture measures the opening pressure, allows 20 to 40 mL of fluid to drain off, then measures the closing pressure. If the brain is normally compliant when the change in volume divided by the change in pressure is ~ 0.62, the closing pressure may be reduced by 0.45 cm of CSF pressure for every 1 mL of CSF removed. Thus removing 30 mL of fluid should reduce closing pressure by ~ 13 cm CSF (10 mm Hg). This is the adult normal pressure–volume index (PVI; 25–30 mL change in volume causes a 10-fold change in pressure in mm Hg). No change in CSF pressure may indicate poor cerebral compliance, low PVI, and increased ICP; a large lowering in CSF pressure may indicate low ICP, herniation, or complete blockage of CSF pathways. Following the lumbar puncture or continuous 3 days of drainage, there should be a repeat cognitive assessment, such as a neuropsychological test, to determine if the quantitative lumbar puncture resulted in clinical improvement. Some clinicians do not rely on this test, whereas others will not shunt questionable cases of NPH without a positive improvement in cognitive assessment after a quantitative lumbar puncture. Treatment of NPH is shunting, either ventricular or, at rare times, lumboperitoneal.

Communicating and noncommunicating hydrocephalus symptoms include nausea, vomiting, gait disturbance, frontal headache (frequently worse in the morning), paresis of upward gaze, disorders of sodium, and papilledema. Temporizing measures for relief may include a ventricular catheter and/or diuretics (acetazolamide or furosemide). Permanent treatment should be directed at the offending pathology; however, frequently, a CSF-diverting procedure, such as a shunt or third ventriculostomy, is required.[17,18,19,20,21] An endoscopic third ventriculostomy is usually reserved for obstructive hydrocephalus. Although there are reports of success for communicating hydrocephalus our experience does not support that it is more likely than not to resolve the communicating hydrocephalus.

Obstructive (noncommunicative) hydrocephalus is blockage of the normal flow of CSF, causing dilatation of the ventricles proximal to the obstruction.

Triventricular hydrocephalus is specifically a stenosis occurring at the sylvian aqueduct, yielding dilatation of both lateral ventricles and the third ventricle.

Common etiologies include edema, mass effect, mass lesion, and congenital abnormality.

Communicating (nonobstructive) hydrocephalus is a disruption of the equilibrium of secretion and absorption of CSF, yielding an increased volume of CSF. It is most commonly caused by malabsorption of the CSF by the arachnoid granulations. Common etiologies include infection, hemorrhage, trauma, and noninfectious meningitis.

Pseudotumor cerebri (idiopathic benign intracranial hypertension) symptoms may include nausea, vomiting, headache, retro-orbital pain, visual changes (including blindness, may be permanent) associated with increased ICP, possible optic atrophy, and, when progressive, papilledema (▶ Table 12.4). A CT scan does not show enlarged ventricles but it does show normal or small ventricles.

Treatment of progressive symptoms includes a low salt diet, weight loss, and medical management with diuretics (acetazolamide or furosemide); if refractory, surgical management is warranted, with optic nerve decompression, serial lumbar punctures, or shunting.[22] Surgical procedures should not be performed for headache but reserved for optic nerve and visual changes.

12.5.2 Leptomeningeal or Arachnoid Cysts

Leptomeningeal cysts are congenital fluid collections between two layers of the arachnoid. They are not related to posttraumatic leptomeningeal cysts due to growing skull fractures. There are two types of arachnoid cysts classified by histological findings: (1) simple, in which the lining of the cyst consists of cells capable of secreting CSF (this is the most common type of middle fossa arachnoid cyst), and (2) complex, in which the lining of the cyst is multicellular, often containing neuroglia and ependyma.

Classic presentation is in early childhood, when there is a sudden onset associated with hemorrhagic conversion or cyst rupture. Symptoms and presentation vary according to location and mass effect; asymptomatic lesions are usually identified incidentally (▶ Table 12.5).

Table 12.4 Four diagnostic criteria for pseudotumor cerebri

Cerebrospinal fluid pressure > 20 cm H_2O
Normal cerebrospinal fluid composition
Symptoms of elevated intracranial pressure without focal deficit
Normal imaging studies (occasionally slit ventricles may be seen)

Table 12.5 Arachnoid cysts: signs and symptoms[2,4,5]

Location	Signs and symptoms
Middle fossa 50% of cysts in adults, 30% of cysts in children	Asymptomatic; unilateral headaches, nausea/vomiting, seizures, mild hemiparesis, present at younger age, male:female ratio 3:1, more in left hemisphere, hemorrhage
Suprasellar 9% of cysts	Increased intracranial pressure, hydrocephalus, craniomegaly, developmental delay, precocious puberty, bobbing head, visual loss

Table 12.6 Treatment of congenital middle fossa arachnoid cysts[2,4,5]

Cyst type	Description	Treatment
Type I	Communicates with subarachnoid space	No treatment, follow-up imaging every 6 months for 18 months
Type II	Large, quadrangular, mass effect; delayed uptake with cisternogram contrast	Surgery if symptoms severe; surgery either cystoperitoneal shunting or cyst marsupial fenestration
Type III	Large, round, mass effect; no communication with subarachnoid space; bone expansion of middle fossa	Surgery if symptoms severe; either cystoperitoneal shunting or cyst marsupial fenestration

Diagnosis is via CT scan or magnetic resonance imaging (MRI). Most cysts are static; however; repeat imaging can be used to rule out cystic changes or enlargement. Treatment is indicated only when the mass effect of the cyst causes seizures or neurological deficit and when other etiologies have been ruled out. Surgical treatment is not recommended for headaches because headaches do not usually respond to surgery. The most common treatments are shunting using a low-pressure valve, which has a low rate of recurrence, marsupialization, or a combination of both (▶ Table 12.6).[4,5]

12.5.3 Infectious and Noninfectious Irritants Causing Meningitis

Posttraumatic meningitis is usually limited to head trauma with an associated skull fracture. Organisms are most commonly gram-positive cocci and gram-negative bacilli. Treatment should be directed at the offending agent (▶ Table 12.7).[2,3,6,7,9,10]

Table 12.7 Treatment of meningitis[2,3,6,7,9,10]

Patient population	Organism	Suggested antibiotics
Neonates (< 1 month)	Group B/D *Streptococcus*, Enterobacteriaceae, *Listeria*	Ampicillin, gentamicin (alt. third-generation cephalosporin)
Newborns (1–3 months)	Pneumococci, meningococci, *Haemophilus influenzae*	Ampicillin, third-generation cephalosporin ± dexamethasone
Children (3 months–7 years)	Pneumococci, meningococci, *H. influenzae*	Third-generation cephalosporin (alt. ampicillin)
Older children (>7 years) and adults	*Streptococcus pneumoniae*, *Neisseria* meningococci	Third-generation cephalosporin, ampicillin (in combination with resistance, add rifampin ± vancomycin
Alcoholics, immunocompromised, and elderly	Pneumococci, Enterobacteriaceae, *Pseudomonas*, *Listeria*	Vancomycin, third-generation cephalosporin
Postprocedural	*Staphylococcus aureus*, Enterobacteriaceae, *Pseudomonas*, pneumococci	Vancomycin, ceftazidime ± gentamicin

12.5.4 Trauma-Related Cerebrospinal Fluid Abnormalities

Infectious

Cerebrospinal fluid (CSF) findings in bacterial meningitis are summarized in Chapter 20, Table 20.2.

Cerebrospinal Leaks

CSF leaks are associated with basal skull fractures and anterior fossa fractures resulting in otorrhea and/or rhinorrhea. Diagnosis is made by clinical exam; however, MRI, contrasted CT scans, and radionuclide cisternograms can help identify the source of the leak. Analysis is required (see ▶ Table 12.1) to confirm the fluid as CSF. Treatment consists of general measures to lower ICP, raising the head of the bed, administering acetazolamide to decrease CSF production, inserting a lumbar drain, and/or surgical repair. Surgical repair is indicated in refractory and recurrent CSF leaks.

Pneumocephalus is evidence of air intracranially. Air can be intraparenchymal, intraventricular, subdural, or epidural. It is associated with a skull defect or injury to the tegmen tympani (congenital/traumatic/ related to pressure changes, e.g., deep-sea diving). The skull defect can be congenital, postprocedural, or posttraumatic. Pneumocephalus must be closely monitored with frequent CT scans to confirm resolution. Prophylactic antibiotic use is controversial. A tension pneumocephalus is the result of expanding trapped gas and can be associated with gas-producing bacterial infection, room temperature air expanding due to increased body temperature after sealing the access, and the continued use of nitrous oxide anesthesia gas after the closure of the dura.

Traumatic Lumbar Puncture

Traumatic lumbar puncture can occur during a procedure to obtain CSF; local trauma or disruption of nearby vascular structures can produce a traumatic tap. The CSF analysis will still be accurate in most pathologies; however, its appearance can complicate the diagnosis of subarachnoid hemorrhage. When a CT scan is negative for subarachnoid hemorrhage, yet the patient history and physical exam are highly suspicious, a lumbar puncture can be used to limit the differential diagnosis. ▶ Table 12.8 itemizes the characteristics of a traumatic tap.

Table 12.8 Traumatic punctures[2,4,5]
Decline in number of RBCs with succeeding tubes
WBCs proportional to blood RBCs
Blood will clot
No xanthochromia if first attempt within 2–12 hours, unless protein > 150 mg/dL or RBCs > 1.5 M/mm^3 or high lipid levels
Xanthochromia appears in the CSF within 2 hours in limited cases, 6 hours 70% of time, and 12 hours 90% of time.
Protein consistent with plasma or increased above-normal CSF levels by 1 mg/1,000 RBCs.
Abbreviations: CSF, cerebrospinal fluid; RBC, red blood cell; WBC, white blood cell.

Case Management

Initially, it is possible that the fluid coming out of her nose was CSF; however, this was less likely because there was no evidence of intradural air on the CT scan. The intracranial air was purely epidural. Furthermore, because of intubation, air sinus congestion can certainly develop. The fluid leaking from the nose can be tested for glucose, but there is a 45–75% chance of a false-positive finding. Any leakage of fluid onto the bed linen can also be observed for a halo sign, which represents central blood and mucus surrounded by a ring of spreading CSF. The best test to determine if the fluid coming from the nose is CSF is beta2-transferrin. Because there was no globe damage, it is unlikely that the fluid is vitreous humor.

During external ventricular drain insertion, it is prudent to test the CSF for the possibility of infection. These tests include color, clarity, glucose level, protein level, and cell count. Any concerns of possible CSF leakage could be initially treated by slightly lowering the drainage bag. The bag should not be dramatically lowered because this may allow air into the intracranial or intradural compartment.

References

[1] Dorland's Illustrated Medical Dictionary. Philadelphia, PA: WB Saunders; 1994
[2] Greenberg MS. Handbook of Neurosurgery. 5th ed. New York, NY: Thieme; 2001
[3] Gilroy J. Basic Neurology. 3rd ed. New York, NY: McGraw-Hill; 2000
[4] Winn HR. Youman's Neurological Surgery. 5th ed. Philadelphia, PA: WB Saunders; 2004
[5] Wilkins RH, Regengachary SS. Neurosurgery. 2nd ed. New York, NY: McGraw-Hill; 1996
[6] Sacher RA, McPherson RA. Widmann's Clinical Interpretation of Laboratory Tests. 11th ed. Philadelphia, PA: FA Davis; 2000
[7] Ropper AH, Brown RH. Adams and Victor's Principles of Neurology. 8th ed. New York, NY: McGraw-Hill; 2005
[8] Kandel ER, Schwartz JH, Jessel TM. Principles of Neural Science. 4th ed. New York, NY: McGraw-Hill; 2000
[9] Layon AJ, Gabrielli A, Friedman WA. Textbook of Neurointensive Care. Philadelphia, PA: WB Saunders; 2004
[10] Rowland LP. Merritt's Neurology. 10th ed. Philadelphia, PA: Lippincott Williams & Wilkins; 2000
[11] Ryall RG, Peacock MK, Simpson DA. Usefulness of beta 2-transferrin assay in the detection of cerebrospinal fluid leaks following head injury. J Neurosurg. 1992; 77(5):737–739
[12] Fransen P, Sindic CJ, Thauvoy C, Laterre C, Stroobandt G. Highly sensitive detection of beta-2 transferrin in rhinorrhea and otorrhea as a marker for cerebrospinal fluid (C.S.F.) leakage. Acta Neurochir (Wien). 1991; 109(3–4):98–101
[13] Pérez-Fígares JM, Jimenez AJ, Rodríguez EM. Subcommissural organ, cerebrospinal fluid circulation, and hydrocephalus. Microsc Res Tech. 2001; 52(5):591–607
[14] Illowsky BP, Kirch DG. Polydipsia and hyponatremia in psychiatric patients. Am J Psychiatry. 1988; 145(6):675–683
[15] Migliore A, Paoletti P, Villani R. The rate of exchange of Na and other ions between plasma and cerebrospinal fluid in normal subjects and in hydrocephalic infants. Dev Med Child Neurol. 1965; 7:310–316
[16] Whitton TL, Lam AM. Neurosurgical Intensive Care. In: Moore AJ and Newell DW, eds. Neurosurgery principles and practice.Spinger;2004:85–86
[17] Mayberg MR. Neurosurgery Clinics of North America. Philadelphia, PA: WB Saunders; 2001
[18] Mori K, Tsutsumi K, Kurihara M, Kawaguchi T, Niwa M. Alteration of atrial natriuretic peptide receptors in the choroid plexus of rats with induced or congenital hydrocephalus. Childs Nerv Syst. 1990; 6(4):190–193
[19] Tsutsumi K, Niwa M, Himeno A, et al. Alpha-atrial natriuretic peptide binding sites in the rat choroid plexus are increased in the presence of hydrocephalus. Neurosci Lett. 1988; 87(1–2):93–98
[20] Diringer MN, Kirsch JR, Ladenson PW, Borel C, Hanley DF. Cerebrospinal fluid atrial natriuretic factor in intracranial disease. Stroke. 1990; 21(11):1550–1554
[21] Milhorat TH. The third circulation revisited. J Neurosurg. 1975; 42(6):628–645
[22] McGirt MJ, Woodworth G, Thomas G, Miller N, Williams M, Rigamonti D. Cerebrospinal fluid shunt placement for pseudotumor cerebri-associated intractable headache: predictors of treatment response and an analysis of long-term outcomes. J Neurosurg. 2004; 101(4):627–632

13 Intracranial Pressure Fundamentals

Tyler Carson, Dan E. Miulli, and Javed Siddiqi

Abstract

The Monro–Kellie hypothesis states that the skull is a solid box within which the volume of all the components—the brain, cerebrospinal fluid, and blood—should remain constant. Alteration in pressure in one of these compartments is compensated by volume changes in the other. The detailed neurologic examination allows the clinician to determine when there is abnormal function. This can be compensated with monitors that provide additional information about the physiological state of the brain, which in turn can be used to prevent or limit ischemia and nervous system damage.

Keywords: AVDO2, cerebral blood volume, CSF dynamics, hemodynamic monitoring, intracranial hypertension, Poiseuille's law, SVI, SVV

Case Presentation

A 42-year-old man is brought to the emergency department after rear-ending another vehicle at a high speed. He was an unrestrained driver and tested positive for ethanol and methamphetamines. His initial Glasgow Coma Scale (GCS) score was 12, but he was combative and was subsequently intubated. He has obvious signs of facial trauma and several scalp lacerations. His paralytics and sedatives have worn off, and he is localizing to central pain, but less on the left side, with no eye opening to verbal or painful stimulus. His pupils are 2 mm and reactive on the left, 4 mm and sluggish on the right. His noncontrast brain computed tomographic (CT) scan shows an 8 mm right subdural hematoma with 11 mm of midline shift at the septum pellucidum. His basilar cistern is effaced. Traumatic subarachnoid hemorrhage is also noted bilaterally in the posterior frontal region, near the vertex.

See end of chapter for Case Management.

13.1 What Is Intracranial Pressure?

Elevated intracranial pressure (ICP) remains a frequently encountered dilemma in the neurosurgical intensive care unit (NICU). Few other pathologies challenge clinicians' insight and vigilance as does intracranial hypertension. Elevated ICP results in secondary brain injury and poor neurologic outcome.[1]

Furthermore, intracranial hypertension is found in 40 to 60% of severe head injuries and is a major factor in the deaths of 50% of all fatalities.[2]

The beneficial effects of removing pieces of the skull in cases of brain swelling have been known since the time of Hippocrates, Galen, and the ancient Egyptians.[2] However, the dynamics governing intracranial pressure were not fully understood until the early 19th century. When Alexander Monro and George Kellie postulated that "anything new or exuberant cannot be intruded" within the cranium "without an equivalent displacement."[2] This would later become known as the Monro–Kellie doctrine or hypothesis, stating that "the sum of volumes of brain, CSF, and intracranial blood is constant."[3]

ICP is therefore a function of the contents of the cranial vault. The sum of the volumes of blood, brain, cerebrospinal fluid (CSF), and other elements (tumor, hematoma, abscess, edema), which are incompressible liquids and solids in the inelastic bony cranial vault together constitute the ICP.

$$V_{CSF} + V_{Blood} + V_{Brain} + V_{Other} = V_{Intracranial\ space} = Constant$$

An increase in any of the intracranial elements causes a concomitant decrease in the other elements. This principle does not apply to children with unfused sutures or to patients with comminuted skull fractures, both of whose cranial vaults are not a fixed space.

13.2 Cerebral Blood Flow, CSF Dynamics, and Intracranial Pressure

Cerebral autoregulation of blood flow has long been studied and is still not completely understood. As far back as 1939 Fog showed pial arteries to demonstrate compensatory dilatation and constriction in reaction to changes in blood pressure.[4,5] Later studies and reviews by Lassen[6] and Kontos et al[7] showed that, despite a wide range of systemic systolic blood pressures (60–140 mm Hg) the cerebral perfusion pressure remained relatively constant. In a more recent review by Koller and Toth it appears that the vasomotor response in cerebral vessels is regulated not only at large vessel on a pressure-sensitive myogenic mechanism but also regionally by flow signal metabolites, such as 20-HETE, nitric oxide, potassium, and transient receptor potential (TRP) channels.[8] Metabolic variables, such as $PaCO_2$, cerebral hyperemia resulting in nitric oxide (NO) production, K^+ and H^+ ion concentrations, and cerebral metabolic activity resulting in elevated adenosine levels have all been shown to affect cerebral blood flow[9] and are available to monitor and manipulate in the neurosurgical intensive care unit (NICU).

Tenets are based on knowledge of the cardiopulmonary system, specifically, cardiac output. In this, adjustments of vasopressors, inotropes, chronotropes, and other medication are made to optimize cerebral perfusion. Though usually requiring invasive monitoring, cardiac output may be approximated with a simple calculation:

$$\text{Cardiac output} = SV \times HR = \frac{VO_2}{AVDO_2 \times 10}$$

where SV is stroke volume, HR is heart rate, VO_2 is oxygen consumption, and $AVDO_2$ is arteriovenous oxygen content difference.

Newer advances in hemodynamic monitoring systems, such as the FloTrac sensor (Edwards), allow continuous monitoring of cardiac output, cardiac index, stroke volume, stroke volume index (SVI), and stroke volume variance (SVV). This is done though monitoring via a standard arterial line connected to the FloTrac sensor, which uses an algorithm to calculate these hemodynamic variables. The physician can direct therapy in terms of preload, afterload, and cardiac contractility to optimize these parameters based on the patient's condition. For example, SVV was shown to be a significantly better predictor of fluid responsiveness as compared to central venous pressure (CVP) and pulmonary capillary wedge pressure (PCWP).[10] The treatment algorithm shown in ▶ Fig. 13.1 can guide therapy in an attempt to improve stroke volume and in turn cardiac output.

The effect of cardiac output (CO) on cerebral blood flow (CBF) is controversial. Deegan et al showed that dynamic autoregulation of CBF remained constant with induced changes in CO via thigh cuff.[11] Bouma and Muizelaar[12] found no relationship between CO and CBF in head-injured patients. Conversely, Ogawa et al[13] showed that increases in CO via saline infusion increased CBF without a change in mean arterial pressure (MAP). Ogawa et al[13] also showed changes in CO via thigh cuff, and albumin infusion showed a linear increase or decrease in CBF without a change in MAP. Ultimately, CO likely has an effect on CBF, especially in cases when autoregulation is impaired.

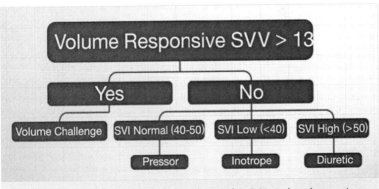

Fig. 13.1 Treatment algorithm. SVI, stroke volume index; SVV, stroke volume variance.

CBF is measurable with neuroimaging modalities, including xenon CT, positron emission tomography (PET) scanning, transcranial Doppler, and functional magnetic resonance imaging (fMRI). These techniques are usually unavailable on a continuous basis to most clinicians. CBF is dependent on cerebral perfusion pressure (CPP). Normal adult CPP is > 50 mm Hg.

CBF is related to CPP via Poiseuille's law. Using this formula, CPP is directly proportional to CBF and also to vessel radius; it is inversely proportional to blood viscosity and vessel length. Shown mathematically, Poiseulle's law is

$$CBF = \frac{8(CPP)r^4}{\pi(n)(l)},$$

where r is vessel radius, n is viscosity, and l is vessel length.

$$CPP = MAP - ICP,$$

where MAP is mean arterial pressure.

$$MAP = DBP \frac{(SBP - DBP)}{3}$$

where DBP is diastolic blood pressure and SBP is systolic blood pressure.

Optimization of CPP at 60 to 70 mm Hg has been more reliably shown to be associated with an improved neurologic outcome.[14] Normal ICP is age dependent (▶ Table 13.1).

Although many definitions for a pathological threshold of ICP have been given, 20 to 25 mm Hg is generally accepted as truly pathological.[3]

Table 13.1 Normal intracranial pressure levels[1,2,3,15,16]

cm CSF × 1.36 = mm Hg	
Dependent upon atmospheric pressure (varies with altitude), hydrostatic pressure, and filling pressure	
CSF pressure needs to be 3–5 mm Hg higher than venous pressure for absorption.	
Adults and older children	5–15 mm Hg
	6.5–19.5 cm CSF
Young children	< 3–7.4 mm Hg
Term infants	< 1.5–5.9 mm Hg
CSF pressure decreases 0.5–1.0 cm CSF for every milliliter of CSF removed. A minor decrease in pressure suggests hydrocephalus, whereas a large drop in pressure may signify tumor.	
Abbreviation. CSF, cerebrospinal fluid.	

13.3 Etiology of and Findings Associated with Intracranial Hypertension

The causes of intracranial hypertension include the following:
- Cerebral edema.
- Hyperemia (loss of autoregulation).
- Hematoma: epidural hematoma (EDH), subdural hematoma (SDH), intracerebral hemorrhage (ICH), foreign body, or combination with depressed skull fracture.
- Hydrocephalus.
  - Communicating from posttraumatic, secondary to aneurysmal subarachnoid hemorrhage (SAH) or arteriovenous malformation (AVM), meningitis.
  - Obstruction from tumor and aqueductal stenosis.
- Hypercarbia (minute ventilation is too low or impaired alveolar gas exchange).
  - Low minute ventilation.
  - Impaired gas exchange: hemothorax, pneumothorax, and pulmonary contusions.
  - Pneumonia.
  - Acute respiratory distress syndrome (ARDS).
- Venous obstruction/thrombosis.
- Agitation (increased intrathoracic and intra-abdominal pressures).
- Status epilepticus (may be without overt tonicoclonic activity).
- Vasospasm.
- Hyponatremia.

The following findings are associated with intracranial hypertension:
- Drowsiness → Somnolence → Obtundation.
- Nausea/vomiting.
- Blurred vision or diplopia.
- Cushing's triad.
  - Hypertension.
  - Bradycardia.
  - Respiratory irregularity.
- Motor or sensory deficits.
- Cranial nerve (CN) palsies: CN III for uncal herniation; CN VI for acute hydrocephalus; CN VI and VII for enlarging cerebellar hemorrhage.[3]

13.4 Monitoring Intracranial Pressure

Previously, much confusion existed regarding which patient populations would benefit from monitoring ICP.[17,18,19] Indications for ICP monitoring were

Table 13.2 Intracranial pressure ventriculostomy monitor

Indications	Contraindications
1. GCS score ≤ 8	1. Coagulopathy
2. Unclear GCS; patient going to operating room for other reason	2. Rapidly improving neurologic exam in patient with GCS score < 8 (6-hour cutoff)
3. Multisystem injury, making fluid management and neurologic exam difficult	3. Patient known to be postictal (and without obvious intracerebral injury)
4. Anticipate prolonged sedation/paralysis from other injuries (that appear more severe than head injury)	4. ICP bolt harmful to patient (i.e., increases shift in patient with trapped ventricle)
	5. Appearance of "brain death"
	6. Intoxication (without good evidence of head injury)

Abbreviations: GCS, Glasgow Coma Scale; ICP, intracranial pressure.

refined in 1995 by Bullock et al.[20] They include GCS score ≤ 8 (postresuscitation) and abnormal noncontrast brain CT or normal brain CT, but with at least two of the following: age > 40 years, SBP < 90, decerebrate or decorticate posturing on motor exam.[14]

Relative contraindications to ICP monitoring include coagulopathy (international normalized ratio [INR] > 1.3), anoxic injury ("postcode"), and metabolic causes of coma, including intoxication[14] (▶ Table 13.2).

13.4.1 Types of Monitors

Various forms of monitoring have been used to assess ICP. Currently, intraventricular catheters are by far the most common. Their usefulness is twofold: proper assessment of ICP with less drift than other modalities, and the ability to treat intracranial hypertension by evacuation of CSF. Other methods include intraparenchymal, subarachnoid, subdural, and epidural bolts and, in infants, fontanometry.

Intraventricular catheters are typically placed at Kocher's point in the frontal lobe. Other sites commonly used for ventriculoperitoneal shunts may be used, including Keen's point, Dandy's point, and Frazier's point. Landmarks exist for frontal lobe placement of intraventricular catheters. Generally, placement is performed on the nondominant side, 1 to 2 cm anterior to the coronal suture.

13.4.2 Procedure

Kocher's point is located 12.5 cm posterior to the nasion in the sagittal plane, then 2.5 cm lateral to midline. A small patch of hair is shaved, and the sterile site is prepped. After infusing lidocaine with epinephrine into the subcutaneous tissue and periosteum, a 1 to 2 cm linear incision is made. The hand drill is introduced in the trajectory of the opposite medial canthus of the eye and approximately 1 cm anterior to the tragus. After bone purchase is made through both tables of the skull, the drill is removed, and the dura is incised in a cruciate manner. A catheter is placed in the same trajectory as the drill, with the catheter advanced approximately 4 to 6 cm. A palpable "pop" through the ependymal surface is often felt, and retrieval of CSF is seen. Depending on the system used, the system is secured into place and attached for monitoring and drainage of CSF. Sterile dressings are then applied.

Intraparenchymal pressure monitors may also be placed with the above described procedure and placement of the parenchymal fiber 2 to 3 cm into the brain substance.

At many locations, triple lumen ventricular catheters are used and are supplemented with microdialysis catheters, temperature, pH, and oxygenation probes. This has provided advanced therapeutic models for optimization of multiple variables.

13.4.3 Waveforms

Normal waveforms are rarely seen due to changes associated with the traumatic population. However, the tallest peak of the ICP wave corresponds to the atrial systolic wave. The smaller peak corresponds to the A wave on the CVP waveform.

Pathological waves are due to alterations of CPP, whether resulting from increased ICP or decreased MAP, or both. An increase in ICP is thought to be associated with a sharpened appearance of the waveforms. An increase in venous pressure, conversely, has a more rounded appearance (▶ Table 13.3).

Table 13.3 Normal and abnormal intracranial pressure waveforms[15]

Increased ICP Waveform		
Peak	Wave	Origin
First large peak	Percussion wave W_1 (pulsatile)	Systolic pressure, large intracranial arteries and choroid plexus CBF
Second small peak	Tidal wave W_2 (pulsatile)	Central venous wave from right atrium, from brain increased elastance/decreased compliance
Inverted	Inverted	Miscalibrated monitor
Third small peak	Dicrotic wave W_3	Arterial pulse
Expiration	Increases overall wave	Increasing central venous pressure
Inspiration	Decreases overall wave	Decreasing central venous pressure

(continued)

Table 13.3 continued

Increased ICP Waveform		
Peak	Wave	Origin
Peak	Change with increased ICP	
First large peak	Increases slightly	
Second small peak	Increases disproportionately to first wave	
Third small peak	Increases disproportionately to first wave	

Abbreviations: CBF, cerebral blood flow; ICP, intracranial pressure.

In 1960, Lundberg described several pathologies and associated changes in waveform characteristics.[16] Lundberg A waves (plateau waves) are usually seen with ICP > 50 mm Hg. It has been postulated that there may be an associated increase in MAP. Lundberg B waves (pressure pulses) are described as an amplitude of 10 to 20 mm Hg and are associated with various types of breathing. Lundberg C waves have a frequency of 4–8/min and have been seen in normal pressures as well as with Lundberg A waves in the premorbid state (▶ Table 13.4).

Table 13.4 Abnormal intracranial pressure waveform analysis[15,16]

Lundberg A wave (plateau wave)
Mean wave > 50 mm Hg
Entire wave lasts 5–20 minutes, then returns to slightly elevated baseline
Increased cerebral blood volume from low CPP, then vasodilation, increasing ICP, lowering CPP, causing ischemia, and resulting in brainstem response
Occurs when ICP exceeds the limits of cerebral compliance; reflects ischemia
Lundberg B wave (pressure wave)
Mean wave > 20–50 mm Hg
Entire wave lasts > 30 seconds to 3 minutes.
Possibly not due to increased ICP; may be due to respiratory changes and variations in CBF
Can be seen in sleep
Suggests that Lundberg A (plateau) waves may form
Lundberg C wave (preterminal wave)
Mean wave < 20 mm Hg
Entire wave increased every 10 seconds
ICP transmission of cyclic variation in SBP

Abbreviations: CBF, cerebral blood flow; CPP, cerebral perfusion pressure; ICP, intracranial pressure; SBP, systolic blood pressure.

Case Management

The patient had a GCS score of 7 upon reexamination after his sedatives and paralytics wore off. The patient has an intracranial hematoma on the right with mass effect, with a larger right pupil (which is observed to be sluggishly reactive to light). This is an acute emergency, and the patient should be taken to the operating room immediately for evacuation of the hematoma. On the way to the operating room, his head of bed should be raised to 30 degrees. He should be hyperventilated to PCO_2 of 30 and given intravenous hypertonic saline or mannitol. After the clot is evacuated, the patient should also have a ventriculostomy/ICP monitor inserted in the operating room for diagnosis and treatment of ICP in the NICU postoperatively.

References

[1] Marmarou A, Anderson RI, Ward JD, et al. Impact of ICP instability and hypotension on outcome in patients with severe head trauma. J Neurosurg. 1991; 75:159–166

[2] Winn R. Youman's Neurological Surgery. 6th ed. Philadelphia, PA: Saunders/Elsevier; 2011

[3] Greenberg MS. Handbook of Neurosurgery. 7th ed. New York, NY: Thieme; 2010

[4] Fog M. Cerebral circulation. II. Reaction of pial arteries to increase in blood pressure. Arch Neurol Psychiatry. 1939; 41:260–268

[5] Fog M. Cerebral circulation. The reaction of pial arteries to a fall in blood pressure. Arch Neurol Psychiatry. 1937; 37:351–364

[6] Lassen NA. Cerebral blood flow and oxygen consumption in man. Physiol Rev. 1959; 39(2):183–238

[7] Kontos HA, Wei EP, Navari RM, Levasseur JE, Rosenblum WI, Patterson JL, Jr. Responses of cerebral arteries and arterioles to acute hypotension and hypertension. Am J Physiol. 1978; 234(4):H371–H383

[8] Koller A, Toth P. Contribution of flow-dependent vasomotor mechanisms to the autoregulation of cerebral blood flow. J Vasc Res. 2012; 49(5):375–389

[9] Peterson EC, Wang Z, Britz G. Regulation of cerebral blood flow. Int J Vasc Med. 2011; 2011:823525

[10] Cannesson M, Musard H, Desebbe O, et al. The ability of stroke volume variations obtained with Vigileo/FloTrac system to monitor fluid responsiveness in mechanically ventilated patients. Anesth Analg. 2009; 108(2):513–517

[11] Deegan BM, Devine ER, Geraghty MC, Jones E, Ólaighin G, Serrador JM. The relationship between cardiac output and dynamic cerebral autoregulation in humans. J Appl Physiol (1985). 2010; 109(5):1424–1431

[12] Bouma GJ, Muizelaar JP. Relationship between cardiac output and cerebral blood flow in patients with intact and with impaired autoregulation. J Neurosurg. 1990; 73(3):368–374

[13] Ogawa Y, Iwasaki K, Aoki K, Shibata S, Kato J, Ogawa S. Central hypervolemia with hemodilution impairs dynamic cerebral autoregulation. Anesth Analg. 2007; 105(5):1389–1396

[14] Bratton SL, Chestnut RM, Ghajar J, et al. Brain Trauma Foundation, American Association of Neurological Surgeons, Congress of Neurological Surgeons, Joint Section on Neurotrauma and Critical Care, AANS/CNS. Guidelines for the management of severe traumatic brain injury. VIII. Intracranial pressure thresholds. J Neurotrauma. 2007; 24 Suppl 1:S55–S58

233

[15] Narayan RK, Kishore PRS, Becker DP, et al. Intracranial pressure: to monitor or not to monitor? A review of our experience with severe head injury. J Neurosurg. 1982; 56(5):650–659

[16] Lundberg N. Continuous recording and control of ventricular fluid pressure in neurosurgical practice. Acta Psychiatr Scand Suppl. 1960; 36(149):1–193

[17] Yuan Q, Wu X, Sun Y, et al. Impact of intracranial pressure monitoring on mortality in patients with traumatic brain injury: a systematic review and meta-analysis. J Neurosurg. 2015; 122 (3):574–587

[18] Mendelson AA, Gillis C, Henderson WR, Ronco JJ, Dhingra V, Griesdale DEG. Intracranial pressure monitors in traumatic brain injury: a systematic review. Can J Neurol Sci. 2012; 39(5):571–576

[19] Heros RC. Surgical treatment of cerebellar infarction. Stroke. 1992; 23(7):937–938

[20] Bullock R, Chestnut RM, Clifton G, et al. Guidelines for the Management of Severe Head Injury. New York, NY: The Brain Trauma Foundation, American Association of Neurological Surgeons, and Joint Section of Neurotrauma and Critical Care; 1995

14 Cerebral Protection Measures

Tyler Carson, Dennis Cramer, Dan E. Miulli, and Javed Siddiqi

Abstract
Once ischemia begins in the brain time becomes critical to recognize and treat the condition. At times the systems of the body cannot be directed by nervous system communication to restore the delivery of vital nutrients or remove the cause preventing the delivery. The neurointensivist can come to the aid of the nervous system and provide augmentation to its structure and function through the judicious use of oxygen, blood pressure, and surgery. However, when those initial interventions are not adequate, when the intracranial pressure is refractory, heroic measures can be considered when adequate survival is possible. These measures are precisely delivered and not without considerable side effects.

Keywords: autoregulation, hypertonic saline, hypotension, hypothermia, hypoxia, ischemia, pentobarbital, refractory ICP

Case Presentation

A 32-year-old man was an unrestrained driver involved in a head-on traffic collision at high speed. The patient was intubated in the field, and his Glasgow Coma Scale (GCS) score on arrival to the emergency room was 6 T. Head computed tomographic scan shows diffuse petechial hemorrhages and left frontal contusion, with no midline shift or surgical hematoma demonstrated. The patient is transferred to the intensive care unit where an intracranial pressure (ICP) monitor and cerebrospinal fluid drainage device is promptly placed. Initial ICP is 20 mm Hg; however, 4 hours later the on-call physician is notified that the ICP has slowly been moving upward and is now at 35 mm Hg.

See end of chapter for Case Management.

14.1 Introduction

The ultimate result of a severe head injury primarily depends on the extent of injury at the time of incident and the extent of secondary injury in the ensuing days after the initial injury. This chapter discusses the therapies for prevention of secondary injury, the only modifiable variable from the neurocritical care standpoint.

A primary brain injury from trauma includes contusions, epidural or subdural hematomas, intracerebral hemorrhage, and diffuse axonal injuries. Secondary brain injuries include edema, ischemia, and hypoxemia, which can result in infarction and/or herniation. Initially, surgical intervention for a space-occupying mass should always be considered before proceeding to neurocritical care management. A space-occupying lesion in itself will result in secondary injury via herniation and brain ischemia if untreated.

Secondary brain injury initiates numerous pathological and chemical changes that significantly impact the patient's neurologic outcome. The mainstay of treating a secondary brain insult is to ensure adequate cerebral oxygenation. Metabolic requirements increase in the damaged brain tissue, and sufficient oxygenation is imperative to prevent cell apoptosis and secondary injury. Oxygen delivery to the brain is governed by (1) cerebral blood flow (CBF) via intracranial pressure (ICP) and cerebral perfusion pressures (CPPs), (2) oxygen carrying capacity of the blood, and (3) arterial partial pressure of oxygen. Many studies indicate that the overall outcome for patients with severe traumatic brain injury (TBI) is directly affected by hypoxia and elevated ICPs.[1,2]

Because CBF is difficult to measure, physicians can easily follow the mean arterial pressure (MAP) and ICP to estimate CPP. CBF is related to MAP and ICP, as shown in the following equations:

$$CBF = CPP/CVR = (MAP - ICP)/CVR,$$

where CVR is cerebrovascular resistance.

The equations show the complex relationship between brain perfusion and blood pressure. The Monro–Kellie hypothesis, which helps to explain the significance of ICP, states that the sum of the intracranial volumes of blood, brain tissue, and cerebrospinal fluid (CSF) are constant and that any increase in one component will be counterbalanced by a decrease in another. The volume of brain tissue is 90%; blood and CSF are 5% each. All of these are contained within the rigid skull. The introduction of additional volume, such as from hemorrhage or edema, must be compensated by changes in the blood or CSF volumes. Failure to counterbalance these changes will result in increased ICP and possibly intracranial shifts (herniation). Increased ICP can be compensated by shifting CSF from the ventricles and subarachnoid space to the spinal canal or by decreasing the intracranial blood volume via collapsing veins and constricting cerebral arteries. Changes in vessel diameter can result in a reduction of cerebral intravascular volume by as much as 70 mL, easily buffering a new volume mass, such as a hemorrhage.[3]

After compensatory mechanisms for increased ICP are exhausted the patient begins suffering from secondary brain insults. Eighty to 90% of patients with TBI who die are found to have histopathological evidence of cerebral ischemia.[4] Studies show that approximately one-third of patients with TBI experience an "ultra-early" period of significantly decreased cerebral blood within 6 hours of injury.[5] The ischemia is characterized by focal reductions in CBF below the threshold of 18 mL/100 g/min, resulting in ischemic neuronal cell death.[6] The hypoxic conditions perpetuate a hypermetabolic rate, resulting in an aerobic to anaerobic metabolism and leading to an increased concentration of lactic acid.[7] Ionic homeostasis is then compromised, leading to a complex process of calcium influx and cellular injury and death.[8]

Therefore strict ICP and CPP management is paramount in prevention of secondary injury. Options available for ICP management start with basic patient positioning—with the head of the bed elevated and the neck straight to improve venous outflow. Emphasis must be placed on normocarbia with a goal of $PaCO_2$ 35–40. Short-term hyperventilation may be beneficial in acute herniation; however, the resultant reduction in CBF has been shown to worsen outcomes in periods of prolonged therapy.[2] In turn, hypercarbia must be avoided as well because it results in vasodilation and increased ICP.

Hyperosmolar agents, such as mannitol and 23.4% hypertonic saline (HTS), can be used to mobilize extravascular water to intravascular space, in turn reducing cerebral edema. Recent studies point to improved results with side-effect profile with HTS versus mannitol[9,10] because mannitol tends to result in a drop in blood pressure and in turn decreased CBF. In addition, with prolonged administration, mannitol tends to have a rebound increase in ICP as it collects in brain tissue where the blood–brain barrier has been disrupted. Serum sodium and osmolarity should be monitored every 6 hours with either bolus hyperosmolar therapy or continuous infusions of 3% hypertonic saline. Serum osmolality > 320 mOsmol/L and serum sodium > 160 mmol/L are associated with an increased risk of nephrotoxicity and should be avoided. Recommended target serum sodium is within the range of 145–155 mmol/L.[11]

Anemia in the setting of brain injury has been shown to result in poor neurologic outcome. Laboratory studies using animal models and healthy human subjects suggest that anemia below a hemoglobin (Hb) concentration of 7 g/dL results in impaired brain function and below 10 g/dL may be detrimental to recovery from TBI. Models indicate impairment in delivery of oxygen (DO_2) with hemoglobin levels < 10 mg/dL. However, it remains controversial as to the minimal threshold for packed red blood cells (PRBC) transfusion in the brain injury patient.[12,13] Some studies point to worse outcomes in TBI patients who receive transfusions but fail to account for severity of disease. It is the standard practice at our institution to transfuse brain injury patients with Hb levels < 10 mg/dL.

New technologies, such as the Licox Brain Oxygen Monitoring System (Integra), which monitors brain tissue oxygenation, have given the neurocritical care physician another tool to guide therapy. Therapy directed specifically at brain tissue oxygenation has shown good results. A 2012 review of patients with TBI showed that 61% of patients with TBI had a favorable outcome with brain tissue oxygen-based therapy compared with 42% of patients who had a favorable outcome with ICP/CPP goal-directed therapy.[14] Brain tissue oxygen tension of < 15 mm Hg is associated with a significantly worse outcome and death compared with patients whose $PBTO_2$ remained > 15 mm Hg.[2] No specific guidelines for brain tissue oxygen monitoring currently exist, but it is a promising and useful adjunctive parameter for management of brain injury patients.

14.2 Pharmacological Cerebral Metabolic Depressants

An estimated 15% of all head-injured patients suffer from refractory ICP.[15] When all other medical and surgical modalities have failed to adequately control elevated ICP, the physician may attempt the use of pharmacological agents to reduce the cerebral metabolic rate (CMR) and hence ICP in a patient who is deemed salvageable. Many pharmacological agents have been used to lower ICP, such as pentobarbital, thiopental, etomidate, propofol, isoflurane, and desflurane, but not enough data exist to recommend one drug over another. Most published information addresses the use of barbiturates, especially pentobarbital.

In 1974, Shapiro et al were the first to report the use of pentobarbital-augmented hypothermia in reducing CMR and ICP.[16] This therapy remains controversial, mainly because of the potential side effects of myocardial hypotension, hypothermia, immunosuppression, hypokalemia, and hepatic and renal dysfunction.[17] Accordingly, the Brain Trauma Foundation, in cooperation with the American Association of Neurological Surgeons, has recommended a guideline using high-dose barbiturate therapy in hemodynamically stable head-injured patients with elevated ICP resistant to maximal medical and surgical treatment modalities.[2]

Because of marked hypotension seen in ~ 50% of patients treated with barbiturates, many will require cardiac inotropes and/or vasopressors to maintain an MAP resulting in a CPP ≥ 70 mm Hg,[18] unless increased secondary risk concerns favor an acceptable lower CPP. Dopamine (primarily a vasoconstrictor) is commonly used starting at 3 µg/kg/min and titrating to a maximum 20 µg/kg/min to maintain CPP ≥ 70 mm Hg. Phenylephrine starting between 100 and 180 µg/min, with a maintenance dosage of 40 to 60 µg/min, or norepinephrine at 8 to 12 µg/min is frequently used for progressively decreasing CPP and/or hypotension. Hemodynamic monitoring via the FloTrac sensor (Edwards) or similar monitoring may be necessary to adjust cardiac medications and to ensure adequate volume status, systemic resistance, and cardiac output.

Many protocols have been used to administer barbiturate therapy. Eisenberg's protocol starts with a loading dose of pentobarbital at 10 mg/kg intravenous (IV) over 60 minutes, followed by 5 mg/kg every hour for 3 hours, with a maintenance dosage of 1 to 3 mg/kg/h.[19] In a study by Cormio et al on 67 patients with severe head injury undergoing treatment for refractory intracranial hypertension, pentobarbital loading doses decreased ICP and MAPs on average by 12 and 9 mm Hg, respectively.[20] A more recent study by Marshall et al using Eisenberg's protocol found response rates to pentobarbital therapy for refractory ICP of 38%, defined as ICP < 25 mm Hg for 24 hours after therapy initiation.[21] It can generally be considered that if the induced pentobarbital coma does not lower the ICP within 1 to 4 hours, it is unlikely to succeed without any other therapy.

Thiopental has been used with good reported outcomes; however, availability has become a limiting factor in the United States. It works by producing cerebral metabolic depression and cerebral vasoconstriction. The loading dose is 5 mg/kg IV over 10 minutes, with a continuous infusion of 5 mg/kg/h (range 3–5 mg) for 24 hours. After 24 hours, the infusion may be decreased to 2.5 mg/kg/h because fat stores have now become saturated.

Propofol is a well-established sedative-hypnotic agent that has been used as an alternative to control elevated ICP, but questions remain regarding the pharmacodynamics of the drug. A study by Oertel et al has suggested a key mechanism responsible for the metabolic suppressive effect is a decrease in CO_2 production, resulting in a global "pharmacological hypocapnia."[22] TBI guidelines[2] recommend propofol for control of ICP, but it has not shown any improvement in mortality or 6-month outcome, and high doses can produce significant morbidity, such as in the case in propofol infusion syndrome.[23] The starting dose is 5 to 10 µg/kg/min and increases by 5 to 10 µg/kg/min every 5 to 10 minutes until ICP is controlled. Like the barbiturates, propofol exhibits hypotensive effects that may require cardiac medications or eventual discontinuation. In addition to the cardiotoxic effects, propofol may cause electrocardiographic changes and discoloration of urine.

A continuous electroencephalogram is recommended to monitor electrocerebral activity. Burst suppression of 1 to 3 bursts/page may not be necessary if control of ICP ≤ 20 to 25 mm Hg is achieved without the use of larger doses of the cerebral metabolic depressant agents.

Pharmacologically induced burst suppression is generally maintained 3 to 7 days; if computed tomography (CT) does not show any new findings, and ICP has been controlled, then therapy can be withdrawn slowly by reducing the infusion rate while monitoring ICP. Because of prolonged high-dose barbiturate therapy and the long half-lives of these drugs, it is difficult to distinguish the residual pharmacological effects from the clinical condition. If a high index of suspicion for brain death is entertained, a nuclear cerebral metabolic test is warranted; if the test is negative, one should proceed with a cerebral angiogram before pronouncing brain death.

The prophylactic use of barbiturates for ICP treatment has shown no benefits in patients with intracranial mass lesions and was even found to be harmful in patients with diffuse injury (mortality of 77% vs. 41% in the mannitol group).[24] A 2000 Cochrane Database review evaluating barbiturate therapy in acute TBI concluded that there was no evidence that barbiturate therapy improves outcome for patients with acute severe brain injuries. The review also demonstrated that barbiturate therapy results in a decrease in blood pressure in one in four patients, and this hypotensive effect will offset any ICP-lowering effect on cerebral perfusion.[25]

Alternative agents to pentobarbital have not been well studied, but they have been used because of easier accessibility. A study comparing etomidate, isoflurane, and thiopental in animals undergoing 3 hours of middle cerebral artery occlusion found injured brain volume largest in the etomidate and isoflurane groups and smallest in the thiopental group.[26]

Surgical management for refractory ICP in the form of decompressive craniectomy should be considered prior to or in conjunction with metabolic depressants or hypothermic therapies. The study by Aarabi et al[27] comparing outcome following decompressive craniectomy for refractory ICP showed a 28% mortality rate postcraniectomy compared to studies by Eisenberg et al and Marshall et al[19,21] on pentobarbital therapy alone in refractory ICP of 62% and 64% mortality, respectively.

14.3 Hypothermia

Control of temperature is of extreme importance in the head-injured patient. Mild induced hypothermia (MIH) has been studied extensively as both a prophylactic neuroprotectant measure and in "late phase" for management of refractory ICP. The benefits of MIH are directed at prevention of secondary injury through reduction of the cerebral metabolic rate of oxygen, reduced cerebral glucose demand, inhibition of excitotoxicity, reduction in thermal pooling, inhibition of early gene expression, and prevention of apoptotic cell death.[28] In a recent review study by Urbano and Oddo[28] 17 controlled trials were evaluated in which patients with severe TBI with refractory intracranial hypertension were treated with MIH therapy. In comparison to normothermia all 17 studies showed a significant reduction in ICP, and 12 of the 17 studies found a significant improvement in patient outcome. Another recent systematic review by Sadaka and Veremakis[29] found significantly lower ICP in patients treated with MIH (range 10–25 mm Hg) than in those assigned to normothermia (range 20–35 mm Hg).

The optimal temperature target for MIH is 35–36°C. Tokutomi and colleagues reported that lowering body temperatures to 35 to 36°C could reduce intracranial hypertension while maintaining CPP without significant cardiac dysfunction or oxygen delivery abnormalities.[30] Temperatures below 35°C have been associated with worse outcomes. Gupta et al showed MIH below 35°C decreases brain tissue oxygenation.[31]

The duration of treatment is directed toward ICP reduction. Typical treatment periods range from 3 to 5 days. A recent meta-analysis by McIntyre et al[32] found MIH therapy > 48 hours to be associated with better outcomes and a study by Jiang et al[33] compared 2-day average time of MIH therapy to 5-day average time of therapy and found a significant improvement in outcome with a 5-day treatment period without increased complications.

Rapid rewarming should be avoided at all costs. Studies have shown not only reversal of the protective effect of MIH with rapid rewarming but also rebound cerebral edema due to hyperemia leading to rebound intracranial hypertension.[34] Slow, controlled ($0.1-0.2°C/h$) rewarming is recommended after MIH to reduce the risk of rebound cerebral edema and intracranial hypertension.[32]

The results for MIH as a prophylactic neuroprotectant therapy, however, have not shown any significant discernible benefit thus far. The recently published National Acute Brain Injury Study: Hypothermia II (NABIS: HII) by Clifton et al[35] enrolled 232 TBI patients across six sites in the United States and Canada. The treatment group of patients had MIH therapy initiated within 2 to 5 hours of injury and were cooled to a temp of 35°C initially, with further cooling to 33°C if criteria were met. Patients were maintained at this temperature for 48 hours and slowly rewarmed. No significant difference in Glasgow Outcome Score (GOS) was noted between those patients who received MIH and normothermic patients and the trial was terminated in June 2009 for futility. Other studies of early MIH therapy have echoed this result. The Sydenham et al[36] review of early MIH therapy evaluated 23 trials with 1,614 patients. There was a slight benefit reducing death and unfavorable outcome in patients treated with MIH; however, when correcting for low-quality trials no significant difference was noted.

Clearly MIH therapy has a benefit in treatment of refractory intracranial hypertension with relatively well defined treatment parameters. Furthermore, there is clear scientific evidence of the benefit of hypothermia in prevention of secondary neuronal injury. Clinical trials, however, have been unable to show any significant quantifiable benefit in the early prophylactic use of hypothermia in TBI; therefore such practice is not standard treatment.

14.4 Blood Glucose Control

TBI leads to numerous neurochemical events and is associated with a catecholamine stress response, including hyperglycemia.[37] Many studies have shown hyperglycemia to correlate with the severity of brain injury and to be a predictor of neurologic outcome.[38,39,40] A study by Young et al showed that patients who had the highest peak admission 24-hour serum glucose level had the worst neurologic outcome at 18 days from injury.[38] The researchers also found that patients with a peak 24-hour serum glucose level > 200 mg/dL had a 2-point decrease in their GOS and that those patients with a serum glucose level < 200 mg/dL experienced a 4-point increase during the 18-day study period. Rovlias and Kotsou also found serum glucose levels > 200 mg/dL in the first 24 hours to be highly predictive of an unfavorable outcome.[41]

Kushner et al found the median initial serum glucose level in patients with acute ischemic cerebral infarction to be 155 mg/dL.[40] Additionally, clinical recovery was significantly poorer in patients with an initial glucose level greater than the median. The researchers reported that serum glucose admission levels correlated with the extent of metabolic brain abnormalities seen on acute positron emission tomography (PET) scanning.

During normal aerobic metabolism, energy in the brain is formed primarily when glucose is oxidized to CO_2 and water. The cellular metabolism of glucose begins with the process of glycolysis, resulting in the generation of pyruvate, the reduced form of nicotinamide adenine dinucleotide (NADH), and adenosine triphosphate (ATP):

$$Glucose + 2ADP + 2P_i + 2NAD^+ \rightarrow 2Pyruvate + 2ATP + 2NADH + 2H^+ + 2H_2O,$$

where ADP is adenosine diphosphate.

Pyruvate can be converted to lactate or to the amino acid alanine, or it can enter the citric acid, or Krebs, cycle (▶ Fig. 14.1). The energy products derived from the citric acid, or Krebs, cycle (tricarboxylic acid) are used in the final step of glucose metabolism as it enters the electron transport chain (ETC; ▶ Fig. 14.2). The end result of glucose breakdown is 38 moles of ATP, which is more efficient than the 6 moles of ATP produced via glycolysis alone. The detrimental effects of hypoxic or ischemic brain injury result from anaerobic metabolism in which glucose is converted to lactate and hydrogen ions, rather than pyruvate. With increased levels of glucose available for lactate production, excessive lactate accumulation leads to greater tissue acidosis and subsequent neuronal damage.[42] There is considerable evidence of TBI patients with serum glucose levels correlated with neurologic outcome. However, further clinical trials are needed to address neurologic outcome with strict glucose control in the acute brain injury.

14.5 Antiapoptotic/Neuromodulators

Development of medications to limit secondary injury caused by inflammatory response leading to cell apoptosis is an intriguing new adjuvant treatment modality. To this point in time no specific medications have any proven utility in the clinical setting of TBI. Simvastatin, which has been shown to improve outcomes and provide a neuroprotective effect in patients with aneurysmal subarachnoid hemorrhage (SAH),[43] is currently being evaluated for use in TBI. Statins inhibit 3-hydroxy-3-methylglutaryl coenzyme A reductase and block the formation of mevalonate, an important precursor for both cholesterol and nonsterol products.[44,45] This mechanism accounts for the neuroprotective

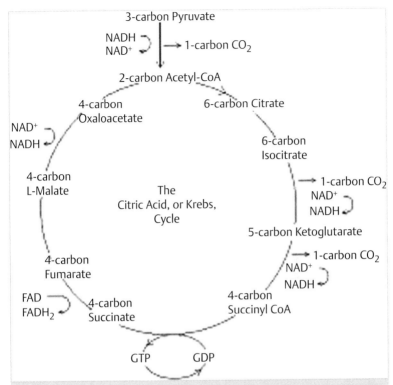

Fig. 14.1 The citric acid, or Krebs, cycle. CoA, coenzyme A; GDP, guanosine diphosphate; GTP, guanosine triphosphate; COQ, coenzyme Q; NAD+, oxidized form of nicotinamide adenine dinucleotide; NADH, reduced form of nicotinamide adenine dinucleotide.

properties of statins by improving endothelial vasomotor function, increasing endothelial cell fibrinolytic activities, reducing thrombogenic potential, blocking platelet activation, and suppressing cytokine responses during cerebral ischemia.[44,46] Animal models have shown that these neuroprotective effects clinically demonstrated in aneurysmal SAH may also apply in TBI. Wu et al[47] showed that in a rat model simvastatin after TBI significantly improved functional recovery by augmenting angiogenesis in the lesion boundary zone via the vascular endothelial growth factor receptor (VEGFR)-2/Akt/endothelial NO synthase signaling pathway. A recent study by Xie et al[48] showed enhanced proliferation and neurogenesis of cultured stem cells from rats treated with simvastatin after TBI.

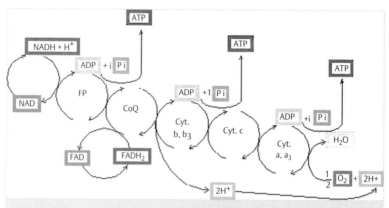

Fig. 14.2 Electron transport chain. ADP, adenosine diphosphate; ATP, adenosine triphosphate; COQ, coenzyme Q; FP, flavoprotein.

Other compounds, such as NNZ-2566, a Glypromate (Neuren) analogue, have also been shown to improve functional recovery and attenuate apoptosis and inflammation in a rat model after TBI.[49] NNZ-2566 has completed phase 2 clinical trial in TBI patients, and final analysis is pending.

The role of neuroprotective pharmacological treatments in TBI is likely to grow in the future with the development of new medications and the results of studies currently under way.

Case Management

In the case of the 32-year-old man, a CT scan should be repeated to identify any surgical hematomas. Efforts to decrease the ICP and increase the CPP should be undertaken. Initially, the physician should ensure that the head-injured patient is well sedated and that his pain is being treated. If elevated ICP issues continue, the physician may consider mannitol and/or hypertonic saline, and possibly starting a vassopressor and/or inotrope to maintain the CPP at the desired goal. If the patient's elevated ICP remains refractory to the previous medications, one may consider placing him into a pharmacologically induced coma.

References

[1] Marmarou A, Anderson RI, Ward JD, et al. Impact of ICP instability and hypotension on outcome in patients with severe head trauma. J Neurosurg. 1991; 75 Suppl 1:S:59–S–66

[2] Bratton SL, Chestnut RM, Ghajar J, et al. Brain Trauma Foundation, American Association of Neurological, Surgeons, Congress of Neurological Surgeons, Joint Section on Neurotrauma and Critical Care, AANS/CNS. Guidelines for the management of severe traumatic brain injury. VIII. Intracranial pressure thresholds. J Neurotrauma. 2007; 24 Suppl 1:S55–S58

[3] Wijdicks E. The Clinical Practice of Critical Care Neurology. New York, NY: Lippincott-Raven; 1997

[4] Graham Dl. The pathology of brain ischaemia and possibilities for therapeutic intervention. Br J Anaesth. 1985; 57(1):3–17

[5] Bouma GJ, Muizelaar JP, Stringer WA, Choi SC, Fatouros P, Young HF. Ultra-early evaluation of regional cerebral blood flow in severely head-injured patients using xenon-enhanced computerized tomography. J Neurosurg. 1992; 77(3):360–368

[6] Schröder ML, Muizelaar JP, Bullock MR, Salvant JB, Povlishock JT. Focal ischemia due to traumatic contusions documented by stable xenon-CT and ultrastructural studies. J Neurosurg. 1995; 82 (6):966–971

[7] Kraig RP, Petito CK, Plum F, Pulsinelli WA. Hydrogen ions kill brain at concentrations reached in ischemia. J Cereb Blood Flow Metab. 1987; 7(4):379–386

[8] Bullock R, Zauner A, Woodward JJ, et al. Factors affecting excitatory amino acid release following severe human head injury. J Neurosurg. 1998; 89(4):507–518

[9] Kamel H, Navi BB, Nakagawa K, Hemphill JC, III, Ko NU. Hypertonic saline versus mannitol for the treatment of elevated intracranial pressure: a meta-analysis of randomized clinical trials. Crit Care Med. 2011; 39(3):554–559

[10] Marko NF. Hypertonic saline, not mannitol, should be considered gold-standard medical therapy for intracranial hypertension. Crit Care. 2012; 16(1):113

[11] Ogden AT, Mayer SA, Connolly ES, Jr. Hyperosmolar agents in neurosurgical practice: the evolving role of hypertonic saline. Neurosurgery. 2005; 57(2):207–215, discussion 207–215

[12] Kramer AH, Zygun DA. Anemia and red blood cell transfusion in neurocritical care. Crit Care. 2009; 13(3):R89

[13] Utter GH, Shahlaie K, Zwienenberg-Lee M, Muizelaar JP. Anemia in the setting of traumatic brain injury: the arguments for and against liberal transfusion. J Neurotrauma. 2011; 28(1):155–165

[14] Nangunoori R, Maloney-Wilensky E, Stiefel M, et al. Brain tissue oxygen-based therapy and outcome after severe traumatic brain injury: a systematic literature review. Neurocrit Care. 2012; 17 (1):131–138

[15] Gudeman SK, Miller JD, Becker DP. Failure of high-dose steroid therapy to influence intracranial pressure in patients with severe head injury. J Neurosurg. 1979; 51(3):301–306

[16] Shapiro HM, Wyte SR, Loeser J. Barbiturate-augmented hypothermia for reduction of persistent intracranial hypertension. J Neurosurg. 1974; 40(1):90–100

[17] Schalén W, Messeter K, Nordström CH. Complications and side effects during thiopentone therapy in patients with severe head injuries. Acta Anaesthesiol Scand. 1992; 36(4):369–377

[18] Rea GL, Rockswold GL. Barbiturate therapy in uncontrolled intracranial hypertension. Neurosurgery. 1983; 12(4):401–404

[19] Eisenberg HM, Frankowski RF, Contant CF, Marshall LF, Walker MD. High-dose barbiturate control of elevated intracranial pressure in patients with severe head injury. J Neurosurg. 1988; 69 (1):15–23

[20] Cormio M, Gopinath SP, Valadka A, Robertson CS. Cerebral hemodynamic effects of pentobarbital coma in head-injured patients. J Neurotrauma. 1999; 16(10):927–936

[21] Marshall G, James R, Landman M, et al. Pentobarbital coma for refractory intra-cranial hypertension after severe traumatic brain injury: mortality predictions and one- year outcomes in 55 patients. J Trauma. 2010; 69(2):275:2–83

[22] Oertel M, Kelly DF, Lee JH, Glenn TC, Vespa PM, Martin NA. Metabolic suppressive therapy as a treatment for intracranial hypertension–why it works and when it fails. Acta Neurochir Suppl (Wien). 2002; 81:69–70

[23] Kelly DF, Goodale DB, Williams J, et al. Propofol in the treatment of moderate and severe head injury: a randomized, prospective double-blinded pilot trial. J Neurosurg. 1999; 90(6):1042–1052

[24] Schwartz ML, Tator CH, Rowed DW, Reid SR, Meguro K, Andrews DF. The University of Toronto head injury treatment study: a prospective, randomized comparison of pentobarbital and mannitol. Can J Neurol Sci. 1984; 11(4):434–440

[25] Roberts I. Barbiturates for acute traumatic brain injury. Cochrane Database Syst Rev. 2000(2): CD000033

[26] Drummond JC, Cole DJ, Patel PM, Reynolds LW. Focal cerebral ischemia during anesthesia with etomidate, isoflurane, or thiopental: a comparison of the extent of cerebral injury. Neurosurgery. 1995; 37(4):742–748, discussion 748–749

[27] Aarabi B, Hesdorffer DC, Ahn ES, Aresco C, Scalea TM, Eisenberg HM. Outcome following decompressive craniectomy for malignant swelling due to severe head injury. J Neurosurg. 2006; 104 (4):469–479

[28] Urbano LA, Oddo M. Therapeutic hypothermia for traumatic brain injury. Curr Neurol Neurosci Rep. 2012; 12(5):580–591

[29] Sadaka F, Veremakis C. Therapeutic hypothermia for the management of intracranial hypertension in severe traumatic brain injury: a systematic review. Brain Inj. 2012; 26(7–8):899–908

[30] Tokutomi T, Morimoto K, Miyagi T, Yamaguchi S, Ishikawa K, Shigemori M. Optimal temperature for the management of severe traumatic brain injury: effect of hypothermia on intracranial pressure, systemic and intracranial hemodynamics, and metabolism. Neurosurgery. 2003; 52(1):102–111, discussion 111–112

[31] Gupta AK, Al-Rawi PG, Hutchinson PJ, Kirkpatrick PJ. Effect of hypothermia on brain tissue oxygenation in patients with severe head injury. Br J Anaesth. 2002; 88(2):188–192

[32] McIntyre LA, Fergusson DA, Hébert PC, Moher D, Hutchison JS. Prolonged therapeutic hypothermia after traumatic brain injury in adults: a systematic review. JAMA. 2003; 289(22):2992–2999

[33] Jiang JY, Xu W, Li WP, et al. Effect of long-term mild hypothermia or short-term mild hypothermia on outcome of patients with severe traumatic brain injury. J Cereb Blood Flow Metab. 2006; 26 (6):771–776

[34] Iida K, Kurisu K, Arita K, Ohtani M. Hyperemia prior to acute brain swelling during rewarming of patients who have been treated with moderate hypothermia for severe head injuries. J Neurosurg. 2003; 98(4):793–799

[35] Clifton GL, Valadka A, Zygun D, et al. Very early hypothermia induction in patients with severe brain injury (the National Acute Brain Injury Study: Hypothermia II): a randomised trial. Lancet Neurol. 2011; 10(2):131–139

[36] Sydenham E, Roberts I, Alderson P. Hypothermia for traumatic head injury. Cochrane Database Syst Rev. 2009(2):CD001048

[37] Rosner MJ, Newsome HH, Becker DP. Mechanical brain injury: the sympathoadrenal response. J Neurosurg. 1984; 61(1):76–86

[38] Young B, Ott L, Dempsey R, Haack D, Tibbs P. Relationship between admission hyperglycemia and neurologic outcome of severely brain-injured patients. Ann Surg. 1989; 210(4):466–472, discussion 472–473

[39] Feibel JH, Hardy PM, Campbell RG, Goldstein MN, Joynt RJ. Prognostic value of the stress response following stroke. JAMA. 1977; 238(13):1374–1376

[40] Kushner M, Nencini P, Reivich M, et al. Relation of hyperglycemia early in ischemic brain infarction to cerebral anatomy, metabolism, and clinical outcome. Ann Neurol. 1990; 28(2):129–135

[41] Rovlias A, Kotsou S. The influence of hyperglycemia on neurological outcome in patients with severe head injury. Neurosurgery. 2000; 46(2):335–342, discussion 342–343

[42] Marsh WR, Anderson RE, Sundt TM, Jr. Effect of hyperglycemia on brain pH levels in areas of focal incomplete cerebral ischemia in monkeys. J Neurosurg. 1986; 65(5):693–696

[43] Chen J, Zhang ZG, Li Y, et al. Statins induce angiogenesis, neurogenesis, and synaptogenesis after stroke. Ann Neurol. 2003; 53(6):743–751

[44] Goldstein JL, Brown MS. Regulation of the mevalonate pathway. Nature. 1990; 343(6257):425–430

[45] Delanty N, Vaughan CJ. Vascular effects of statins in stroke. Stroke. 1997; 28(11):2315–2320

[46] Vaughan CJ, Delanty N. Neuroprotective properties of statins in cerebral ischemia and stroke. Stroke. 1999; 30(9):1969–1973

[47] Wu H, Jiang H, Lu D, et al. Induction of angiogenesis and modulation of vascular endothelial growth factor receptor-2 by simvastatin after traumatic brain injury. Neurosurgery. 2011; 68 (5):1363–1371, discussion 1371

[48] Xie C, Cong D, Wang X, et al. The effect of simvastatin treatment on proliferation and differentiation of neural stem cells after traumatic brain injury. Brain Res. 2015; 1602:1–8

[49] Lu XC, Chen RW, Yao C, et al. NNZ-2566, a glypromate analog, improves functional recovery and attenuates apoptosis and inflammation in a rat model of penetrating ballistic-type brain injury. J Neurotrauma. 2009; 26(1):141–154

15 Neuropharmacology

John Ogunlade, Nicholas Qandah, and Dan E. Miulli

Abstract

The neurointensivist's expertise in medical management is equivalent to the expertise in surgical management of the nervous system. Not only are systemic conditions treated to improve the organs of the body, the systemic conditions are treated to ensure that the brain and spinal cord receive the optimal delivery of nutrients. Treating one organ does not preclude understanding how the treatment affects the brain. Some medications, although excellent for the heart, might harm the brain and lead to a less desirable overall outcome. Neuropharmacology allows the clinician to meticulously calculate the treatment of the nervous system injury and prevent other primary and secondary injuries.

Keywords: ACE, alpha agonist, beta blocker, calcium channel blocker, hemodynamic agents, magnesium, nitrogen, vasopressors

> ## Case Study
>
> A 45-year-old man was an unrestrained driver of a motorcycle that was involved in an accident. He is taken to the trauma center with a Glasgow Coma Scale score of 8; his pupils are sluggish and reactive. He is intubated. He has multiple fractures and an elevated intracranial pressure of 30 mm Hg and cerebral perfusion pressure of 55 mm Hg.
>
> *See end of chapter for Case Management.*

15.1 Introduction

Treating the neurosurgical patient requires forethought and very close attention to detail, and therefore each form of treatment, whether surgical or medical management, must be meticulously calculated, as even the simplest decisions can drastically change the patient's outcome. In patients who have suffered a primary injury to the brain, once the initial insult has been addressed, the role of treatment shifts to the prevention of secondary injury caused by hypotension, hypoxia, hyperemia, hypertension, electrolyte imbalances, or infection, just to name a few. This chapter examines the medications used in the prevention and treatment of primary and secondary brain injuries.

15.2 Hemodynamic Agents

15.2.1 Hypertension

Hypertension is a chronic disease that can cause a severe acute neurological injury or can exponentially exacerbate secondary injury to the central nervous system (CNS). Treatment of chronic hypertension and/or transient hypertension is based on understanding the underlying cause. In a patient with traumatic brain injury, blood pressure is tightly regulated to allow a therapeutic range of cerebral perfusion pressure (CPP), normalize intracranial pressure (ICP) and prevent rebleeding or hemorrhagic stroke in dead necrotic brain parenchyma. In patients with ischemic stroke "permissive hypertension is allowed to a systolic blood pressure limit (usually 160–180 mm Hg) to allow profusion to penumbra. Though there are many pharmaceutical agents that can be used to treat hypertension, knowing each agent's mechanism of action can yield favorable results and prevent unintended outcomes from inherent side effects of these agents. Always remember to order blood pressure and heart rate parameters when writing for a drug.[1,2] Furthermore, it is vitally important that when blood pressure control is paramount not to order blood pressure medication as "BID," "TID," and so forth, but to write for the specific times ordered. This will also allow staggering of the blood pressure medication and prevent the large swings of blood pressure that can occur if multiple antihypertensives are given at the same time.

15.2.2 Nitrogen

Nitrogen-based drugs react with oxyhemoglobin to produce nitrous oxide, which causes vasodilation, reducing systemic resistance and in turn reducing systolic blood pressure. In patients with suspected elevated ICP (e.g., hemorrhagic stroke, traumatic brain injury, or malignant cerebral edema) this class of antihypertensives should not be used due to its mechanism of action, vasodilation, which would also occur in the cranium.[3] According to the Monro–Kellie doctrine this increase in intravascular blood volume would cause an increasing ICP, thus decreasing CPP and leading to secondary injury. This class of drug also has the side effects of coronary steal syndrome, headache, hypotension, rebound hypertension, and methemoglobinemia, which can result in undesirable patient outcome. However, there may be a role for vasodilation during times of increased cardiac output.

Sodium Nitroprusside (Nipride)

Action: Reacts with oxyhemoglobin to form cyanide and nitric oxide (NO). NO stimulates cyclic guanosine monophosphate (cGMP) production, causing potent vasodilation (arterial > venous) and hepatic and renal metabolism.[1,4]

Contraindications: Increased ICP, intracranial mass lesion (raises ICP), pregnancy.[1,3]

Rx: Intravenous (IV) drip 0.25 to 8 µg/kg/min. To prepare: 50 mg in 500 mL dextrose 5% in water (D5W) = 100 µg/mL; can be double concentrated to reduce fluid or glucose load.[1,5]

Side effects: "Cerebral and coronary steal" phenomenon due to preferential peripheral vasodilation before cerebral vasodilation. Thiocyanate/cyanide toxicity causes neurologic deterioration and hypotension (cover bottle with foil: light sensitive). Nausea, diuresis, platelet inhibition; may increase ICP.[1,3,4]

Nitroglycerin (Tridil)

Action: Releases NO, resulting in guanylyl cyclase stimulation of cGMP synthesis. This medication acts predominantly on venous capacitance vessels, affecting arterial vascular smooth muscle at higher concentrations. Primarily venodilation without reflex tachycardia.[1,4]

Contraindication: Increased ICP or decreased cerebral perfusion[1,2,3]

Rx: IV drip 10 to 20 µg/min (increase by 5–10 µg/min every 5–10 min).[1,4,5]

Side effects: Does not cause "coronary steal"; can cause transient increase in ICP, headache, hypotension, rebound hypertension, and methemoglobinemia.[1,2,3,4,5]

Hydralazine (Apresoline)

Action: Direct arteriolar smooth muscle vasodilator; may act through NO or calcium.[1,4]

Contraindication: Liver metabolism; slow acetylators should not receive > 200 mg/d—may induce lupus-like syndrome.[1,4]

Rx: 10 to 20 mg every 15 to 20 minutes, maximum 40 mg; repeat as needed.[1,4,5]

Side effects: Nausea/vomiting, headache, increased intracranial blood flow, reflex tachycardia.[1,4]

15.2.3 Beta Blockers

Beta blockers are a first-line drug in traumatic brain injury and hemorrhagic stroke as they have been associated with a significant reduction in mortality.

Beta blockers should not be used in patients with a history of cocaine or methamphetamine abuse due to the potential of inciting drug-induced coronary artery vasoconstriction.[6,7,8] The combination of beta blockers and stimulants, such as cocaine and methamphetamines, can cause systemic vasoconstriction and paradoxical hypertension. This is due to the release of norepinephrine in excess (from stimulant use) compounded with blockade of β-adrenergic receptors (β_2 causes vasodilation) causing unopposed α_1-adrenergic receptor stimulation. The end result is vasoconstriction, which can exacerbate hemorrhagic stroke and cause increased ICP, cerebral ischemia, myocardial infarction, and death.

Labetalol (Normodyne)

Action: Blocks α_1 selective, β nonselective; hepatic glucuronide conjugation; may lower ICP.[1,4,8]

Contraindications: Asthma, pregnancy.[1]

Rx: Give each dose by slow intravenous push (IVP) (over 2 minutes) every 10 minutes until desired blood pressure (BP) is achieved; dose sequence: 20, 40, 80, 80, then 80 mg (300 mg total). Once controlled, use = same total dose IVP every 8 hours. Alternative: IV drip: add 40 mL (200 mg) to 160 mL of intravenous fluids (IVF) (result 1 mg/mL). Run at 2 mL/minute (2 mg/min) until desired BP (usual effective dose 50–200 mg) or until 300 mg given, then titrate the rate. Bradycardia limits dose; increase slowly because the effect takes 10 to 20 minutes. Oral dose: start with 200 mg twice a day if converting from IV; otherwise, start 100 mg orally twice a day and increase 100 mg/dose every 2 days, maximum 2,400 mg/d.[1,2,4,5]

Side effects: Fatigue, dizziness, orthostatic hypotension.[1,4]

Esmolol (Brevibloc)

Action: Short-acting selective β_1 antagonist; metabolized by red blood cell esterase, urinary excretion; may lower ICP.[1,4,8]

Contraindication: Avoid in congestive heart failure (CHF).[1]

Rx: Mix 5 g/500 mL normal saline (NS), give IV 500 µg/kg loading dose over 1 minute, follow with 4-minute infusion starting with 50 µg/kg/min. Repeat the loading dose and increment the infusion rate by 50 µg/kg/min every 5 minutes. Rarely > 100 µg/kg/min is required. Doses > 200 µg/kg/min add little benefit.[1,2,5]

Side effects: Dose-related hypotension; resolves within 30 minutes of discontinuation. Less bronchospasm than with other beta blockers.[1,2]

15.2.4 Calcium Channel Blockers

Nimodipine has been identified as a standard of care in prevention and treatment of vasospasms in patients who have subarachnoid hemorrhage from ruptured aneurysm. Though the mechanism of action in preventing vasospasm is unclear, it was concluded from a double-blinded, randomized clinical trial that nimodipine significantly reduces the occurrence of cerebral arterial spasm.

Nimodipine (Nimotop)

Action: Inhibits calcium ion influx in vascular smooth muscle and neurons, resulting in increased collateral circulation and prevention of neuronal calcium overload.[1]

Contraindications: Hypersensitivity to drug class, parenteral use, caution if there is hepatic disease.[1,4]

Rx: 60 mg oral/nasogastric (NG) every 4 hours × 21 days. May dose at 30 mg oral/NG every 2 hours × 21 days if patient's blood pressure is hypotensive and patient is not tolerating 60 mg dosing.[1]

Side effects: Hypotension, rash, headache, flushing, gastrointestinal bleeding, thromboembolism, CHF, thrombocytopenia anemia, ileus, intestinal obstruction.[1,4]

Diltiazem (Cardizem)

Action: Slow calcium-channel antagonist; relaxes vascular smooth muscle without reflex tachycardia.[1]

Contraindications: Sick sinus syndrome, wide complex tachycardia, Wolff–Parkinson–White (WPW) syndrome, second-degree or greater atrioventricular (A-V) block and concurrent beta blockers.[1,4]

Rx: 20 mg IV over 2 minutes; 0.25 mg/kg. May repeat 1 × in 15 minutes if response is inadequate. Not suggested as a drip for neurosurgical patients.[1]

Side effects: Hepatitis, edema, blurred vision, flushing, injection site reaction.[1,4]

Nifedipine (Procardia)

Action: Short-acting calcium-channel blocker. Decreases systemic vascular resistance; increases cardiac index, cerebral blood flow (by 10–20%), glomerular filtration rate, and Na^+ retention.[1,4]

Contraindications: Hypersensitivity, acute myocardial infarction.[1,4]

Rx: Oral 10 to 20 mg, faster onset with sublingual/buccal administration (puncture capsule) or if chewed. If no response after 20 to 30 minutes, give additional 10 mg.[1,4,5]

Side effects: Flushing, headache, palpitation, edema, reflex tachycardia.[1,4]

Nicardipine (Cardene)

Action: The only second-generation IV dihydropyridine calcium channel blocker.

Contraindications: Can often cause neurologic worsening in patients with stroke, intracerebral hemorrhage, and subarachnoid hemorrhage. Nicardipine IV drip is the relative large volume of fluid needed (up to 150 mL/h). This calcium channel blocker has been shown to increase ICP in some limited animal and human studies.

Rx: Nicardipine drip 25 mg/250 mL in 250 mL NS, on a pump for a concentration of 0.1 mg/mL induction at a rate of 0.2 µg/kg/min, or 5 mg/h (50 mL/h), and may be increased in increments of 2.5 mg/h every 5 to 15 minutes, depending on the need to rapidly or gradually control blood pressure, to a maximum of 15 mg/h (150 mL/h). Once the desired level is achieved decrease the rate to 3 mg/h (30 mL/h). Nicardipine drip is not compatible with sodium bicarbonate injection or lactated Ringer's solution.

Side effects: Dizziness, fainting, unusual weakness, lightheadedness, headache, flushing, nausea, vomiting, tiredness, swelling of the ankles/feet, frequent urination, shortness of breath, irregular heartbeat, joint/muscle pain, tingling of the hands/feet, mood changes, ringing in the ears.

15.2.5 Angiotensin II Receptor Blockers

Angiotensin II receptor blockers (ARBs) are medications that block the action of angiotensin II by preventing it from binding to its receptors on the smooth muscles on blood vessels. As a result, blood vessels dilate, reducing blood pressure. Examples of ARBs include candesartan cilexetil, eprosartan, irbesartan, losartan, mesylate, olmesartan, telmisartan, valsartan.

Action: Allow blood vessel wall relaxation and dilation, reducing blood pressure and increasing release of sodium and water into urine.

Contraindications: Hypersensitivity, pregnancy.

Rx: The oral dosage depends on the specific medication used.

Side effects: Headache and dizziness. Other side effects may be diarrhea, stomach problems, muscle cramps, back and leg pain, insomnia, nasal congestion, cough, sinus problems, and upper respiratory infection. This class of drug is less likely to cause a cough when compared to angiotensin–converting enzyme blockers.

15.2.6 Angiotensin-Converting Enzyme Inhibitors

Angiotensin-converting enzyme (ACE) inhibitors are used as first-line drugs in the treatment of hypertension because they have been proven to reduce the risk of primary stroke beyond their blood pressure lowering capacity. It is believed that their effects on the renin–angiotensin–aldosterone system are their primary mechanism of action in the reduction of stroke risk. In addition, early use of ACE inhibitors immediately after stroke has been associated with improved cerebral perfusion.[9,10] This is thought to be a result of their effect on improving vascular compliance by reducing proliferation of vascular smooth muscle, enhancing endogenous fibrinolysis, and inhibiting plaque rupture and vascular occlusion. ACE inhibitors are also used in the treatment of traumatic brain injury because they have no deleterious effect on ICP.

Enalaprilat (Vasotec)

Action: ACE inhibitor; may lower ICP.[1,4,9,10]
   Contraindication: Pregnancy.[1]
   Rx: Titrate to effect, starting with IV 1.25 mg slowly over 5 minutes, followed by 1.25 to 5 mg IV every six hours depending on response within 15 minutes; may repeat 0.625 mg IV in one hour if response is inadequate, but maximum 6 hour dose should not exceed 5 mg.[1,4,5]
   Side effects: Hyperkalemia ~ 1%; can cause renal insufficiency, angioedema, agranulocytosis.[1,4]

15.2.7 Alpha Agonist

In treating hypertension, clonidine is the most widely used α-adrenergic receptor agonist. It is a centrally acting presynaptic α_2-adrenergic receptor agonist that causes a decrease in peripheral vascular resistance and a decrease in sympathetic tone. This gives clonidine its antihypertensive and sedative properties. In the neurosurgical intensive care unit (NICU), clonidine is effective in treating patients with cocaine and methamphetamine abuse as its mechanism of action is antagonistic to these stimulants by decreasing presynaptic calcium levels, thus inhibiting the release of norepinephrine. This reduces hypertension created by systemic vasoconstriction and agitation created by overstimulation.

Clonidine (Catapres)

Action: Inhibits sympathetic outflow by acting on cardiovascular control receptors in the medulla oblongata.[1,4]
   Contraindication: Hypersensitivity.[1]

Rx: Rapid control: 0.2 mg orally, then 0.1 mg orally every hour; stop at 0.8 mg total or if orthostatic. Maintenance dose: 0.1 mg orally two or three times a day; increase slowly to maximum 2.4 mg/d (usual 0.2–0.8 mg/d). Patch 0.1 mg, 0.2 mg, 0.3 mg/wk titrate to desired effect; maximum 0.6 mg/wk.[1,4,5]

Side effects: Tachycardia rare; mild confusion/sedation; fluid retention, dry mouth, constipation, rebound hypertension.[1]

15.2.8 Hypotension

It is important to prevent hypotensive episodes in the neurologically compromised patient because it is associated with an increase in morbidity and mortality. The first step in treating hypotension is identifying the cause, such as volume loss, heart failure, infection, or shock. Treatment of the underlying cause will correct the hypotension; however, symptomatic treatment must be initiated with volume resuscitation and vasopressor support.

Dopamine (Intropin)

Action: Primarily a vasoconstrictor; 25% of dopamine given is rapidly converted to norepinephrine. At doses > 10 µg/kg/min, α, β, and dopaminergic effect (essentially giving norepinephrine). At 2 to 10 µg/kg/min, primarily β_1, positive inotrope. At 0.5 to 2.0 µg/kg/min, primarily dopaminergic, vasodilating renal, mesenteric, coronary, and cerebral vessels, positive inotrope.[1,4]

Contraindication: Pregnancy class C.[1,4]

Rx: Mix 800 mg/250 mL NS, central line. Start with 2 to 5 µg/kg/min and titrate for response; maximum 20 µg/kg/min.[1,2,4,5]

Side effects: Tachycardia, peripheral vasoconstriction, arrhythmias, hyperglycemia.[1,4]

Dobutamine (Dobutrex)

Action: Racemic mixture: L-isomer is alpha agonist, D-isomer nonspecific; beta agonist comparable to dopamine and nitroprusside.[1,4]

Contraindication: Hypertrophic cardiomyopathy.[1]

Rx: Mix 500 mg/250 mL NS. Usual range 2.5 to 10.0 µg/kg/min; rarely, doses up to 40 µg used. To prepare: Put 50 mg in 250 mL D5 W to yield 200 µg/mL.[1,2,4,5]

Side effects: Tachycardia, possibly platelet function inhibition.[1,4]

Norepinephrine (Levophed)

Action: β_1- and α_1-adrenergic receptor agonist.[1]

Contraindications: Hypertrophic obstructive cardiomyopathy, tetralogy of Fallot (right ventricular outflow tract obstruction).[1,4]

Rx: Mix 4 mg/250 mL NS. Initial rate 0.5 to 1.0 μg/min. Average 4 to 16 μg/min; maximum 30 to 47 μg/min.[1,4]

Side effects: Vasoconstriction (splanchnic and renal), arrhythmias.[1]

Phenylephrine (Neo-Synephrine)

Action: Pure alpha vasoconstrictor; causes reflex increase in parasympathetic tone with resultant slowing of pulse. Useful in hypotension associated with tachycardia.[1,4]

Contraindication: Spinal cord injuries.

Rx: Mix 40 mg/500 mL NS to yield 80 μg/mL; rate of 8 mL/h = 10 μg/min. Vasopressor range: Initial 100 to 180 μg/min; maintenance 40 to 60 μg/min.[1,4]

Side effects: Cardiac output and renal blood flow may decrease.[1]

Inamrinone (Inocor)

Action: Inotrope-vasodilator; inhibits phosphodiesterase III; resembles dobutamine hemodynamically with less tachyphylaxis.[1,4]

Contraindication: Thrombocytopenia.[1,4]

Rx: 0.75 mg/kg IV slow bolus over 2 to 3 minutes, then 5 to 30 μg/kg/min infusion. May rebolus 0.75 mg/kg IV slow 30 minutes after starting therapy.[1,4,5]

Side effects: Vasodilation hypotension, 2% thrombocytopenia, and hepatotoxicity.[1,4]

Epinephrine (Adrenaline)

Action: Nonspecific adrenergic agonist has β_2 activity unlike norepinephrine and twice as potent ionotrope.[1,4]

Contraindications: Hypertrophic obstructive cardiomyopathy, tetralogy of Fallot (right ventricular outflow tract obstruction).[1,4]

Rx: 0.5 to 1.0 mg of 1:10,000 solution IVP; may repeat every 5 minutes (may bolus per endotracheal tube). Drip: Start at 1 μg/min; titrate up to 8 μg/min (to prepare: put 1 mg in 100 mL NS).[1,4,5]

Side effects: Vasoconstriction (splanchnic and renal), arrhythmias.[1]

Isoproterenol (Isuprel)

Action: Nonselective β-adrenergic receptor agonist, potent inotrope (β_1), and peripheral vasodilator (β_2); second-line agent after dopamine for bradycardia unresponsive to atropine.[1,4]

Contraindications: Digitalis bradycardia, angina.[1]

Rx: Mix 1 mg/500 mL NS = 2 μg/mL; start at 2 μg/min, titrate up to 10 μg/min.[1,5]

Side effects: Tachycardia, vasodilation, increased myocardial oxygen demand.[1,4]

15.3 Electrolytes/Intravenous Fluids

The optimal fluid status in patients with neurologic disease is euvolemia. Electrolytes function within a narrow therapeutic range to promote health and ameliorate disease. Increasing amounts of electrolytes are needed at times of stress but still less than would cause further harm.

15.3.1 Sodium and Intravenous Fluids

Phosphorus

Hyper: Phos-Lo (calcium acetate) 2 tablets NG/oral three times a day with meals.[1,4]

Action: Combines with dietary phosphate to form insoluble calcium phosphate.[1]

Contraindications: Hypersensitivity to components, hypercalcemia, renal calculi.[1]

Side effects: Hypercalcemia.[1]

Hypo: Potassium phosphate 1 to 2 g three times a day divided NG/IV three times a day.[1,5]

Action: Elevates serum phosphorus and serum potassium levels.[1]

Contraindications: Hyperphosphatemia, hyperkalemia, hypocalcemia, hypomagnesemia, renal failure.[1]

Side effects: Diarrhea, nausea, stomach pain.[1]

Calcium

Hyper: Treat aggressively with 0.9 NS infusion to correct volume deficit. Follow with loop diuretic (i.e., furosemide 20–40 mg IV/oral every 2–4 hours). May use zoledronate 4 mg IV over 15 minutes four times a day if unresponsive to loop diuretic.[1,5]

Hyper: Calcium gluconate 2.25 to 14 mEq slow IVP or 500 to 2000 mg orally two or three times a day. Calcium chloride 500 to 1,000 mg slow IVP every 1 to 3 days.[1,5]

Action: Elevation of serum calcium.[1,4]

Contraindications: Hypersensitivity, hypercalcemia.[1,4]

Side effects: Extravasation necrosis, hypotension.[1,4]

Magnesium

Hypo: Magnesium sulfate 1 g of 20% solution intramuscularly (IM) every 6 hours × 4 doses or 2 g IVP over 1 hour (note: monitor for hypertension); 1 g will raise serum magnesium 0.4 mEq/dL.[1,5]

    Action: Elevation of serum magnesium.[1]

    Contraindications: Heart block, serious renal impairment, myocardial damage, hepatitis, Addison's disease.[1]

    Side effects: Hypotension, asystole, CNS depression, diarrhea, decreased neuromuscular transmission.[1]

Potassium

Hyper: Treat with D5W, IV calcium, and insulin administration if severe. Kayexalate (sodium polystyrene) 1 g/kg up to 15 to 60 g orally every 6 hours as needed.[1,5]

    Action: Exchanges sodium ions for potassium ions in the intestines.[1]

    Contraindications: Hypersensitivity, hypernatremia.[1]

    Side effects: Hypokalemia, hypocalcemia, hypomagnesemia, sodium retention.[1]

    Hypo: Potassium chloride 20 to 40 mEq orally twice a day or 10 to 20 mEq IVP over 1 hour (note: monitor for cardiac arrhythmias).[1,5]

    Action: Elevation of serum potassium and serum chloride.[1]

    Contraindications: Severe renal impairment, untreated Addison's disease, hyperkalemia, severe tissue trauma.[1]

    Side effects: Diarrhea, nausea and vomiting, bradycardia, hyperkalemia, weakness, dyspnea.[1]

15.4 Blood Products

Patients in the NICU should have a complete blood count (CBC) checked daily. Blood products should be administered as needed to keep hemoglobin at ~ 10.0 mg/dL. Platelets and plasma should be administered on a case-by-case basis. Generally, the international normalized ratio (INR) should be kept equal to or less than 1.4, platelet count should be kept greater than 100,000.[2]

15.4.1 Packed Red Blood Cells

Each unit of packed red blood cells will raise hemoglobin by 0.8 mg/dL.

15.4.2 Fresh Frozen Plasma

Plasma transfusion is indicated in patients with documented coagulation factor deficiencies and active bleeding, or who are about to undergo an invasive procedure with suspected coagulation factor deficiencies. Deficiencies can be secondary to congenital or acquired diseases, such as liver disease, warfarin anticoagulation, disseminated intravascular coagulation, or massive replacement with red blood cells and crystalloid/colloid solutions.

One unit is approximately 250 mL and must be ABO compatible but not Rh factor compatible. The usual dose is 4 units to improve coagulation status by increasing factor levels of at least 10%. However, the amount will vary depending on the patient's size and clotting factor levels.

15.4.3 Platelets

Platelets are indicated in patients with disorders of hemostasis. Platelets are collected from pooled random donors or from a single donor. If given pooled platelets, the dosage is 4 to 6 units, whereas if given from a single donor a standard pack is equivalent to 4 pooled units and a large pack is equivalent to 6 pooled units. Functional platelet count should be maintained above 100,000/µL for patients undergoing neurosurgical procedures. Abnormal platelet function can be seen with medications such as aspirin, and with kidney disease, liver disease, malignancy, sepsis, and tissue trauma. If platelet dysfunction is present, the patient will require higher levels of platelets to achieve hemostasis. The number of units required to increase the number of platelets is dependent upon weight, being anywhere from 5,000/µL per unit for a 200 lb/91 kg patient to 22,000/µL per unit for a 50 lb/23 kg patient.

15.4.4 Cryoprecipitate

Cryoprecipitate contains fibrinogen, von Willebrand factor, factor VIII, factor XIII, and fibronectin. It comes in concentrates of 6 units. Each unit provides about 350 mg of fibrinogen. Usually 6 bags or 1 pooled bag is given, which raises the fibrinogen by 1,560 mg or 45 mg/dL. Cryoprecipitate is also used to make fibrin glue.

15.5 Antiepileptic Medications

15.5.1 Phenytoin (Dilantin)

Action: Modulates voltage-gated Na and Ca neuron channels and enhances Na/K adenosine triphosphatase (ATPase) neuronal and glial activity. Reduced repetitive firing in neurons caused by slowing in the rate of recovery of channels due to enhanced inactivation of Na CNS depressant, reduces seizure propagation, induces cerebellar-vestibular dysfunction; also weak antiarrhythmic, inhibits insulin release.[1,2,4]

Contraindication: Hypersensitivity to medication; class C pregnancy.[1,4]

Rx: Loading dose 15 to 20 mg/kg IV. Do not exceed 50 mg/min IV. Usual 1 g load IV slow over 1 hour, then maintenance of 100 mg IV three times a day. Always check levels after 3 days. Fosphenytoin formulation can be given faster IV because it does not contain propylene glycol. Before infusion, it should be diluted in D5 W or 0.9% NS to a concentration of 1.5 to 25.0 mg/mL (phenytoin equivalents; PE). To avoid hypotension, do not exceed 150 mg PE/min. For seizure prophylaxis, loading dose is 16 to 18 mg/kg IV or IM. Daily maintenance dose is 4 to 6 mg PE/kg/d IV or IM, divided into 2 or more doses.[1,2,4,5]

Side effects: Hypotension, hyperglycemia, arrhythmia, peripheral neuropathy, gingival hyperplasia, megaloblastic anemia (rare), hepatotoxicity (rare), Stevens–Johnson syndrome.[1]

15.5.2 Valproic Acid (Depakene)

Action: Inhibitor of γ-aminobutyric acid (GABA) transaminase and glutamate decarboxylase.[1,4]

Contraindication: Pregnancy.[1]

Rx: 600 to 3,000 mg/d; start at IV/oral 10 to 15 mg/kg/d. If dose > 250 mg/d, it should be divided.[1,5]

Side effects: Gastrointestinal upset, pancreatitis, liver failure if < 2 years of age, teratogenic, drowsiness, hyperammonia, hair loss, weight gain, tremor.[1]

15.5.3 Carbamazepine (Tegretol)

Action: Blocks voltage-dependent Na channel in neuronal cell membrane; hepatic metabolism. Before starting, check CBC, platelet count, and serum Fe. Do not start or stop if white blood cell count < 4, hematocrit < 32, platelet count < 100, reticulocyte < 3, Fe > 150.[1,4]

Contraindication: Hepatic failure or insufficiency[1]

Rx: 200 to 400 orally twice to four times a day.[1,5]

Side effects: Aplastic anemia, ataxia, drowsiness, transient diplopia, Stevens–Johnson syndrome, syndrome of inappropriate antidiuretic hormone, hepatitis.[1]

15.5.4 Phenobarbital (Luminal)

Action: Opens postsynaptic Cl ion channels, decreasing Na and Ca influx.[1,4]

Contraindication: Multiple drug interactions.[1,4]

Rx: IV/oral/IM loading 20 mg/kg/d; slow maintenance 30 to 250 mg/d divided twice or three times a day; therapeutic level 15 to 30 μg/mL.[1,4,5]
Side effects: Cognitive impairment, paradoxical hyperactivity.[1,4]

15.5.5 Primidone (Mysoline)

Action: Same as phenobarbita.l[1,4]
   Contraindication: Multiple drug interactions.[1]
   Rx: Start 125 mg/d × 1 week; increase slowly to avoid sedation, 250 to 1,500 mg/d, divide twice a day.[1]
   Side effects: Fewer side effects, more significant in seizure control; loss of libido.[1]

15.5.6 Ethosuximide (Zarontin)

Action: Antiseizure.[1]
   Contraindication: Hypersensitivity to succinimides; use with caution in pregnancy.
   Rx: Oral/NG only 500 to 1,500 mg/d. In children, start at 250 mg/d, titrate up to 500 mg/d divided twice a day.[1]
   Side effects: Lethargy, hiccoughs, headache, Stevens–Johnson syndrome, systemic lupus erythematosus–like syndrome, psychotic behavior.[1]

15.5.7 Clonazepam (Klonopin)

Action: Benzodiazepine used short term in acute setting; not for long-term use.[1,4]
   Contraindication: Long-term use.[1]
   Rx: Start IV/NG at 1.5 mg/d, divided three times a day, increased by 0.5 mg every 3 days. Usual dosage range 1 to 12 mg/d; maximum 20 mg/d.[1,5]
   Side effects: Ataxia, drowsiness behavior changes.[1]

15.5.8 Gabapentin (Neurontin)

Action: Unknown.[1,4]
   Contraindication: Hypersensitivity.[1]
   Rx: Start 300 mg oral/NG at bedtime, and increase slowly over 3 days to 600 mg until therapeutic; hold for loose stools.[1]
   Side effects: Dizziness, ataxia, fatigue, nystagmus, viral infection.[1,4]

15.5.9 Lamotrigine (Lamictal)

Action: Inhibits release of glutamate and voltage-sensitive Na channels.[1,4]

Contraindication: Hypersensitivity to pregnancy class C.[1]

Rx: Start 50 mg orally four times a day × 2 weeks, then twice a day × 2 weeks.[1,2,4,5]

Side effects: Headache, fatigue, nausea/vomiting, pancreatitis, peripheral neuropathy.[1]

15.5.10 Levetiracetam (Keppra)

Action: Unknown.[1,4]

Contraindication: Hypersensitivity.[1]

Rx: Oral/NG 500 mg twice a day, titrate to effective maximum 3,000 mg daily.[1]

Side effects: Somnolence, weakness.[1]

15.5.11 Pentobarbital (Nembutal)

Action: Short-acting barbiturate, depressing cortical activity.[1,4]

Contraindications: Hypersensitivity, hepatic impairment, dyspnea, porphyria, pregnancy.[1,4]

Rx: For induction of coma: Loading dose of 10 mg/kg IV over 30 minutes, then 5 mg/kg every hour × 3 doses, then maintenance 1 mg/kg/h titrating to 1 to 2 burst per page. For status epilepticus: IV start at 65 to 95 mg/min, titrate up to 1,400 mg total dose.[1,2,5]

Side effects: Bradycardia, hypotension, syncope, rash, exfoliative dermatitis, Stevens–Johnson syndrome.[1]

15.6 Corticosteroids

Many animal models have demonstrated that corticosteroids stabilize cell membrane structures, stabilize the blood–spinal cord barrier reducing vasogenic edema, enhance blood flow in the spinal cord, inhibit endorphin release, prevent free radical accumulation, and moderate the inflammatory response. However, corticosteroids have many side effects and must be used with caution. These side effects include sepsis, pneumonia, death due to respiratory complications, and other complications (▸ Table 15.1).

15.6.1 Dexamethasone (Decadron)

Action: Decreases inflammation by suppressing immune response, inhibiting polymorphonuclear neutrophil leukocyte migration.[1,4]

Contraindications: Hypersensitivity, active untreated infections.[1,4]

Rx: Brain tumor protocol for cerebral edema: 10 to 20 mg loading dose, then 4 to 10 mg every 6 hours. Minimal 10-day taper for weaning.[2]

Table 15.1 Corticosteroids[1,2,4,5]

Name	Approximate equivalent dose (mg)	Relative anti-inflammatory potency	Relative miner-alocorticoid potency	Biologic half-life (hours)
Betamethasone	0.6–0.75	20–30	0	36–54
Cortisone	25	0.8	2	8–12
Dexamethasone	0.75	20–30	0	36–54
Fludrocortisone	–	10	125	18–36
Hydrocortisone	20	1	2	8–12
Methylpredniso-lone	4	5	0	18–36
Prednisolone	5	4	1	18–36
Prednisone	5	4	1	18–36
Triamcinolone	4	5	0	12–36

Side effects: Cushing's syndrome, hypersensitivity reactions, immunosuppression, insomnia, agitation, vertigo, psychosis, delirium, pseudotumor cerebri, increased appetite.[1,4]

Methylprednisolone (Solu-Medrol)

Action: Decreases inflammation by suppressing immune response, inhibiting polymorphonuclearneutrophil leukocyte migration[1,4]

Contraindications: Hypersensitivity, active untreated infections.[1]

Rx: Spinal shock protocol: 30 mg/kg IV over 15 minutes, followed 45 minutes later by infusion of 5.4 mg/kg/h × 23 hours.[1,2]

Side effects: Cushing's syndrome, hypersensitivity reactions, immunosuppression, insomnia, agitation, vertigo, psychosis, delirium, pseudotumor cerebri, increased appetite.[1,4]

15.7 Nonsteroidal Anti-inflammatory Drugs

Nonsteroidal anti-inflammatory drugs (NSAIDs) inhibit isoforms of the enzyme cyclo-oxygenase (COX 1–3) blocking prostaglandin synthesis. NSAIDs alone may be given for pain that is 4 or less. They should be withheld back for 4 to 10 days after mild bleeding and not given at all with severe bleeding, and they should be given with a stomach protectant and adequate hydration to help prevent side effects. NSAIDs belong to multiple drug groups with each group affecting individual patients differently. Therefore, if one group of NSAIDs does not work consider treatment with another. When pain is 4 to 8, NSAIDs can be given with other pain-altering medications (▶ Table 15.2).

Table 15.2 Nonsteroidal anti-inflammatory drugs[1,2,4,5]

Generic name	Dose	Frequency (hours)	Maximum daily dose	Class
Acetamino-phen	10–75 mg/kg/d	4–6	4,000 mg	Para-amino-phenol, COX–3 inhibitor
Aspirin	5–100 mg/kg/d	4–6	8,000 mg	Salicylate
Celecoxib	200–400 mg	12–24	800 mg	COX-2 inhibitor
Choline mag-nesium trisali-cylate	30–60 mg/kg/d	8–12	4,500 mg	Salicylate
Diclofenac	25–75 mg	6–8	200 mg	Pyrroleacetic acid
Diflunisal	250–500 mg	8–12	1,500 mg	Salicylate
Flurbiprofen	50–100 mg	6–8	300 mg	Propionic acid
Ibuprofen	5–50 mg/kg/d	4–6	3,200 mg	Propionic acid
Indomethacin	25–75 mg	8	200 mg	Indoleacetic acid
Ketoprofen	12.5–75.0 mg	6–8	300 mg	Propionic acid
Ketorolac	30–60 mg	IV, oral 6–8	150 mg	Pyrroleacetic acid
Meloxicam	7.5–15 mg	24	15 mg	Benzothiazine
Naproxen	250–500 mg	6–8	1,500 mg	Propionic acid
Oxaprozin	600–1200 mg	8–12	1,800 mg	Propionic acid
Piroxicam	10–20 mg	24	20 mg	Benzothiazine

Abbreviations: COX-2, cyclo-oxygenase-2; COX-3, cyclo-oxygenase-3; IV, intravenous.

15.8 Sedatives

15.8.1 Propofol

Action: Enhances synaptic inhibition mediated by GABA.[1,4]

Contraindications: Allergy to egg or soybean. Reduce doses for elderly, hypovolemic, or those with concomitant use of narcotics.[1,4]

Rx: Sedation: IV bolus 0.1 to 1.0 mg/kg, titrate slowly to the desired effect (onset of slurred speech); infusion 20 to 75 µg/kg/min, monitoring respiratory/cardiac function continuously. Anesthetic induction: IV 2 to 4 mg/kg (give slowly over 30 seconds in 2–3 divided doses). Anesthetic maintenance: IV bolus 25 to 50 mg, then infuse at 100 to 200 µg/kg/min. Antiemetic: 10 mg IV.[1,2,4] May also be used for burst suppression but ability to provide neuronal protection is controversial. The patient should be on ventilator support when this medication is used.

Side effects: Hypotension from myocardial depression, decreases systemic vascular resistance. Depresses laryngeal reflexes more than barbiturates or etomidate. Pain on injection into small veins, histamine release with rapid injection, anaphylaxis.[1,4]

15.8.2 Midazolam (Versed)

Action: Binds to GABA receptors containing gamma subunits, half-life 1.5 to 3 hours.[1,4]

Contraindications: Hypersensitivity, narrow-angle glaucoma, pregnancy.[1]

Rx: Conscious sedation: Slow IVP 1 to 2 mg over 2 minutes (do not exceed 2.5 mg with initial dose), wait 2 to 3 minutes, repeat up to total of 0.1 to 0.15 mg/kg. IM preop: 0.07 to 0.08 mg/kg (5 mg/70 kg) ~ 1 hour preop. Induction general anesthesia: Initial dose slow IVP. For nonpremedicated average adult age < 55 years: 0.25 mg/kg; for > 55 years, American Society of Anesthesiologists (ASA) class I or II 0.2 mg/kg; for ASA class III or IV, 0.15 mg/kg. To maintain, repeat 25% initial dose.[1,4] May also be used for burst suppression but ability to provide neuronal protection is controversial.

Side effects: Decreased tidal volume/respiratory rate, hypotension, drowsiness, oversedation, nausea and vomiting.[1]

15.8.3 Lorazepam (Ativan)

Action: A benzodiazepine with antianxiety, sedative, and anticonvulsant effects, which interacts with the GABA–benzodiazepine receptor complex.

Contraindications: Hypersensitivity to benzodiazepines or their vehicles (polyethylene glycol, propylene glycol, and benzyl alcohol). It should not be used in patients with acute narrow-angle glaucoma, or in nonintubated patients with sleep apnea syndrome or severe respiratory insufficiency. The use of Ativan injection intra-arterially is contraindicated because, as with other injectable benzodiazepines, inadvertent intra-arterial injection may produce arteriospasm resulting in gangrene, which may require amputation.

Rx: Mild sedation: IV 0.5 to 2 mg (0.044 mg/kg). Conscious sedation: up to a total of 4 mg (0.05 mg/kg). Can also be used IM, reaching peak concentration in 3 hours. Orally 0.5 to 1 mg two to three times per day. Can also be used for burst suppression but ability to provide neuronal protection is controversial.

As with benzodiazepines, its action can be reversed with flumazenil (Romazicon) but resedation may occur. Flumazenil action begins less than 2 minutes after administration and peaks in 6 to 10 minutes. The initial dosage is 0.2 mg IV repeated at 1-minute intervals to a maximum of 1 mg.

Side effects: Respiratory depression, fetal damage.

15.8.4 Pentobarbital (Nembutal)

Action: Fast-acting barbiturate with 3- to 4-hour duration of action.

Contraindications: Hypersensitivity, status asthmaticus, severe cardiovascular disease, porphyria.

Rx: Load IV 10 mg/h. Give as 2.5 mg/kg/h slowly every 15 minutes for 4 doses. Hold if blood pressure drops inappropriately. Then continue at 10 mg/kg/h for 3 additional hours. Next continue maintenance dose at 1 to 3 mg/kg/h. Titrate for 1 to 2 burst per page. If the loading dose achieves burst suppression then continue at maintenance dose. Watch for inadequate blood pressure/cerebral perfusion pressure. If using to salvage brain function, ICP should decrease within the hour after burst suppression has occurred. Check daily CBC and blood cultures to monitor for infection and sepsis. Check pentobarbital level 1 hour after completing loading dose and daily thereafter. May also be used for burst suppression but ability to provide neuronal protection is controversial.

Side effects: Hypotension, inability to rapidly diagnose infection.

15.8.5 Haloperidol (aka Haldol)

Action: Blocks postsynaptic D_1 and D_2 receptors in the brain; depresses reticular activating system; depresses hypothalamic hormones.[1,4]

Contraindications: Hypersensitivity, Parkinson's disease, severe cardiac or hepatic disease, bone marrow suppression, coma.[1]

Rx: Sedation: This medication should be titrated for effect, as overdosing can be a problem. Oral dosing is 0.5 to 2.0 mg every 8 to every 12 hours, initially; severe disease may need 3.0 to 5 mg every 8 to 12 hours initially, but not to exceed 20 mg/d.

IM dosing (haloperidol lactate formulation) is prompt acting, and 2 to 5 mg every 4 to 8 hours should suffice, but repeated dosing may be necessary every hour; not to exceed 20 mg/d.[1]

In September 2007, the U.S. Food and Drug Administration (FDA) strengthened label warnings for IV haloperidol regarding QT prolongation and torsades de pointes in response to adverse event reports. IV use of haloperidol lactate is technically *off label*, and haloperidol decanoate should not be used. IV dosages should be checked in the most current sources. If IV administration of Haldol lactate in a large single dose or large cumulative dose is required for ICU delirium and patient safety, an electrocardiograph should be placed and monitored prior to administration and for a minimum of 4 hours after administration of IV.[11]

Side effects: Hypotension/hypertension, anxiety, extrapyramidal and dystonic reactions, pseudoparkinsonian reactions, tardive dyskinesia, neuromalignant syndrome, akathisia,[1] and decreased neurological outcome after head injury.[12]

15.8.6 Thiopental (Pentothal)

Action: Short-acting barbiturate.[1,4]

Contraindications: Hypersensitivity, status asthmaticus, severe cardiovascular disease, porphyria.[1,4]

Rx: Adults: Initial concentration should not exceed 2.5%. Give 50 mg test dose moderately rapid IVP; if tolerated, give 100 to 200 mg IVP over 20 to 30 seconds (500 mg may be required in a large patient).[1,4,5] May also be used for burst suppression but ability to provide neuronal protection is controversial.

Side effects: Dose-related respiratory depression, myocardial depression, hypotension in hypovolemic patients, irritation if extravasated, intra-arterial injection—necrosis, agitation if injected slowly.[1]

15.8.7 Etomidate

Action: Potentiates GABA and depresses reticular activating system.[1,4]

Contraindication: Hypersensitivity.

Rx: IV induction: 0.1 to 0.6 mg/kg. Infusion: 0.25 to 1.00 mg/min (5 to 20 mg/kg/min). Continuous infusion not recommended. Rectal: In children 6 months to 6 years old, 6.5 mg/kg produces reliable hypnosis in 4 minutes but maintains a rapid recovery without any untoward effects.[1] May also be used for burst suppression but ability to provide neuronal protection is controversial.

Side effects: Pain on injection into small veins, high incidence of thrombophlebitis (24% compared with thiopental 4%), myoclonus. Lowers seizure threshold, nausea and vomiting, adrenocortical suppression.[1]

15.8.8 Ketamine

Action: Direct effect on the cortex and limbic system, producing cataleptic-like state, dissociated from surroundings.[1]

Contraindications: Increased ICP, hypertension, hypersensitivity, aneurysms, thyrotoxicosis, CHF, angina.[1,4]

Rx: 1 to 2 mg/kg IV over 1 to 2 minutes or 4 mg/kg IM induces 10- to 20-minute dissociative state.[1] May also be used for burst suppression but ability to provide neuronal protection is controversial.

Side effects: Concurrent atropine minimizes hypersalivation; hallucinations, vivid dreams, hemodynamic instability.[1]

15.9 Anticoagulants

Most NICU patients are immobilized for one reason or another. Deep venous thrombosis prophylaxis should be implemented as soon as possible. Always begin with sequential compression devices and thigh-high compression stockings. Patients who will be long-term immobilized should be considered for anticoagulation drugs. Depending on the pathology, patients with traumatic intracranial hemorrhage with no sequelae 72 hours posthemorrhage may be started on anticoagulation drugs.[2]

15.9.1 Heparin

Action: Prevents the conversion of fibrinogen to fibrin.[1,4]

Contraindications: Hypersensitivity, severe thrombocytopenia, uncontrolled bleeding.[1]

Rx: 5,000 units subcutaneous three times a day.[1,4,5]

Side effects: Bleeding, vasospasm, thrombocytopenia, bruising.[1,4]

15.9.2 Lovenox

Action: Prevents the conversion of fibrinogen to fibrin.[1,4]

Contraindications: Hypersensitivity to pork products, uncontrolled bleeding.[1]

Rx: Prevention: 40 mg SC once daily. Treatment of deep venous thrombosis or pulmonary embolus: 1 mg/kg twice a day.[1,4,5]

Side effects: Bleeding, fever, bruising.[1,4]

15.10 Pain Medications

The most commonly prescribed medications for severe pain are opioids, which stimulate mu, kappa, delta, and the nociceptin receptor (NOP) also known as the nociceptin/orphanin FQ (N/OFQ) receptor. The first and most widely used opioids are the group that stimulates the mu receptor; these include morphine, Demerol, Dilaudid, and fentanyl. Clinically, the effect of opioids is to raise the pain threshold, increasing the minimal intensity needed to feel pain. At the anatomical level, opioids act by inhibiting nociceptive transmission to the spinal cord, activating descending inhibitory pathways, and altering higher-center activity of pain perception. Just as NSAIDs belong to different groups with considerable variability in efficacy, opioid groups vary in ability to treat pain, even in the same individual.

15.10.1 Lidocaine Patch (Lidoderm 5%)

Action: Topical analgesic.[1]

Contraindications: Hypersensitivity, broken skin barrier; but still can place adjacent to incision.[1]

Rx: Place one to three patches 12 hours per day (12 hours on, 12 hours off); when using on fresh surgical incision, apply both sides but not over.[1]
Side effects: Local edema, erythema, urticaria, anaphylaxis.[1,4]

15.10.2 Acetaminophen (Tylenol)

Action: Suspected to be cyclo-oxygenase-3 (COX-3) inhibitor at very high doses.[1,4]

Contraindications: Hypersensitivity, chronic alcohol abuse, impaired liver function.[1,4]

Rx: Adults: 650 to 1,000 mg oral/PR (far point of accommodation) every 4 to 6 hours, not to exceed 4,000 mg/d; children: 10 to 15 mg/kg oral/PR every 4 to 6 hours.[1,4,5]

Side effects: Hepatic toxicity.[1,4]

Equianalgesic Doses for Severe Pain (▶ Table 15.3).

Table 15.3 Equianalgesic dose for severe pain[1,2,4,5]

Drug	Receptor agonist or antagonist	Route	Dosage	Dosage frequency (hours)	Half-life (hours)
Morphine	Mu	IV	0.1 mg/kg	3–4	2.1–2.6
		IM	0.2 mg/kg	3–4	
		Oral	0.3 mg/kg	3–4	
Ketamine	Mu	IV	5 µg/kg/min	3–4	
Hydromor-phone	Mu	IV, IM	0.015 mg/kg 0.5–1.0 mg/ h	3–6	2.6–3.2
		Oral	0.06 mg/kg	3–6	
Fentanyl	Mu	IV	25–50 µg/h		3.7
		TC	25–100 µg/ h, 600– 7,200 µg	72 hour patch	3.7
Oxycodone	Mu	Oral	0.2 mg/kg	3–4	
Hydrocodone	Mu	Oral	0.2 mg/kg	3–4	
Meperidine	Mu	IV	0.75 mg/kg	2–3	3
		IM	75 mg		3
		Oral	300–400 µg	4–6	3
Levorphanol	Mu	IM	0.02 mg/kg	6–8	11
		Oral	0.04 mg/kg	6–8	11
Buprenorphine	Mu	IV	0.4 mg/kg	6–8	5
		SL	2–24 mg	6–8	5

(continued)

Table 15.3 continued

Drug	Receptor agonist or antagonist	Route	Dosage	Dosage frequency (hours)	Half-life (hours)
Codeine	Mu	IV	1 mg/kg	6–8	3
		IM	1 mg/kg	6–8	3
		Oral	1 mg/kg	3–4	
Tramadol	Mu	Oral	50–100 mg	6	
Nalbuphine	Kappa agonist, mu antagonist	IV	0.15–2.50 mg/kg	3–6	5
Butorphanol	Kappa agonist, mu agonist and antagonist	IV, IM	2 mg 0.5–4.0 mg 0.25–32.0 mg/day maximum	3–4	3
		IN	1 mg spray, 1–4 mg/d	3–6	
Thyrotropin-releasing hormone		IV			
Naloxone	Binds mu receptor without stimulation; also binds kappa and delta	IV	0.4 mg every 2–3 minutes		1
Pentazocine	Kappa; mu agonist and antagonist	Oral	50 mg	4–6	4
Propoxyphene hydrochloride	Mu	Oral	65 mg	4–6	9

Abbreviations: IM, intramuscularly; IN, intranasal; IV, intravenous; SL, sublingual; TC, transcutaneous.

15.10.3 Ketorolac (Toradol)

Action: Inhibits prostaglandin synthesis; only parenteral NSAID approved for use in pain control in the United States.[1,4]

Contraindication: Hypersensitivity to NSAIDs, active peptic ulcer disease, recent gastrointestinal perforation, renal impairment, bleeding. Do not use prophylactically before major surgery.[1,4]

Rx: 10 mg orally every 4 to 6 hours; IM/IV 30 to 60 mg every 6 to 8 hours, do not use for more than 72 hours. Acute pain after surgery when bleeding is controlled: 120 mg in 500 mL normal saline to run at 10 mL/h until completed over 50 hours. Must have initial loading dose of 30 to 60 mg IV. Stomach protectants must be given.[1,4]

Side effects: Bleeding time prolonged by platelet function inhibition, gastric mucosal irritation, and erosion, even though given in IV or IM form. Side effects are worse in the elderly and with prolonged use.[1,4]

15.10.4 Nalbuphine (Nubain)

Action: Kappa agonist, mu antagonist.[1,4]

Contraindications: Hypersensitivity, head injury, impaired pulmonary or liver function, pregnancy, elderly patients.[1]

Rx: IV 0.15 to 2.5 mg/kg every 3 to 6 hours.

Side effects: Respiratory depression, severe bradycardia, severe hypotension, sedation, headache, dysphoria.[1,4]

15.10.5 Butorphanol (Stadol)

Action: Kappa agonist, mu agonist and antagonist.[1,4]

Contraindications: Hypersensitivity; substance abuse; impaired liver, renal, and pulmonary function. Use caution in head-injured patients and CNS depression.[1,4]

Rx: IV 2 mg, IM 0.5 to 4.0 mg every 3 to 4 hours, 0.25 to 32.0 mg/d maximum; intranasal 1 mg spray every 3 to 6 hours.[1]

Side effects: Respiratory depression, substance abuse, severe hypotension, severe bradycardia, sedation, nausea/vomiting.[1,4]

15.10.6 Tramadol (Ultram)

Action: Affects mu opioid receptors.[1,4]

Contraindications: Hypersensitivity, ethanol intoxication, substance abuse history. Use caution with head-injured patients, those with CNS infections or lesions, and patients with elevated ICP.[1,2,4]

Rx: 50 to 100 mg orally every 4 to 6 hours as needed.[1]

Side effects: Hypoventilation, constipation, bradycardia. Large dose given rapidly may cause chest wall rigidity, dysconjugate gaze, headaches.[1,4]

15.10.7 Codeine

Action: Weak opioid.[1]

Contraindications: Hypersensitivity, respiratory depression, paralytic ileus. Use caution in patients with elevated ICP, seizure disorder, or head injury.[1]

Rx: Adults: 30 to 60 mg IM/oral every 3 hours; children: 0.5 to 1 mg/kg/dose every 4 to 6 hours.[1]

Side effects: Respiratory depression, CNS depression, hypotension, bradycardia, syncope, cardiac arrest, elevated ICP, seizures, paralytic ileus, dependency, shock, anaphylactoid reactions. More common side effects include dizziness, nausea and vomiting, sedation, and constipation.[1]

15.10.8 Hydrocodone

Action: Moderate opioid.[1,4]

Contraindications: Hypersensitivity, respiratory depression, paralytic ileus, CNS depression, head injury, elevated ICP, seizure disorder.[1,4]

Rx: Available in 5.0, 7.5, and 10.0 mg doses with acetaminophen dose, 1 or 2 tablets orally every 4 to 6 hours; not to exceed 60 mg hydrocodone in 24 hours, not to exceed 4,000 mg acetaminophen per 24 hours.[1,4]

Side effects: CNS depression, respiratory depression, dependency, paralytic ileus, increased ICP, hypotension, nausea and vomiting, sedation.[1,4]

15.10.9 Fentanyl

Action: Binds to mu opiate receptor in the CNS, inhibits pain pathway. Opiate potency 100 × morphine. In small doses, lasts 20 to 30 minutes. Supplied in concentration 50 µg/mL Increases cerebral blood flow.[1,4]

Contraindications: Hypersensitivity, increased ICP, respiratory depression, pregnancy.[1,4]

Rx: 25 to 100 µg (0.5–2.0 mL) IVP, repeat as needed. Also available as transdermal patch, which is changed every 72 hours, delivering 25, 50, 75, or 100 µg/h.[1]

Side effects: Hypoventilation, constipation, bradycardia. Large dose given rapidly may cause chest wall rigidity, dysconjugate gaze.[1]

15.10.10 Morphine

Action: Binds to mu opiate receptor in the CNS; inhibits pain pathway, increases cerebral blood flow.[1,4]

Contraindications: Hypersensitivity, increased ICP, respiratory depression.[1,4]

Rx: Drip: mix 100 mg/100 mL NS, start 2 mg every hour, titrate to effect maximum 10 mg every hour. IVP: start 2 mg every 1 to 2 hours, increase as needed.[1,2,4,5]

Side effects: Respiratory depression, miosis, hypotension, bradycardia, apnea, pulmonary edema, dysconjugate gaze.[1,4]

15.11 Antiemetics

Nausea and vomiting are frequent problems for patients in the NICU due to stimulation of the chemoreceptor trigger zone (CRTZ). Phenothiazine derivatives, such as Phenergan, should be avoided in general, due to a lowering of the seizure threshold.[2]

15.11.1 Ondansetron (Zofran)

Action: Selective 5-hydroxytryptamine (5HT)-receptor antagonist; blocks serotonin on vagus nerve terminals and in the CRTZ.[1,4]

    Contraindication: Hypersensitivity to ondansetron.[1]

    Rx: 4 to 8 mg IV every 6 to 8 hours as needed for nausea/vomiting.[1,2]

    Side effects: Malaise, fatigue, headache.[1]

15.11.2 Granisetron (Kytril)

Action: Selective 5-HT-receptor antagonist. Blocks serotonin both peripherally and centrally at CRTZ.[1,4]

    Contraindication: Hypersensitivity to granisetron.[1]

    Rx: 1 mg orally every 12 hours or 2 mg orally every 24 hours.[1]

    Side effects: Headache, constipation, dizziness, insomnia, anxiety.[1,4]

15.11.3 Trimethobenzamide (Tigan)

Action: Inhibits CRTZ.[1,4]

    Contraindications: Hypersensitivity to trimethobenzamide or benzocaine. Injection contraindicated in children.[1,4]

    Rx: 250 to 300 mg orally three or four times a day, 200 mg IM/PR three or four times a day.[1]

    Side effects: Hypotension, depression, coma, disorientation, jaundice, muscle cramps, blurred vision.[1,4]

15.12 Reversal Agents

15.12.1 Flumazenil

Action: Competitively inhibits benzodiazepine at receptor sites.[1,4]

    Contraindications: Pregnancy, patients chronically treated with benzodiazepines where antagonism may provoke a withdrawal syndrome and/or seizures. May provoke a panic attack.[1]

    Rx: 0.2 mg IV every minute × 1 to 5 doses; maximum dose 1 mg, 3 mg/h.[1]

Side effects: Seizures—high risk in patients on benzodiazepines for long-term sedation, hypoventilation, arrhythmias, and resedation.[1,4]

15.12.2 Naloxone

Action: Oxymorphone derivative, competitively binds to opioid receptors, half-life (t½) ~ 4 to 60 minutes.[1,4]

Contraindication: Hypersensitivity; may cause acute withdrawal from opioids in individuals who are physically dependent.

Rx: Load: 1 to 4 μg/kg, infuse at rate of 5 to 15 μg/kg/h. Titrate IV in small doses 20 to 40 μg.[1,5]

Side effects: Severe unmasked pain can lead to sympathetic and cardiovascular stimulation: hypertension, dysrhythmias, pulmonary edema, and cardiac arrest.[1,4]

15.12.3 Naltrexone

Action: Oxymorphone derivative, competitively binds to opioid receptors, t½ > 10 hours.[1]

Contraindication: See naloxone.

Rx: Oral: 100 mg or greater.[1,4]

Side effects: See naloxone.

Case Management

The patient must be fully resuscitated with 0.9% normal saline. Initially attempts should be made to increase his cerebral perfusion pressure with fluids, and if not successful, with vasopressive medications. A chemistry panel, complete blood count, and coagulation profile should be obtained. After resuscitation, if the patient's GCS score remains 8 or less and the coagulation profile is in the normal range with or without the use of blood products, an ICP monitor and drain should be inserted. There is no indication for steroids in the treatment of isolated severe head injury. Sedation could be administered to help control respiratory rate if necessary. Pain medication must be administered when appropriate. An antiepileptic medication could be started if the patient is at a higher risk of seizures and if a seizure event would likely worsen brain injury.

References

[1] Lacy CF, Armstrong LL, Goldman MP. Lance LL. Drug Information Handbook. 25th ed. Hudson, OH: Lexi-Comp; 2016

[2] Greenberg MS. Handbook of Neurosurgery. 8th ed. New York, NY: Thieme; 2016

[3] Turner JM, Powell D, Gibson RM, McDowall DG. Intracranial pressure changes in neurosurgical patients during hypotension induced with sodium nitroprusside or trimetaphan. Br J Anaesth. 1977; 49(5):419–425

[4] Murray L, ed. Physician's Desk Reference. 69th ed. Montvale, NJ: Thompson PDR; 2015

[5] Green SM, ed. Tarascon Pocket Pharmacopoeia. Lompoc, CA: Tarascon Publishing; 2005

[6] Lange RA, Cigarroa RG, Flores ED, et al. Potentiation of cocaine-induced coronary vasoconstriction by beta-adrenergic blockade. Ann Intern Med. 1990; 112(12):897–903

[7] Allen GS, Ahn HS, Preziosi TJ, et al. Cerebral arterial spasm–a controlled trial of nimodipine in patients with subarachnoid hemorrhage. N Engl J Med. 1983; 308(11):619–624

[8] Cotton BA, Snodgrass KB, Fleming SB, et al. Beta-blocker exposure is associated with improved survival after severe traumatic brain injury. J Trauma. 2007; 62(1):26–33, discussion 33–35

[9] Hilleman DE, Lucas BD, Jr. Angiotensin-converting enzyme inhibitors and stroke risk: benefit beyond blood pressure reduction? Pharmacotherapy. 2004; 24(8):1064–1076

[10] Padma MV. Angiotensin-converting enzyme inhibitors will help in improving stroke outcome if given immediately after stroke. Ann Indian Acad Neurol. 2010; 13(3):156–159

[11] Haldol Dosing Indications. http://reference.medscape.com/drug/haldol-decanoate-haloperidol-342974. Accessed June 13, 2016

[12] Parikh S, Koch M, Narayan RK. Traumatic brain injury. Int Anesthesiol Clin. 2007; 45(3):119–135

16 Nutrition

Jerry Noel, Silvio Hoshek, Rosalinda Menoni, and Dan E. Miulli

Abstract
Nutritional management is medical treatment. Nutrition should be considered equal to all other medical managements, for its proper use can optimize nervous system recovery and prevent further injury. Once the brain is injured, even to the point of coma, brain metabolism is increased and should be treated as early as possible. Withholding nutrition is dangerous, leading to decreased gastrointestinal mucosa integrity, depression of the immune response, and other abnormalities, which in turn leads to increased morbidity and mortality. The amount of nutrition, the type of nutrition, the additives to the nutrition, and the method of delivery of the nutrition are specific for patients with central nervous system injuries.

Keywords: catabolic cascade, catecholamines, enteral feeding, GI mucosa integrity, Harris–Benedict formula, Hypermetabolism, MVI, nitrogen loss

---

Case Presentation

A 60-year-old man (154 lb [70 kg], 5 ft 5 in [166 cm]) was in a motor vehicle accident and suffered a traumatic subarachnoid hemorrhage. His Glasgow Coma Scale score is 7. The patient was in the neurosurgical intensive care unit for 2 days, intubated, with a heart rate of 90.
   See end of chapter for Case Management.

16.1 Nutritional Requirements

Only half of neurologic injury occurs at the time of the ictus, with the remaining damage occurring as secondary damage. The biggest impact on avoidable exacerbations can be made in the neurosurgical intensive care unit (NICU). The survival for patients with severe head injury depends largely on critical management, including, but not limited to, oxygenation, blood pressure, intracranial pressure/cerebral perfusion pressure, and optimal nutrition.[1]

Adequate nutrition is critical to maintaining internal systems, meeting the metabolic demands of increased activity in illness, and helping in the repair and healing of wounds. Considering all the secondary insults occurring in the patient while in the NICU, nutrition may play an even larger role than once imagined, especially if nutrition is considered not as an adjunct but as a necessary therapy.[2,3,4]

Supplements, such as vitamin C, zinc, selenium, and multivitamin concentrate infusions (MVIs), among others, are also necessary to promote wound healing.

Nutritional management of the neurosurgical patient is a high priority in the NICU setting. Central nervous system (CNS) injury can stem from trauma, metabolic disorders, stroke, ischemia, neoplasm, and neuromuscular dysfunction, all of which in the acute stage can significantly increase metabolic needs. Adequate nutrition is critical to sustaining body systems, meeting the increased metabolic demands of illness, and supporting healing. Yet nutritional support has not been considered a primary treatment modality; subsequently the incidence of malnutrition in ICU patients may be as high as 50%.[5] Thus, in all admissions to the NICU, nutrition must be promptly and adequately addressed in the management of patients with CNS injury.

Contrary to what was once thought, after neurologic injury there is a severe profound systemic hypermetabolic reaction that results in the rapid depletion of whole-body energy stores. If not attended to, a catabolic injury cascade results in the loss of gastrointestinal (GI) mucosa integrity, reductions in body muscle mass, reductions in systemic protein stores and synthesis, and the compromise of both humoral and cellular immune competence.[6] Nutrition can help the patient with neurologic injury fight infections, improve ventilator function, and promote wound healing.

16.2 Undernutrition

Inadequately feeding patients results in the following:

- Loss of GI mucosa integrity.
- Reductions in body muscle mass.
- Reductions in systemic protein stores and synthesis.
- Compromise of both humoral and cellular immune competence.
- Decrease in the absolute number of circulating T cells.
- Promotion of cutaneous anergy.
- Depressed production of new antibodies in response to a novel antigen.

Suboptimal nutrition is dangerous; it has been shown to decrease the absolute number of circulating T-cells, promote cutaneous anergy, and depress the production of new antibodies in response to a novel antigen. The depression of the immune response caused by undernutrition can significantly increase the probability and virulence of infectious complications in surgical patients.

Energy stores and fat stores allow the body to function for a long time without devastating effects. The earliest studies show that a 30% preoperative weight loss led to a 10-fold increase in morbidity and mortality of gastric surgery. By extrapolation, using fuzzy logic, there is the assumption that a 15% weight loss in the bedridden patient is of little consequence, bearing in mind that a 30% weight loss is potentially very deleterious. Nutritional problems are usually discussed only after visual signs of weight loss, which is the reason nutrition during the first several days to as much as 2 weeks has not been studied. Three randomized class I studies have evaluated the relationship between caloric intake and patient outcomes.[7,8,9,10] Rapp et al[9] showed that the consequence of severe undernutrition for a 2-week period after injury was an increased mortality rate when compared to those individuals that had full caloric replacement by 7 days. In Young et al's study,[10] there was no difference in those patients that were fed parenterally at 3 days when compared to those fed enterally at 9 days.

It is necessary to know how to determine weight in order to determine if there is weight loss. The ideal body weights for people with a medium frame are the following:

- *Men*: 106 lb. for 5 ft, then add 6 lb for each additional inch.
- *Women*: 100 lb for 5 ft, then add 5 lb for each additional inch.
- *For both*: Subtract 10 lb for small frame and add 10 lb for large frame.

When protein calorie malnutrition occurs there is a depletion of skeletal muscle and visceral muscle in a 30:1 ratio. The measured level of the serum protein albumin can approximate visceral muscle stores. Mortality risk increases by about 37% for each gram deficit of serum albumin. Decreased albumin is also responsible for altering colonic resorption of water and salt, manifested by edema and ascites, and it causes gastric stasis, prolonged small bowel retention, delayed wound healing, and increased wound infection. When a patient has not been fed or when a patient has been hypermetabolic because of neurologic injury, a nutritional blood test panel should be obtained that includes albumin, prealbumin, transferrin, total iron-binding capacity, and serum creatinine. To further help with nutritional assessment there should be strict monitoring of total input and output and daily weights (▸ Table 16.1).

Table 16.1 Nutritional assessment[2,3,4]

Test for nutrition	Normal values	Meaning of low value
Serum albumin	3.5–5.5 g/dL	<3.5 compromised protein status, fluid overload, stress
Prealbumin (transthyretin)	14.0–42 mg/dL, 20% lower after 60 years of age	<14.0 protein depletion
Transferrin	215–415 mg/dL	<200 md/dL malnutrition
Total iron binding capacity	270–400 mcg/dL	Compromised protein status
Serum creatinine	0.6–1.6 mg/dL	<0.6 muscle wasting due to calorie deficiency
Total input and output	Euvolemic to slight hypervolemic	Dehydration and resultant hypotension
Daily weights		Loss of fluid or undernutrition

Nutrition must not be thought of as preventing large stores of excess fat from being lost but as a form of therapy. At the same time nutrition must not be haphazardly given, for it has side effects just as any drug does. The nutritional formula must be beneficial and should aid in treatment of the neurologically injured patient.

16.3 Hypermetabolism following Central Nervous System Injury

Patients have an inflated hypermetabolic response to neurologic injury. Hadley et al[7,8] demonstrated a mean resting energy expenditure 46% above the normal predicted basal metabolic rate in a study of 45 head injury patients. Most other investigators who measured metabolic expenditure in the rested comatose patient also demonstrate a metabolic rate that is approximately 120 to 250% of the predicted normal basal metabolic rate. During these times, in order to meet the needs of the increased energy production, there is a marked increase in gluconeogenesis, hepatic protein synthesis, and use of protein, carbohydrate, and fat. The increased use of fats, carbohydrates, and proteins not only makes supplying nutrition difficult, it accelerates the development of malnutrition in patients who are not being fed. In the CNS-injured patient there is a change in the ratio of nutrients required; there is an increased demand for protein and lipid calories and a relative decrease in carbohydrate needs. These requirements must be taken into account when designing a nutritional formula for the CNS-injured patient.

The basic requirements in neurologic injury include the following:

- Increased metabolism.
- Increased protein.
- Increased lipid.
- Decreased carbohydrate.

The adaptive response to CNS injury is an increase in catecholamines, cortisol, and glucagons and a subsequent increase in metabolism and hyperglycemia.[8] Both gluconeogenesis and lipolysis continue. Even with hyperglycemia, 75 to 90% of energy is still supplied by fat oxidation. In moderation, fat oxidation is not a major problem; however, when there is decreased blood return and continued fat oxidation there is free radical production and further neurological damage. Although protein is required for the repair of injured brain, the changes in catecholamines, cortisol, and glucagon lead to proteolytic metabolism. Catecholamines are released and in turn stimulate the release of adrenocortictropic hormone, growth hormones, glucagon, and insulin. Catabolic hormones, such as glucagons, cortisol, and catecholamines, cause use of alternate energy sources when there are no further nutrients supplied. As the injury continues, stress increases and proteolysis persists, making it impossible to achieve a positive nitrogen balance in the early period after CNS injury. Even if CNS-injury patients are paralyzed or put into barbiturate comas, they still require 100 to 120% of the resting energy expenditure.[11] A major part of the increase in resting energy expenditure in comatose patients is due to muscle tone.[12]

The following are normal responses to CNS injury:
• Increased catecholamines.
• Increased cortisol.
• Increased glucagons.
• Proteolysis.
• Gluconeogenesis.
• Lipolysis.
• Increased adrenocortictropic hormone, growth hormones, and insulin.

In addition to the loss of protein stores throughout the body, injury results in other changes, such as electrolytes being lost from GI tract secretions. Just as protein stores must be replaced, electrolytic losses must be replaced in nutritional therapy (▶ Table 16.2).[2]

16.4 How Much Nutrition Is Needed?

The average normal calorie requirement is 30 kcal per kg per day for a Glasgow Coma Scale (GCS) score > 12, 35 kcal per kg per day for a GCS score from 8 to 12, and 40–45 kcal per kg per day for a GCS score from 3 to 7. However, indirect calorimetry performed with the aid of a portable metabolic cart once a day for the first several days is the most accurate way to determine the patient's resting energy expenditure and nutrition requirements. This method is unnecessary since the general energy requirements are known using the Harris–Benedict formula (▶ Table 16.3), although the Harris–Benedict equation contains systematic error of 5 to 15% overestimation.

Table 16.2 Gastrointestinal losses following central nervous system injury[2,3,4,5]

GI Loss	Sodium mEq/L	Chloride mEq/L	Potassium mEq/L
Gastric	60	100	10
Bile	140	100	10
Pancreas	140	75	10
Small bowel	100	100	20
Diarrhea	60	45	30

Table 16.3 Harris–Benedict equation for determining general energy requirements[2,3,4,5,7, 8,9]

Part I—Men [66.47 + 13.75 × weight in kilogram + 5.0 × height in centimeters − 6.76 × age in years] = basal calories.
Part II—Multiply basal calories by adjusted activity factor and then by injury factor = the required energy expenditure in total calories per day.
Part I—Women [655.10 + 9.65 × weight in kilograms + 1.85 × height in centimeters − 4.68 × age] = basal calories.
Part II—Multiply basal calories by adjusted activity factor and then by injury factor = the required energy expenditure in total calories per day.

Note: Activity factors: confined to bed 1.2 and out of bed 1.3. Injury factors: minor surgery 1.1, major surgery 1.2; infection mild 1.2, moderate 1.4, and severe 1.8; trauma skeletal 1.35, head injury with steroids 1.6, blunt 1.35; and burns 40% 1.5, 100% 1.95.

Reproduced with permission from Page CP, Hardin TC. Nutritional Assessment and Support: A Primer. Baltimore, MD: Williams & Wilkins; 1989.

Clifton et al[13] simplified the adjustment factors correcting the Harris–Benedict overestimation. They showed that the required percentage of resting energy expenditure of total calories calculated from part I of the Harris–Benedict formula can be estimated accurately using GCS score, heart rate, and days since the injury. The Clifton equation is

$$152 - [14 \times \text{the Glasgow Coma Score}] + 0.4 \times \text{the heart rate} + 7$$
$$\times \text{ the days since injury}$$
$$= \text{percentage of required energy expenditure}.$$

In the first 2 weeks after injury energy expenditure rises regardless of neurological course, but its extent beyond this is unknown. The hypermetabolic response is also prolonged in patients who have other major organ system trauma. This hypermetabolism can be exaggerated for up to a year in severe head injury patients; however, this should not be thought of as the norm.

In the neurologically injured patient the resting energy requirements will be supplied by muscle breakdown or other body stores of proteins, fats, and carbohydrates (► Table 16.4).

Table 16.4 Resting energy requirements[2,3,4]

Substrate providing calories	Kcal per gram
Muscle	1
Carbohydrate	4
Protein	4
Fat	9

Initially in the neurologically injured patient, the hypermetabolic state often is combined with undernutrition and compromising protein synthesis, resulting in lean muscle mass catabolism for essential amino acids. As the hypermetabolism hypercatabolic process continues, nitrogen is lost through the urine and feces. There is essentially no nitrogen gained through normal levels of nutrition, and a great deal of nitrogen is lost, leading to a negative nitrogen balance. For each gram of nitrogen in the urine and feces, 6.25 grams of protein have been catabolized. Nonfed patients with severe brain injury continue to lose 14 to 25 grams of nitrogen per day. The maximum excretion occurs during the second week. The average nitrogen loss of a head injury patient is 0.2 grams of nitrogen/kg/d, which will result in a 10% loss of lean mass in 7 days.[8] This is about double or triple the loss in the normal person. Unlike the Studley paper that showed that a 30% preoperative weight loss led to an increased morbidity and mortality of gastric surgery by 10-fold there are no studies that examine nitrogen loss or nitrogen replacement with outcome; therefore nitrogen balance may not be a major issue. Nonetheless, a study by Clifton et al[14] examined two matched groups of comatose head injury patients and determined that the level of nitrogen intake should be 20% of the core composition of a 50 kcal/kg/d feeding protocol. For the hypermetabolic patient 20% is the maximal protein content of most enteral feedings and 20% is the maximal amino acid content of most parenteral formulations.

Any feeding has to take into consideration fluid requirements, which averages 35 mL per kilogram per 24 hours, more in athletes and less in the elderly. The following is an additional way to measure normal fluid requirements (average 35 mL/kg, elderly 30 mL/kg):

- 100 mL per kilogram for the first 10 kg in 24 hours then
- 50 mL per kilogram for the next 10 kg in 24 hours then
- 20 mL per kilogram for remainder weight in kg in 24 hours age < 60
- 50 mL per kilogram for the next 10 kg in 24 hours

The protein content of the fluid should be 1, 1.5, or 2 kcal/mL in order to meet partial nutritional needs and to continue a fluid euvolemic state. There are many physiological circumstances that require increased fluids from the normal amount. Fever increases fluid requirements by 12.5% for each 1°C above normal, sweating 10–25%, and hyperventilation 10–60%.[15]

Fluid types must also be used judiciously. The deleterious effects of hypotonic intravenous solutions on brain injury have been known since 1919;[16] therefore, immediately after neurological problems, intravenous fluid such as lactated Ringer's (Na = 130 mEq/L; 273 mOsm/L), dextrose 5% in water, and 0.45 normal saline should be avoided. Decreasing intravenous fluids 1 mEq/L decreases osmotic pressure 38.6 mm Hg[16] and can lead to brain edema. On the other hand, it is also known that hypertonic saline solutions lower intracranial pressure.[17,18]

There have been multiple class I investigations of the amount of feeding, the route of feeding, the use of steroids, and nitrogen balance, but none of these studies have looked at patient outcome or complications. Even the evidence of what to feed the CNS-injured patient remains unclear. The formulas must be specifically tailored; even the ingredients once thought to be the foundation of nutritional therapies need to be reexamined. High osmolar total parenteral nutrition (TPN) increases brain edema after cryogenic injury in animals[19] because of changes in serum osmolarity. The increased edema does not occur with lower osmolarity TPN. Besides hyperosmolar nutrition causing worse outcome after CNS injury, hyperglycemia is well recognized as worsening outcome after CNS injury and must be avoided.[20,21,22,23] It has even been suggested that hypoglycemia may be neurocytoprotective.[23,24] Hyperglycemia is common in trauma patients even without supplementation and is exacerbated by the administration of any TPN, hyper- or iso-osmolar.[10] Therefore, TPN should not be given during the first 48 hours after CNS injury, and serum glucose concentrations must be closely monitored and treated vigorously and kept below 110 mg/dL.[25,26]

Nutritional treatments should not deliver less than the minimal daily requirements, and as nutritional science matures nutritional requirements in specific diseased states will be developed.

16.5 The Gut Benefits from Nutrition

Early nutritional support increases CD4 cells, the CD4:CD8 ratio, and the T-lymphocyte responsiveness to concanavalin-A, which assists immune function in patients sustaining CNS injury.[27] For nutrition delivery to the body to optimally occur in a physiological manner, the GI tract cells must be functioning. A functioning GI tract is necessary to protect against infection and sepsis from its own bacteria, particularly after neurologic injury or surgical stress. If the gut is maintained there will be no bacterial overgrowth, no proliferation of specific pathogens within the bowel, and no penetration of the pathogens into the bowel wall. Furthermore, with nutrition, the GI tract will remain the principal organ in the regulation of interorgan amino acid exchange, with glutamine being the most important amino acid available to the GI cells. After CNS injury, the GI tract cells' uptake of glutamine increases despite decreased oral intake and decreased delivery of glutamine to the intestinal mucosa. Glutamine is the most abundant amino acid in the blood, possibly because it is a precursor for purines and pyrimidines. When there is no added nutrition available, glutamine must come from another source; it originates from the muscle catabolism.

In summary, the primary benefits of maintaining GI mucosa glutamine nutrition are as follows:

- Protects against infection and sepsis from its own bacteria.
- Prevents the proliferation of specific pathogens within the bowel.
- Enables the GI tract to remain the principal organ in the regulation of inter-organ amino acid exchange.
- Enables protein production.
- Enables nitrogen transport and ammonia excretion.
- Prevents muscle degradation.
- Decreases hypermetabolism.

In undernutrition, muscle undergoes proteolysis and releases essential glutamine into the circulation, supplying the basic requirements for GI enterocytes and for renal aminogenesis. However, the GI cells quickly use the glutamine from the muscle, thereby decreasing the circulating glutamine level available to other cells of the body for protein production, nitrogen transport, and ammonia excretion. In functioning cells throughout the body, glutamine is catabolized by mitochondrial glutaminase to glutamate and ammonia, and once released into the circulation and across the blood–brain barrier, it can destroy brain cells. However, not all glutamine by-products are neurotoxic; alanine is used by the liver for gluconeogenesis, and ammonia is converted to urea. Circulating glutamine is necessary for the gut to prevent infection, necessary to cells for protein synthesis, important for nitrogen and carbon transport and for ammonia excretion, the major substrate for gluconeogenesis, the substrate for renal angiogenesis, and a fuel source for rapidly replicating cells, but too much glutamine can be a problem. Although the by-products of glutamine metabolism can cause neurological problems, there is no evidence that an exogenous supply to the gut increases neurologic injury when the kidneys and liver are functioning. Therefore, the net overall requirement is for glutamine to be provided during CNS injury as soon as possible at appropriate levels to maintain homeostasis.

16.6 How to Feed CNS-Injury Patients

Patients can be fed using the stomach, using the intestines, and using the veins. Each venue has its advantages and disadvantages. Multiple issues affect each type of feeding. Enteral feeding in the neurologically impaired patient is often complicated by medications such as phenobarbital, morphine, and other narcotics that delay gastric emptying. Ott et al[28] found that, for a mean of 15 days, more than 50% of head-injured patients did not tolerate enteral feedings because of delayed gastric emptying. However, gastric feeding does not have to be the method of choice when using the GI tract. There has been one class I report and one class II report indicating better tolerance of enteral feeding with jejunal rather than gastric administration. Enteral feedings do have advantages over intravenous feedings. If the gut works, use it. It is more cost-effective, safer, has fewer complications, and is more physiological than parenteral nutrition.

Indications for enteral nutrition include the following:
- Malnourished patients expected to be unable to eat > 5–7 days.
- Nourished patients not able to eat for 7–9 days.
- Patients that are unable to consume adequate amounts of kilocalories to prevent macronutrient and micronutrient deficiencies.

Contraindications to enteral nutrition include the following:
- Severe acute pancreatitis.
- High output proximal fistula.
- Inability to gain access.
- Patients expected to eat within 5–7 days.
- Intractable vomiting and diarrhea.
- Aggressive therapy not indicated.

Using the GI tract has physiological superiority in terms of stimulating gut hormones, gastric acid buffering, low cost, and buffering supplements into the blood. The advantages of enteral feeding are decreased hyperglycemia, decreased infection and sepsis, and decreased cost. Enteral feeding does maintain the gut mucosa integrity, prevent infection, promote protein synthesis, transport toxins, and decrease hypermetabolism. The only advantage of parenteral nutrition can be seen when enteral feeding cannot be tolerated, immediately preoperatively, when there is a need for intentional bowel rest, and when there is bowel dysfunction; then the intravenous route must be used for a short time. Intravenous nutrition can also supplement enteral nutrition when not enough calories and proteins are being provided. Parenteral nutrition does aggravate brain edema in laboratory animals and may cause elevated liver or pancreatic enzymes. Lebkowski[29] showed that neither parenteral nor enteral nutrition in severe head injury patients made any difference in outcome. However, the same study also demonstrated that no nutrition made any difference in outcome.

The neurologically injured patient is often treated in the flat bed position, especially if spinal injuries have occurred or vasospasms are present. Most of the time the patient has the head of the bed at 30–45 degrees or is titrated to the best intracranial pressure. When the head of the bed is flat the patients are at risk for aspiration. If aspirations are suspected, tube feedings should be held until the feeding tube can be placed into the small intestine. Intubation does provide a degree of protection, especially if a subglottic suction endotracheal tube is used. However, recent literature demonstrated ulcers in an animal model; therefore its use cannot be recommended.[30] When there is a concern about possible aspiration, gastric reflux, or a tracheoesophageal fistula, food coloring can be added for 24 hours to feedings for investigation. In the past, blue food coloring and methylene blue have been added to enteral feedings to detect aspiration. Increased absorption and systemic levels of drugs such as methylene blue can occur when there is increased intestinal permeability. The blue dye then interferes with normal adenosine triphosphate production and ultimately inhibits mitochondrial respiration, leading to shock, metabolic acidosis, and cell death;[31] therefore its use cannot be recommended.

Severe head injury patients who remain comatose and those with spinal cord injury have swallowing difficulties and may be fed either parenterally or enterally. Prolonged use of a nasogastric or orogastric tube should be avoided because of the risk of mucosal ulceration and sinus disease. Patients who are expected to have feeding difficulties for 1 month or more should have a percutaneous endoscopic gastrostomy tube placed.

Eventually, established feedings should approximate the normal bolus manner of feeding instead of continuous feedings, although initially, continuous feedings[32,33] are better tolerated in the critically injured patient.[34] If given the choice of gastric or duodenal feeding versus jejunostomy the more proximal area should be used because a patient receives fewer calories via the more distal jejunostomy tube. This was exemplified by Opeskin and Lee[35] in the case of a healthy 16-year-old patient with severe head injury being fed by jejunostomy tube who died because of malnutrition. She had hyperperistalsis that caused the jejunostomy tube to migrate even more distal, resulting in less nutrition being absorbed.

The gut may provide the most efficient and safe route of fluid administration and should be used as the first choice when there are no contraindications. For example, when diabetes insipidus is suspected, an enteric feeding tube can be used to provide the patient water when intravenous water would never be considered.

Once again no class I studies have looked at patient outcome, but there are multiple class II–IV studies that provide evidence of outcome. Borzotta et al[36] demonstrated that neither enteral nutrition nor TPN was effective in changing outcome. In the past, when compared to enteral nutrition, TPN was thought of as a superior means of nutrition because of the misconception that the bowel was atonic. However, Hadley et al[7] demonstrated that aggressive enteral feeding could be accomplished early and effectively despite bowel atony. Grahm et al[37] added support to using enteral routes when they demonstrated that enteral-fed patients had statistically significant lower rates of hospital-acquired infection and sepsis and shorter stays in the intensive care unit than patients receiving the same caloric and nitrogen supplements by TPN. Grahm et al passed a malleable nasojejunal feeding tube directly into the proximal jejunum with the aid of bedside fluoroscopy. They used the nasojejunal feeding tube in spite of a history of blunt abdominal trauma, the use of barbiturates, narcotics, and other agents and compared the results to TPN. The minor differences that tended to favor enteral nutrition were less hyperglycemia, less of a difference in osmolarity loads causing edema, and lower cost. Enteral nutrition preserved gut mucosa, stimulated complex circulatory hormonal mechanisms that are intrinsic to the human digestive system, and preserved the secretion of the immunoglobulin A immune system. Thus the use of enteral nutrition tends toward improved efficacy. Furthermore, enteral feedings are best accomplished if the tube is placed in the jejunum, decreasing chances of aspiration and improving GI tract motility.

Postpyloric enteral feeding requires the following:

- Bowel sounds must be present.
- Bowel movements or flatus is not necessary.
- Placement of a nasoduodenal feeding tube.
- Confirmation of certain feeding tubes by abdominal X-ray.
- Maintaining the head of the bed at 30 degrees or greater.
- Checking the gastric residuals by oral gastric tube.
- The feeding tube must be flushed with a bolus of at least 30 mL water every 4 hours to prevent clogging.

Small intestinal feedings can reduce the risk of aspiration. In addition to a decrease in infection rates with early enteral feedings, the occurrence of bacterial translocation (the passage of bacteria across the intestinal wall) is also decreased.

When starting tube feedings determine that there are bowel sounds, confirm the placement of certain tubes by abdominal X-ray, place the head of the bed at 30 degrees or more, then determine the total amount of calories or the goal calories and the amount of liquid, in milliliters, to be given per hour for 24 hours. Begin tube feedings at 10–50 mL per hour, full strength. Check for gastric residuals after the first 2 hours, then after every 4 hours for three cycles. If the amount of feeding formula residual is greater than 50% of the feedings delivered during the cycle checked, hold the feedings for 1 hour and recheck every hour until there is less than 50% of the feedings delivered during the last cycle. It is often difficult as well as inaccurate to measure residuals with pliable feeding tubes. If feedings are tolerated increase the amount 20–40 mL every 8 hours until the goal is reached. Make sure that the feeding tube is flushed with 30 mL of water every 4 hours to prevent clogging.

When tube feedings have reached the goal amount and are well tolerated bolus feeding may begin. Give feedings during normal waking hours every 4 hours. Start with double the hourly rate of the continuous tube feedings. Flush with at least 30 mL of water after every bolus, then clamp the feeding tube. Next follow the same guidelines for checking residuals with continuous feedings. Check for gastric residuals after the first 2 hours, then after every 4-hour cycle. The cycles of bolus feedings may be increased to every 6 hours if fluid requirements dictate. If the amount of residual feeding formula in the gut is greater than 50% of the feedings delivered during the cycle, hold the feedings for 1 hour and recheck every hour until there is less than 50% of the feedings delivered during the last cycle; resume when appropriate.

Discontinue enteral feedings only when oral intake is appropriate. If possible wean the tube feedings to oral intake; this is often easier with bolus-type delivery. However, some patients do not tolerate oral intake if a nasal feeding tube is in place.

Occasionally diarrhea occurs with tube feedings. Likely causes are elixir medications containing sorbitol, magnesium-containing antacids, oral antibiotics, phosphorus supplements, cimetidine, metopramide, lactulose, pseudomembranous colitis, and GI disorders. When diarrhea starts measure stool *Clostridium difficile* titers, especially if the stool is very malodorous. Then increase fiber by considering the addition of pectin or psyllium; however, psyllium will clog the feeding tube. When treating diarrhea do not initially give antidiarrheal agents before the cause is known, it will slow down the elimination of the offending agent and prolong the diarrhea. Do not stop the tube feedings for any length of time and do not change formulas.

16.7 What Should CNS-Injury Patients Be Fed?

Nutrition is a form of therapy. Nutrition must be safe, it must prevent secondary injury, and it should improve outcome. Nutrition decreases the risk of infection, maintains the gut mucosa integrity, promotes protein synthesis, transports toxins, prevents muscle degradation, and decreases hypermetabolism. To decrease complications nutrition should be made slightly acidic since gastric alkalinization significantly increases the risk of nosocomial ammonia in patients ventilated long term.[38] The brain requires about 20% of the body's resting energy expenditure, and although dependent on glucose it will use ketones under conditions of significant deprivation. Ritter et al[39] randomized 20 severe head injury patients to receive osmolite high nitrogen HN or carbohydrate-free tube feeds. The experimental tube feed contained 2,060 kcal/L, 129 g/L of protein and 175 g/L of fat. In these patients blood glucose was lower, blood lactate was lower, arterial ketones were higher, and daily nitrogen loss was lower. Unfortunately the investigators did not measure outcome. To be well rounded, in addition to proteins, enteral nutrition must contain fat and possibly some carbohydrates. Each should be added in moderation; carbohydrates should not be overused because hyperglycemia leads to worse outcomes in neurologic injury. Large amounts of administered carbohydrates/glucose have several negative effects. First, they will raise the carbon dioxide production due to its relatively high respiratory quotient of 1. The respiratory quotient of protein oxidation is 0.8 and of fat oxidation is 0.7. The higher respiratory quotient of carbohydrates will result in increased ventilation needs and decreased ability to be weaned. High serum glucose levels will also stimulate lipogenesis and result in hepatic steatosis. Additionally, high glucose increases the resting energy expenditure due to thermic effect of the large doses of administered carbohydrates.

The use of tight glucose control 80–110 mg/dL improves mortality and morbidity. This can be accomplished with a humulin regular sliding scale IV dosage or much more accurately with an insulin continuous infusion. Continuous infusion of insulin has been shown to provide more steady states, approximating physiological conditions.[40,41,42,43,44]

16.7.1 Fats

In addition to an amount of carbohydrates, fats must be included in feedings. Although Roth et al[45] described how a fat emulsion containing 20% intralipid caused life-threatening hemophagocytosis, hypertriglyceridemia, and creaming plasma after a 3-day period of parenteral nutrition in a 21-year-old patient, fats are important. They provide 8 kilocalories per gram of fat and normally make up 10% or less of the consumed calories in the modern diet. Diets should contain medium-chain fatty acids because they are well tolerated and do not increase deleterious plasma lipoproteins. Essential fatty acids are required, with each type having advantages and disadvantages. Diets rich in omega-6 polyunsaturated fatty acids, such as those obtained from corn, safflower, and sunflower oils, diminish the immune response to infection, trauma, or tumor growth as documented by Alexander and Peck.[46] Arachidonic acid, a by-product of fats, breaks down and stimulates oxygen free radicals and further damage. On the other hand, diets abundant in omega-3 polyunsaturated fatty acids, such as found in cold water fish oils, stimulate the immune response to infection and trauma and activate the rejection of foreign bodies.

16.7.2 Proteins

Proteins are very important in nutrition and must supply the enormous need for specific amino acids. Saito et al[47] demonstrated that arginine is important in neurologic injury. When arginine made up 2% of the total nonprotein calories in burn-injured animals it increased survival, improved delayed hypersensitivity, and reduced susceptibility to infection. Arginine is thymotrophic and improves cellular immunity by increasing thymic lymphocyte sensitivity. Arginine also improves wound healing and decreases nitrogen release.[8] Amino acids are vital for neurological healing, such as inosine, which has been shown to stimulate axonal growth.[48] However, not all amino acids benefit head-injury patients. Theoretically, glutamine and glutamate from the diet can cross a disrupted blood–brain barrier and exacerbate glutamate neurotoxicity immediately after primary injury or during secondary injury and lead to the loss of cells in the ischemic penumbra. This has not been proven in human subjects. In general, after injury, protein catabolism leads to increased nitrogen levels and an increased production of ammonia. However, the levels of nitrogen that lead to increased ammonia and neuronal damage are not known. It is recommended that the ratio of nitrogen to nonprotein calories in the human diet range from 1:75 to 1:185. Enteral feedings should contain at least 15% of calories as protein by the seventh day after injury. The optimal amount of protein per kilogram of body weight in the neurologically injured patient is unknown. Normal nutrition suggests 1.5 grams per kilogram; studies suggest 2.5 grams per kilogram[49] but it may be as high as 4.5 grams per kilogram. Proteins, electrolytes, and dextrose add osmolarity. Most feedings should have an osmolarity around 300 so that it does not add to edema at lower osmolarities nor leak across the damaged blood–brain barrier as higher osmolarity would.

In addition to the main building blocks of carbohydrates, fats, and protein, the neurologic injury nutritional formula should contain 1 to 2 calories per milliliter to decrease the fluid load. The formula should be high in zinc, which is associated with an improved neurologic recovery rate and improved protein levels in patients with severe closed head injury.[50] The formulas should also be low in iron and high in desferrioxamine. Desferrioxamine prevents the damage associated with free radical generation and reperfusion injury. It inactivates the iron-dependent enzyme ribonucleotide reductase, which has been shown to decrease infarct size and improve functional recovery.[51] Creatine-enriched formula can help prevent secondary neurologic energy in an animal model.[52] The formula must contain vitamins and other elements. Glucose loads should be low because of problems with hyperglycemia, and large doses of glucose will suppress lipolysis and prevent mobilization of stored linoleic acid. It may also be prudent to add human growth hormone.[53] This has no effect on nitrogen imbalance in highly stressed immobilized patients after severe head injury, but it significantly enhances serum protein concentrations.

16.7.3 Disease-Specific Formulas

Immune-enhancing formulas with glutamine, arginine, omega-3 fatty acids, and nucleotides have been recently used in critically ill patients. Glutamine and arginine have been shown to decrease infection rates and promote wound healing in the critically ill[54] but are contraindicated in patients with hepatic and renal failure. Arginine supplementation has immune-enhancing benefits, including increased rate of protein repletion, improved collagen synthesis, wound healing, and enhanced T-cell function.

The goal of pulmonary formulas is to reduce carbon dioxide production. These formulas are low in carbohydrates and have a high (50%) fat content. Care must be taken to avoid overfeeding. Total calorie intake has more of an impact on respiratory function than specialized pulmonary formulas.

Hepatic formulas are low in protein to minimize ammonia production. These formulas contain large amounts of the branched-chain amino acids valine, leucine, and isoleucine, and low amounts of aromatic amino acids. These formulas assist in treating encephalopathy, especially from ammonia.

Special diabetic formulas contain high fiber, low carbohydrate, and high fat to provide nutritional support to patients with hyperglycemia and may be considered in all neurologically injured patients. However, due to delayed gastric emptying in a head trauma patient, close monitoring of tube feeding tolerance is recommended. Absorption may be enhanced with the use of elemental formulas if intestinal atrophy or loss of absorptive surface has occurred.

Characteristics of an optimal nutritional formula in the treatment of an acute neurologic injury are as follows:[55,56,57,58]

- 1–2 calories per milliliter, depending on the need for euvolemia or hypervolemia.
- Slightly acidic.
- Small intestine placement.
- Osmolarity 300.
- High protein, containing arginine, inosine, and glutamine.
- Fatty acids with medium-chain and omega-3 and polyunsaturated fatty acids.
- Very low or absent carbohydrates.
- Fiber 25–35 g/d.
- High magnesium initially.
- High zinc.
- Desferrioxamine.
- Creatine.
- Low potassium initially.
- Low calcium, 800–1,500 mg/d initially.
- Low iron.

16.8 Total Parenteral Nutrition

The only advantage of parenteral nutrition can be seen when enteral feeding cannot be tolerated, immediately preoperatively, with the need for intentional bowel rest, and proven severe bowel dysfunction; then the intravenous route must be used for a short time. Intravenous nutrition can also supplement enteral nutrition when not enough calories and proteins are being provided.

TPN is drug therapy delivered to the intravenous system without the benefit of the GI buffering system. TPN must contain the appropriate medications to provide optimal nutrition. Electrolytes, protein, fats, and vitamins are required for health and are provided in most nutritional supplements but must be added to intravenous TPN. The amount that the physician prescribes is

dependent on sex, age, organ losses, and diseased states. The normal requirements thus vary by the same criteria, but general guidelines are given in
▸ Table 16.5.

Often electrolytes are prescribed in different units, and the conversion must
be known. Intravenous fluids are given in milliequivalents and dietary supplements are given in milligrams (▸ Table 16.6).

Table 16.5 General guidelines to normal nutritional requirements[2,3,4,5,15]

Nutrient	Recommended daily allowance	Nutrient	Recommended daily allowance
Sodium	60–150 mEq/d 1– 1.7 mEq/kg/d	Zinc	15 mg/d RDA 2.5–5 mg/d IV
Potassium	70–150 mEq/d 0.9– 1.3 mEq/kg/d	Copper	2–3 mg/d RDA 0.5–1.5 mg/d IV
Chloride	60–150 mEq/d 1–1.7 mEq/kg/d	Chromium	55–70 µg/d RDA 10–15 mg/d oral
Magnesium	0.35–0.45 mEq/kg/d	Manganese	2–5 mg/d RDA 0.15–0.8 mg/d IV
Calcium	800–1500 mg/d 0.2–0.3 mEq/kg/d	Selenium	55–70 µg/d RDA 125 µg/d IV
Phosphorus	7–30 mmol/ 1,000 kcal 3–4 g/d	Iron	10–15 mg/d RDA
Vitamin A	3,300 IU/d	Fatty Acids	0.1 g/kg/d
Vitamin D	200–400 IU/d	Protein	0.8–4 g/kg/d
Vitamin E	10 IU/d	Glucose	100 cal/day
Vitamin C	100 mg/d	Fiber	25–35 g/d
Vitamin K	64–80 µg/d	Cystine	13 mg/kg/d
Folacin	400 µg/d	Isoleucine	23 mg/kg/d
Niacin	40 mg/d	Leucine	40 mg/kg/d
Riboflavin	3.6 mg/d	Lysine	30 mg/kg/d
Thiamine	3 mg/d	Methionine	13 mg/kg/d
Vitamin B6	4 mg/d	Phenylalanine	39 mg/kg/d
Vitamin B12	3–5 µg/d	Tyrosine	39 mg/kg/d
Pantothenic acid	15 mg/d	Threonine	15 mg/kg/d
Biotin	60 µg/d	Tryptophan	6 mg/kg/d
		Valine	20 mg/kg/d

Abbreviations: IU, international unit; IV, intravenous.

Table 16.6 Electrolyte requirements in different units[2,3,4,5,15]

Electrolyte	mEq	mmol	Mg
Sodium	1	1	23
NaCl (1 g)	43	43	1,000
	17 Na	17 Na	393 Na
Potassium	1	1	39
	26	26	1,000
Calcium	1	0.5	20
	50	25	1,000
Magnesium	1	0.5	12
	82	41	1,000
Phosphorus	2	1	31
Chloride	1	1	35
	29	29	1,000

Table 16.7 Recommended electrolyte requirements in total parenteral nutrition[a] [2,3,4,5,15]

Electrolyte	mEq
Sodium	5–10
Potassium	20–40
Phosphorus	10–15
Magnesium	8
Calcium	5

[a] For each 1,000 kcal of TPN add milliequivalents of electrolyte.

The requirements in the average healthy individual are not the same as in the debilitated individual. When providing TPN the amount of electrolytes must be adjusted for 1,000 kcal of TPN (▶ Table 16.7).

Typical central intravenous TPN must be adjusted for the disease state, determining the beneficial compounds to be added. The fluid requirements must also be obtained according to the disease state and whether euvolemia or hypervolemia is beneficial. Peripheral administration requires adjustment to prevent peripheral vein injury. As such the amount of amino acids in peripheral intravenous feedings should be 35 grams, dextrose 70 grams, sodium chloride 15 mEq, and heparin 200 units (▶ Table 16.8).

Prior to beginning TPN make sure that the central venous access line has one port labeled for only TPN. Central line TPN usually contains 70% dextrose, 10% amino acids, and 20% fat emulsion. If peripheral access is chosen the amount of dextrose is decreased to 20%, amino acids to 8.5%, and fats to 10%. As with the administration of all intravenous medication the TPN must be delivered at a constant rate. The TPN delivery system must be maintained sterile. Document the patient's height, weight, age, sex, heart rate, GCS score, days since the injury, total caloric goal, and the fluid desired. There are specific TPN formulas commercially available. Start TPN at 50 mL per hour and increase every 8 hours until the goal can be reached in 24 hours. When discontinuing the TPN taper the infusion rate by 50% every 30 minutes for 1 hour to prevent hypoglycemia.

TPN is a direct assault on the liver and pancreas and bypasses the stomach, providing electrolytes directly to the bloodstream. TPN causes fatty liver, cholestasis, GI atrophy, and gastric hyperacidity. Therefore, multiple tests should be monitored when delivering TPN (▶ Table 16.9).

Table 16.8 Typical central total parenteral (IV) nutrition formula (not peripheral administration)[2,3,4,5,14,15]

Ingredients	Average amount (per liter
Carbohydrate dextrose	250 g
Lipids 20%	250 mL
Amino acids	60 g
Sodium acetate	60 mEq
Sodium chloride	60 mEq
Sodium phosphate	60 mEq
Potassium acetate	60 mEq
Potassium chloride	60 mEq
Potassium phosphate	60 mEq
Magnesium sulfate	16–24 mEq/d
Calcium gluconate	10–15 mEq/d
Multivitamins	10 mL
Vitamin C	1,000 mg
Vitamin K	10 mg/wk
Trace elements	4 mL
Insulin	At least 15 units/d
Zinc extra	10 mg
Heparin	1,000 units

Table 16.9 Tests for patients receiving total parenteral nutrition[2,3,4,5,14,15]

Tests	Frequency
Serum electrolytes, glucose, BUN, Creatinine, calcium, magnesium, phosphorus	Daily
Albumin, prealbumin, transferrin, total iron binding capacity, hepatic enzymes, bilirubin, triglycerides, prothrombin time, WBC	Weekly

Abbreviations: BUN, blood urea nitrogen; WBC, white blood cell count.

16.9 Changing Metabolic Conditions

Formulas must have the ability to change under different metabolic conditions. For example, magnesium is important early in injury for preventing vasospasms and for preventing the spread of glutamate neurotoxicity; however, it is not beneficial after 7–10 days when recovery is expected, when cell transmission is needed.

16.10 Additional Concerns for Nutrition

Nutritional therapy must be customized for clinical conditions (▶ Table 16.10).

At times the neurologically injured patient may not have been fed for 1–3 days, is inactive, and may often receive narcotics, all which individually can result in decreased gut motility. Therefore, initial admitting orders for the NICU should include a stool softener, such as docusate sodium or the combination capsule casanthranol/docusate sodium. Appropriate bowel movement prevents abdominal distension, pain, anxiety, nausea, and vomiting. Therefore, treat constipation appropriately. Always consider abdominal injury in the multitrauma patient and if not present and if stool softeners do not result in regularly scheduled bowel movements, then bisacodyl suppositories and enemas should be given every other day unless a bowel movement has occurred.

There is no benefit to initially give metoclopramide in patients with severe neurological injury to stimulate gastric motility; it does not prophylactically improve gastric tolerance and it can cause CNS effects, such as neuroleptic malignant syndrome, parkinsonian symptoms, dystonic reactions, restlessness, and others.[59]

Table 16.10 Different nutritional requirements in clinical conditions

Clinical condition	Nutritional requirement
Syndrome of inappropriate antidiuretic hormone	Decreased fluids
Cerebral salt wasting	Increased salt
Diabetes insipidus	Decreased salt and increased fluids
Ventilators	Increased phosphorus
Initial head injury	Increased magnesium
Vasospasms	Increased magnesium

16.11 Conclusion

Neurologic injury initiates a cascade of local and systemic metabolic responses. Patients become hypermetabolic, hypercatabolic, and hyperglycemic and develop decreased immune competence and altered GI function. New methods of enteral feeding, such as percutaneous placements of tubes or fluoroscopic placements of proximal jejunostomy tubes, allow early feeding and adequate nutrition. Evidence indicates that early small bowel feeding of patients with acute head injury results in decreased incidence of infection and shorter NICU stays. Optimal nutritional support for improving neurologic recovery continues to be established. It is more likely that this will be a dynamic state, changing from person to person, and over time, depending on the clinical circumstances. There are many advantages to early feeding. Early feeding should not be based on preventing a loss of weight, but should be based on using the nutrition as a form of therapy. However, nutrition should not have detrimental effects; it must not cause secondary injury. Nutritional formulas cannot contain hyperosmotic hyperglycemic solutions, omega-6 polyunsaturated fatty acids, irons, glutamate, as well as an abundance of amino acids that will be converted into ammonia. These formulas should not be administered. Early feedings favors better outcomes.

Case Management

A 60-year-old, 70 kg, 66 cm man was in a motor vehicle accident with a traumatic subarachnoid hemorrhage. His GCS score is 7. The patient was in the ICU for 2 days, intubated, with a heart rate of 90. A soft nasal feeding tube should be placed into the proximal small intestine because the patient is expected to have a decreased mental status for an extended time but will be able to orally feed in less than 30 days. An enteral nutritional formula with continuous feedings should be used days 1 through 7 after neurologic injury. The formula should have water content 110% of normal or 35 mL/kg/d. The general caloric requirements for 70 kg with a GCS score of 7 is 40 kcal/kg yielding 2,800 kcal/d. The Harris–Benedict equation predicted required calories would be $6.47 + 13.75 \times 70\,kg + 5.0 \times 66\,cm - 6.76 \times 60 = 1,547.37$ calories. Then the 1,547.37 calories would be multiplied by the activity bedridden factor 1.2 and then trauma factor 1.35, yielding a total 2,506.74 calories. Adjusted instead by the Clifton equation the percentage of resting energy requirement is $152 - [14 \times$ the GCS score of $7] + 0.4 \times$ the heart rate of $90 + 7 \times$ the second day since injury, giving a predicted increased metabolism of 104% of normal, yielding 1,609 kcal. The nutritional therapy should have an osmolarity of 300 mOsm, and pH 7.5–7.8. The patient should have frequent finger-stick glucose checks and a continuous insulin drip to keep blood glucose less than 110 mg/d.

References

[1] Guidelines for the Management of Severe Head Injury, 1995, 2000, 2007. https://www.brain-trauma.org/uploads/11/14/Guidelines_Management_2007w_bookmarks_2.pdf Brain Trauma Foundation

[2] Page CP, Hardin TC. Nutritional Assessment and Support: A Primer. Baltimore, MD: Williams and Wilkins; 1989

[3] Morgan SL, Weinsier RL. Fundamentals of Clinical Nutrition. 2nd ed. St. Louis, MO: Mosby; 1998

[4] Heimburger DC, Weisner BL. Handbook of Clinical Nutrition. 3rd ed. St. Louis, MO: Mosby; 1997

[5] Christman JW, McCain RW. A sensible approach to the nutritional support of mechanically ventilated critically ill patients. Intensive Care Med. 1993; 19(3):129–136

[6] Studley HO. Percentage of weight loss: a basic indicator of surgical risk in patients with chronic peptic ulcer. JAMA. 1936; 106:458–460

[7] Hadley MN, Grahm TW, Harrington T, Schiller WR, McDermott MK, Posillico DB. Nutritional support and neurotrauma: a critical review of early nutrition in forty-five acute head injury patients. Neurosurgery. 1986; 19(3):367–373

[8] Hadley MN. Hypermetabolism following head trauma: nutritional considerations. In: Barrow D, ed. Complications and Sequelae of Head Injury. New York, NY: Thieme American Association of Neurological Surgeons; 1992: 161–168

[9] Rapp RP, Young B, Twyman D, et al. The favorable effect of early parenteral feeding on survival in head-injured patients. J Neurosurg. 1983; 58(6):906–912

[10] Young B, Ott L, Haack D, et al. Effect of total parenteral nutrition upon intracranial pressure in severe head injury. J Neurosurg. 1987; 67(1):76–80

[11] Magnuson B, Hatton J, Zweng TN, Young B. Pentobarbital coma in neurosurgical patients: nutrition considerations. Nutr Clin Pract. 1994; 9(4):146–150

[12] Clifton GL, Robertson CS, Choi SC. Assessment of nutritional requirements of head-injured patients. J Neurosurg. 1986; 64(6):895–901

[13] Clifton GL, Robertson CS, Grossman RG, Hodge S, Foltz R, Garza C. The metabolic response to severe head injury. J Neurosurg. 1984; 60(4):687–696

[14] Clifton GL, Robertson CS, Contant CF. Enteral hyperalimentation in head injury. J Neurosurg. 1985; 62(2):186–193

[15] Matarese LE, Gottschlich MM. Contemporary Nutrition Support Practice: A Clinical Guide. Philadelphia, PA: WB Saunders; 1998

[16] Weed, LH,, McKibben, PS.. Pressure changes in the cerebro-spinal fluid following intravenous injection of solutions of various concentrations. Am J Physiol. 1 919; 48:512–531

[17] Prough DS, Whitley JM, Taylor CL, Deal DD, DeWitt DS. Regional cerebral blood flow following resuscitation from hemorrhagic shock with hypertonic saline. Influence of a subdural mass. Anesthesiology. 1991; 75(2):319–327

[18] Schmoker JD, Zhuang J, Shackford SR. Hypertonic fluid resuscitation improves cerebral oxygen delivery and reduces intracranial pressure after hemorrhagic shock. J Trauma. 1991; 31 (12):1607–1613

[19] Waters DC, Hoff JT, Black KL. Effect of parenteral nutrition on cold-induced vasogenic edema in cats. J Neurosurg. 1986; 64(3):460–465

[20] Chopp M, Welch KM, Tidwell CD, Helpern JA. Global cerebral ischemia and intracellular pH during hyperglycemia and hypoglycemia in cats. Stroke. 1988; 19(11):1383–1387

[21] Kalimo H, Rehncrona S, Söderfeldt B, Olsson Y, Siesjö BK. Brain lactic acidosis and ischemic cell damage: 2. Histopathology. J Cereb Blood Flow Metab. 1981; 1(3):313–327

[22] Myers RE.A unitary theory of causation of anoxic and hypoxic brain pathology. In: Fahn S, Davis JN, Rowlands LP, eds. Cerebral Hypoxia and Its Consequences. New York, NY: Raven Press; 1979:195–213

[23] Pulsinelli WA, Waldman S, Rawlinson D, Plum F. Moderate hyperglycemia augments ischemic brain damage: a neuropathologic study in the rat. Neurology. 1982; 32(11):1239–1246

[24] Marie C, Bralet AM, Gueldry S, Bralet J. Fasting prior to transient cerebral ischemia reduces delayed neuronal necrosis. Metab Brain Dis. 1990; 5(2):65–75

[25] Siemkowicz E, Hansen AJ. Clinical restitution following cerebral ischemia in hypo-, normo- and hyperglycemic rats. Acta Neurol Scand. 1978; 58(1):1–8

[26] Strong AJ, Miller SA, West IC. Protection of respiration of a crude mitochondrial preparation in cerebral ischaemia by control of blood glucose. J Neurol Neurosurg Psychiatry. 1985; 48(5):450–454

[27] Sacks GS, Brown RO, Teague D, Dickerson RN, Tolley EA, Kudsk KA. Early nutrition support modifies immune function in patients sustaining severe head injury. JPEN J Parenter Enteral Nutr. 1995; 19(5):387–392

[28] Ott L, Young B, Phillips R, et al. Altered gastric emptying in the head-injured patient: relationship to feeding intolerance. J Neurosurg. 1991; 74(5):738–742

[29] Lebkowski WJ. Does hyperalimentation improve outcome in patients with severe head injury? Rocz Akad Med Bialymst. 1994; 39:117–120

[30] Berra L, Panigada M, De Marchi L, et al. New approaches for the prevention of airway infection in ventilated patients. Lessons learned from laboratory animal studies at the National Institutes of Health. Minerva Anestesiol. 2003; 69(5):342–347

[31] Maloney J, Metheny N. Controversy in using blue dye in enteral tube feeding as a method of detecting pulmonary aspiration. Crit Care Nurse. 2002; 22(5):84–85

[32] Pender SM, Courtney MG, Rajan E, McAdam B, Fielding JF. Percutaneous endoscopic gastrostomy-results of an Irish single unit series. Ir J Med Sci. 1993; 162(11):452–455

[33] Kiel MK. Enteral tube feeding in a patient with traumatic brain injury. Arch Phys Med Rehabil. 1994; 75(1):116–117

[34] Rhoney DH, Parker D, Jr, Formea CM, Yap C, Coplin WM. Tolerability of bolus versus continuous gastric feeding in brain-injured patients. Neurol Res. 2002; 24(6):613–620

[35] Opeskin K, Lee KA. Failure of a feeding jejunostomy. Med Sci Law. 1993; 33(3):263–266

[36] Borzotta AP, Pennings J, Papasadero B, et al. Enteral versus parenteral nutrition after severe closed head injury. J Trauma. 1994; 37(3):459–468

[37] Grahm TW, Zadrozny DB, Harrington T. The benefits of early jejunal hyperalimentation in the head-injured patient. Neurosurgery. 1989; 25(5):729–735

[38] Tryba M, Cook DJ. Gastric alkalinization, pneumonia, and systemic infections: the controversy. Scand J Gastroenterol Suppl. 1995; 210:53–59

[39] Ritter AM, Robertson CS, Goodman JC, Contant CF, Grossman RG. Evaluation of a carbohydrate-free diet for patients with severe head injury. J Neurotrauma. 1996; 13(8):473–485

[40] Finney SJ, Zekveld C, Elia A, Evans TW. Glucose control and mortality in critically ill patients. JAMA. 2003; 290(15):2041–2047

[41] Mesotten D, Van den Berghe G. Clinical potential of insulin therapy in critically ill patients. Drugs. 2003; 63(7):625–636

[42] Van den Berghe G, Wouters PJ, Bouillon R, et al. Outcome benefit of intensive insulin therapy in the critically ill: Insulin dose versus glycemic control. Crit Care Med. 2003; 31(2):359–366

[43] Preiser JC, Devos P, Van den Berghe G. Tight control of glycaemia in critically ill patients. Curr Opin Clin Nutr Metab Care. 2002; 5(5):533–537

[44] van den Berghe G, Wouters P, Weekers F, et al. Intensive insulin therapy in critically ill patients. N Engl J Med. 2001; 345(19):1359–1367

[45] Roth B, Grände PO, Nilsson-Ehle P, Eliasson I. Possible role of short-term parenteral nutrition with fat emulsions for development of haemophagocytosis with multiple organ failure in a patient with traumatic brain injury. Intensive Care Med. 1993; 19(2):111–114

[46] Alexander JW, Peck MD. Future prospects for adjunctive therapy: pharmacologic and nutritional approaches to immune system modulation. Crit Care Med. 1990; 18(2) Suppl:S159–S164

[47] Saito H, Trocki O, Wang SL, Gonce SJ, Joffe SN, Alexander JW. Metabolic and immune effects of dietary arginine supplementation after burn. Arch Surg. 1987; 122(7):784–789

[48] Chen P, Goldberg DE, Kolb B, Lanser M, Benowitz LI. Inosine induces axonal rewiring and improves behavioral outcome after stroke. Proc Natl Acad Sci U S A. 2002; 99(13):9031–9036

[49] Wilson RF, Dente C, Tyburski JG. The nutritional management of patients with head injuries. Neurol Res. 2001; 23(2–3):121–128

[50] Young B, Ott L, Kasarskis E, et al. Zinc supplementation is associated with improved neurologic recovery rate and visceral protein levels of patients with severe closed head injury. J Neurotrauma. 1996; 13(1):25–34

[51] Hershko C. Control of disease by selective iron depletion: a novel therapeutic strategy utilizing iron chelators. Baillieres Clin Haematol. 1994; 7(4):965–1000

[52] Scheff SW, Dhillon HS. Creatine-enhanced diet alters levels of lactate and free fatty acids after experimental brain injury. Neurochem Res. 2004; 29(2):469–479

[53] Behrman SW, Kudsk KA, Brown RO, Vehe KL, Wojtysiak SL. The effect of growth hormone on nutritional markers in enterally fed immobilized trauma patients. JPEN J Parenter Enteral Nutr. 1995; 19(1):41–46

[54] Bower RH, Cerra FB, Bershadsky B, et al. Early enteral administration of a formula (Impact) supplemented with arginine, nucleotides, and fish oil in intensive care unit patients: results of a multicenter, prospective, randomized, clinical trial. Crit Care Med. 1995; 23(3):436–449

[55] Chiang YH, Chao DP, Chu SF, et al. Early enteral nutrition and clinical outcomes of severe traumatic brain injury patients in acute stage: a multi-center cohort study. J Neurotrauma. 2012; 29 (1):75–80

[56] Marcus HE, Spöhr FA, Böttiger BW, Grau S, Padosch SA. [Nutritional therapy in traumatic brain injury : Update 2012]. Anaesthesist. 2012; 61(8):696–702

[57] Malakouti A, Sookplung P, Siriussawakul A, et al. Nutrition support and deficiencies in children with severe traumatic brain injury. Pediatr Crit Care Med. 2012; 13(1):e18–e24

[58] Costello LA, Lithander FE, Gruen RL, Williams LT. Nutrition therapy in the optimisation of health outcomes in adult patients with moderate to severe traumatic brain injury: findings from a scoping review. Injury. 2014; 45(12):1834–1841

[59] Marino LV, Kiratu EM, French S, Nathoo N. To determine the effect of metoclopramide on gastric emptying in severe head injuries: a prospective, randomized, controlled clinical trial. Br J Neurosurg. 2003; 17(1):24–28

17 Fluid Management

Samir Kashyap, Robert Dahlin, Raed Sweiss, James Berry, and Dan E. Miulli

Abstract
Edema develops at times of brain injury. The edema occurs as fluids and nutrients cross a broken blood–brain barrier or cross a cell membrane. It was once thought appropriate that the restriction of fluid would decrease the brain or spinal cord edema. However, it is now recognized that the meticulous use of the proper fluids can ameliorate edema, improve ischemia, and improve neurologic outcome. Hypotension should be avoided at all cost. Fluids are regulated in the body and brain through numerous factors, including hormones, fluid osmolality, osmolarity, tonicity, and specific cellular water receptors. Because fluids are used for medical treatment, the monitoring of the fluid volume may be required through devices other than the skin tone, mucosal dryness, urine color, blood pressure, and electrolyte concentrations in the serum and urine.

Keywords: ADH, aquaporin, colloids, hormones, hypervolemia, intravenous fluids, osmolality, osmolarity

Case Presentation

A 60-year-old woman presents with a loss of consciousness, right-sided weakness, and a Glasgow Coma Scale score of 9. Her husband found her in the morning on the kitchen floor. She was wearing her nightclothes, and her husband does not know when or if she made it into the bedroom to sleep. She has a past medical history of mild chronic obstructive pulmonary disease and hypertension. She was and still is intubated because of mild respiratory difficulties. In the field, intravenous fluids (dextrose 5% in water) were started because of presumed dehydration.

See end of chapter for Case Management.

17.1 Need for Intravenous Fluids

The body is composed of 50 to 70% water and requires euvolemia to survive optimally and to overcome illness. Intravenous fluids are administered to preserve the extracellular volume and preserve electrolyte balance—allowing for adequate tissue perfusion in the critical care setting, such as severe sepsis or traumatic brain injury (TBI).[1] The understanding of sodium and water balance is key to managing the patient in the neurosurgical intensive care unit (NICU). Although water content is different among individuals, in general, men have a higher percentage of body fluid, and, in either sex, the amount decreases with age. Fifty-five to 75% of the body's total fluid is intracellular, and 25 to 45% is extracellular. The extracellular fluid is located in intravascular plasma (25%) and interstitial spaces (75%). Therefore, in a 70 kg man, of the 48 L of total body fluid, 67% is intracellular (32 L), 25% is interstitial (12 L), and 8% is intravascular (4 L).

Fluid balance is extremely complicated, governed by antidiuretic hormone (ADH) (also known as arginine vasopressin [AVP]), aldosterone, and the natriuretic peptides: brain (BNP), atrial (ANP), and C-type (CNP). The main control of fluid balance is the tonicity made mostly by sodium, with the minor constituents chloride and bicarbonate ions of the extracellular fluid adding to the remainder. Potassium, magnesium, and phosphate constitute intracellular ions and tonicity. The hormones mentioned react to as little as a 1 to 2% change in vascular tonicity.

17.2 Hormone Control of Fluids

ADH/AVP is made in the magnocellular part of the supraoptic nuclei of the hypothalamus and conveyed to the posterior pituitary, where it is secreted. It binds to the distal renal collecting tubules to stimulate water reabsorption and to make concentrated urine in response to opioids, barbiturates, and carbamazepine, as well as high osmolality, hypovolemia, stress, hypoglycemia, and pain. ADH/AVP is a potent vasoconstrictor. In addition to affecting renal tubule cells, it affects brain cells. ADH/AVP V receptors appear to control fluid entry into the brain cell by activation of aquaporin-2, allowing fluid into the cell, which, if increased excessively, increases brain edema and infarction.[2]

Aldosterone is released in response to baroreceptors sensing hemorrhage, decreased intravascular volume, or decreased blood pressure. The baroreceptors stimulate renin angiotensin, leading to aldosterone release and causing sodium resorption followed by water retention.

Natriuretic peptides not only cause renal sodium loss and fluid loss but they also reduce water and sodium in areas of brain edema by directly reducing brain cell water and brain capillary permeability.[3,4] ANP increases cerebral blood flow and causes significant cerebral vasodilation. It is also produced in the hypothalamus and is found in the median eminence, midbrain, choroid plexus, and spinal cord.[5] BNP fibers are found along the carotid, middle cerebral, posterior communicating, and anterior cerebral arteries (▶ Table 17.1).[6]

Normally, a person is able to drink and will become thirsty when the osmoreceptors in the anterior hypothalamus become stimulated at approximately 295 mOsm/kg. However, when the patient is comatose from stroke, trauma, tumor, infection, or other devastating neurologic disease, the physician must prescribe appropriate fluids. The average dose of intravenous fluids (IVFs) can be approximated several ways using a general or graduated, weight-based formula (▶ Table 17.2). There are several physiological circumstances that require increased fluids above the normal amount (▶ Table 17.3).

Table 17.1 Hormone control of fluids[6,7,8,9,10]

Hormone	Fluid action	Vessel action
ADH/AVP	Water reabsorption increased	Vasoconstriction
Aldosterone	Sodium reabsorption increased	Vasoconstriction
Natriuretic peptide	Renal sodium loss	Vasodilation
ANP, BNP, CNP	Renal and brain water loss	

Abbreviations: ADH, antidiuretic hormone; ANP, atrial natriuretic peptide; AVP, arginine vasopressin; BNP, brain natriuretic peptide; CNP, C-type natriuretic peptide.

Table 17.2 Daily and hourly fluid requirements: graduated, weight-based formulas[5,7,8,9,10]

Daily Fluid Requirements[a]

100 mL/kg for the first 10 kg in 24 hours, then

50 mL/kg for the next 10 kg in 24 hours, then

20 mL/kg for remainder weight in kg in 24 hours age < 60 years

15 mL/kg for remainder weight in kg in 24 hours age > 60 years

[a] For 70 kg male, age 55: (1,000 + 500 + 1,000)/24 = 104 mL/h

Hourly Fluid Requirements[a]

4 mL/h for the first 10 kg

2 mL/h for the next 10 kg

1 mL/h for remainder weight in kg

[a] For 70 kg male, age 55: 110 mL/h

Daily Fluid Requirements, Average[a]

Average 35 mL/kg, elderly 30 mL/kg

[a] For 70 kg male, age 55: 2,450/24 = 102 mL/h

Table 17.3 Increased fluid requirements, by percent[a,5,7,8,9,10]

Fever: 12.5% for each 1°C above normal

Sweating: 10 to 25%

Hyperventilation: 10 to 60%

[a] A 70 kg male, age 55, requiring 110 mL/h who has an elevated temperature 1°C and is sweating may require 135 to 151 mL/h.

If these conditions are not taken into consideration, a patient will become hypovolemic. Volume status can be approximated using the following clinical criteria:

- Heart rate: > 110 beats/min.
- Systolic blood pressure (SBP): < 90 mm Hg.
- Dry mucosal surface.
- Crackling heard in lungs.
- Evidence of skin edema or turgor.
- Central venous pressure: < 6 to 8 mm Hg.
- Urine specific gravity: < 1.010 or > 1.030.
- Urine color: clear or amber.
- Urine output: < 0.5 mL/kg/h.
- Daily weight change: increase or decrease of 1 kg.
- Input and output, 8 hours: < 500 mL (24 hours: < 1,500 mL).

Each value by itself may not be diagnostic, but when weighted, it can lead to a clearer idea of fluid balance.

17.3 Osmolality, Osmolarity, and Tonicity

Just knowing the fluid balance of the patient or even the cell will not allow proper maintenance. The amount of solutes concentrated in fluid is also vital. Osmolality is a measure of the number of osmotically active particles measured in osmoles or milliosmoles per kilogram of solvent (mmol/kg or mOsm/L). A highly concentrated osmotic solution will have a high osmolality. That is, it will have more osmotically active particles per unit of solvent than a solution with a low osmolality.

Osmolarity is the total quantity (concentration) of dissolved substances in a solution both penetrating and not penetrating the semipermeable membrane.

Tonicity reflects only the concentration of nonpenetrating solutes in the extracellular space compared with the nonpenetrating solute concentration inside the cell.

The intracellular space is a large reservoir, accounting for 67%, or 32 L, of fluid, and can easily control the solutes in the extracellular volume of 25%, or 12 L An iso-osmotic cell has an osmolarity of 300 mOsm; that is, it contains 300 mOsm of penetrating and nonpenetrating solutes. When the extracellular fluid also contains 300 mOsm of penetrating and nonpenetrating solutes, the extracellular solution is isotonic, and the cell will not change fluid volume. When the extracellular solution contains 250 mOsm (equivalent to lactated Ringer's solution) of penetrating and nonpenetrating solutes, the extracellular fluid is hypotonic, and the cell will swell as the fluid rushes into the large cellular reservoir in an attempt to make the extracellular space isotonic. If the extracellular solution contains 921 mOsm concentration (equivalent to 3% saline) of penetrating and nonpenetrating solutes, the extracellular solution is hypertonic, and the cell will shrink; fluid will rush out in an attempt to make the extracellular space isotonic.

In reality, the cell contains different amounts of penetrating and nonpenetrating solutes compared with the interstitial and intravascular fluid. A cell may have 300 mOsm of nonpenetrating solutes and 20 mOsm of penetrating solute, such as urea, causing it to be hyperosmotic (320 mOsm). If the extracellular fluid has 300 mOsm of nonpenetrating solutes, the extracellular solution is isotonic, and the cell will not change fluid volume. The tonicity is always the relationship of the nonpenetrating solutes across the cellular membrane. Even though the cell's osmolarity is 320 mOsm (300 mOsm nonpenetrating and 20 mOsm penetrating solutes), the extracellular solution is isotonic because it has the same concentration of nonpenetrating solutes as the cell. There are multiple osmotically active components, or osmoles, of solute concentrated in body fluid, expressed as mOsm/L. The intracellular penetrating solute concentration, such as urea and ethanol, does not affect fluid movement because the penetrating solutes will equilibrate across the semipermeable membrane.[11]

The nonpenetrating particles or solutes making up the tonicity of the intravascular fluid are inorganic ions of sodium, chloride, bicarbonate, and potassium, as well as organic osmolytes of amino acids, sorbitol, and methylamines, among others. These osmoles do not easily cross the cell membrane, are restricted to the extracellular or intracellular compartments by the semipermeable cellular membrane, and therefore drive the fluid shifts or the tonicity of the fluid. Compounds such as ethanol, urea, and other solutes easily cross the intravascular boundary and therefore do not significantly add to the tonicity of the fluid, although they do add to the osmolarity.

Sodium is the major component of intravascular fluid whose regulation is closely tied to the volume of the same intravascular fluid. It is the main determinant of tonicity or effective osmolality, which determines where fluid will move. The normal plasma osmolality is 280 to 290 mOsm/L (although some sources suggest as low as 275 to as high as 295 mOsm/L) and is closely controlled by thirst osmoreceptors in the anterolateral hypothalamus. Intracellular components consist of potassium and other tightly regulated anions, leading to an osmolality of 300 mOsm/L, driving fluid into the cell. Tonicity affects fluid movement. The normal concentrations of intra- and extracellular components in osmoles are given in ▶ Table 17.4.

Table 17.4 Normal concentrations of components in intra- and extracellular fluid[5,7,8,9,10]

Component	Intracellular fluid (mOsm/L)	Extracellular fluid (mOsm/L)
Sodium	5–15	135–145
Potassium	140–150	3.5–5.0

Table 17.5 Average daily requirements of extracellular components (for 70 kg [154 lb] man)[5,7,8,9,10]

Component	mEq/L	mEq/kg	Change in mEq
Sodium	60–150	1.0–2.0	80–120
Potassium	55–80	0.5–1.3	50–100
Chloride	60–150	1.0–1.7	80–120
Calcium		0.2–0.3	6–10
Magnesium			20
Phosphorus			30
Glucose			100–200

From the average extracellular concentrations, the daily requirements of those same constituents can be deduced (▶ Table 17.5).

17.4 The Blood–Brain Barrier and Intravenous Fluids

The blood–brain barrier (BBB) has an effective pore size of 8 angstroms (Å) and is impermeable to sodium, ions, water-soluble compounds, and protein, but is permeable to lipophilic substances and gases. The BBB is unique in that it separates the central nervous system environment from the rest of the body. This is accomplished via tight junction-connected endothelial cells and specialized transporter proteins that ensure only select molecules cross the barrier.[12] The majority of substances are actively transported across the brain capillary endothelial cell to the brain interstitial space. The cerebrospinal fluid (CSF) flows along a gradient to the ventricle and is absorbed through the arachnoid villi, where a pressure differential allows it to pass into the venous sinus. Likewise, the larger reservoir, the cellular fluid, is actively transported into the brain interstitial space and follows the same pathway. Ninety-one percent of the circulating fluid is in the intracellular and interstitial spaces; this is the area where fluid and solute need to be regulated.

The optimal treatment would be to actively remove solutes out of the cell into the brain interstitial space, through the ventricles, and into the blood. This would be accomplished with high-tonicity, low-osmolality fluid flowing from the brain capillary endothelial cell into the interstitium, increasing the tonicity of the interstitial fluid with nonpermeable sodium. Low molecular weight solutes would then leave the damaged swollen brain cell, followed by water. The damaged cell contains increased osmoles of H^+ and K^+. Therefore, if ion exchange mechanisms are functioning, lower interstitial solutes of H^+, K^+, and others would simultaneously draw the cellular toxins out of the cell into the

CSF, followed by water, then drained out of the ventricle into the venous system; simulating CSF ventricular dialysis.

Inhibiting CSF formation or decreasing intravascular volume does not decrease intracellular and interstitial edema. Decreasing edema is accomplished by removing CSF.

The microvascular endothelial cells are highly susceptible to hypoxia and are prone to destabilization in certain conditions. During times of trauma and disease, the cell may be swollen in an initial response to dilute the solute toxins. Severe TBI is a condition that predisposes the BBB to such a state.[13] There is additional swelling when fluid increases in the brain interstitial space in an attempt to dilute those increased solutes that entered through the broken BBB. If the interstitial fluid does not drain out of the ventricle, the brain will swell, compressing blood vessels and leading to further ischemia.

The brain initially attempts dialysis by opening the BBB, allowing water and solutes to enter the brain interstitium, attempting to have a hypo-osmolar, hypertonic solution, so that solutes may leave the cell, followed by the increased cellular water.

The BBB, which is formed by the cerebral capillary endothelial cells, contains channels regulated by aquaporins through which water flows somewhat passively down an osmotic gradient. The cerebral capillary endothelial cells are different in function and regulation from those of the brain arteriole or venule. The other brain fluid barrier, albeit much smaller in area, is between the blood and CSF and consists of the choroid plexus epithelium. Tight gap junctions, low pinocytic activity, and specific energy-dependent membrane transporters regulate the passage of substances into and through the capillary endothelial cells to the brain interstitial fluid. Substances can freely diffuse into the capillary endothelial cells if they are gases, lipid soluble, and have a molecular weight less than 400 to 600 daltons (Da). However, most substances, such as choline, glucose, glutamate, and lactate, are associated with either a carrier-mediated transport system or solutes, such as cationized albumin, insulin, insulin-like growth factor, and transferrin. Others are associated with a receptor-mediated transport system. Both systems transport substances through the capillary endothelial cell into the brain interstitial space.

The intact BBB only mildly restricts the passive diffusion of water from a cellular hypotonic solution to an interstitial hypertonic space through aquaporin-regulated channels. In the adult, the BBB regulates most common IVF types. However, the brain damaged by trauma, ischemia, tumors, and increased pressure does not have an intact BBB, nor is the barrier intact with changes in normal brain homeostasis that occur with edema, hyperventilation, mannitol infusion, hyperthermia, hypotension, hypertension, or tumor necrosis factor secretion. During these times of stress, when the BBB is open, vasogenic edema has begun, and the brain is at further risk of damage if the incorrect therapeutic fluids are used. The damaged brain does not benefit from dehydration hypovolemia but from a euvolemic to slightly hypertonic state.[14,15] *During times of initial brain injury systolic blood pressure spikes above 140 mm Hg must be avoided at all costs, as well as hypotonic fluid, and hyperthermia.*

In addition to vasogenic edema from an opened BBB, the more common cellular cytotoxic edema forms in an effort to combat further injury, diluting the cellular toxins accumulated because of decreased blood and plasma flow (e.g., hydrogen ions and potassium). Therefore, dehydration hypovolemia becomes deleterious for combating cytotoxic edema. Euvolemia must be maintained to flush the toxins from the cell. The cell must maintain an osmotic gradient in the brain interstitial space, which allows the transport of solutes and water out of the cell.

Since 1919, the deleterious effects of hypotonic solution have been known.[16] Decreasing the IVF 1 mEq/L will decrease the osmotic pressure 38.6 mm Hg; likewise, decreasing the IVF 5 mEq/L (10 mOsm/kg) will decrease the osmotic pressure 193 mm Hg. This change in fluid drive is minimal under normal homeostasis but will aggravate the swelling and increase the intracranial pressure (ICP) in an opened BBB, a condition that occurs with tumors, ischemia, and trauma. The best fluid approximates or is slightly above normal sodium concentration and normal tonicity without having an additional glucose load. The calculated mOsm/L of individual fluids is shown in ▶ Table 17.6; however, it should be noted that the actual measured osmolality is ~ 20 mOsm/kg water fewer[17] Administering hypertonic saline decreases intracellular volume from 32.0 to 30.6 L, increases interstitial volume from 12.0 to 13.2 L, and increases intravascular volume from 4.0 to 4.4 L. Normal saline has no significant effect on intracellular volume, increases interstitial volume from 12.00 to 14.25 L, and increases intravascular volume from 4.00 to 4.75 L. Dextrose 5% in water (D5W) increases intracellular volume from 32 to 34 L, increases interstitial volume from 12.00 to 12.75 L, and increases intravascular volume from 4.00 to 4.25 L.[18] Therefore, normal saline should be used for resuscitation and any time there is brain damage or the potential for brain damage. D5W, half-normal saline, and lactated Ringer's solution should be avoided as they can exacerbate cerebral edema resulting in increased ICP. Hypertonic saline must be considered during times of increasing cerebral edema (▶ Table 17.6).

Prescribing additives to IVFs must be done with care. Hyperglycemia at the time of primary or secondary injury aggravates ischemic insults and worsens neurologic outcome by increasing lactic acidosis. The condition is not from previously unknown or untreated hyperglycemia; rather, it is usually from reaction to trauma, stress, glucocorticoid administration, sepsis, or other causes.

Table 17.6 Concentration of sodium, osmolarity, osmolality, and glucose of available intravenous fluids[17,18]

Intravenous fluid	Sodium (mEq/L, or mmol/L)	Osmolarity calculated tonicity (mOsm/L)	Measured osmolality	Glucose (g/L)
Normal body fluids	142	280–290	280–290	
0.9 normal saline NaCl	154	308	282	
0.45 half-normal saline NaCl	77	154		
D5W	0	252	259	50
D5 W, 0.45% NaCl	77	406		50
D5 W, 0.9% NaCl	154	560		50
Lactated Ringer's solution	130	273	250	
Normosol	40	363		50
Plasmanate plasma protein fraction (human), 5% USP	145	300		
3% NaCl	513	1030	921	
Albumin 5%	130–160	330		
Albumin 25%	130–160	330		
Hetastarch 6%	145	310	307	

Abbreviation: D5 W, dextrose 5% in water.

Hyperglycemia causes a dose-dependent increase in the severity of ischemic and severe head injury. In one study, glucose > 150 mg/dL had worse outcome than glucose < 150 mg/dL.[19] Hyperglycemia-induced lactic acidosis increases neurologic damage, increases infarct size, and causes secondary injury, a condition that appears to be a major cause of decreased outcome in patients with severe head injury.[20,21]

Therefore, under conditions of suspected brain injury, as seen with ischemia, tumors, and trauma, do not give IV solutions that would worsen edema, such as those containing dextrose, low tonicity, and low sodium.[22] Start fluid maintenance with IV normal saline to keep the patient euvolemic to slightly hypervolemic.

17.5 Hypovolemia

Hypotension must be avoided at all costs. Per the *Brain Trauma Foundation Guidelines*, even one episode of hypotension (SBP < 90 mmHg) doubles morbidity and mortality. Hypovolemia decreases cardiac output and nervous tissue perfusion. It may be seen with a blood urea nitrogen/creatinine (BUN:Cr) ratio greater than 15/20:1 or any other number of clinical conditions. Also, it does not improve outcome after brain injury.

The body attempts to correct hypovolemia by upregulation of norepinephrine, ADH, renin-angiotensin II, and aldosterone, each increasing sodium reabsorption and water retention. Sodium absorption is increased in the renal proximal tubule cells by rennin-angiotensin II, and reabsorption of sodium occurs at the distal tubule and collecting duct by the stimulation of aldosterone. Norepinephrine decreases glomerular filtration rate–enhancing sodium reabsorption at the proximal tubule. However, these hormones also affect brain cell water absorption in a similar fashion, further increasing water retention in the brain interstitium and cell. Therefore, not only trauma patients but also patients with cerebral ischemia, vasospasms, and spinal cord injuries require fluid resuscitation. Euvolemia to slight hypervolemia improves outcomes in head trauma. Each effect of hypotension further worsens the effects of trauma. Daily maintenance fluids should be administered to compensate for the normal loss, for example, in a 70 kg man of 1,200 to 1,500 mL/d and to maintain a urine output of 0.5 to 1.0 mL/kg/h. If there are questions concerning volume status that cannot be determined using clinical and laboratory data presented in this chapter, then a FloTrac sensor (Edwards Lifesciences), a Pulse Contour Continuous Cardiac Output, PiCCO (GE Healthcare), or a Swan-Ganz catheter (Edwards Lifesciences) should be inserted to attempt to obtain normal[23,24] or optimal values in the management of head injury (▶ Table 17.7).[25]

Patients with spinal cord injury have decreased sympathetic tone, leading to vasodilation, bradycardia, hypotension, and decreased perfusion. These patients must have adequate fluid resuscitation with euvolemia and vasopressors to restore sympathetic tone. They should not be overhydrated, which would cause hyponatremia, pulmonary edema, and worsening of spinal cord edema.

Table 17.7 Invasive hemodynamic monitoring[25]

	Normal values	Optimal values (mm Hg)
Central venous pressure	0–8	6–8
Pulmonary artery diastolic pressure	6–16	12–16
Pulmonary capillary wedge pressure	6–14	10–14

17.6 Intravenous Fluids in Extremes of Pathological Conditions

When intensive care management of the neurologically injured patient begins to fail with standard fluids and treatment, additional or different IVFs may be required. When ICP or edema remains elevated, despite initial measures, hypertonic saline or less often mannitol may be needed.

Hypertonic solutions have been shown to lower ICP[26,27,28] and improve cerebral perfusion pressure,[29,30,31,32] whereas isotonic fluids do not improve ICP, as can be deduced from changes in intracellular, interstitial, and intravascular volumes, as already noted.[33] In a study by Vassar et al,[34] hypertonic saline reduced ICP in patients with severe head injury. Furthermore, 7.5% sodium chloride (NaCl) improved survival when compared with standard treatment in patients with a Glasgow Coma Scale score of 3 to 8. Wade et al[35] performed a meta-analysis of patients with severe head injury who receive hypertonic saline and demonstrated that they are twice as likely to survive as those who receive standard therapy. Hypertonic saline is more beneficial than mannitol in refractory intracranial hypertension[36,37] by creating a driving force that pulls water out of the brain cells and interstitium. In a recent study, Eskandari et al demonstrated that boluses of 14.6% hypertonic saline, rather than a single dose, could be used to effectively treat refractory intracranial hypertension without significant cardiovascular adverse effects.[38] Hypertonic saline has an increased concentration of sodium and chloride. In an attempt to decrease hyperchloremic metabolic acidosis, the hypertonic solution may be made with a balanced mixture of sodium chloride and sodium acetate.

There is growing evidence that lactate administration may be beneficial in severe TBI patients. Lactate is an alternative to glucose in providing energy for the brain. Rodent models have demonstrated improved cognitive dysfunction and a diminished reduction of adenosine triphosphate. In a multicenter study by Ichai et al, administration of 0.5 mL/kg/h of sodium lactate versus 0.9% saline solution over a period of 48 hours resulted in a 50% decrease in episodes of elevated ICP and a 30% reduction in patients who experienced increased ICP (36% vs. 66%).[38,39]

There is considerable debate regarding resuscitation with colloids. However, if a 1 to 2 L fluid bolus of normal saline does not stabilize the patient, or 20 mL/kg in children per Advanced Trauma Life Support (ATLS) guidelines, then colloid should be given. Crystalloids such as normal saline remain intravascular for a maximum of 2 hours, and their effect on pulmonary wedge pressure and cardiac index is small. Colloids contain high molecular weight solutes that do not readily cross the capillary wall, remain intravascular for longer periods of time, and require smaller infused volumes. Some investigators have demonstrated that colloids exacerbate pulmonary edema, decrease cardiac output, and compromise the immune system. Others believe that colloids reduce secondary brain injury. Of the colloids, blood may be the best alternative for fluid resuscitation, attempting to maintain a hemoglobin and hematocrit of 10 and 33%, respectively.[40,41,42,43,44,45] This allows maximum oxygen-carrying capacity and the best viscosity.[46,47,48,49] Hemodilution to a hemoglobin and hematocrit of 10 and 33%, respectively, has been studied in the management of cerebral vasospasms, in an attempt to improve viscosity and oxygen-carrying capacity as well as cerebral blood flow.[50,51] Hematocrit lower than 30% decreases oxygen-carrying capacity beyond the improvements made because of increased viscosity. Even in ischemic stroke patients, a hematocrit of 30% optimizes infarct volume, being worse for values > 35% and < 26%.[52,53] Anemia, where the hematocrit is less than 25 to 30%, increases cerebral vasodilation, ICP, and edema.[54]

Several substances in addition to blood have been used to increase volume, such as albumin, Plasmanate (Bayer Pharmaceuticals), Normosol (Abbott Laboratories), and hetastarch. Each volume expander has risks; however, the best expander remains blood. Plasmanate appears to be better than lactated Ringer's solution and causes fewer lung problems when compared with other fluids.[55,56] Normosol may have better red blood cell protection than Plasmanate.[57] Hetastarch, although it expands volume well, does have the side effect of bleeding, significantly elevating partial thromboplastin time. It therefore should not be used when hemorrhage has occurred or may occur.[58] Albumin 5, 20, or 25% may[59,60] or may not improve outcome when used in the trauma patient and may in fact increase pulmonary extravascular fluid.[61] Although 5% albumin is oncotically and osmotically equivalent to plasma, its use remains controversial. The Saline Versus Albumin Fluid Evaluation (SAFE) study[62] concluded that, in patients in the NICU, use of 4% albumin or normal saline for fluid resuscitation results in similar outcomes at 28 days. The authors looked at 6,997 randomized patients. For the entire study population, there were no significant differences in deaths and number of days spent in the NICU, hospital, on ventilator, or in renal replacement therapy. However, the subgroup analysis of patients with trauma and brain injury trended toward an increased relative risk of death. There was insufficient power to make significant claims. The actual number of patients (59 of 241) receiving albumin with trauma and head injury compared with those receiving saline (38 of 251) was small ($p = 0.009$). In the analysis of death in all patients with trauma, 81 of 596 were in the albumin group, and 59 of 590 deaths were in the saline group ($p = 0.06$); however, once again, the power was too low to support significant claims. Patients with head injury constituted only 7% of the study population. The investigators concluded that there needs to be further study of trauma and head injury patients.

Mannitol has been in the neuroscience armamentarium for some time. Mannitol improves viscosity and therefore circulation. It does, however, open the BBB and, with multiple doses, will cross into the interstitial space and increase its osmotic pull of fluids into the tissue, causing hypotonicity, contrary to the intended desire of therapy. It works on the microvasculature in several minutes, vasoconstricting, decreasing viscosity, increasing cerebral blood flow,[63,64,65,66,67,68] and acting as a free radical scavenger. Mannitol works best at high ICP, low cerebral perfusion pressure at vasodilation when autoregulation is preserved. Its plasma expansion is equal to 7.5% NaCl. The systemic capillary is permeable to water, which moves into the intravascular space to dilute mannitol, while an intact brain is not freely permeable to water to the same extent as the systemic capillary or the damaged BBB. As an osmotic diuretic, mannitol draws in systemic water, causing hemodilution and improving shear rate and red blood cell deformity. The osmotic effect is delayed 15 to 30 minutes, and persists 90 minutes to 6 hours. Mannitol has a small osmotic effect in the brain, only changing the brain water content 2 to 6%. It becomes less effective after multiple doses, such as more than three or four doses in 24 hours. If given at higher rates, mannitol moves across the defective BBB into tissue, exacerbating edema.[69,70] Mannitol can be used when there is suspected increased ICP, such as in the emergency room. When given, there must be adequate fluids to support blood pressure because hypotension doubles morbidity and mortality rates associated with severe head injury. On occasion, mannitol can demonstrate an increase in ICP and a transient short-term decrease in sodium, magnesium, phosphorus, and potassium. Mannitol increases intravascular osmolality; therefore, when there is reasonable concern about osmolality, a measured recording of osmolality must be made, not a calculated recording.

Guidelines for the Management of Severe Head Injury[71] states that

[m]annitol is effective therapy for the control of increased ICP. Intermittent bolus is probably better than continuous infusion therapy. Dose ranges are 0.25–1 g/kg.

Option: Where mannitol is being used prior to ICP monitoring, where it is not titrated, evidence of raised ICP should be present (e.g., signs of transtentorial herniation or progressive neurologic deterioration). Serum osmolarity should be kept < 320 mOsm, because when greater the incidence of renal failure is increased. Euvolemia should be maintained and a Foley catheter inserted.

17.6.1 Diuretics

Mannitol may be the most appropriate agent for diuresis in the short term. Another agent is furosemide, which acts by inhibiting distal tubule reabsorption of sodium and water. It can also reduce ICP and CSF production. The dose varies with the degree of diuresis required, from as little as 5 mg IV every 4 to 6 hours to as high as 80 to 160 mg every 6 hours. The use of furosemide should be exercised with caution as severe head injury patients are prone to dumping urine due to cerebral salt wasting or syndrome of inappropriate diuretic hormone (SIADH). Oftentimes, a low-dose Lasix (5–10 mg IV) is sufficient to achieve euvolemia for a selected period in these specific patients. Acetazolamide is a carbonic anhydrase inhibitor reducing CSF production from the choroid plexus while vasodilating. It can be used during conditions of excess CSF production, which by itself causes an increased ICP. It should not be used during times of intracellular and interstitial edema. The usual dose is 125 to 250 mg three or four times a day to a maximum of 2 g/d. Side effects include metabolic acidosis that should be checked with a chemistry panel or arterial blood gases. Other side effects include paresthesia, altered taste, renal calculi, and nausea.

17.7 Calculation of Fluid Balance and Hemodynamic Monitoring

Fluid balance determination may be a difficult task in the NICU because of medications and concomitant injuries. It is important to determine fluid input and output exactly because severe TBI patients experience a loss of cerebral autoregulation and may be prone to fluid overload. The patient must be weighed daily using the same scale and the same clutter of material, such as sheets, blankets, pillows, sequential compression devices, and monitors. Although bothersome to the nursing staff, the most exact measurement would be to weigh without these items.

There is no concrete means to determine fluid balance; however, technologies are evolving. The fluid balance can be determined from clinical exam and laboratory tests, but continuous monitoring of cardiac output parameters helps guide management of fluids. Swan-Ganz catheters have long been a mainstay of this type of monitoring, but FloTrac and PiCCO continuous cardiac output monitoring have become more favored in recent years due to their ease of setup and reliable data.

The FloTrac system extracts its data from an arterial line. This makes use of the FloTrac system convenient as many patients in the NICU will have an arterial line placed for blood pressure management. It provides many parameters that can inform clinical decision making in regard to fluid management. The primary parameters for assessing fluid responsiveness are as follows:
- Stroke volume variation (SVV) *Normal (< 13%).*
  - The measurement of the beat to beat variation in stroke volume per each breathing cycle. It is a reliable method of determining fluid responsiveness in a 100% mechanically ventilated patient. If a patient has an SVV < 13%, they have little variation between cycles and are likely fluid replete. If a patient has an SVV > 13%, they most likely will be fluid responsive.

- Stroke volume index (SVI) *Normal 35–50.*
  - This parameter is a complement to SVV. It is especially useful in patients with an SVV of 10–13%, sometimes referred to as a gray zone. If an individual has an SVV > 13% and does not respond to fluids, SVI can help determine the next appropriate step. If SVI is low (< 35), a pressor would be indicated; normal (35–50), an inotrope is indicated; high (> 50), diuresis would be indicated.

The PiCCO (Pulse Index Continuous Cardiac Output) monitoring system functions similarly to the FloTrac; however, it delivers information from venous blood flow in addition to arterial blood flow. The system uses a central line and an arterial line, preferably inserted into a large artery such as the femoral or axillary artery. The hemodynamic measurements are acquired by a thermodilution technique. A selected volume of cold saline is injected through the central line, and the system uses the temperature gradient and dissipation curve to measure the global end diastolic index (GEDI), extravascular lung water index (ELWI), intrathoracic blood volume (ITBV), cardiac index (CI), stroke volume variation (SVV), stroke volume index (SVI), and systemic vascular resistance (SVR).

- Global end diastolic index (GEDI) *Normal (680–800)*—Measurement of end diastolic volume—a marker of preload.
- Extravascular lung water index (ELWI) *Normal(< 10)*—Measurement of fluid in the lungs—a marker of pulmonary edema.
- Cardiac index (CI) *Normal (3–5).*[72]

The use of PiCCO and FloTrac is especially helpful in subarachnoid hemorrhage patients as correct and judicious fluid management is paramount in preventing delayed cerebral ischemia (DCI) while avoiding the adverse effects of fluid overload. A recent study performed by Tagami et al showed that optimizing GEDI helped to prevent DCI. In this study, a GEDI of less than 822 mL/m^2 was found to be the threshold that was associated with DCI. This study had several limitations. GEDI was only measured once daily and the effects of ELWI as well as cardiac dysfunction were not taken into account. Patients in this study also did not exhibit a typical pattern of DCI according to their SAH grade. Therefore, the results of this study should be implemented with caution.[73] A similar study performed by Obata et al evaluated the utility of PiCCO in identifying pulmonary edema and its occurrence in the time course of an SAH patient.[74] The PiCCO monitoring system helped predict the onset quickly and accurately. The time course of its development (early vs. delayed) helped to inform the etiology (cardiogenic vs. noncardiogenic) so the appropriate management could be implemented.[75]

Although ▶ Table 17.8 simplifies the calculation of fluid balance, the true determination is not simple. A simplified method of fluid administration is to determine a patient's weight (kg) and add 40 mL/h. If the patient is ventilated, experiencing fever, or severely brain injured, an extra 10% should be added for each, respectively. The clinical exam for volume status must be part of the daily examination of the NICU patient.[8,9,10]

Table 17.8 Calculation of fluid balance[7,8,9,10]

Component (absolute value or daily change)	Positive overload (value or lose [L] pts)	Negative dry (value or gain [G] pts)
Hgb (12–16)	<10 or L1.5 or>	>15 or G1.5 or>
HCT (37–54)	<30 or L4 or>	>50 or G4 or>
Na (134–145)	<134 or L5 or>	>145 or G5 or>
BUN (7–18) **or (only give 1 or 2 pts)**	<10 or L4 or>	>18 or G4 or>
BUN (7–18)	<5 or L7 (2 pts)	
Creatinine (0.7–1.3)	<0.7 or L0.3 or>	>1.3 or G0.3 or>
Serum osmolarity (280–300)	<280 or L15 or>	>300 or G15 or>
Heart rate		>110 or G30 or>
SBP		<90 or L35 or>
Orthostatics		Positive
Mucosa		Mucosa dry
Lungs	Crackles	
Skin	Edema	Turgor (2 pts)
CVP (0–8 mm Hg) ([a]▽ = 6–8)	>9 or G5 or>	<4 or L5 or>
Urine specific gravity (1.010–1.030)	<1.010 or L0.020 or>	>1.030 or> G0.020 or>
Urine color	Clear	Amber
Urine output		<0.5 mL/kg/h (2 pts)
Weight change daily	Gain >2.2 lb	Lose >2.2 lb
I&Os 8 hours	+500	–500
I&Os 24 hours **or**	+1,000 **or**	–1,000 **or**
(only give 1 or 2 pts)	+1,500 or >(2 pts)	–1,500 or >(2 pts)
Current hemodynamic parameters		
Cardiac output 4–7	Cardiac index 2.8–4.2	MAP

(continued)

Table 17.8 continued

Component (absolute value or daily change)	Positive overload (value or lose [L] pts)	Negative dry (value or gain [G] pts)
PCWP 6–14[a] 10–14 ▽	PAD 6–16[a] 12–16 ▽	SVR 770–1,500

Abbreviations: BUN, blood urea nitrogen; CVP, central venous pressure; HCT, hematocrit; Hgb, hemoglobin; I&Os, inputs and outputs; MAP, mean arterial pressure; Na, sodium; PAD, pulmonary artery diastolic pressure; PCWP, pulmonary capillary wedge pressure; SBP, systolic blood pressure; SVR, systemic vascular resistance; ▽, optimal value for the treatment of head injury.[25]

Note: Of a total of + 17 points for positive overload, overload occurs at greater than 5 points. Of a total of – 22 points for negative dry, dry occurs at less than – 5 points. To determine fluid status, add positive values in column 2 and negative values in column 3.

[a] Average values.[23,24]

Assuming no significant effects of vasoconstrictors or severe cardiopulmonary changes, the values of pulmonary artery diastolic pressure (PAD) below may be used to adjust fluids. Numbers preceded by + or – indicate change from previous reading.

If PAD > 17 or > + 5, decrease fluids 25%. If PAD < 10 or < – 5, increase fluids 50%.

If PAD > 20 or > + 8, decrease fluids 50%. If PAD < 8 or < – 8, increase fluids 100%.

If PAD > 23 or > + 10, give diuretic, and decrease fluids 75%.

If PAD < 6 or < – 10, increase fluids 100%, and give fluid bolus 300% over 1 hour; if no response, give 100% bolus colloid.

17.7.1 Specific States of Fluid and Electrolyte Imbalance

Specific states of fluid and electrolyte imbalance can be calculated using the following equation:

$$Osmolality(mOsm/L) = 2 \times (Na\ mEq/L + K\ mEq/L) + (BUN/2.8) + (glucose/18)$$

17.7.2 Hyponatremia

There are three states of hyponatremia (Na < 135 mmol/L), the most common being hypotonic hyponatremia and the least common being isotonic and hypertonic (▶ Table 17.9). A specific paradigm can be followed to determine the etiology and appropriate treatment for the disease state. It is especially important in neurosurgical patients because hyponatremia is associated with increased morbidity and mortality.[76]

Table 17.9 States of hyponatremia

State (Na < 135 mEq/L or mmol/L)	Subtypes	Clinical condition	Treatment
Isotonic (serum mOsm 280–290)		Hyperproteinemia, hyperlipidemia	Correct underlying disorder
Hypertonic (serum mOsm > 290)		Glucose, mannitol load	Correct underlying disorder
Hypotonic (mOsm < 280)	Isovolemic	Water intoxication	Fluid restriction
		K+ loss, diuretics, carbamazepine	Fluid restriction
		TB, cirrhosis	Fluid restriction
		SIADH	Fluid restriction
	Hypervolemic	CHF, liver disease	Fluid restriction, loop diuretic, 3% NaCl, NaCl tablets
		TURP	Multiple
	Hypovolemic	CSW	Increase volume, 3% NaCl, NaCl tablets
		D5W, 0.45% NaCl	Increase volume with 0.9% NaCl

Abbreviations: CHF, congestive heart failure; CSW, cerebral salt wasting; D5W, dextrose 5% in water; SIADH, syndrome of inappropriate antidiuretic hormone; TB, tuberculosis; TURP, transurethral prostatic resection.

Isotonic hyponatremia (serum mOsm 280–290) is caused by hyperlipidemia and hyperproteinemia that increase plasma volume and dilute sodium. The expected amount of sodium reduction is equal to the current protein concentration minus 8 g/dL multiplied by 0.25. A very large protein concentration is needed to change the sodium concentration significantly. Treatment consists of correcting the underlying disorder.

Hypertonic hyponatremia (serum mOsm > 290) is more commonly seen with diseases of hypertonicity, such as hyperglycemia, or after hypertonic administration of glucose, mannitol, or glycine, causing dilution of sodium. The expected amount of sodium reduction is equal to 1.45 mmol/L for each 100 mg/dL increase in blood glucose above 200 mg/dL. Treatment consists of correcting the underlying disorder.

Hypotonic hyponatremia (serum mOsm < 280) is the most common type seen in the NICU patient and itself consists of three subtypes: isovolemic, hypovolemic, and hypervolemic.

Isovolemic hypotonic hyponatremia occurs after consumption of large amounts of water in patients with mild renal impairment, potassium loss from diuretics, or gastrointestinal loss, as well as in those with tuberculosis, bronchogenic tumors, cirrhosis, aspergillosis, stress, severe pain, acute intermittent porphyria, and those receiving positive pressure ventilation. It is also associated with the use of carbamazepine, phenothiazines, antidepressants, chlorpropamide, oxytocin, thiazide diuretics, sulfonylureas, and opiates, and with SIADH. (Information regarding the diagnosis, symptoms, and treatment of SIADH is given later in the chapter.) Increasing intrathoracic pressure causes aortic baroreceptors to sense hypotension and respond with water retention. Most causes are treated with fluid restriction of 800 to 1,500 mL/d. Lower sodium levels can be treated with sodium tablets (2 g) three or four times per day or 3% NaCl IV solution. The use of each depends on the clinical condition.

Hypervolemic hypotonic hyponatremia is the subtype of edema seen in congestive heart failure, cirrhosis, and transurethral prostatic resection. Most causes are treated with fluid restriction of 800 to 1,500 mL/d and can be augmented with loop diuretic because of the higher afterload. Lower sodium levels can be treated with sodium tablets 2 g three or four times per day or 3% NaCl IV solution. The use of each depends on the clinical condition.

Hypovolemic hypotonic hyponatremia occurs when loss of fluids rich in sodium, such as bile, sweat, and fluids found in the pancreas, small intestine, and lung, are replaced with D5 W or 0.45% NaCl. The most common clinical condition of this subtype seen in the NICU patient is the syndrome of cerebral salt wasting (CSW). (Information regarding the diagnosis, symptoms, and treatment of CSW is given later in the chapter.) Renal loss of sodium and low volume in CSW are opposite the condition of SIADH. CSW is seen in subarachnoid hemorrhage (SAH) of any type and is possibly due to the brain releasing natriuretic factor from the hypothalamus in an attempt to increase cerebral blood flow and cause cerebral vasodilation during times of vasospasm. Natriuretic peptides not only cause renal sodium loss and fluid loss, they also reduce water and sodium in areas of brain edema. Natriuretic peptide fibers are found along the carotid, middle cerebral, posterior communicating, and anterior cerebral arteries, areas of highest vasospasm. CSW occurs 3 to 7 days after initial SAH, concomitant with a time of vasospasm occurrence.

Diagnosis of SIADH

The diagnosis of SIADH includes the following parameters:
• Normal or elevated intravascular volume.
• Serum sodium < 134 mEq/L.
• Low serum osmolality (< 280 mOsm/L).
• High urine osmolality, high or normal urinary sodium (> 18 mEq/L).
• Normal renal, adrenal, and thyroid function.

Hyponatremia in SIADH occurs due to bronchogenic tumors, meningitis, trauma, increased ICP, tumors, and craniotomy.

Symptoms of SIADH

Symptoms of SIADH include headache, confusion, lethargy, nausea/vomiting, muscle cramps, depressed deep tendon reflexes, and seizures; these can lead to coma and death.

Treatment of SIADH

Treatment of SIADH involves slowly elevating the sodium level and restricting fluids to an amount less than urine output. In the adult, fluid intake should be restricted to 800 to 1,500 mL/d. If severe SIADH is present, use 3% NaCl and furosemide. (The furosemide causes excretion of dilute urine.) If there is chronic SIADH, as seen in some alcoholics, then elevate the sodium level slowly, 8 to 10 mEq/L per 24 hours, to prevent osmotic demyelination syndrome of the pons or other areas. In a chronic alcoholic patient, stop 3% NaCl when the serum sodium level reaches 125 mEq/L to prevent a relative hyperosmolar condition in this specific type of patient. The rebound relative hyperosmolar state may be the pathophysiology involved in central myelinolysis. Other treatments include phenytoin or demeclocycline 150 to 300 mg orally every 6 hours to inhibit ADH.

Diagnosis of CSW

The diagnosis of CSW includes the following parameters:
- Serum sodium < 134 mEq/L.
- Low serum osmolality (< 280 mOsm/L).
- Urine osmolality normal or elevated.
- High urinary sodium (> 18 mEq/L).
- Low CVP, pulmonary capillary wedge pressure, and pulmonary artery diastolic pressure.
- Low vascular volume.
- Dehydration.

Symptoms of CSW

The symptoms of CSW include headache, confusion, lethargy, nausea/ vomiting, muscle cramps, depressed deep tendon reflexes, and seizures; these can lead to coma and death.

Treatment of CSW

In treating CSW, volume replacement should include 3% NaCl IVF at 10 to 50 mL/h and, if appropriate, salt tablets 2 to 3 g three or four times a day. Fludrocortisone acetate increases sodium absorption but usually is not needed.

CSW usually ends within 2 to 3 weeks, at which time salt replacement should be discontinued.

17.8 Hypernatremia

Hypernatremia occurs when serum sodium is > 150 to 155 mEq/L. However, symptoms do not present until later, when serum sodium is > 160 mEq/L and serum osmolality is > 330 mOsm/L. At this point, the patient may exhibit confusion, lethargy, and seizure. Serum sodium > 180 mEq/L can be associated with increased rates of mortality, but the mortality may be the result of a life-ending process, not necessarily of the hypernatremia.

To determine the amount of fluid needed to correct the hypernatremia, the total body water (TBW) deficit should be calculated. Normal TBW averages 60% but ranges from 50 to 70%, more in younger men and less in older women.

Fluid deficit in liters = (Na current − Na normal 140 mEq/L/140 mEq/L × (TBW : normal 60% of body weight[kg])

If current sodium in, for example, a 70 kg man is 170 mEq/L, the free water deficit would be

$$(170 - 140)/140 \times (0.6 \times 70)$$

$$30/140 \times 42 = 8.99 \text{ L}$$

The deficit of free water must be replaced slowly, usually one-half over 24 hours and the remainder over 1 or 2 days.

As with hyponatremia, there are three states: isovolemic, hypervolemic, and hypovolemic. Isovolemic hypernatremia is seen with sweating, use of isotonic fluids to replace hypotonic losses, and diabetes insipidus (DI) with sufficient fluid replacement. DI occurs most commonly after pituitary surgery and less commonly TBI. Severe head injury can cause damage to the posterior pituitary, resulting in decreased secretion of ADH. It manifests primarily as excessive loss of large volumes of inappropriately dilute urine. In DI, there is an 85% loss of ADH capacity. In posttraumatic DI, the condition is transient in nature and often lasts 3–5 weeks, but symptoms can persist up to 1 year. A recent study showed that approximately 21% of posttraumatic DI patients will experience persistent DI, although the authors concede that this may be a slight overestimation.[77] It is seen as a familial condition; occurs idiopathically, posttrauma, and with craniopharyngioma, lymphoma, neurosarcoidosis, meningitis, autoimmune diseases, and aneurysm; is linked to the administration of mannitol, phenytoin, furosemide, hydrochlorothiazide, and ethanol; is seen in brain death or impending brain death; and is associated with Wegener's granulomatosis and lymphocytic hypophysitis.

Hypervolemic hypernatremia results from the use of hypertonic solutions and mineralocorticoid excess. Hypervolemic hypernatremia is seen in hypotonic fluid loss, such as in burn patients, and with diarrhea, vomiting, and nasogastric suctioning. It is also seen in adrenal insufficiency, chronic renal failure, and after DI has started without correction. The osmotic diuresis from mannitol use or with hyperglycemia results in urine that is iso-osmotic or hyperosmotic, not hypo-osmotic as in DI.

When administering mannitol, the amount of osmolarity added to the serum from mannitol can be determined from the difference of the calculated serum osmolarity [mOsm/L = 2 × (Na mEq/L + K mEq/L) + (BUN/2.8) + (glucose/18)] compared with the measured serum osmolality.

17.8.1 Therapeutic Hypernatremia

In severe TBI patients, hypernatremia is not necessarily pathological. The use of hypertonic saline solution to drive serum sodium concentration of 145–155 mEq/L is useful in reducing ICP. As mentioned previously, the administration of hypertonic saline results in an increase in intravascular volume and a decrease in intracellular volume.

17.8.2 Diagnosis of Hypernatremia

The diagnosis of hypernatremia includes the following parameters:

- High urine output (> 250 mL/h more than input fluids).
- Large water loss in urine relative to sodium loss, with resultant high normal or above normal serum sodium.
- Low urine specific gravity (< 1.005).
- Low urine osmolarity (50–150 mOsm/L).
- High serum osmolality (> 290–295 mOsm/L).

After craniopharyngioma or pituitary surgery, there can be different types of DI. For example, there can be a transient phase, which occurs 12 to 36 hours postop; a prolonged phase, in which sodium remains abnormal for months or permanently; and a triphasic phase, in which injury to the pituitary reduces ADH for 4 to 5 days. This is then followed by cell death, liberating ADH for 4 to 5 days, during which time the DI resolves. The final phase is defined by the absence of ADH, either short-term or prolonged.

17.8.3 Symptoms of Hypernatremia

Symptoms of hypernatremia include confusion, loss of consciousness, tonico-clonic seizures, and rhabdomyolysis. There is no evidence that it causes intra-cranial hemorrhage.

17.8.4 Treatment of Hypernatremia

Treatment of hypernatremia includes the following:
- • Desmopressin (DDAVP) IV 1 to 5 µg (works for 8–20 hours) or
- • Arginine vasopressin intramuscularly, subcutaneously 12.5 µg (works for 4–8 hours)
- • Desmopressin (DDAVP) intranasally 1 to 5 µg (works for 12–20 hours).

Check laboratory tests and urine specific gravity every 6 hours.

Replace urine output greater than input with 0.45 normal saline, or use gastrointestinal system through a feeding tube to replace with free water. Do not give free water IV if it can be avoided. The rapid correction can cause cerebral edema and permanent neurologic damage. One half of the water deficit as calculated above should be corrected in 24 hours and the remainder over 1 to 2 days; the rate of correction should not exceed 10 to 12 mmol/L/24 h in an attempt to prevent further cerebral edema.

17.9 Other Electrolyte Imbalances

17.9.1 Magnesium

This cation occurs both as protein bound and as a free divalent ion. Magnesium is lost with acidosis, diuresis, extracellular fluid expansion, diarrhea, alcoholism, and phosphate depletion. Low magnesium (< 1.5 mg/dL) is associated with seizures, confusion, and cardiac disturbances.[7] It is thought to be consumed blocking the N-methyl-D-aspartate channel as a response to brain insult. Treatment consists of 25% magnesium sulfate 2 g every 4 hours given within the first 4 hours after brain injury to maintain therapeutic levels. Treatment should not result in extensive vasodilation and decreased blood pressure, which lead to poor outcomes due to episodes of ischemia. Magnesium in the setting of TBI is typically low and its correction in multiple studies in rats and one human study[78] demonstrated improved outcome, but in other studies using higher dosages and possibly episodes of hypotension has not been found to correlate with improved outcomes.[79] In a randomized, double-blind trial of continuous infusions of magnesium at two doses versus placebo for 5 days within 8 hours of injury to maintain magnesium ranges of 1.0–1.85 mmol/L or 1.25–2.5 mmol/L, patients receiving magnesium did not benefit.[78] Magnesium in the setting of aneurysmal subarachnoid hemorrhage has been considered historically to decrease poor outcomes by decreasing the risk for vasospasm. The magnesium for Aneurysmal Subarachnoid Hemorrhage (MASH-2) trial was a large phase III randomized, placebo-controlled trial involving 1,204 patients where 26.2% of patients receiving magnesium experienced a poor outcome versus 25.3% in the placebo group.[80] Their conclusion being that magnesium sulfate does not improve clinical outcomes.

17.9.2 Calcium

Free ionized calcium is controlled by the parathyroid hormone and vitamin D. Parathyroid hormone stimulates the release of calcium from the bones, reabsorption from the kidneys, and absorption from the gastrointestinal tract. Hypocalcemia (<8.5 mEq/L) may be seen with phenytoin use, albumin, alkalosis, low magnesium, sepsis, pancreatitis, vitamin D deficiency, hypoparathyroidism, and rhabdomyolysis. Low serum albumin will decrease total calcium but will not affect ionized calcium. Therefore, ionized calcium should be measured, not calculated. Low calcium is associated with neuronal irritability, such as seizures, confusion, paresthesia, hypotension, arrhythmias, sinus tachycardia segment prolongation, apnea, stridor, and no response to norepinephrine or dopamine. If calcium is suspected to be low, then the magnesium level should be checked and, if low, corrected. Ionized calcium levels must be checked, and low levels should be treated with 100 to 200 mg in 50 to 100 mL D5W bolus, followed by 1 to 2 mg/kg/h infusion for 6 to 12 hours.

17.9.3 Potassium

Potassium is an intracellular cation whose release by the kidney is controlled by aldosterone. Only 0.4% of total body potassium is present in the plasma; therefore, intracellular stores can effectively replenish extracellular pools. During times of brain damage, cellular acidosis causes potassium to leave the cell for the intravascular space. Other causes include diabetic ketoacidosis, angiotensin-converting enzyme inhibitors, beta blockers, digoxin, heparin, nonsteroidal anti-inflammatory drugs, trimethoprim-sulfamethoxazole, rhabdomyolysis, and rewarming after hypothermia.

Hyperkalemia (K+ > 5.5 mmol/L) produces paralysis, muscle weakness, dysesthesia, and cardiac disturbances due to neuroexcitability of cellular membranes. Treatment of symptomatic hyperkalemia consists of 10 mL calcium gluconate 10% solution containing 93 mg of elemental calcium. Calcium antagonizes the cardiac muscle toxicity for 20 to 60 minutes. Sodium bicarbonate, as well as insulin and glucose infusion, causes enhanced activity of Na^+-K^+ adenosine triphosphatase, moving K^+ into the cell. This helps stabilize the neurological and neuromuscular toxicity. However, sodium bicarbonate may bind calcium, making its action ineffective. Cation exchange resins, such as polystyrene sulfonate (Kayexalate) removes 1 mEq K^+ from the body for each gram given. The usual dose is 20–50 g dissolved in 100–200 mL 20% sorbitol given every 3 hours, up to five doses per day. However, should there be any suggestion of renal failure, hemodialysis should be instituted as soon as possible.

Hypokalemia is defined as a $K^+ < 3.5$ mmol/L. It is most relevant in patients with cardiac arrhythmias, which is a common comorbidity in patients treated in the NICU. Potassium is important in stabilization of the cardiac rhythm. Patients with hypokalemia are at a higher risk for the development of atrial fibrillation.[81] Currently it is recommended that patients with atrial fibrillation maintain a potassium level of greater than 4.0. To adequately replete low potassium levels it may be necessary to correct magnesium levels as low magnesium can increase potassium excretion in the kidneys.[82,83]

Case Management

This patient should have the IVF switched to normal saline at 35 mL/kg/d, plus a 10% increase for presumed hyperventilation. She should have a computed tomographic scan and laboratory tests to include a chemistry panel and arterial blood gases.

References

[1] Moritz ML, Ayus JC. Maintenance Intravenous Fluids in Acutely Ill Patients. N Engl J Med. 2015; 373(14):1350–1360

[2] Vakili A, Kataoka H, Plesnila N. Role of arginine vasopressin V1 and V2 receptors for brain damage after transient focal cerebral ischemia. J Cereb Blood Flow Metab. 2005; 25(8):1012–1019

[3] Rosenberg GA, Scremin O, Estrada E, Kyner WT. Arginine vasopressin V1-antagonist and atrial natriuretic peptide reduce hemorrhagic brain edema in rats. Stroke. 1992; 23(12):1767–1773, discussion 1773–1774

[4] Naruse S, Takei R, Horikawa Y, et al. Effects of atrial natriuretic peptide on brain oedema: the change of water, sodium, and potassium contents in the brain. Acta Neurochir Suppl (Wien). 1990; 51:118–121

[5] Andrews BT. Fluid and electrolyte disorders in neurosurgical intensive care. Neurosurg Clin N Am. 1994; 5(4):707–723

[6] Edvinsson L, Krause DN. Neuropeptides. In: Edvinsson L, Krause DN, eds. Cerebral Blood Flow and Metabolism. 2nd ed. Philadelphia, PA: Lippincott Williams & Wilkins; 2002:273

[7] Ropper A, Gress D, Diringer M, et al. Fluid and metabolic derangements. In: Neurological and Neurosurgical Intensive Care. 4th ed. Philadelphia, PA: Lippincott Williams & Wilkins; 2004:105–112

[8] Layon AJ, Gabrielli A, Friedman WA. Textbook of Neurointensive Care. Philadelphia, PA: WB Saunders; 2004

[9] Suarez JI. Critical Care Neurology and Neurosurgery. Totowa, NJ: Humana Press; 2004

[10] Wijdicks EF. The Clinical Practice of Critical Care Neurology. 2nd ed. Oxford: Oxford University Press; 2003

[11] w3.ouhsc.edu/human_physiology/Cell%20Fiz%20Discussion%20questions.htm. Accessed July 2005

[12] Bynoe MS, Viret C, Yan A, Kim DG. Adenosine receptor signaling: a key to opening the blood-brain door. Fluids Barriers CNS. 2015; 12:20

[13] Engelhardt S, Huang SF, Patkar S, Gassmann M, Ogunshola OO. Differential responses of blood-brain barrier associated cells to hypoxia and ischemia: a comparative study. Fluids Barriers CNS. 2015; 12:4

[14] Rosner MJ, Becker DP. Origin and evolution of plateau waves. Experimental observations and a theoretical model. J Neurosurg. 1984; 60(2):312–324

[15] Rosner MJ, Daughton S. Cerebral perfusion pressure management in head injury. J Trauma. 1990; 30(8):933–940

[16] Weed LH, McKibben PS. Experimental alteration of brain bulk. Am J Physiol. 1919; 48:531–555

[17] Gravenstein D, Gravenstein N. Intraoperative and immediate postoperative neuroanesthesia. In: Layon AJ, Gabrielli A, Friedman WA, eds. Textbook of Neurointensive Care. Philadelphia, PA: WB Saunders; 2004

[18] Chernow B. The Pharmacologic Approach to the Critically Ill Patient. 3rd ed. Baltimore, MD: Williams & Wilkins; 1994:272–290

[19] Lam AM, Winn HR, Cullen BF, Sundling N. Hyperglycemia and neurological outcome in patients with head injury. J Neurosurg. 1991; 75(4):545–551

[20] Wass CT, Lanier WL. Glucose modulation of ischemic brain injury: review and clinical recommendations. Mayo Clin Proc. 1996; 71(8):801–812

[21] Cherian L, Hannay HJ, Vagner G, Goodman JC, Contant CF, Robertson CS. Hyperglycemia increases neurological damage and behavioral deficits from post-traumatic secondary ischemic insults. J Neurotrauma. 1998; 15(5):307–321

[22] Zornow MH, Prough DS. Fluid management in patients with traumatic brain injury. New Horiz. 1995; 3(3):488–498

[23] Darovic GO. Hemodynamic Monitoring Invasive and Noninvasive Clinical Application. 3rd ed. Philadelphia, PA: WB Saunders; 2002

[24] Lefor AT. Critical Care on Call. New York, NY: Lange Medical Books; 2002:354

[25] Narayan RK, Wilberger JE, Polishock JT. Neurotrauma. New York, NY: McGraw-Hill; 1996:87–89, 315–317

[26] Prough DS, Whitley JM, Taylor CL, Deal DD, DeWitt DS. Regional cerebral blood flow following resuscitation from hemorrhagic shock with hypertonic saline. Influence of a subdural mass. Anesthesiology. 1991; 75(2):319–327

[27] Schmoker JD, Zhuang J, Shackford SR. Hypertonic fluid resuscitation improves cerebral oxygen delivery and reduces intracranial pressure after hemorrhagic shock. J Trauma. 1991; 31 (12):1607–1613

[28] Bayir H, Clark RS, Kochanek PM. Promising strategies to minimize secondary brain injury after head trauma. Crit Care Med. 2003; 31(1) Suppl:S112–S117

[29] Simma B, Burger R, Falk M, Sacher P, Fanconi S. A prospective, randomized, and controlled study of fluid management in children with severe head injury: lactated Ringer's solution versus hypertonic saline. Crit Care Med. 1998; 26(7):1265–1270

[30] Khanna S, Davis D, Peterson B, et al. Use of hypertonic saline in the treatment of severe refractory posttraumatic intracranial hypertension in pediatric traumatic brain injury. Crit Care Med. 2000; 28(4):1144–1151

[31] Munar F, Ferrer AM, de Nadal M, et al. Cerebral hemodynamic effects of 7.2% hypertonic saline in patients with head injury and raised intracranial pressure. J Neurotrauma. 2000; 17(1):41–51

[32] Horn P, Münch E, Vajkoczy P, et al. Hypertonic saline solution for control of elevated intracranial pressure in patients with exhausted response to mannitol and barbiturates. Neurol Res. 1999; 21 (8):758–764

[33] Fisher B, Thomas D, Peterson B. Hypertonic saline lowers raised intracranial pressure in children after head trauma. J Neurosurg Anesthesiol. 1992; 4(1):4–10

325

[34] Vassar MJ, Perry CA, Holcroft JW. Prehospital resuscitation of hypotensive trauma patients with 7.5% NaCl versus 7.5% NaCl with added dextran: a controlled trial. J Trauma. 1993; 34(5):622–632, discussion 632–633

[35] Wade CE, Grady JJ, Kramer GC, Younes RN, Gehlsen K, Holcroft JW. Individual patient cohort analysis of the efficacy of hypertonic saline/dextran in patients with traumatic brain injury and hypotension. J Trauma. 1997; 42(5) Suppl:S61–S65

[36] Vialet R, Albanèse J, Thomachot L, et al. Isovolume hypertonic solutes (sodium chloride or mannitol) in the treatment of refractory posttraumatic intracranial hypertension: 2 mL/kg 7.5% saline is more effective than 2 mL/kg 20% mannitol. Crit Care Med. 2003; 31(6):1683–1687

[37] Mirski AM, Denchev ID, Schnitzer SM, Hanley FD. Comparison between hypertonic saline and mannitol in the reduction of elevated intracranial pressure in a rodent model of acute cerebral injury. J Neurosurg Anesthesiol. 2000; 12(4):334–344

[38] Eskandari R, Filtz MR, Davis GE, Hoesch RE. Effective treatment of refractory intracranial hypertension after traumatic brain injury with repeated boluses of 14.6% hypertonic saline. J Neurosurg. 2013; 119(2):338–346

[39] Ichai C, Payen JF, Orban JC, et al. Half-molar sodium lactate infusion to prevent intracranial hypertensive episodes in severe traumatic brain injured patients: a randomized controlled trial. Intensive Care Med. 2013; 39(8):1413–1422

[40] Allcock JM, Drake CG. Ruptured intracranial aneurysm: the role of arterial spasm. J Neurosurg. 1965; 22:21–29

[41] von Kummer R, Scharf J, Back T, Reich H, Machens HG, Wildemann B. Autoregulatory capacity and the effect of isovolemic hemodilution on local cerebral blood flow. Stroke. 1988; 19(5):594–597

[42] Mead CO. A study of cerebral blood flow in experimental head injury: the beneficial effects of hemodilution. Proc Inst Med Chic. 1970; 28(5):173–179

[43] Jurkiewicz J, Mempel E, Szumska J, Czernicki Z. Use of haemodilution in the treatment of craniocerebral injuries (author's transl.) [in French]. Neurochirurgie. 1979; 25(2):122–123

[44] Cole DJ, Drummond JC, Osborne TN, Matsumura J. Hypertension and hemodilution during cerebral ischemia reduce brain injury and edema. Am J Physiol. 1990; 259(1 Pt 2):H211–H217

[45] Shin'oka T, Shum-Tim D, Jonas RA, et al. Higher hematocrit improves cerebral outcome after deep hypothermic circulatory arrest. J Thorac Cardiovasc Surg. 1996; 112(6):1610–1620, discussion 1620–1621

[46] Hassler W, Chioffi F. CO2 reactivity of cerebral vasospasm after aneurysmal subarachnoid haemorrhage. Acta Neurochir (Wien). 1989; 98(3–4):167–175

[47] Hint H. The pharmacology of dextran and the physiological background for the clinical use of rheomacrodex and macrodex. Acta Anaesthesiol Belg. 1968; 19(2):119–138

[48] Ekelund A, Reinstrup P, Ryding E, et al. Effects of iso- and hypervolemic hemodilution on regional cerebral blood flow and oxygen delivery for patients with vasospasm after aneurysmal subarachnoid hemorrhage. Acta Neurochir (Wien). 2002; 144(7):703–712, discussion 712–713

[49] Duebener LF, Sakamoto T, Hatsuoka S, et al. Effects of hematocrit on cerebral microcirculation and tissue oxygenation during deep hypothermic bypass. Circulation. 2001; 104(12) Suppl 1:I260–I264

[50] Korosue K, Heros RC. Mechanism of cerebral blood flow augmentation by hemodilution in rabbits. Stroke. 1992; 23(10):1487–1492, discussion 1492–1493

[51] Ohtaki M, Tranmer BI. Role of hypervolemic hemodilution in focal cerebral ischemia of rats. Surg Neurol. 1993; 40(3):196–206

[52] Lee SH, Heros RC, Mullan JC, Korosue K. Optimum degree of hemodilution for brain protection in a canine model of focal cerebral ischemia. J Neurosurg. 1994; 80(3):469–475

[53] Shimoda M, Oda S, Tsugane R, Sato O. Intracranial complications of hypervolemic therapy in patients with a delayed ischemic deficit attributed to vasospasm. J Neurosurg. 1993; 78(3):423–429

[54] Gravenstein D, Gravenstein N. Intraoperative and immediate postoperative neuroanesthesia. In: Layon AJ, Gabrielli A, Friedman WA, eds. Textbook of Neurointensive Care. Philadelphia, PA: WB Saunders; 2004:696–700

[55] Laks H, O'Connor NE, Anderson W, Pilon RN. Crystalloid versus colloid hemodilution in man. Surg Gynecol Obstet. 1976; 142(4):506–512

[56] Shires GT, III, Peitzman AB, Albert SA, et al. Response of extravascular lung water to intraoperative fluids. Ann Surg. 1983; 197(5):515–519

[57] Brown WJ, Kim BS, Weeks DB, Parkin CE. Physiologic saline solution, Normosol R pH 7.4, and Plasmanate as reconstituents of packed human erythrocytes. Anesthesiology. 1978; 49(2):99–101

[58] Trumble ER, Muizelaar JP, Myseros JS, Choi SC, Warren BB. Coagulopathy with the use of hetastarch in the treatment of vasospasm. J Neurosurg. 1995; 82(1):44–47

[59] Belayev L, Alonso OF, Huh PW, Zhao W, Busto R, Ginsberg MD. Posttreatment with high-dose albumin reduces histopathological damage and improves neurological deficit following fluid percussion brain injury in rats. J Neurotrauma. 1999; 16(6):445–453

[60] Chorny I, Bsorai R, Artru AA, et al. Albumin or hetastarch improves neurological outcome and decreases volume of brain tissue necrosis but not brain edema following closed-head trauma in rats. J Neurosurg Anesthesiol. 1999; 11(4):273–281

[61] Bunn F, Lefebvre C, Li Wan Po A, Li L, Roberts I, Schierhout G. Human albumin solution for resuscitation and volume expansion in critically ill patients. The Albumin Reviewers. Cochrane Database Syst Rev. 2000; 2(2):CD001208

[62] Finfer S, Bellomo R, Boyce N, French J, Myburgh J, Norton R, SAFE Study Investigators. A comparison of albumin and saline for fluid resuscitation in the intensive care unit. N Engl J Med. 2004; 350(22):2247–2256

[63] Andrews RJ, Muto RP. Retraction brain ischaemia: mannitol plus nimodipine preserves both cerebral blood flow and evoked potentials during normoventilation and hyperventilation. Neurol Res. 1992; 14(1):19–25

[64] Andrews RJ, Bringas JR, Muto RP. Effects of mannitol on cerebral blood flow, blood pressure, blood viscosity, hematocrit, sodium, and potassium. Surg Neurol. 1993; 39(3):218–222

[65] Johnston IH, Harper AM. The effect of mannitol on cerebral blood flow. An experimental study. J Neurosurg. 1973; 38(4):461–471

[66] Mendelow AD, Teasdale GM, Russell T, Flood J, Patterson J, Murray GD. Effect of mannitol on cerebral blood flow and cerebral perfusion pressure in human head injury. J Neurosurg. 1985; 63 (1):43–48

[67] Meyer FB, Anderson RE, Sundt TM, Jr, Yaksh TL. Treatment of experimental focal cerebral ischemia with mannitol. Assessment by intracellular brain pH, cortical blood flow, and electroencephalography. J Neurosurg. 1987; 66(1):109–115

[68] Shirane R, Weinstein PR. Effect of mannitol on local cerebral blood flow after temporary complete cerebral ischemia in rats. J Neurosurg. 1992; 76(3):486–492

[69] Kaufmann AM, Cardoso ER. Aggravation of vasogenic cerebral edema by multiple-dose mannitol. J Neurosurg. 1992; 77(4):584–589

[70] Wise BL, Perkins RK, Stevenson E, Scott KG. Penetration of 14C-labelled mannitol from serum into cerebrospinal fluid and brain. Exp Neurol. 1964; 10:264–270

[71] Guidelines for the Management of Severe Head Injury. New York, NY: Brain Trauma Foundation; 2000

[72] Gantner D, Moore EM, Cooper DJ. Intravenous fluids in traumatic brain injury: what's the solution? Curr Opin Crit Care. 2014; 20(4):385–389

[73] Pulsion Medical Inc. Advanced Hemodynamic Monitoring. Irving, TX; 2009

[74] Obata Y, Takeda J, Sato Y, Ishikura H, Matsui T, Isotani E. A multicenter prospective cohort study of volume management after subarachnoid hemorrhage: circulatory characteristics of pulmonary edema after subarachnoid hemorrhage. J Neurosurg. 2015; 125(2):254–263

[75] Tagami T, Kuwamoto K, Watanabe A, et al. SAH PiCCO Study Group. Optimal range of global end-diastolic volume for fluid management after aneurysmal subarachnoid hemorrhage: a multicenter prospective cohort study. Crit Care Med. 2014; 42(6):1348–1356

[76] Rahman M, Friedman WA. Hyponatremia in neurosurgical patients: clinical guidelines development. Neurosurgery. 2009; 65(5):925–935, discussion 935–936

[77] Capatina C, Paluzzi A, Mitchell R, Karavitaki N. Diabetes Insipidus after Traumatic Brain Injury. J Clin Med. 2015; 4(7):1448–1462

[78] Gennarelli T, Cruz J, McGinnis G, Jaggi J. Development of Methods to Evaluate New Treatments for Acute Head Injury. Atlanta, GA: Centers for Disease Control and Prevention; 1997:R49/CCR303687

[79] Stippler M, Fischer MR, Puccio AM, et al. Serum and cerebrospinal fluid magnesium in severe traumatic brain injury outcome. J Neurotrauma. 2007; 24(8):1347–1354

[80] Temkin NR, Anderson GD, Winn HR, et al. Magnesium sulfate for neuroprotection after traumatic brain injury: a randomised controlled trial. Lancet Neurol. 2007; 6(1):29–38

[81] Dorhout Mees SM, MASH-II study group. Magnesium in aneurysmal subarachnoid hemorrhage (MASH II) phase III clinical trial MASH-II study group. Int J Stroke. 2008; 3(1):63–65

[82] Krijthe BP, Heeringa J, Kors JA, et al. Serum potassium levels and the risk of atrial fibrillation: the Rotterdam Study. Int J Cardiol. 2013; 168(6):5411–5415

[83] Huang CL, Kuo E. Mechanism of hypokalemia in magnesium deficiency. J Am Soc Nephrol. 2007; 18(10):2649–2652

18 Ventilator Management

Justen Watkins, Dan E. Miulli, James Berry, Glenn Fischberg, and Javed Siddiqi

Abstract
A single episode of hypotension or hypoxia doubles the morbidity or mortality associated with severe brain injury. The neurointensivist has available the mechanical means to lessen the risk of hypoxia, and the ventilator should be used timely and appropriately to prevent ischemia. In the setting of central nervous system disease quick timing to restore oxygenation can prevent the neurons in the ischemic penumbra from dying and is required to prevent surrounding cells from infarction. However, it should never be thought that giving oxygen through the ventilator is the only means to restore oxygenation to the central nervous system tissue. Delivering oxygen is dependent upon a functional airway and is the first consideration. Once intubated, the meticulous control of the oxygen levels, carbon dioxide levels, and airway pressures both in the patient and in the ventilator can improve brain tissue oxygenation as long as the act of breathing and moving the oxygen across the alveoli into the circulation can be accomplished.

Keywords: cricothyroidectomy, hyperoxygenation, intubation, nondepolarizing paralytic, PCO2, pneumonia, preoxygenation, rapid sequence intubation

---

Case Presentation

A 43-year-old man presents after a motor vehicle accident with obvious contusions to his chest, abdomen, and head. At the scene he easily makes quick swallow breaths, he does not follow commands nor open his eyes to pain, he makes incomprehensible sounds and has flexor/decorticate posturing. His pupils are equal and briskly reactive. There is no obvious asymmetry of chest movement or chest deformity, and the abdomen is slightly distended but not hard. Should the patient be intubated?

See end of chapter for Case Management.

18.1 Reasons for Intubation

The Brain Trauma Foundation's *Guidelines for the Management of Severe Traumatic Brain Injury (4th edition)* address blood pressure and oxygenation as follows:

Guideline: *hypotension (systolic blood pressure < 90 mm Hg) or hypoxia (apnea or cyanosis in the field, PaO_2 < 60 mm Hg, or SpO_2 < 90%) must be scrupulously avoided, if possible, or corrected immediately.*

The brain and spinal cord require constant adequate blood flow for oxygen and energy substrates. Ischemia must be prevented at all costs to prevent or minimize secondary injury. Depending upon the severity and onset of central nervous system tissue hypoxia, glucose and glycogen are depleted in 4 minutes. In the setting of brain injury, hypoxia exacerbates the primary injury and leads to secondary injury. This is because, in addition to the general lack of energy substrates, there is a demand for additional energy from the injured brain as demonstrated by an increased metabolism and an increased brain temperature in the layer surrounding the penumbra. When the brain tissue partial pressure of oxygen (PbO_2) is less than 20 mm Hg, anaerobic respiration becomes the predominant energy exchange mechanism. This leads to glucose-store-dependent lactic acidosis, decreased pH, vasodilatation, mitochondrial damage, and cell death (aka secondary injury).

Intubation may help prevent significant secondary brain injury from hypoxia, which is oxygen saturation less than 90%, PaO_2 less than 60 mm Hg, apnea, or cyanosis. Stocchetti et al[1] demonstrated that hypoxic patients without hypotension had three times the mortality rate and 20 times the severe morbidity rate of the nonhypoxic patients. Furthermore, prehospital intubation of severe trauma victims significantly reduced mortality.[2] Systematic withholding of endotracheal intubation in patients with severe head injury is not recommended.

18.2 Requirements for Intubation

The patient in our case study has a Glasgow Coma Scale (GCS) score of 6; 3 for decorticate/flexor posturing, 2 for incomprehensible sounds, and 1 for not opening his eyes. The definition of severe head injury is a GCS score of 8 or less, and according to the *Guidelines for the Management of Severe Traumatic Brain Injury* initial management and resuscitation should include intubation: GCS ≤ 8 intubate.

Careful and rigorous neurologic examination, including assessment of brainstem reflexes, might help to identify patients with a very high probability of death despite mechanical ventilation.[3]

Considerable national variation in the care of severely head injured patients still persists even though the *Guidelines for the Management of Severe Traumatic Brain Injury* were first published in 1995. Those that actively follow those management strategies have an associated decreased mortality rate for patients with severe head injury, with no significant difference in functional status at discharge among survivors.[4]

In addition to data supporting intubation for severe head injury the literature does support intubation for stroke as well. However, intubation in the face of stroke still remains somewhat controversial. Magi et al[5] concluded that the overall prognosis of patients with acute stroke intubated and ventilated at presentation in hospital for deterioration is severe, but the observed survival rate is sufficient to justify this treatment, even in cases not requiring other invasive procedures such as neurosurgery or angiography. The severity of the ischemic event often leads to mechanical ventilation, and in two-thirds of those individuals, death in the hospital; the remainder are severely disabled. In a study of a multiethnic urban population, survival was unlikely if patients were deeply comatose or deteriorated clinically after intubation. However, the authors concluded that mechanical ventilation for stroke was relatively cost-effective for extending life but not for preserving quality of life.[6]

18.3 Methods of Intubation

18.3.1 Preintubation

Prior to intubation the patient is preoxygenated with 100% oxygen to maintain the arterial oxygen percent saturation (O_2 saturation) at the highest level. Maintaining cervical spine precautions, with previous placement of a cervical collar, a jaw thrust technique keeps the airway open for oxygenation. Do not use a head tilt technique in a patient with any suspected spinal injuries. After suctioning the upper airway using spinal immobilization the patient then undergoes rapid sequence intubation with in-line orotracheal, blind nasotracheal, esophageal-tracheal (ET) Combitube (Moore Medical), or laryngeal mask airway. The equipment must be available, and tube cuffs checked prior to delivering the paralytics. If tracheal intubation cannot be performed because of facial fractures then intubation after cricothyrotomy or tracheotomy must be considered.

Preintubation:
- Maintain C-spine precautions.
- Preoxygenate with 100% oxygen.
- Check ET-tube cuff inflation and deflation.
- Suction patient.
- Do not use head tilt in trauma patient.
- Rapid sequence sedation and paralysis.
- Intubate.
  - Orotracheal.
  - Blind nasotracheal.
  - Esophageal-tracheal Combitube.
  - Laryngeal mask.
  - Cricothyrotomy or tracheotomy.

18.3.2 Rapid Sequence Intubation

Medications in order of use for rapid sequence intubation are as follows: (1) Preoxygenate with 100% oxygen by mask. (2) Premedicate with lidocaine 1.5 to 2 mg/kg intravenous (IV) over 30 to 60 seconds to help prevent a spike in increased intracranial pressure (ICP), if the latter is an active issue. Maximal effect requires allowing approximately 3 minutes prior to attempted intubation. (3) Use of a sedating agent (see later discussion) if there is any semblance of alertness or awareness prior to paralyzing a patient. (4) The use of a nondepolarizing paralytic, such as rocuronium, may be considered at the 10% intubating dose of 0.06–0.1 mg/kg to lessen fasciculations from the next drug, the depolarizing agent succinylcholine, at 1.5 mg/kg IV push, which acts in 30 seconds to 1 minute. While intubating, raise the head of the bed to 30 degrees when possible as one would in general to control elevated ICP. Attempt tracheal intubation with cricoid pressure if needed. If unable to intubate within 20–30 seconds stop and ventilate with a bag-mask for 30–60 seconds before once again attempting orotracheal intubation. After the tube is visualized passing through the vocal cords confirm placement by listening to breath sounds over the lateral chest, watching the chest rise and fall, not just the abdomen, seeing a mist in the tracheal tube with expiration, and using a CO_2 detector after five to six breaths or an esophageal detector device. Treat intubation-induced bradycardia with atropine 0.5 mg IV push in adults or 0.1 mg minimum in children (0.01 mg/kg).

Rapid sequence intubation:[7,8,9]

- Preoxygenate with 100% oxygen.
- Lidocaine 1.5–2 mg/kg IV.
- Rocuronium 0.06–0.1 mg/kg.
- Succinylcholine 1.5 mg/kg intravenous push (IVP).
- Intubate.
- If unsuccessful bag-mask ventilate for 30–60 seconds.
- Reattempt.

To determine whether the intubation has been successful, perform the following:
- Listen for breath sounds over lateral chest.
- Watch chest, not abdomen, rise and fall.
- Observe mist in ET tube.
- Use CO_2 detector after five or six breaths.
- Treat intubation-induced bradycardia with atropine.

Premedication/induction/sedation in head injury patients may prevent the increased ICP that can occur from pain or suctioning. Use drugs depending upon the time requirement for intubation and the need to assess the neurologic exam again after intubation. Agents include those listed in ▶ Table 18.1.

Table 18.1 Drugs used in rapid sequence intubation

Drug	Dosage IV push	Onset	Duration
Lidocaine	1.5–2 mg/kg IV	30–60 s	5–10 min
Atropine	0.01 mg/kg IV children (min. 0.1 mg)	30–60 s	3–5 min
Fentanyl	2–3 µg/kg IV over 2–3 minutes	60 s	30–60 min
Midazolam	0.02–0.04 mg/kg	2 min	1–2 h
Etomidate	0.2–0.6 mg/kg	60 s	3–5 min
Ketamine	2 mg/kg	30–60 s	15 min
Thiopental	3–5 mg/kg	20–40 s	5–10 min

Abbreviation: IV, intravenous.

Paralytic prophylaxis prior to succinylcholine or paralytics in place of succinylcholine are shown in ▶ Table 18.2. Use an alternative agent if there are significant risk factors against succinylcholine. These include hyperkalemia or high risk of hyperkalemia that may result from prolonged immobilization, myopathies, renal failure, or extensive burn injury or muscle crush injury, as well as already dangerously elevated ICP, or personal or family history of malignant hyperthermia.[7,8,9] Cisatracurium may be preferred in those with renal or liver failure or very advanced age, due to organ-independent Hofmann degradation, thus avoiding prolonged effects.[10,11] Remember after intubation the patient will need to have a neurological exam. Sometimes the patient may need to be examined for brain death as the intubation was a reaction to a code or simply finding the patient. It is best to decide quickly prior to intubation the neurologic status. However, the GCS score should be determined after resuscitation and not in place of resuscitation.

Table 18.2 Paralytic agents

Drug	Paralytic (mg/kg)	Prophylaxis (mg/kg)	Onset	Duration (min)
Succinylcholine	1–2	–	30–60 s	4–6
Rapacuronium	1.5	–	60–90 s	15
Rocuronium	0.6–1.2	0.06	2 min	30–90
Vecuronium	0.15–0.25	0.01	2–5 min	25–40
Cisatracurium	0.15–0.2	–	1.5–3 min	44–81
Atracurium	0.4	0.04	3–5 min	20–35
Pacuronium	0.1	0.01	3–5 min	45–60

Side effects of commonly administered drugs include the following:
- Succinylcholine: depolarizing effect may cause fasciculations and increase ICP or cause muscle pain—give with prophylaxis. May cause dysrhythmia and hyperkalemia. May cause cardiac arrest in healthy children and adolescents. May cause malignant hyperthermia.
- Pancuronium: vagolytic; can increase cardiac output, ICP, and pulse rate. Reversible with neostigmine and other anticholinesterases.[12]

Ochs et al[13] evaluated the ability of paramedic rapid sequence intubation to facilitate intubation of patients with severe head injuries in an urban out-of-hospital system. They examined adult severe head injury patients more than 10 minutes away from the hospital. The patients were premedicated with midazolam, paralyzed with succinylcholine, and given rocuronium after tube placement was confirmed. The Combitube was used as a salvage airway device. Outcome measures included intubation success rates, preintubation and post-intubation oxygen saturation values, arrival arterial blood gas values, and total out-of-hospital times for patients intubated en route versus on scene. Of the 114 enrolled patients, 84% underwent successful endotracheal intubation, and 15% required Combitube intubation, with only 1 (0.9%) airway failure. There were no complications and blood gases were superb with paramedic-performed rapid sequence intubation of patients with severe head injuries.

18.3.3 Emergent Cricothyroidotomy

Emergent cricothyroidotomy should only be performed by individuals familiar with the anatomy after unsuccessful or unavailable endotracheal intubation in upper airway obstruction. The procedure requires a knife blade and handle, antiseptic solution, and a tracheostomy tube, and a pediatric ET tube or 14-gauge catheter over needle. Palpate the cricothyroid membrane between the thyroid and cricoid cartilages; it is the soft space between the "Adam's apple" and the first hard ring toward the chest. A vertical incision is made in the skin and then the cricothyroid membrane is incised horizontally. Next the knife handle is inserted into the opening and rotated 90 degrees. The tube is passed through the opening and the cuff inflated. If a 14-gauge catheter-over-needle is available it may be used to puncture the cricothyroid membrane, removing the needle and mounted with a 12-mL syringe, which will serve as a connector for ventilation. The cricothyrotomy may be converted under controlled conditions in the operating room by a skilled person to a tracheostomy once the airway has been secured. Tracheostomies are not appropriate procedures for urgent situations.[14]

Emergent cricothyroidotomy:
- Palpate the first space between Adam's apple and hard ring.
- Make vertical incision in skin.

- Make horizontal incision in cricothyroid membrane.
- Insert knife handle and turn 90 degrees.
- Pass tube through opening and inflate cuff.

18.4 Hyperventilation after Intubation

Normal ventilation is currently the goal for severe TBI patients in the absence of cerebral herniation and normal partial pressure of carbon dioxide in arterial blood (PaCO2) ranges from 35–45 mm Hg.[15]

Guideline: The use of prophylactic hyperventilation PaCO2 less than or equal to 25 mm Hg is not recommended.

Brain tissue oxygenation is dependent upon cerebral blood flow, or the related measurement of cerebral perfusion pressure. Therefore, treatment modalities that cause vasoconstriction and decrease cerebral blood flow, such as aggressive hyperventilation, must be questioned and modified in the management armamentarium.

Hyperventilation works by decreasing plasma PCO_2, which causes an increase in the ambient pH in or around the brain cerebrovasculature, leading to cerebral vasoconstriction decreasing the cerebral blood flow and in some cases decreasing ICP. Early after closed head injury cerebral blood flow is low. Cerebral blood flow during the first day after injury is less than half that of normal individuals; it then increases for at least 3 days thereafter, except in those patients who have uncontrollable ICP.

Cerebral blood flow is generally less than 30 mL/100 g/min during the first 8 hours after injury and may be less than 20 mL/100 g/min during the first 4 hours after injury in patients with the worst trauma. The cerebral blood flow around contusions is lower than the global blood flow. The blood flow in punctate hemorrhages may be even lower. Individuals with severe head injury may actually have increased oxygen extraction for 24–36 hours, requiring at least baseline blood flow, and possibly higher.

Cerebral blood flow has been measured with hyperventilation, and there are significant differences in and around contusions, even having local variability secondary to hyperventilation-induced steal. Cerebral blood flow does change with hyperventilation; there is a 3 to 4% change in cerebral blood flow per millimeter change in PCO_2, as demonstrated by Obrist et al.[16]

When cerebral blood flow is decreased, the level at which irreversible ischemia or infarction takes place is not precisely known. The same study by Obrist et al suggested that, in patients with severe head injury, there is a depression of normal cerebral metabolism, and the reduced cerebral blood flow that occurs may in many cases be appropriate for the metabolic needs of the brain.

Cerebral blood flow is lowest in patients with subdural hematomas, diffuse injuries, and hypotension, and highest in those with epidural hematomas or normal computed tomographic scans. There is a direct correlation between cerebral blood flow and Glasgow Coma Scale score during the first 4 hours after injury, as demonstrated by Bouma et al,[17] and therefore the consequences of cerebral blood flow reducing hyperventilation become more apparent.

Aggressive hyperventilation to a PCO_2 of 25 or less has been the cornerstone in the management of severe head injury for more than 20 years because it can cause a rapid reduction of ICP. However, there are no studies showing an improvement in outcome in neurologic patients with severe head injury using hyperventilation empirically. Hyperventilation reduces ICP by causing cerebral vasoconstriction and a subsequent reduction in cerebral blood flow. As stated earlier, cerebral blood flow is reduced by 50% during the first day after severe head injury and, therefore, hyperventilation can only exacerbate this already deadly condition. Raichle et al[18] looked at a group of healthy individuals treated with hyperventilation. When these individuals had their PCO_2 decreased by 15 to 20 mm Hg from normal, there was a 40% decrease in cerebral blood flow after 30 minutes. Four hours later, despite continued hyperventilation, the cerebral blood flow increased to 90% of baseline, even though the PCO_2 was still decreased, demonstrating that hyperventilation to reduce ICP may only be a temporary phenomenon. This suggests that hyperventilation, if necessary, should only be used in short bursts.

In the same study when the original PCO_2 was quickly restored the cerebral blood flow was increased to 31% above baseline. The quick restoration increases cerebral blood volume and in turn can increase ICP. Therefore, when elevating PCO_2 from below normal levels, gradually increase the PCO_2.

In the autoregulatory intact individual, there is a 3–4% change in cerebral blood flow per mm Hg change in PCO_2. This decrease in cerebral flow occurs less when cerebral blood flow is already reduced, and this lower CO_2 vasoresponsivity is associated with a poorer outcome. Local CO_2 responsivity can differ from values by more than 50%. Cold et al[19] demonstrated that in some patients cerebral autoregulation is preserved with normocapnia and lost with hypocapnia. Others have found varying responses with hyperventilation. Crockard et al[20] found an increase in ICP associated with a decrease in PCO_2, and Obrist found a decrease in ICP in only half of the patients treated with hyperventilation; however, over 90% of those patients also had a decrease in cerebral blood flow.

In a landmark class I study Muizelaar et al[21] published the results of a prospective randomized clinical study in which 77 patients were randomized to a group treated with chronic prophylactic hyperventilation for 5 days after injury (PCO_2 of 25, ± 2 mm Hg) or to a group that was kept normocapnic (PCO_2 35 ± 2). Those patients who were treated with prophylactic hyperventilation had a significantly worse outcome than those in the normocapnic group at 3 and 6 months. They did say that hyperventilation may be beneficial with hyperemia, and hyperventilation is needed in signs of acute herniation. Multiple studies demonstrate that aggressive hyperventilation causes secondary injury of decreased brain tissue oxygen.[22,23,24,25]

The literature is replete with documentation of improved survival for severe head injury using modern treatment paradigms. The majority of physicians who are exposed to head trauma patients, explicitly the emergency department doctors, are managing severe head injury patients in accordance with the *Guidelines for the Management of Severe Traumatic Brain Injury*, with the exception of avoiding prophylactic hyperventilation. However, it is hoped that more education and exposure to the evidence regarding prophylactic hyperventilation of severely head injured patients may improve adherence to the hyperventilation guidelines as well.[26]

18.5 Measuring Cerebral Blood Flow

At times hyperventilation should be used. It should be used with caution in appropriate settings. A patient with a simple cold should not get 1 g of penicillin eight times a day for 3 weeks. However, a simple *Staphylococcus aureus* infection may require 500 mg four times a day for 10 days. In the same way, hyperventilation has a role. As the guidelines for the management of severe head injury state, "Hyperventilation therapy may be necessary for brief periods when there is acute neurological deterioration or for longer periods if there is intracranial hypertension refractory to sedation, paralysis, cerebral spinal fluid drainage and osmotic diuretics. SjO_2 and $AVdO_2$ and cerebral blood flow monitoring may help to identify cerebral ischemia if hyperventilation, resulting in PCO_2 that is less than 30 mmHg, is necessary."

18.5.1 Arteriovenous Differences in Oxygen

Not all facilities have the ability to measure cerebral blood flow directly; therefore, they choose to measure it indirectly using $AVdO_2$ or SjO2. The arteriovenous difference in oxygen is indirectly a manifestation of metabolism and cerebral blood flow. The brain makes up approximately 2% of the body weight and uses 20% of the cardiac output and 25% of the resting body glucose. It has a very small energy reserve; therefore, metabolism is tightly coupled to cerebral blood flow. Normally metabolism is 1.5 µg/g/min, or 3.4 mL/100 g/min; this is the cerebral metabolic rate of oxygen. Approximately 19 mL/dL of O_2 is delivered to the brain on the arterial side and approximately 12 to 13 mL/dL of O_2 is the value on the venous side, yielding approximately 35% oxygen extraction, leaving an AVdO$_2$ of 6.5 mL/dL.

The brain uses 90% aerobic and 10% anaerobic respiration. This occurs through the citric acid cycle. Approximately half the energy is used for cell maintenance and half the energy is used for brain function. Normally there is a very small amount of lactate produced.

Isolated severe head injury patients were studied keeping systolic blood pressure, hematocrit, and temperature normal.[27] These patients were divided into two groups. One group had mass lesions requiring surgery and the other did not. Both were treated according to protocol, meaning they were intubated, sedated, and paralyzed; their PCO$_2$ was kept greater than 30 mmHg; and they were given mannitol if the ICP was elevated. Patients had jugular venous catheters inserted, and the arteriojugular differences of oxygen (AVdO$_2$) were calculated before treatment and 30 minutes after treatment. In those patients who underwent evacuation of a mass lesion their perfusion pressure was termed adequate to prevent ischemia; however, some individuals still demonstrated infarction by computed tomographic scan. ICP and cerebral perfusion pressure were normal. The closer the AVdO$_2$, the less likely chance there was of having an infarction. Likewise in the nonsurgical group those patients who developed an infarction also had adequate ICP and cerebral perfusion pressure after treatment, but they had a larger AVdO$_2$, suggesting they required more oxygen for energy maintenance. There was a change in AVdO$_2$ in both groups that predicted the outcome. An elevated arteriovenous difference in oxygen signifies increased oxygen extraction, which is consistent with ischemia. It would seem that the failure of the AVdO$_2$ to improve with treatment was the one factor that was consistent with infarction. The ideal monitor, therefore, would give reliable continuous readings, would be portable, and would suggest a cause and appropriate therapy.

18.5.2 Jugular Venous Oxygen Saturation

SjO$_2$ is the reciprocal of AVdO$_2$. If oxygen extraction increases, the AVdO$_2$ will increase but the SjO$_2$ will decrease. This measurement assumes that cerebral metabolism and hemoglobin are constant, and the effective dissolved oxygen is negligible. There are limitations to SjO$_2$ measurement. It is contraindicated with C-spine injuries, coagulopathy, and tracheostomies. It measures hemispheric flow, which may not be constant from one side to the other, and even on one side it will give measurements of general hypoxia but will not allow region-specific treatment. Changes in SjO$_2$ can occur after herniation has taken place. There are artifacts associated with catheter movement, and placement has to be precise—not too proximal and not against a vessel wall. SjO_2 less than 50% is consistent with ischemia. Profound or prolonged episodes of desaturation are associated with a poor outcome. Desaturations are most common with low cerebral blood flow. SjO_2 less than 50% is the equivalent of $AVdO_2$ exceeding 9 mL/dL.

18.6 Oxygen Level

The question of what level to keep the PO_2 and oxygen saturation is even more controversial than hyperventilation, leading to many debates between the pulmonologist and the neurosurgeon. The reason for the debate stems from the discussion between the hemoglobin molecule and the measurements of brain tissue oxygen. In whole blood the hemoglobin molecule has an oxygen carrying capacity of 17–21 mL O_2/100 mL blood, when oxygen is bound to its four hemoglobin sites. However, that figure does not reflect the additional, albeit small, amounts of oxygen dissolved in the blood. That amount, the PaO_2, also reflects free oxygen molecules dissolved in plasma and not just those bound to hemoglobin. Likewise oxygen saturation SaO_2 alone does *not* reveal how much total oxygen is in the blood.

The oxygen saturation and the partial pressure of oxygen in the blood can be most readily adjusted by increasing the inspired oxygen (FIO_2). Oxygen saturation and partial pressure of oxygen are also affected by perfusion, such as with cerebral blood flow. In general without concomitant disease the hemoglobin molecule is 100% saturated at a PO_2 of 80 mm Hg, 75% saturated at a PO_2 of 40 mm Hg, and 50% saturated at a PO_2 of 27 mm Hg. In addition to the fact that blood plasma carries additional oxygen it is important to remember that red blood cells only reach 85% of the brain cells, the remainder being dependent upon the circulating plasma. Oxygen does not always bind to the hemoglobin molecule in the same manner; there is a decreased affinity of hemoglobin for oxygen with increasing temperature, increasing PCO_2 and 2,3-DPG and decreasing pH. This makes it harder for the hemoglobin to bind to oxygen (requiring a higher partial pressure to achieve the same oxygen saturation), but it makes it easier for the hemoglobin to release bound oxygen.

Therefore, the debate hinges on the following: Arterial hemoglobin saturation of 100% is the upper limit of usefulness; increasing the FIO_2 to past the maximal saturation of hemoglobin only increases the dissolved O_2 in plasma, which represents 2–3% of overall O_2 transport. Use of FIO_2 levels higher than 60% may be harmful when used for longer than 24 hours in adults.

However, that is only half the story; the other half rests upon studies that actually measure brain tissue oxygenation and predict outcome. In these studies, increasing PO_2 to higher levels than necessary to saturate hemoglobin, as performed in the O_2-treated cohort, improved the O_2 supply in brain tissue ($PBtO_2$). During the early period after severe head injury increased lactate levels in brain tissue were reduced by increasing FIO_2.[28] Other studies have demonstrated improved mortality using hyperbaric oxygen. Measurements demonstrated reduce mortality by 50% and improved aerobic metabolism.[29,30,][31] The treatment PO_2 varied some from keeping PO_2 150 mm Hg[32] to a simple approach of ventilation with 100% O_2 for at least the first 6–18 hours after any severe head injury (SHI) when metabolic demand is greatest.[28]

18.7 Measuring $PbtO_2$

There are two favored technologies for measuring brain tissue oxygen, the Neurotrend[33] (Codman and Shurtleff) and the Licox[34] sensor (Integra Neurosciences). The small probe, approximately 0.5 mm in diameter, can be inserted through a standard twist drill hole into a nonlesion where there should be a steady $PBtO_2$ or into a lesion area with a low but dynamic $PBtO_2$. The cerebral tissue monitoring system measures four areas of brain metabolism, physiological information about progression of secondary injury at the cellular level that may indicate the onset of ischemic injury, as observed in 80% of trauma-related deaths. These measurements have shown that by increasing the inspired oxygen beyond 80% there continues to be an increase in $PBtO_2$.[25,35,36,37] Specifically increasing inspired oxygen from 30 to100% increased $PBtO_2$ to a steady state of 40 mm Hg.[38] Not only does the $PBtO_2$ improve, the outcome improves.[39,40,41,42,43]

Finally when investigating hyperventilation using the cerebral metabolism sensor a PCO_2 of 27–32 mm Hg decreases $PBtO_2$ in patients with severe head injury.[24,44,45] Increasing the PaO_2 to levels higher than needed to fully saturate hemoglobin apparently can increase PO_2, especially when it is low, and this effect can continue over a period of several hours.

18.8 Pulmonary Problems

There are many patients on the neurology and neurosurgery service that may come to the intensive care unit without a severe head injury and without a severe cerebral vascular accident. The patients may develop abnormal breathing patterns from masses, inflammation, or infections. There are some typical abnormal breathing patterns (▶ Table 18.3).

Cheyne–Stokes respirations occur when there is diffuse forebrain injury. At that time the patient hyperventilates low PCO_2, stops breathing, which normalizes PCO_2. This results in hyperventilation and apnea, with the hyperventilation being longer than the apnea; therefore the patient becomes alkalotic. In the rare central neurogenic hyperventilation there can be a midbrain lesion, such as in the thalamus.[46] However, because of its unlikely presentation, the physician when seeing continuous hyperventilation should instead consider a

Table 18.3 Abnormal breathing patterns and location[24,46,47]

Type	Pattern	Location
Cheyne–Stokes	Hyperventilation, short apnea, hyperventilation	Diffuse forebrain injury
Central neurogenic	Hyperventilation	Midbrain, thalamus
Apneustic pontine, brainstem	Prolonged pause at full inspiration	Pontine, brainstem
Ataxic	Random deep and shallow	Medulla
Cluster	Irregular breath and pause	Low medulla

Table 18.4 Types of pulmonary dysfunction in neurologic patients

Acute congestive heart failure	Chronic obstructive pulmonary disease/asthma	Neurogenic pulmonary edema
Acute respiratory distress syndrome	Diaphragm rupture	Pneumonia
Airway obstruction	Diaphragm paralysis	Pneumothorax
Apnea	Fat/brain emboli	Pulmonary contusion
Aspiration	Hemothorax	Pulmonary edema
Atelectasis	Hyper-/hypoventilation	Tracheobronchial
Chest wall injury	Injury	Ventilation/perfusion mismatch

cause of pulmonary edema or aspiration. With the also rare apneustic breathing, which is demonstrated by a prolonged pause at full inspiration, there may be a mid to caudal pontine lesion, brainstem stroke, or basilar artery occlusion. In ataxic breathing there is very irregular breathing, with random deep and shallow breaths randomly mixed. Ataxic breathing is a terminal stage usually pointing to a medullary lesion. Finally, the patient may have a cluster pattern consisting of clusters of breaths in irregular sequence with varying pauses, indicative of end-stage lower medullary failure or lesion. Each breathing pattern should be associated with a clinical condition verifying the level of the lesion. When there is no confirmatory exam, think of the many other causes of pulmonary dysfunction in the neurologic patient (▶ Table 18.4).

Patients with severe neurologic problems such as severe head injury develop secondary problems, such as electrolyte derangements, 59% of the time, pneumonia 41% of the time, and coagulopathy 18% of the time. These secondary problems usually occur 2–4 days after the injury and affect approximately 3% of the outcomes.[47] Therefore, the neurocritical care specialist should be most cognizant of ways to prevent and treat such issues. Pneumonia can be attenuated early by ensuring airway protection, utilizing chest physiotherapy, and understanding the nosocomial infection. Other nonpreventable associations with pneumonia include neutralization of gastric pH.

Pneumonia can initially be mistaken for pulmonary embolism, acute respiratory distress syndrome, very early neurogenic pulmonary edema, or, in the nonintubated patient, airway obstruction. Upper airway obstruction is common in the first 24 hours after stroke, especially if patients remain in the supine position. The risks for obstruction prior to intubation are the same risk factors for typical obstructive sleep apnea (body mass index and neck circumference), and appear to be the best predictors of its occurrence.[48]

The incidence of neurogenic pulmonary edema is unknown. It should be differentiated from pneumonia, aspiration, cardiac failure, and pulmonary contusion. Neurogenic pulmonary edema may occur in relation to epilepsy, meningitis, severe head injury, subarachnoid hemorrhage, or neoplasms. Early in its course there may be dyspnea, chest pain, minor hemoptysis, tachypnea, tachycardia, fever, hypoxia, elevated systolic blood pressure/pulmonary pressure, and rales (not gallops or murmurs). The chest X-ray may show bilateral central fluffy infiltrates. The etiology may be due to hydrostatic forces and permeability changes or to the release of catecholamines. If the pulmonary edema is due to increased ICP then lower the ICP and provide supportive care. At times, there may be difficulty differentiating neurogenic pulmonary edema from that due to heart failure or fluid overload, or in what combination this may be occurring. Aid in assessment of cardiac function, fluid status, and pulmonary pressures may be obtained via pulmonary artery catheter use. Lesser invasive devices may be used for assessment of cardiac output and fluid status via bioimpedance/bioresistance, applied Fick principle, pulsed Doppler, and pulse contour analysis.[49]

18.9 Ventilator Management

Newer techniques of mechanical ventilation allow the neurocritical care specialist an increased number of mechanisms not previously available. In a very large study Esteban et al[50] inquired into 412 medical/surgical units from the Americas and Europe, the patients requiring ventilation were on assist control (AC) 47%, synchronized intermittent mandatory ventilation (SIMV) 46%, or a combination of both. The median tidal volume was 9 mL/kg in AC and a median pressure support of 18 cm H_2O. Positive end expiratory pressure was not used in 31% of the patients.

Ventilator types consist of volume-cycled ventilation, pressure-cycled ventilation, and time-cycled pressure-limited ventilation. In each type, the tidal volume (Vt) would be: (1) constant with inspiratory pressure limits dependent upon applied pressure and the compliance of the lung and chest wall with incomplete exhalation; or (2) limiting, when there is incomplete exhalation and the respiratory rate increases to compensate (used mostly in infants and small children); or (3) dependent, maintaining airway pressure at a preset maximum for a preset time with an added inspiratory pause, used where there is a problem with lung and chest wall compliance.

Ventilator modes consist of controlled mechanical ventilation (CMV), AC, SIMV pressure support, and high frequency jet ventilation (HFJV) (▶ Table 18.5). CMV is independent of patient breathing; it delivers a minute ventilation determined by a preset Vt and rate. It is frequently used in the pharmacologically paralyzed patient; if the patient is not paralyzed he or she may not be able to synchronize with the ventilator and therefore may become quite agitated. AC mode, in addition to a preset rate of volume-controlled breaths, delivers only full breaths through preset Vt when patients initiate a breath by creating negative pressure. Consequently, this assists spontaneously initiated ventilations, and any anxious patients would hyperventilate. This would not be a method of limiting alkalosis. The sensitivity would have to be set at a level that could be adequate for needed breaths in someone who could not muster adequate volumes as well. This would have to be adjusted by lowering Vt, lowering the set rate or by initiating sedation, if this mode is to be continued. SIMV modes have a preset rate and Vt; however, the patient can breathe spontaneously but with assistance by a set pressure support in lieu of an automatic Vt between ventilator breaths. In pressure support (PS) the ventilator provides a constant pressure once a negative inspiratory force or initial inspiratory flow is initiated, assisting the patient's own inspiration. By itself PS does not provide a minimum minute ventilation, allowing the patient to work at breathing and demonstrate capacity to breathe adequately as pressure is reduced to that which only compensates for the resistance of the tubing. Minute ventilation may be changed by increasing or decreasing pressure support. HFJV delivers a minute ventilation at 50–300 breaths per minute at reduced mean airway pressure and therefore reducing increased ICP. It is used when there is high peak inspiratory pressure greater than 70–80 cm H_2O. HFJV can cause problems due to the quick movement of air at high pressures, such as dryness and mucosal injury.

Table 18.5 Types of ventilators[13,14,16,48]

Ventilator mode	Patient control	Parameters
CMV preset Vt and rate	Machine driven	Preset Vt and rate
AC preset Vt, minimum rate	Patient driven, machine backup full breath	Preset Vt
SIMV	Patient driven, machine backup full breath	Preset Vt and rate
PS preset pressure	Patient driven	Preset pressure
HFJV preset minute ventilation	Machine driven	Preset minute ventilation

Abbreviations: AC, assist control; CMV, controlled mechanical ventilation; HFJV, high-frequency jet ventilation; PS, pressure support; SIMV, synchronized intermittent mandatory ventilation; Vt, tidal volume.

In addition to the modes of ventilation, PS and positive end expiratory pressure (PEEP) can be added. PEEP maintains the opening of small airways at end expiration to improve PaO_2 so that a lower concentration of oxygen can be used. PEEP also increases pleural pressure, intrathoracic pressure, and central venous pressure while decreasing cardiac output if not volume-repleted, systolic blood pressure, free water clearance, urine, and urine sodium; therefore, amounts of PEEP should be increased or decreased slowly. The increased end expiratory pressure can cause barotrauma. Since PEEP increases pulmonary vascular resistance and central venous pressure its usage in patients with severe neurologic problems has been questioned. Studies determined that the adverse effects of PEEP are dependent upon intracranial compliance. Patients who require artificial ventilation can be safely ventilated using PEEP or an inverse inspiration/expiration ratio, if the blood pressure is monitored and a possible drop of the arterial blood pressure is treated.[51] As far as the amount of PEEP, in humans 10 cm H_2O of PEEP had no effect on ICP,[52] whereas 15 cm H_2O of PEEP in normal dogs had mild effects that became worse if the ICP was elevated their own.[53]

18.10 Extubation versus Tracheostomy

The decision to extubate neurosurgical patients carries important consequences. The goal is to extubate these patients as soon as they are able to ventilate on their own and are able to sufficiently protect their own airway. Many providers traditionally base readiness for extubation in part on a patient demonstrating the capacity to follow commands. Applying this to the neurologic and neurosurgical population is frequently not valid, and may shortchange many who are ready for ventilator liberation. A late-stage Alzheimer's patient, for example, may not follow commands, engage in activity, nod to questions, or speak a word, yet can sit in a chair comfortably all day with no hint of respiratory difficulties. Patients do not need to be interactive, only reactive, for airway protection. A patient may become ventilator dependent as a result of remaining on mechanical support over several days or even weeks; thus arbitrary prolongation of mechanical ventilation should be avoided. However, commonly in the neurosurgical intensive care setting, patients may be suffering from neurologic injury that keeps them in a state which precludes sufficient protection of their own airway.

As soon as it becomes apparent that the patient will likely require mechanical ventilation for a prolonged period, tracheostomy should be pursued.

There are many advantages of tracheostomy over endotracheal intubation, not the least of which being improved ventilator weaning times.

Advantages of the tracheostomy include the following:[54]
- More comfort.
- Easier cleaning of the mouth and face.

- May allow swallowing and the ability to eat and drink.
- May allow speech with the help of a speaking device.
- May help weaning from the ventilator.
- May reduce swelling in the airway and mouth caused by having an endotracheal tube in place for a long time.

The reasons for improved ventilator weaning with a tracheostomy over an endotracheal tube have been delineated in studies and include decreased work of breathing as the main factor.[55,56]

It should be noted that there is some evidence showing early tracheostomy in neurosurgical intensive care patients who exhibit poor GCS scores is associated with decreased complications associated with mechanical ventilation;[57] thus long-term strategies for ventilation must be considered early on in the course of a neurosurgical patient's intensive care unit stay.

18.11 Conclusion

Patients with severe head injury should be assessed for airway, breathing, and circulation. They should have rapid sequence intubation in the field utilizing spinal precautions. Once intubated, patients should initially be placed on 100% FIO_2 and ventilated at a rate to maintain a PCO_2 of 35 mm Hg. Any episode of hypoxia and hypotension must be avoided to maintain optimal cerebral blood flow and brain tissue oxygenation. Prophylactic hyperventilation should not be used unless there is evidence of increasing ICP despite all other acceptable measures. Then mild hyperventilation can be used for brief periods of time. Long-term ventilator strategy should be considered early on in the course of the neurosurgical patient's ICU stay, with early consideration of tracheostomy if the patient presents with a poor GCS score or has early predictable long-term ventilator needs.

Case Management

The patient presents with a GCS score of 5 (eyes 1, verbal 1, motor 3). Thus this patient should be intubated for airway protection.

References

[1] Stocchetti N, Furlan A, Volta F. Hypoxemia and arterial hypotension at the accident scene in head injury. J Trauma. 1996; 40(5):764–767

[2] Hsiao A, Michaelson S, Hedges J. Emergent intubation and CT scan pathology of blunt trauma patients with Glasgow Coma Scale scores 3–13. Prehosp Disaster Med. 1998; 32:26–32

[3] Santoli F, De Jonghe B, Hayon J, et al. Mechanical ventilation in patients with acute ischemic stroke: survival and outcome at one year. Intensive Care Med. 2001; 27(7):1141–1146

[4] Bulger EM, Nathens AB, Rivara FP, Moore M, MacKenzie EJ, Jurkovich GJ, Brain Trauma Foundation. Management of severe head injury: institutional variations in care and effect on outcome. Crit Care Med. 2002; 30(8):1870–1876

[5] Magi E, Recine C, Patrussi L, Becattini G, Nannoni S, Gabini R. Prognosis of stroke patients undergoing intubation and mechanical ventilation [in Italian]. Minerva Med. 2000; 91(5–6):99–104

[6] Mayer SA, Copeland D, Bernardini GL, et al. Cost and outcome of mechanical ventilation for life-threatening stroke. Stroke. 2000; 31(10):2346–2353

[7] Reynolds SF, Heffner J. Airway management of the critically ill patient: rapid-sequence intubation. Chest. 2005; 127(4):1397–1412

[8] Martyn JA, Richtsfeld M. Succinylcholine-induced hyperkalemia in acquired pathologic states: etiologic factors and molecular mechanisms. Anesthesiology. 2006:158–169

[9] Blanié A, Ract C, Leblanc PE, et al. The limits of succinylcholine for critically ill patients. Anesth Analg. 2012; 115(4):873–879

[10] Atherton DPL, Hunter JM. Clinical pharmacokinetics of the newer neuromuscular blocking drugs. Clin Pharmacokinet. 1999; 36(3):169–189

[11] Cope TM, Hunter JM. Selecting neuromuscular-blocking drugs for elderly patients. Drugs Aging. 2003; 20(2):125–140

[12] Cummins RO. ACLS Provider Manual. Dallas, TX: American Heart Association; 2002

[13] Ochs M, Davis D, Hoyt D, Bailey D, Marshall L, Rosen P. Paramedic-performed rapid sequence intubation of patients with severe head injuries. Ann Emerg Med. 2002; 40(2):159–167

[14] Lyerly HK, Gaynor JW. The Handbook of Surgical Intensive Care. 3rd ed. St. Louis, MO: Mosby Year Book; 1992

[15] Guidelines for the Management of Severe Traumatic Brain Injury, 4th Edition, Brain Trauma Foundation, September 2016. https://braintrauma.org/uploads/03/12/Guidelines_for_Management_of_Severe_TBI_4th_Edition.pdf. Accessed December 30, 2016

[16] Obrist WD, Langfitt TW, Jaggi JL, Cruz J, Gennarelli TA. Cerebral blood flow and metabolism in comatose patients with acute head injury. Relationship to intracranial hypertension. J Neurosurg. 1984; 61(2):241–253

[17] Bouma GJ, Muizelaar JP, Choi SC, Newlon PG, Young HF. Cerebral circulation and metabolism after severe traumatic brain injury: the elusive role of ischemia. J Neurosurg. 1991; 75(5):685–693

[18] Raichle ME, Posner JB, Plum F. Cerebral blood flow during and after hyperventilation. Arch Neurol. 1970; 23(5):394–403

[19] Cold GE, Christensen MS, Schmidt K. Effect of two levels of induced hypocapnia on cerebral autoregulation in the acute phase of head injury coma. Acta Anaesthesiol Scand. 1981; 25(5):397–401

[20] Crockard HA, Coppel DL, Morrow WF. Evaluation of hyperventilation in treatment of head injuries. BMJ. 1973; 4(5893):634–640

[21] Muizelaar JP, Marmarou A, Ward JD, et al. Adverse effects of prolonged hyperventilation in patients with severe head injury: a randomized clinical trial. J Neurosurg. 1991; 75(5):731–739

[22] Obrist WD, Martin NA. Arteriovenous oxygen difference in head injury. J Neurosurg. 1998; 88 (6):1122–1124

[23] Dings J, Meixensberger J, Amschler J, Roosen K. Continuous monitoring of brain tissue PO2: a new tool to minimize the risk of ischemia caused by hyperventilation therapy. Zentralbl Neurochir. 1996; 57(4):177–183

[24] Kiening KL, Härtl R, Unterberg AW, Schneider GH, Bardt T, Lanksch WR. Brain tissue pO2-monitoring in comatose patients: implications for therapy. Neurol Res. 1997; 19(3):233–240

[25] van Santbrink H, Maas AI, Avezaat CJ. Continuous monitoring of partial pressure of brain tissue oxygen in patients with severe head injury. Neurosurgery. 1996; 38(1):21–31

[26] Huizenga JE, Zink BJ, Maio RF, Hill EM. Guidelines for the management of severe head injury: are emergency physicians following them? Acad Emerg Med. 2002; 9(8):806–812

[27] Le Roux PD, Newell DW, Lam AM, Grady MS, Winn HR. Cerebral arteriovenous oxygen difference: a predictor of cerebral infarction and outcome in patients with severe head injury. J Neurosurg. 1997; 87(1):1–8

[28] Menzel M, Doppenberg EM, Zauner A, Soukup J, Reinert MM, Bullock R. Increased inspired oxygen concentration as a factor in improved brain tissue oxygenation and tissue lactate levels after severe human head injury. J Neurosurg. 1999; 91(1):1–10

[29] Sukoff MH. Effects of hyperbaric oxygenation. J Neurosurg. 2001; 95(3):544–546

[30] Rockswold SB, Rockswold GL, Vargo JM, et al. Effects of hyperbaric oxygenation therapy on cerebral metabolism and intracranial pressure in severely brain injured patients. J Neurosurg. 2001; 94(3):403–411

[31] Jain KK, Sukoff MA. Textbook of Hyperbaric Medicine. 3rd ed. Seattle, WA: Hogrefe & Huber; 1999:351–371

[32] Zauner A, Doppenberg EM, Woodward JJ, Choi SC, Young HF, Bullock R. Continuous monitoring of cerebral substrate delivery and clearance: initial experience in 24 patients with severe acute brain injuries. Neurosurgery. 1997; 41(5):1082–1091, discussion 1091–1093

[33] Codman Neurotrend ®. Codman and Shurtleff, Inc. 325 Paramount Drive Rayham, MA 02767. Telephone: 508–880–8100

[34] LICOX ®. Integra Neuro Sciences. 311 Enterprise Drive, Plainsboro, New Jersey 08536 Telephone: 800–654–2873

[35] Sarrafzadeh AS, Kiening KL, Bardt TF, Schneider GH, Unterberg AW, Lanksch WR. Cerebral oxygenation in contusioned vs. nonlesioned brain tissue: monitoring of PtiO2 with Licox and Paratrend. Acta Neurochir Suppl (Wien). 1998; 71:186–189

[36] Schaffranietz L, Heinke W, Rudolph C, Olthoff D. Effect of normobaric hyperoxia on parameters of brain metabolism [in German]. Anaesthesiol Reanim. 2000; 25(3):68–73

[37] Manley GT, Pitts LH, Morabito D, et al. Brain tissue oxygenation during hemorrhagic shock, resuscitation, and alterations in ventilation. J Trauma. 1999; 46(2):261–267

[38] Zauner A, Doppenberg E, Soukup J, Menzel M, Young HF, Bullock R. Extended neuromonitoring: new therapeutic opportunities? Neurol Res. 1998; 20 Suppl 1:S85–S90

[39] Menzel M, Doppenberg EM, Zauner A, et al. Cerebral oxygenation in patients after severe head injury: monitoring and effects of arterial hyperoxia on cerebral blood flow, metabolism and intracranial pressure. J Neurosurg Anesthesiol. 1999; 11(4):240–251

[40] Charbel FT, Hoffman WE, Misra M, Hannigan K, Ausman JI. Cerebral interstitial tissue oxygen tension, pH, HCO3, CO2. Surg Neurol. 1997; 48(4):414–417

[41] van den Brink WA, van Santbrink H, Steyerberg EW, et al. Brain oxygen tension in severe head injury. Neurosurgery. 2000; 46(4):868–876, discussion 876–878

[42] Zhi DS, Zhang S, Zhou LG. Continuous monitoring of brain tissue oxygen pressure in patients with severe head injury during moderate hypothermia. Surg Neurol. 1999; 52(4):393–396

[43] Schneider GH, Sarrafzadeh AS, Kiening KL, Bardt TF, Unterberg AW, Lanksch WR. Influence of hyperventilation on brain tissue-PO2, PCO2, and pH in patients with intracranial hypertension. Acta Neurochir Suppl (Wien). 1998; 71:62–65

[44] Imberti R, Bellinzona G, Langer M. Cerebral tissue PO2 and SjvO2 changes during moderate hyperventilation in patients with severe traumatic brain injury. J Neurosurg. 2002; 96(1):97–102

[45] Carmona Suazo JA, Maas AI, van den Brink WA, van Santbrink H, Steyerberg EW, Avezaat CJ. CO2 reactivity and brain oxygen pressure monitoring in severe head injury. Crit Care Med. 2000; 28 (9):3268–3274

[46] Johnston SC, Singh V, Ralston HJ, III, Gold WM. Chronic dyspnea and hyperventilation in an awake patient with small subcortical infarcts. Neurology. 2001; 57(11):2131–2133

[47] Piek J, Chesnut RM, Marshall LF, et al. Extracranial complications of severe head injury. J Neurosurg. 1992; 77(6):901–907

[48] Turkington PM, Bamford J, Wanklyn P, Elliott MW. Prevalence and predictors of upper airway obstruction in the first 24 hours after acute stroke. Stroke. 2002; 33(8):2037–2042

[49] Alhashemi JA, Cecconi M, Hofer CK. Cardiac output monitoring: an integrative perspective. Crit Care. 2011; 15(2):214–222

[50] Esteban A, Anzueto A, Alía I, et al. How is mechanical ventilation employed in the intensive care unit? An international utilization review. Am J Respir Crit Care Med. 2000; 161(5):1450–1458

[51] Schwarz S, Georgiadis D, Schwab S, Aschoff A, Hacke W. Current concepts of intensive care of space-occupying middle cerebral artery infarct [in German]. Nervenarzt. 2002; 73(6):508–518

[52] Cooper KR, Boswell PA, Choi SC. Safe use of PEEP in patients with severe head injury. J Neurosurg. 1985; 63(4):552–555

[53] Cotev S, Paul WL, Ruiz BC, Kuck EJ, Modell JH. Positive end-expiratory pressure (PEEP) and cerebrospinal fluid pressure during normal and elevated intracranial pressure in dogs. Intensive Care Med. 1981; 7(4):187–191

[54] Shirawi N, Arabi Y. Bench-to-bedside review: Early tracheostomy in critically ill trauma patients Critical Care 2005, 10:201 doi:10.1186/cc3828. 17 October 2005

[55] Davis K, Jr, Campbell RS, Johannigman JA, Valente JF, Branson RD. Changes in respiratory mechanics after tracheostomy. Arch Surg. 1999; 134(1):59–62

[56] Diehl JL, El Atrous S, Touchard D, Lemaire F, Brochard L. Changes in the work of breathing induced by tracheotomy in ventilator-dependent patients. Am J Respir Crit Care Med. 1999; 159(2):383–388

[57] Teoh WH, Goh KY, Chan C. The role of early tracheostomy in critically ill neurosurgical patients. Ann Acad Med Singapore. 2001; 30(3):234–238

19 Seizure Disorders: Diagnosis and Management

Vivek Ramakrishnan, Margaret Wacker, Dan E. Miulli, and Glenn Fischberg

Abstract

Seizure disorder is due to irritation of the brain from edema, compression, metabolic derangements, or other circumstances affecting the neurophysiology of the brain tissue. The irritation leads to abnormal electrical discharges of the neurons, which requires additional energy and resources. If the continuous discharge is not halted quickly the brain will not be able to replenish its resources, leading to the failure of normal brain cell homeostasis and eventual cell death. When seizures occur, adequate airway, breathing, and circulation should be maintained in order to help with the brain nutrient delivery to prevent ischemia. The seizure must be stopped as soon as possible and steps should be taken to prevent recurrence.

Keywords: ABCs, anticonvulsants, generalized seizures, seizure prophylaxis, status epilepticus, stroke, trauma, tumors

Case Study

A 23-year-old woman underwent a subfrontal craniotomy for craniopharyngioma. She developed transient diabetes insipidus. Several days later, her sodium level dropped abruptly from the 150 s to 131 after a dose of 1-deamino-8-D-arginine vasopressin (DDAVP, or desmopressin) as the diabetes insipidus was resolving. At the same time, her phenytoin level was found to be subtherapeutic, though this was not immediately corrected because she appeared to be doing well clinically and had no seizures. Later in the evening, her family noticed some staring spells and decreased responsiveness. This persisted, and later she was noted to have some seizure activity witnessed by the nurse. This continued, and the patient then developed nonconvulsive status epilepticus. A follow-up computed tomographic scan was obtained, which showed increased edema in the region of the tumor consistent with hypoxic injury. Despite efforts to correct the electrolytes and control the seizure activity, she went on to brain death.

See end of chapter for Case Management.

19.1 Classification of Seizures

Seizures may occur in patients in the neurosurgical intensive care unit (NICU) as evidence of either a primary or secondary neurologic disease process. In addition, seizure thresholds may be lowered due to metabolic derangements or fever, as was the case in the case study. Seizures may also add to the injury to the brain, especially if they are recurrent, through the imposition of increased metabolic demand or hypoxia due to the suppression of respirations during the seizure episodes. Untreated or unrecognized status epilepticus can be fatal or cause permanent neurologic injury. Hence efforts must be made to reduce the risk of seizures in the already neurologically compromised NICU patient.

Because many of the treatments for epilepsy are more effective for one or another seizure type, a brief review of types of seizures is necessary for choosing appropriate treatment. The International Classification of Epileptic Seizures (▶ Table 19.1) is included here as a basis for understanding different types of seizures.[1] Generalized seizures, including those that have secondarily generalized, may affect respiration and thus be more dangerous to the patient, especially if they are recurrent.

Table 19.1 International classification of epileptic seizures[1,3]

1. Generalized seizures (bilaterally symmetrical and without local onset)
   - a) Tonic, clonic, or tonicoclonic (grand mal)
   - b) Absence (petit mal)
     1. Simple—loss of consciousness only
     2. Complex—with brief tonic, clonic, or automatic movements
   - c) Lennox–Gastaut syndrome
   - d) Juvenile myoclonic epilepsy
   - e) Infantile spasms (West's syndrome)
   - f) Atonic (astatic, akinetic) seizures (sometimes with myoclonic jerks)
2. Partial, or focal, seizures (seizures beginning locally)
   - a) Simple (without loss of consciousness)
     1. Motor (tonic, clonic, tonicoclonic; Jacksonian; benign childhood epilepsy; epilepsia partialis continua)
     2. Somatosensory or special sensory (visual, auditory, olfactory, gustatory, vertiginous)
     3. Autonomic
     4. Psychic
   - b) Complex (with impaired consciousness)
     1. Beginning as simple partial seizures and progressing to impairment of consciousness
     2. With impairment of consciousness at outset
3. Special epileptic syndromes
   - a) Myoclonus and myoclonic seizures
   - b) Reflex epilepsy
   - c) Acquired aphasia with convulsive disorder
   - d) Febrile and other seizures of infancy and childhood
   - e) Hysterical seizures

19.2 Treatment of Seizures

Anticonvulsant medications should be selected by optimizing the drug for the type of seizures the patient has or for which the patient is at risk. For partial-onset seizures, including those with secondary generalization, the preferred agents are carbamazepine and phenytoin. Alternative agents include valproate and many of the newer anticonvulsant agents, including levetiracetam. For absence seizures, first-choice agents are ethosuximide and valproate. Valproate is the first choice for atypical absence or atonic seizures. An alternative is lamotrigine for either absence or atypical absence/atonic seizures. Valproate is also the first choice for myoclonic seizures, with the alternatives of lamotrigine, clonazepam, and clorazepate. For generalized tonicoclonic seizures, valproate, carbamazepine, and phenytoin are preferred agents, though newer antiepileptic drugs, such as topiramate, lamotrigine, and zonisamide, may also be useful. In general, one agent should be chosen and increased to the maximum tolerated dose before beginning polypharmacy for the treatment of seizures. Carbamazepine is contraindicated in primary generalized epilepsy due to possible exacerbation, but may be effective for secondarily generalized epilepsy.

In the setting of the NICU, the mode of administration of agents needs to be considered because many patients are unable to take medications orally. Agents currently available in the United States for intravenous (IV) administration include lorazepam (Ativan), diazepam (Valium), phenytoin (Dilantin), fosphenytoin (Cerebyx), phenobarbital, levetiracetam (Keppra), and valproate (Depacon). In addition, diazepam is available for rectal administration.

Newer antiepileptic agents in wide use over the last several years include levetiracetam and lacosamide (Vimpat). Levetiracetam (Keppra) has a mechanism of action that is unclear; however, it is suggested that the medication might work on presynaptic calcium channels, inhibiting synaptic firing. Lacosamide (Vimpat) has been shown to work on voltage-gated sodium channels and has been approved as an adjunctive therapy for partial seizures as well as neuropathic pain syndromes.

19.3 Status Epilepticus

Status epilepticus is a special case of seizure activity historically thought of as without recovery of consciousness between seizures lasting for more than 30 minutes. It is now generally considered ≥ 5 minutes of continuous clinical and/or electrographic seizure activity, or occurrence of more than one seizure without recovery to clinical baseline between.[2]

There are approximately 100,000 cases per year in the United States.[3,4] In half of the cases, it is the initial manifestation of a seizure disorder. The most commonly affected groups are young children and patients over 60 years of age.

Status epilepticus can be either generalized or partial. Generalized status can be convulsive and nonconvulsive.

Convulsive status includes (1) generalized: may be tonic, tonicoclonic, myoclonic (atonic would be an unusual form of generalized seizure; though without convulsions, still not generally considered either part of the nonconvulsive status epilepticus realm) and (2) focal motor status or epilepsia partialis continua.

Nonconvulsive status includes altered mentation, and despite its designation is still allowed to have subtle movements, such as some facial twitches or eye blinking or automatisms, such as lip smacking. Symptoms may be negative, such as aphasia, catatonia, or lethargy, or positive, such as, crying, laughter, or psychosis. Generalized convulsive status is the most frequent type of status epilepticus, of which 75% of cases are secondarily generalized. There are a variety of causes for status epilepticus, including febrile seizures; cerebrovascular accidents; infection, such as meningitis; idiopathic, epilepsy, or subtherapeutic anticonvulsants; electrolyte imbalance; drug intoxication, especially cocaine; alcohol or benzodiazepine withdrawal; traumatic brain injury; anoxia; and tumors.

Treatment of status epilepticus is directed to stabilizing the patient by stopping seizure activity and addressing the underlying cause of the status epilepticus. Any recurrent seizures without interval return to baseline should be treated aggressively. Historically, mortality from status epilepticus has been reported to be as high as 50%, although more recent data suggest it is on the order of 10 to 12%, to perhaps as high as 20%, of which only ~ 2% of deaths are directly attributable to the status epilepticus.[3,4] Morbidity and mortality may be due to central nervous system (CNS) injury caused by repetitive electrical discharges, systemic stress from the seizure (cardiac, respiratory, renal, or metabolic), or CNS damage from the insult that caused the status epilepticus.

Initial treatment should address airway, breathing, and circulation (ABC). This should include maintaining the airway with an oral airway or possibly intubation, the administration of supplemental oxygen, and cardiac and blood pressure monitoring. Once this has been accomplished, priorities must be to stop further seizure activity and to correct its cause.[1,2,3,4,5,6,7] An IV of normal saline should be started as soon as possible, and both a benzodiazepine, such as lorazepam or diazepam, and phenytoin loading dose should be administered. Intramuscular midazolam has been shown to be as effective as IV lorazepam.[8] Lorazepam and midazolam have the most data, and diazepam should be used if it is the first available as rectal medication. Emergent treatment for status is Class I, Level A evidence for lorazepam and midazolam and Class IIa, Level A for diazepam.[2] The role of valproate is not yet defined for use in status epilepticus, although it is a potential additional anticonvulsant that may be used. In general, except in the case of cocaine-induced seizures, a benzodiazepine alone should not be used; rather, it should be used in conjunction with a longer-acting anticonvulsant.

Concurrently, efforts should be started to identify and correct the underlying cause. This workup should include blood work consisting of electrolytes, glucose, magnesium, calcium, anticonvulsant level, and arterial blood gas. If there is any consideration of CNS infection, a lumbar puncture should be performed unless it is contraindicated. If the patient is hypoglycemic or if glucose cannot immediately be measured, 25 to 50 mL of dextrose 50 (D50) should be given. Fifty to 100 mg of thiamine should be given immediately prior to the D50 in patients in whom thiamine deficiency might be present. Likewise, naloxone (Narcan 0.4 mg IV push [IVP]) should be given in the case of patients who might have taken narcotics. An electroencephalography (EEG) monitor is helpful if available. Paralytic agents will stop the visible manifestation of the seizures, but they do not stop the dangerous electrical activity in the brain that can lead to permanent neurologic damage. Thus they should be avoided in patients with status epilepticus and those without EEG monitoring, except for the use of short-acting agents for intubation. In some cases of prolonged seizure activity, paralytic agents may be helpful in reducing the lactic acidosis and rhabdomyolysis caused by the seizure activity. In these cases, continuous EEG monitoring is necessary to determine whether electrical seizures are continuing and possibly causing further damage to the brain. In addition, narcotics and phenothiazines should be avoided in status epilepticus because they lower the seizure threshold (▶ Table 19.2).

Table 19.2 Protocol for the management of status epilepticus[1,3,4]

1. Lorazepam (Ativan) 0.1 mg/kg IV up to 4 mg (average adult dose) at rate of < 2 mg/min
OR
Diazepam (Valium) 0.2 mg/kg (10 mg average adult dose) IV at 5 mg/min
OR
Valproic acid 20 mg/kg diluted in water or vegetable oil administered rectally in pediatric patients with frequent seizures and no IV access
2. Phenytoin (Dilantin) or fosphenytoin (Cerebyx) load of 20 mg/kg IV at a maximal rate of 50 mg/min. If phenytoin is used, cardiac monitoring should be performed and the rate slowed should arrhythmias occur.
3. If seizures continue, additional phenytoin may be given up to a total of 30 mg/kg
OR
Phenobarbital IV up to a total load of 20 mg/kg. (Because phenobarbital may lower blood pressure and suppress respirations, these need to be monitored during its administration.)
OR
Paraldehyde 0.3–0.5 mg/kg in a 1% solution diluted 1:1 in vegetable oil administered rectally

(continued)

Table 19.2 continued

4. If seizures continue, the patient should be intubated and general anesthesia instituted with pentobarbital to induce burst suppression. This should be started with a load of 15 mg/kg IV and continued at a rate of ~ 2.5 mg/kg/h. Blood pressure should be closely monitored, and pressors may be needed to maintain an adequate blood pressure.

OR

Propofol can be used as an alternative to pentobarbital to induce burst suppression. A load of 40 mg is given and repeated to an induction dose of 2.0–2.5 mg/kg and maintenance of 0.1–0.2 mg/kg/min. Similar to pentobarbital, blood pressure must be closely monitored, and pressors may be needed.

OR

Midazolam (Versed) 5–10 mg bolus at less than 4 mg/min, followed by a 0.05–0.40 mg/kg/h drip

By this stage, continuous electroencephalographic monitoring should be used to titrate either pentobarbital or propofol to provide burst suppression. It should also be used to monitor the effect of treatment and should be instituted as early as is feasible in those patients with refractory status epilepticus who do not rapidly return to baseline function.

19.4 Prophylaxis of Seizures

Evidence-based medicine guidelines are available for prophylaxis of seizures in the setting of both traumatic brain injury and brain tumors.[9,10] Recommendations for prophylaxis in trauma remain more uniform than in neoplastic processes; however, some minor variations exist among institutions.

19.5 Treatment of Trauma

Guidelines for the Management of Severe Traumatic Brain Injury (4th edition), published by the Brain Trauma Foundation in 2016, does not recommend prophylactic use of anticonvulsants for the prevention of late seizures, though it may be useful in preventing early posttraumatic seizures.[11] Current practice based on these guidelines is to treat patients who have suffered severe head injury for 7 days to prevent early posttraumatic seizures. At that point, anticonvulsants are routinely discontinued unless the patient requires treatment for a documented seizure disorder.

The treatment of choice for antiepileptic prophylaxis in the setting of trauma has not been completely defined in current practice; however, the landmark 1990 study by Temkin, et al[12] specifically used phenytoin as the antiepileptic of choice in trauma patients. Levetiracetam is also widely used in the trauma setting as there are fewer side effects than with phenytoin and it is better tolerated by patients. Differences between the two medications do exist, however, particularly in the context of the speed to reach a therapeutic level in the

CNS. Studies have shown that, although levetiracetam levels are detectible in cerebrospinal fluid within 15 minutes after administration, peak levels took approximately 2 hours to appear. Phenytoin, when given as a loading IV dose, can reach therapeutic levels much faster and has become the initial treatment of choice for severe traumatic brain injury in the emergency room setting. In our institution, phenytoin has become the preferred initial antiepileptic in severe traumatic brain injury due to its faster therapeutic onset. One could consider a one-time phenytoin loading dose for a bridging effect in high-risk situations, followed closely by initial levetiracetam regularly scheduled dosing, so that there will be earlier coverage. It should be kept in mind, in particular in those with borderline low blood pressure or shock, that the IV phenytoin may cause hypotension and/or bradycardia. Fosphenytoin may be infused more rapidly with greater avoidance of these adverse effects, though it does require conversion in vivo to phenytoin, and thus the onset of efficacy is not necessarily faster.

Patients who have had a decompressive craniectomy from traumatic brain injury have been shown to have the same rate (and risk) of posttraumatic seizure as any other trauma patient and only require the usual 7-day course.[13]

19.6 Tumors

Prophylaxis guidelines for brain tumors remain less uniform than in the trauma setting, with much variation in length and type of treatment. The American Academy of Neurology published guidelines for the treatment of patients with brain tumors, which recommended against long-term prophylactic use of anticonvulsants, though it did not address the issue in the early perioperative period.[11] If patients are known to have suffered seizures as a result of their tumor, anticonvulsants are indicated for treatment of the seizure disorder. The common practice at our institution for seizures with large intra-axial or extra-axial tumors in the supratentorial compartment include 4 weeks of antiepileptic prophylaxis after surgery followed by an appropriate weaning process.

In tumors and other disease processes, such as aneurysmal subarachnoid hemorrhage, there is variation in the practice of neurosurgeons. We have tended to treat these patients with prophylactic anticonvulsants for a period of 1 week from surgery or bleed until surgery, analogous to the treatment of head injury patients. Long-term use of anticonvulsants is limited to those patients who have had seizures, as treatment of a seizure disorder rather than prophylaxis.

19.7 Stroke

Seizure prophylaxis for stroke patients remains relatively unstudied. Patients with hemorrhagic stroke in the basal ganglia, thalamus, or posterior fossa are routinely not placed on antiepileptics due to the fact that these areas are not epileptogenic. Cortical intraparenchymal hemorrhages or hemorrhages in other areas with significant mass effect and midline shift do have the propensity to cause seizure activity and should be treated appropriately. Guidelines do not exist; however, at our institution we follow similar guidelines as those for trauma patients treating for 7 days after an intraparenchymal hemorrhage.

Patients with large ischemic strokes causing mass effect also fall into the above category as likely benefiting from a short course of antiepileptic prophylaxis.

Case Management

The patient was found to have a subtherapeutic phenytoin level that should have been immediately corrected with a partial reloading of phenytoin. Although a computed tomographic scan was necessary to rule out intracranial hemorrhage after surgery, EEG should have been performed as well. The vital signs may have demonstrated tachycardia and hypertension, even in the face of nonconvulsive status epilepticus. If the seizures were not controlled with lorazepam and phenytoin, then the patient should have been intubated and the seizures treated with general anesthesia.

References

[1] Adams RD, Victor M, Ropper AH. Principles of Neurology. 6th ed. New York, NY: McGraw-Hill; 1997

[2] Brophy GM, Bell R, Claassen J, et al. Neurocritical Care Society Status Epilepticus Guideline Writing Committee. Guidelines for the evaluation and management of status epilepticus. Neurocrit Care. 2012; 17(1):3–23

[3] Bassin S, Smith TL, Bleck TP. Clinical review: status epilepticus. Crit Care. 2002; 6(2):137–142

[4] Greenberg MS. Handbook of Neurosurgery. Lakeland, FL: Greenberg Graphics; 1997

[5] Bleck TP. Management approaches to prolonged seizures and status epilepticus. Epilepsia. 1999; 40 Suppl 1:S59–S63, discussion S64–S66

[6] Brown LA, Levin GM. Role of propofol in refractory status epilepticus. Ann Pharmacother. 1998; 32(10):1053–1059

[7] Scottish Intercollegiate Guidelines Network. Diagnosis and Management of Epilepsy in Adults. Edinburgh, UK: Author; 2003

[8] Silbergleit R, Durkalski V, Lowenstein D, et al. NETT Investigators. Intramuscular versus intravenous therapy for prehospital status epilepticus. N Engl J Med. 2012; 366(7):591–600

[9] Bullock R, Chesnut RM, Clifton G, et al. Guidelines for the management of severe traumatic brain injury. J Neurotrauma. 2000; 17:451–553

[10] Glantz MJ, Cole BF, Forsyth PA, et al. Practice parameter: anticonvulsant prophylaxis in patients with newly diagnosed brain tumors. Report of the Quality Standards Subcommittee of the American Academy of Neurology. Neurology. 2000; 54(10):1886–1893

[11] Brain Trauma Foundation. Guidelines for the Management of Severe Traumatic Brain Injury, 4th edition.. September 2016. https://braintrauma.org/uploads/03/12/Guidelines_for_Management_of_Severe_TBI_4th_Edition.pdf. Accessed December 30, 2016

[12] Temkin NR, Dikmen SS, Wilensky AJ, Keihm J, Chabal S, Winn HR. A randomized, double-blind study of phenytoin for the prevention of post-traumatic seizures. N Engl J Med. 1990; 323 (8):497–502

[13] Ramakrishnan V, Dahlin R, Hariri O, et al. Anti-epileptic prophylaxis in traumatic brain injury: A retrospective analysis of patients undergoing craniotomy versus decompressive craniectomy. Surg Neurol Int. 2015; 6:8

20 Infections

Marc Cabanne and Dan E. Miulli

Abstract

Rapid diagnosis and appropriate treatment of nervous system infections are paramount to preventing death and limiting neurologic disability. Infections of the central nervous system can spread rapidly through the cerebrospinal fluid and its spaces but spread more slowly through the substance of the brain, at times being present for months. The nervous system has a well-developed immune system, which can be compromised by a persistent attack of bacteria, viruses, fungal, and other foreign organisms in the adjacent structures of the blood, skull, ear, and mouth. Once symptomatic, as determined by the neurologic exam and constitutional signs, the infection must be treated empirically after a specimen is obtained through an invasive procedure and prior to the return of a definitive organism.

Keywords: bacterial, empyema, encephalitis, fungal, meningeal signs, meningitis, ventriculitis, viral

Case Study

A 14-year-old, right-handed girl is brought to the emergency room by paramedics with complaints of flulike symptoms over the past 3 or 4 days, followed by an abrupt change in mental status on the day of evaluation. The patient does not have any significant past medical or surgical history. Additionally, she does not have a history of recent travel. On initial evaluation, the patient is observed to be lethargic but arousable with deep stimulation. Her core temperature is 102.7°F. The remaining vital signs are normal. No nuchal rigidity is present. The patient's Glasgow Coma Scale score is 8 without any focal neurologic deficits noted. Routine laboratory tests as well as blood cultures are drawn, with the only abnormality being a mildly elevated white blood cell count with many mononuclear cells. A computed tomographic scan of the brain was interpreted as normal. What is the patient's diagnosis? What are the possible etiologies? What studies are needed to complete a thorough workup? What is the appropriate treatment?

See end of chapter for Case Management.

20.1 Introduction

Infections of the central nervous system (CNS) are relatively infrequent occurrences due to the protection of the blood–brain barrier and innate immune cells; however, when infections occur, they can cause significant morbidity and mortality. Rapid diagnosis and appropriate treatment are paramount to preventing death and limiting disability, particularly in immunocompromised patients.[1,2,3,4] This chapter provides information needed for prompt and accurate diagnosis and treatment of nervous system infections in the intensive care setting. The chapter will focus on the diagnosis and treatment of community-acquired infections of the nervous system, with a section near the end for the discussion of iatrogenic, or hospital-acquired, infections.

Nervous system infections can be divided into two broad categories: infection of the structures surrounding the nervous system (meningitis), and infection of the parenchyma of the brain and/or spinal cord (encephalitis, abscess).

The main and subtypes of infection are discussed here, along with the information necessary for the neurologic intensive care unit.

20.2 Bacterial Infections of the Skull, Meninges, and Brain

20.2.1 Bacterial Meningitis

Bacterial meningitis is an inflammatory response to bacterial invasion of the pia-arachnoid surrounding the CNS. Meningitis following neurosurgical procedures tends to be less severe than community acquired meningitis. Septic meningitis is more severe, with a greater risk for causing persistent neurologic deficits.[1,2,3,4] The result of infection is stagnant blood flow and cerebral ischemia.

Epidemiology: In 1998–1999 the overall incidence of bacterial meningitis in the United States was 2.0 per 100,000. In 2006–2007 this decreased to 1.38 per 100,000.[5]

Risk factors: Alcoholism, splenectomy, human immunodeficiency virus (HIV), diabetes, immunosuppression, malignancy, dialysis, and sickle cell disease.[6,7,8,9]

Predisposing conditions: Otitis media, mastoiditis, sinusitis, bacteremia, pneumonia, and bacterial peritonitis.[6,7,8,9]

Most common organisms: Dependent on age; most spread by respiratory transmission (▶ Table 20.1).

Clinical presentation: Headache, fever, nuchal rigidity, nausea/vomiting, neck or back pain; can have focal neurologic signs, altered level of consciousness, or seizures; onset of symptoms over hours to days.[6,7,8,9]

Table 20.1 Most common organisms in bacterial meningitis[1,2,3,4,5,6,7]

Organisms and characteristics	Age
Streptococcus pneumoniae: Most common organism in all age groups (40–50% of cases); most common organism causing meningitis in patients with cerebrospinal fluid leakage	>7 years
Neisseria meningitidis: 20 to 30% of cases; associated with close living quarters	3–7 years
Haemophilus influenzae: Prior to *Haemophilus influenzae* type B vaccination, most common organism in children <5 years of age; now <5% of cases	3 months–3 years
Group B Streptococcus (agalactiae): Most frequent cause of neonatal meningitis; usually transmitted to infant during delivery; 10 to 15% of cases	<3 months
Escherichia coli: 15% of neonatal cases; 3% of all cases	<3 months
Listeria monocytogenes: 5 to 10% of cases of meningitis in neonates <1 month; fecal–oral transmission: transmitted via mother at the time of birth from genital or gastrointestinal tract colonization	<1 month or >50 years + immuno-suppression

Physical exam signs: Indicative of meningeal irritation.

Brudzinski's sign: Passive flexion of the neck causes involuntary flexion of the knees and hips.

Kernig's sign: Resistance to passive extension of the hip and knee.

Differential diagnosis: Includes viral meningitis, fungal meningitis, viral encephalitis, parenchymal abscess, epidural/subdural empyema, parasitic infection, neuroleptic malignant syndrome, and subarachnoid hemorrhage.

Diagnosis and studies: Cerebrospinal fluid (CSF) findings in bacterial meningitis: Opening pressure elevated, turbid, cloudy in appearance, red blood cell count >200/mm^3 with predominance of neutrophils, glucose decreased, and protein elevated (▶ Table 20.2).

Imaging: Has little role in the diagnosis of meningitis; is necessary to rule out hemorrhage, mass lesions, elevated intracranial pressure (ICP), or other nervous system infections

Lumbar puncture: If ICP is elevated, then the risk of herniation after lumbar puncture is significantly increased; however, it may be valuable for the evaluation of clinical sequelae of infection, such as subdural empyema, hydrocephalus, and infarction, because a lumbar puncture will be one of the most important tools in diagnosing meningitis.

Treatment: Duration of treatment 10 to 14 days, depending on clinical response. Dexamethasone can be used to reduce meningeal inflammation and pain associated with nuchal rigidity, as well as the incidence of hearing loss in patients with *Streptococcus pneumoniae* or *Haemophilus influenzae* type B meningitis (▶ Table 20.3).

Table 20.2 Cerebrospinal fluid analysis[1,2,3,4,5,6,7]

Parameter	Value
Opening pressure	4–15 mm Hg or 5.0–19.5 cm HO
Clarity	Cloudy: indicative of bacterial infection; WBC > 200/mm³ for turbid CSF
Color	Reddish: subarachnoid hemorrhage via traumatic tap; RBC > 6000/mm³ to appear red
	Yellowish: increased protein levels—usually > 150 mg/dL Xanthochromia: spin sample in centrifuge
Cell count and differential	WBC < 5/mm³; may be higher in neonates ↑ neutrophils = bacterial infection ↑ lymphocytes = viral or fungal etiology RBC measured in successive tubes to differentiate subarachnoid hemorrhage from traumatic tap with clearing of CSF and decrease in the number of RBCs
Biochemistry: glucose and protein levels	Glucose ²/₃ blood glucose; CSF = normal values 45–60 mg/dL Glucose ↓ bacterial or fungal infections; normal in viral infections; protein = 15–40 mg/dL; ↑ not specific for type of meningitis
Gram stain/culture and bacterial antigen panels	Gram stain identifies the type, or identity of, the bacteria present in the CSF.[8,9]

Abbreviations: CSF, cerebrospinal fluid; RBC, red blood cell count; WBC, white blood cell count.

Table 20.3 Treatment of bacterial meningitis[1,2,3,4,5,6,7]

Empirical antibiotic treatment based on most common organisms for a particular age group		
Treatment group	Antibiotic	Dosage
Initial treatment	Ceftriaxone or cefotaxime	2 g IV every 12 hours
	and	2 g IV every 6 hours
	Vancomycin	
		2–3 g IV every 8–12 hours (covers penicillin-resistant Streptococcus pneumoniae)
Penicillin allergy	Vancomycin or meropenem	2 g IV every 8 hours
	or	
	Trimethoprim/sulfamethoxazole (use in place of cephalosporin)	5 mg/kg every 6–8 hours
Chronic diseases, immunosuppression, or alcoholism	Add ampicillin	2 g IV every 4 hours
Neonates group B: Streptococcus is suspected	Ampicillin and gentamicin or cefotaxime	
Focused antibiotic treatment based on culture results		

(continued)

Table 20.3 continued

Empirical antibiotic treatment based on most common organisms for a particular age group

Treatment group	Antibiotic	Dosage
Streptococcus pneumoniae	Penicillin	4 million units IV every 4 hours
Neisseria meningitidis	Ceftriaxone	2 g IV every 12 hours
Haemophilus influenzae	Ceftriaxone (peds)	50 mg/kg IV every 12 hours
Group B *Streptococcus*	Penicillin	4 million units IV every 6 hours
Listeria monocytogenes	Ampicillin ± gentamicin	2 g IV every 12 hours 2 mg/kg loading dose then 1.7 mg/kg every 8 hours

Abbreviation: IV, intravenous.

20.2.2 Osteomyelitis of the Skull

Most infections are due to direct extension from infected sinuses, penetrating trauma, or intracranial empyema.

Most common organisms: *Staphylococcus aureus, Staphylococcus epidermidis*, and gram-negative bacilli—*Escherichia coli* must be considered in neonates.

Clinical presentation: Focal pain, fever, scalp erythema, swelling, and tenderness.

Differential diagnosis: Tumor, trauma, and epidural/subdural empyema.

Diagnosis and studies: Skull X-ray will occasionally show inflammation and edema in infected area (Pott's puffy tumor). Computed tomographic (CT) scan can demonstrate infectious changes of the skull as well as associated areas of infection.

Treatment: Consists of a combination of surgical debridement and antibiotic therapy. Surgery involves a craniectomy of the infected skull, replacing it with mesh or acrylic cranioplasty ~ 6 to 12 months postoperatively if there are no signs of infection. Antibiotics are routinely given, such as vancomycin 1 g intravenous (IV) every 12 hours plus ceftazidime 2 g IV every 8 hours. The antibiotics are given for 6 to 12 weeks and are adjusted based on culture and sensitivities.

20.2.3 Subdural Empyema

Subdural empyema is usually the result of direct extension of local infection (e.g., sinus infection), spread via diploic veins in the skull.[10] It represents 15–20% of all intracranial infections. In children meningitis is an important predisposing condition, with subdural empyema occurring in 2–10% of patients.[1] It can be seen in the epidural space and can be associated with osteomyelitis of the skull. Associated cerebral abscess is present in 20–25% of cases.[2] It may also be postoperative, posttraumatic, or related to prior subdural hematoma. There is a 50 to 60% morbidity rate and a 10 to 20% mortality rate.[11]

Most common organisms: Aerobic and anaerobic *Streptococcus* species, *S. aureus,* and gram-negative bacilli.

Clinical presentation: Fever, headache, nuchal rigidity, focal neurologic deficits, mental status changes, seizures, and nausea/vomiting. Symptoms can be similar to other CNS infections, however more rapidly progressive with subdural empyema.

Differential diagnosis: Bacterial meningitis, viral meningitis, fungal meningitis, parasitic infection, viral encephalitis, parenchymal abscess, subarachnoid hemorrhage, HIV, and neuroleptic malignant syndrome.

Diagnosis and studies: CT/magnetic resonance imaging (MRI) with contrast shows fluid collection with a typical crescent shape as well as a degree of mass effect or the presence of midline shift. Lumbar puncture is not recommended due to suspected increased ICP and risk of herniation. When CSF is obtained, the findings are consistent with parameningeal infection. Usually there is an intraoperative culture swab (aerobic and anaerobic cultures).

Treatment: Emergent surgical evacuation via craniotomy; however, burr holes can be used in critically unstable patients if purulent material is liquefied. Antibiotics consist of vancomycin 1 g IV every 12 hours plus ceftazidime 2 g IV every 8 hours plus metronidazole 500 mg IV every 6 hours. The 4- to 6-week course of antibiotics is adjusted depending on culture and sensitivities. Antiepileptics can be given prophylactically and should be used if seizures are present.

20.2.4 Brain Abscess

Brain abscess is a localized suppurative infection of the brain parenchyma,[12] with a male predominance. There is a slightly higher rate in children 5 to 9 years and adults > 60 years, with 25% of cases occurring in children. The infection is usually due to hematogenous spread from the chest or as a result of direct extension; in 25% of cases no source is identified.

Predisposing conditions: Otitis media, sinusitis, mastoiditis, oral infections, lung abscess, pulmonary abnormalities, cyanotic heart disease, bacterial endocarditis, penetrating trauma, and HIV.[13,14,15] Hematogenous spread will typically lead to multiple foci of infection versus a solitary lesion from contiguous spread from local infection.[1]

Most common organisms: *Streptococcus* species—aerobic, anaerobic, microaerophilic; *Staphylococcus aureus* most common secondary to trauma, surgery, or endocarditis[16]; *Staphylococcus epidermidis, Pseudomonas aeruginosa, Enterococcus, Bacteroides, Actinomyces*, and *Nocardia* associated with immunosuppression due to HIV disease[17]; *Mycobacterium tuberculosis* (TB)—most common cause of brain abscess in some developing countries; *Cryptococcus*—usually seen with meningitis; *Aspergillus*—seen in immunosuppressed patients from transplant; and *Toxoplasma gondii*.

Clinical presentation: Headache, fever, altered level of consciousness, visual changes, focal neurologic deficits—specific symptoms depending on location of lesion. Hemiparesis and seizures occur in 30–50% of patients.

Differential diagnosis: Bacterial meningitis, viral meningitis, fungal meningitis, parasitic infection, viral encephalitis, epidural/subdural empyema, intracerebral hemorrhage, subarachnoid hemorrhage, tumor, venous sinus thrombosis, and migraine headache.

Diagnosis and studies: Routine laboratory tests (complete blood count, basic chemistry panel) are usually not helpful. However, erythrocyte sedimentation rate (ESR) is usually elevated and can be used to follow the therapeutic response to antibiotics. C-reactive protein is also very sensitive and may be added as a test. Lumbar puncture is not usually indicated unless meningitis is suspected. When CSF is obtained, the findings are similar to those for other parameningeal infections, such as elevated white blood cell (WBC) count, normal glucose, and elevated protein. Cultures are usually negative.

Imaging: Contrast-enhanced CT or MRI scans show a characteristic rim-enhancing lesion with necrotic center surrounded by white matter edema. It can be difficult to differentiate from primary glial and metastatic tumors. Magnetic resonance spectroscopy can improve diagnostic accuracy.[18] The precise diagnosis of specific organisms requires pathological tissue from biopsy or resection.

Treatment: See ▶ Table 20.4, ▶ Table 20.5

Table 20.4 Differentiating treatment for brain abscess: medical versus surgical[1,2,3,13,14,15,16,17,18,19,20,21]

Indications for medical treatment	Indications for surgical treatment
Multiple lesions	Solitary lesion
Lesions < 3 cm	Lesions > 3 cm
Deep lesions	Proximity to ventricle
Poor surgical candidate	Significant mass effect or midline shift > 0.5 cm
	Altered mental status
	Progressive neurologic deficit

Table 20.5 Brain abscess management[1,2,3,13,14,15,16,17,18,19,20,21]

Antibiotics	Vancomycin 1 g IV every 12 hours + ceftazidime 2 g IV every 8 hours + metronidazole 500 mg IV every 6 hours if anaerobes suspected
Duration	6–12 weeks
Repeat imaging	2–4 weeks after beginning antibiotic therapy
Surgery	Consider if no change in size of the lesion or if neurologic deterioration
Surgical options	Stereotactic biopsy via craniotomy for resection

Abbreviation: IV, intravenous.

20.3 Viral Infections of the Meninges and Brain

20.3.1 Viral Meningitis

Viruses are obligate intracellular parasites that can replicate only within a cell. They contain either deoxyribonucleic acid (DNA) or ribonucleic acid (RNA), and infection occurs via hematogenous spread as part of a systemic infection, usually from a respiratory (measles, mumps, varicella), gastrointestinal (enteroviruses), or oral/genital mucosa (herpes simplex) source or neuronal spread via nerve cells.

Most common organism: *Enterovirus*, consisting of echovirus, coxsackievirus, and nonparalytic poliovirus, is the most common viral meningitis infection type in the United States. It is transmitted by fecal–oral spread. Peak incidence occurs in August–September.

Clinical presentation: Headache, fever, nausea/vomiting, nuchal rigidity, photophobia. However, patients are usually not as ill as with bacterial meningitis.

Differential diagnosis: Bacterial meningitis, fungal meningitis, viral encephalitis, parenchymal abscess, epidural/subdural empyema, severe frontal or sphenoid sinusitis, vaccination, intrathecal administration of drugs, HIV, subarachnoid hemorrhage, migraine headache, parasitic infections, sarcoidosis, and neuroleptic malignant syndrome. The diagnosis of viral meningitis is usually one of exclusion.

Diagnosis and studies: CSF findings in viral meningitis: Opening pressure usually normal; CSF usually clear/colorless; WBC elevated but usually < 200/ mm^3. There is initially a predominance of neutrophils with a shift toward mononuclear cells after 12 to 24 hours. The glucose is normal, and the protein is elevated. Gram's stain and routine cultures are negative; for this reason, viral meningitis is also referred to as aseptic meningitis. Viral cultures for *Enterovirus* are positive in 30 to 50% of cases; therefore, serological testing for the diagnosis of *Enterovirus* is not recommended. Polymerase chain reaction (PCR) can be used for diagnosis, but it is available only in specialized laboratories and is expensive.

Imaging: Usually unremarkable.

Treatment: Currently there is no treatment for enteroviruses, and treatment is symptomatic. Only if varicella-zoster or herpesvirus is suspected is acyclovir usually recommended.

20.3.2 Viral Encephalitis

Most common organisms: The majority of epidemic cases of encephalitis are caused by arboviruses with spread by vector transmission (infected mosquitoes).

Arbovirus types are St. Louis encephalitis, California encephalitis, western equine encephalitis, eastern equine encephalitis, West Nile virus, and La Crosse encephalitis. Encephalitis from arbovirus will peak in August and September when mosquitoes are most active.

Herpes simplex virus is a latent virus found in dorsal root ganglion; it is spread via the neuronal route. The majority of cases are caused by type I virus. CNS infection involves the mesial temporal lobes bilaterally, with one side affected worse than the other. Autopsy studies show a predilection of the olfactory and limbic systems.[19]

Clinical presentation: Most common presentation is altered level of consciousness in the setting of acute febrile illness with possible focal neurologic signs, usually meningeal involvement. Between 5 and 15% of patients with acute viral encephalitis will die, with persistent neurologic deficit occurring in 20–35% of patients.[1]

Differential diagnosis: Bacterial meningitis, viral meningitis, fungal meningitis, parasitic infection, epidural/subdural empyema, parenchymal abscess, tumor, subdural hematoma, HIV, lupus cerebritis, adrenal leukodystrophy, Reye's syndrome, and neuroleptic malignant syndrome

Diagnosis and studies: CSF analysis similar to aseptic meningitis; viral cultures of arboviruses and herpes simplex virus are available only at a specialized laboratory. Electroencephalogram (EEG) can show characteristic periodic lateralizing epileptiform discharges in the case of herpes simplex encephalitis.

Imaging: Critical for diagnosis of encephalitis. Focal hyperintense lesions seen in inconsistent distribution on T2-weighted images and FLAIR (fluid attenuated inversion recovery) sequences on MRI, especially in eastern equine encephalitis, asymmetric bitemporal distribution possibly with hemorrhage in herpes simplex encephalitis.

Treatment: No known treatment for arbovirus infections; herpes simplex encephalitis can be treated with acyclovir 10 mg/kg IV every 8 hours for 14 to 21 days and should be started as soon as possible to attempt to avoid long-term neurologic sequelae. If viral encephalitis is suspected, empirical treatment with acyclovir is indicated, as better outcomes are seen with early institution of antiviral therapy.

20.4 Fungal Infections of the Meninges and Brain

20.4.1 Fungal Meningitis

Most common organisms: Blastomyces, Coccidioides, Cryptococcus, and Histoplasma.

Most common organisms (immunocompromised): Aspergillus, Candida, and Mucorales.

Cryptococcus meningitis

Most common fungal pathogen of CNS; increased incidence of infection with increasing immunosuppression, especially when CD4 < 200. Initial transmission is respiratory that subsequently disseminates into many organ systems, including CNS. Remains latent.

Clinical presentation: Two- to three-week history of headache, fever, nuchal rigidity combined with lethargy, confusion, nausea/vomiting, and rarely focal neurologic defects.

Differential diagnosis: Bacterial meningitis, viral meningitis, viral encephalitis, parasitic infection, subarachnoid hemorrhage, and neuroleptic malignant syndrome.

Diagnosis and studies: CSF analysis consistent with fungal etiology (e.g., elevated WBC with lymphocytic predominance, glucose decreased, and protein elevated). India ink stain; latex agglutination tests are ~ 95% diagnostic.

Imaging: Not usually helpful with diagnosis, but can rule out mass lesions or intracranial hemorrhage.

Treatment: Amphotericin B 0.5 to 0.8 mg/kg/d IV with flucytosine 37.5 mg/kg orally every 6 hours. Treat for 6 weeks. After treatment is completed, use fluconazole as maintenance 400 mg/d for 2 to 3 months. If HIV present, Flucytosine dose is reduced to 25 mg/kg orally every 6 hours.

Histoplasma meningitis

Mostly found in Ohio and Mississippi river valleys; widely disseminated in soil. Respiratory transmission. Disseminated disease can be seen in immunosuppressed patients due to HIV, lymphoma, or iatrogenic cause. May cause mass lesions in parenchyma (histoplasmosis).[20]

Clinical presentation: Similar to *Cryptococcus.*

Differential diagnosis: Similar to *Cryptococcus.*

Diagnosis and studies: CSF consistent with fungal meningitis; serology positive in 60 to 90% with CNS disease, cultures positive < 30%.

Treatment: Amphotericin B 0.7 to 1.0 mg/kg/d IV. Treat for 8 to 12 weeks. In patients with HIV, after treatment with amphotericin B is completed, use itraconazole 200 mg/d indefinitely. Despite aggressive treatment, there is ~ 20% mortality.

Coccidioides immitis meningitis

Endemic in the San Joaquin Valley in central California, where it occurs in soil. There is respiratory transmission. It can present as a mass lesion in the brain parenchyma. Patients can also present with hydrocephalus, often with loculated ventricles, which can be challenging to treat because this infection causes the ependymal surface to become friable and hemorrhagic, leading to high mortality.

Predisposing factors: Pregnancy, immunosuppression, and HIV.

Clinical presentation: Similar to *Cryptococcus* and *Histoplasma.*

Differential diagnosis: Similar to *Cryptococcus* and *Histoplasma.*

Diagnosis and studies: CSF consistent with fungal etiology. The most reliable method of diagnosis is detection of complement-fixing antibody in CSF.[21] Culture is usually negative.

Treatment: Fluconazole 400 to 800 mg/d; if no clinical response, then amphotericin B 0.1 to 0.3 mg/d intrathecal via Ommaya reservoir. Treat for ~ 2 years after CSF is normalized. For HIV patients, treatment is lifelong. Without treatment, *Coccidioides* meningitis is uniformly fatal within 2 years.[22]

Blastomyces dermatitidis meningitis

Distributed along the Mississippi River; exists in moist soil. There is respiratory transmission. Most cases have evidence of systemic infection. CNS is involved in 6 to 33% of patients with disseminated disease.[21,23] A mass lesion forms in the brain parenchyma more frequently than in other fungal infections.

Clinical presentation: Fever, cough, myalgias, arthralgias, and pleuritic chest pain.

Differential diagnosis: Bacterial meningitis, viral meningitis, bacterial abscess, and parasitic infection.

Diagnosis and studies: Culture from pulmonary secretions or tissue biopsy.

Imaging: CT/MRI is not usually helpful unless a mass lesion is present..

Treatment: For pulmonary infection, use itraconazole 200 to 400 mg/d; if infection is severe, use amphotericin B 0.7 to 1.0 mg/kg/d. Treatment is for 6 months. CNS disease requires treatment with maximal dose amphotericin B.

20.4.2 Mucormycosis: Rhizopus, Mucor, and Rhizomucor

Mucormycosis invade the CNS by hematogenous spread or direct invasion. CNS mucormycosis can cause infarction, abscess formation, and mycotic aneurysms.

Predisposing factors: Diabetes and neutropenia.

Clinical presentation: Headache, fever, sinus pain; rhinitis symptoms can progress to cellulitis, proptosis, and cavernous sinus thrombosis.

Diagnosis and studies: Culture of surgical specimen/swab.

Treatment: Surgical debridement combined with amphotericin B 1 mg/kg/d.

Aspergillus

Majority of cases occur in immunosuppressed transplant patients with prolonged neutropenia. It begins as pulmonary disease and disseminates to CNS via hematogenous spread. There can be direct extension from maxillary and ethmoid sinuses. It is associated with cavernous sinus thrombosis and the formation of mycotic aneurysms.

Treatment: Surgical debridement and high-dose amphotericin B.

20.5 Tuberculosis of the Meninges and Brain

20.5.1 Tuberculosis Meningitis

Respiratory transmission: Latent organisms reactivate to cause infection months to years after primary infection. There is hematogenous spread to the meninges and brain parenchyma, preferentials involving optic chiasm, pons, and cerebellum.

Predisposing conditions: Consists of immunosuppression, alcohol abuse, intravenous drug abuse (IVDA), and HIV.

Clinical presentation: Slowly progressive fever, headache, and meningismus. Can also cause lethargy, mental status changes, seizures, and cranial nerve palsies.

Differential diagnosis: Bacterial meningitis, fungal meningitis, viral meningitis, parasitic infection, viral encephalitis, lupus cerebritis, and neuroleptic malignant syndrome.

Diagnosis and studies: Purified protein derivative (PPD) skin testing[24]; chest X-ray may show active or chronic TB infection. CSF analysis is the most useful diagnostic test[25]; it can demonstrate WBC elevation with lymphocytic predominance. Glucose is decreased, protein is elevated. Acid-fast smear positive < 23% of the time; cultures positive in 40 to 70% of cases. Serological test to detect mycobacterial antigens and PCR to detect antibodies in CSF should be performed.

Imaging: Contrast-enhanced CT/MRI can demonstrate meningeal inflammation as well as TB exudate around the basal cisterns. Magnetic resonance angiography can detect vasculitic changes common with TB meningitis.

Treatment: If TB meningitis is suspected, start antibiotic therapy empirically consisting of isoniazid 300 mg daily, rifampin 600 mg daily, ethambutol 15 to 25 mg/kg/d, pyrazinamide 25 mg/kg/d plus pyridoxine. Treat for 1 year. Can supplement with dexamethasone in patients with extreme neurologic compromise.[26] In patients with neurologic compromise, 70 to 80% survival rate; ~ 50% will have neurologic morbidity, including seizures, hemiparesis, hydrocephalus, and organic brain syndrome.

20.5.2 Tuberculoma

Mass lesions in brain parenchyma caused by *Mycobacterium tuberculosis*. Autopsy studies have shown ~ 70% to have multiple lesions. Mass lesions involving brain parenchyma are more frequent in HIV-associated CNS tuberculosis, with the pattern of pathology affected by degree of immunosuppression; less granuloma formation with lower CD4 + counts.[27]

Predisposing factors: Immunosuppression and HIV disease. The mortality of AIDS-associated tuberculous infections has been found to be as high as 33%, depending on degree of immunosuppression.[27]

Clinical presentation: Fever, headache, seizures, and focal neurologic deficits.

Differential diagnosis: Bacterial abscess, fungal abscess, parasitic infection, subdural/epidural empyema, viral encephalitis, lymphoma, toxoplasmosis, tumor, intracerebral hemorrhage, and subarachnoid hemorrhage.

Diagnosis and studies: PPD skin test, CSF analysis consistent with parameningeal infection; pathological tissue needed to rule out malignancy or other infectious conditions. Acid-fast bacilli stain positive in ~ 60%, whereas ~ 60% will grow in culture.

Imaging: Contrast-enhanced CT/MRI can show single or multiple homogeneously enhancing lesions.

Treatment: As for TB meningitis, tuberculomas can be followed with serial imaging if there is no presence of life-threatening mass effect. If lesions enlarge despite appropriate therapy, biopsy to detect resistant organisms or concurrent opportunistic infections should be considered.[27]

20.5.3 Spinal Tuberculosis

Also known as Pott's disease, may accompany meningitis or exist alone. Less frequent than bacterial spinal infections; however, it can cause destruction of bone, fractures, and spinal instability. Ultimately TB exudate surrounds the spinal cord, causing symptoms due to cord compression and infarction due to vasculitic changes of vessels. Spinal TB most often affects the lumbar and thoracic spine and accounts for 50% of extrapulmonary musculoskeletal cases of TB.[1]

Clinical presentation: Symptoms can be sudden or indolent, but typically progress over weeks to months. Back pain associated with muscle spasms and movement can induce a rigid posture with short deliberate steps described as an "aldermanic gait."[1] Other symptoms can include localized pain, weakness, paresthesia, radiculopathy. Sensory level is demonstrated in about two-thirds of patients.[28]

Differential diagnosis: Spinal epidural abscess, spinal cord tumor, spinal stenosis, disk herniation, spondylotic myelopathy, HIV, myelopathy, and multiple sclerosis.

Diagnosis and studies: PPD skin test. CSF consistent with parameningeal infection. Blood cultures are negative; however, biopsy/culture swab is necessary for definitive diagnosis.

Imaging: MRI is the modality of choice; it will show epidural or subdural exudate surrounding and compressing the spinal cord. Imaging characteristics of spinal TB are similar to those seen for neoplasm and can be differentiated from a pyogenic infection if sparing of the disk space and involvement of the posterior elements are present.

Treatment: Surgical decompression of the spinal cord; incision and drainage of abscess with tissue culture for targeted antibiotic therapy, and spinal stabilization. Antibiotic treatment for 1 year with usual anti-TB medications.

20.6 Parasitic Infections

Most common organisms: *Taenia solium* (cysticercosis), *Echinococcus multilocularis* (echinococcus), *Plasmodium falciparum* (malaria), and *Treponema pallidum* (syphilis).

20.6.1 Cysticercosis

Widespread in Central and South America; infection of brain with larval cysts of *Taenia solium* (pork tapeworm). There are two mechanisms of infection: (1) fecal–oral spread with ingestion of eggs and (2) ingestion of cysticerci in undercooked pork followed by self-inoculation with eggs from feces.

Clinical presentation: Headache, nausea/vomiting, seizures, altered level of consciousness, focal neurologic signs, and visual changes.

Classification: (1) Racemose form—cysts found at base of brain in basal cisterns; associated with formation of hydrocephalus; and (2) *Cysticercus cellulosae* form—with parenchymal cysts; associated with seizures.

Differential diagnosis: Bacterial abscess, fungal abscess, *Cryptococcus*, *Coccidiodes*, and tumor.

Diagnosis and studies: Serological testing with immunoblotting and biopsy of surgical specimen are the most accurate. CSF may be normal with parenchymal lesions, with a lymphocytic pleocytosis, increased protein and normal glucose seen with ventricular and subarachnoid forms.

Imaging: Contrast-enhanced CT/MRI can show T1 hypointense single or multiple rim-enhancing cysts. Can occasionally see head of scolex in parenchymal cyst. May see calcifications from old "burned out" cysts.

Treatment: Praziquantel 50 to 100 mg/kg/d for 15 to 30 days; alternative: albendazole 10 to 15 mg/kg/d for 8 days. Some include steroids to help decrease the inflammatory response in the brain parenchyma as the cysts die.

20.6.2 *Echinococcus* (Hydatid [cyst] Disease)

Organism is tapeworm that infects carnivorous animals (dog is primary definitive host). It is common in the Mediterranean; spread by fecal–oral route. CNS is involved in only 2% of cases.[29] *E. multilocularis* is most the common pathogen of the species.

Clinical presentation: Headache, nausea/vomiting, seizures, hemiparesis, papilledema, cranial nerve palsies, and dysarthria.

Diagnosis and studies: Serological tests; however, some immunologic tests might not be accurate due to cross-reactions with other parasitic diseases (e.g., enzyme-linked immunosorbent assay [ELISA], enzyme-linked immunoelectrotransfer blot [EITB] assay).[1]

Imaging: CT/MRI can show a cyst with sharp borders, without enhancement or associated edema. Some lesions may be calcified. Lesions can be found in brain parenchyma, ventricular system, epidural space, subarachnoid space, and orbits.

Treatment: Surgical excision; cyst must be removed intact to prevent spilling contents. Treat with albendazole 400 mg twice a day.

20.6.3 Malaria

All serious infections are caused by *Plasmodium falciparum*; infects over 2.5 billion people worldwide, causing 1 million to 3 million deaths annually. It has been eradicated in North America and Europe. Vector transmission is via female *Anopheles* mosquito. Infection causes capillary vascular obstruction with resultant brain edema and small ring hemorrhages in the subcortical white matter.

Clinical presentation: Fever, chills, anemia, altered level of consciousness, renal failure, jaundice, thrombocytopenia, and seizures.

Diagnosis and studies: Examination of blood smear with Giemsa stain. CSF studies are normal but should be examined to rule out other sources of infection. Cerebral malaria is defined by (1) unarousable coma, (2) evidence of acute *P. falciparum* infection, and (3) no other source of coma.[1]

Treatment: Quinine sulfate 650 mg every 8 hours for 7 days plus doxycycline 100 mg twice a day for 7 days or clindamycin 10 mg/kg IV load and then 5 mg/kg IV every 8 hours for 7 days. Despite treatment, there is a 20% mortality.

20.6.4 Syphilis

Caused by *Treponema pallidum*; transmitted by sexual contact. CNS infection develops in 8 to 40% of cases. If left untreated, ~ 25% will develop tertiary syphilis in 5 to 40 years. Syphilitic gummas are tumorlike lesions primarily involving skin and mucous membranes; can involve the brain.

Neurosyphilis is divided into four syndromes: syphilitic meningitis, meningovascular syphilis, tabes dorsalis, and general paresis. Tabes dorsalis is atrophy of the dorsal columns in the spinal cord leading to loss of sensation and proprioception, mostly in the lower extremities. It is associated with Argyll–Robertson pupil (no pupillary reaction to light, but accommodation is preserved). General paresis (also referred to as general paralysis of the insane) is the gradual deterioration of mental function with loss of motor control and seizures.

Diagnosis and studies: VDRL test in CSF and rapid plasma regain in serum.

Treatment: Penicillin G 12 million to 24 million units IV/d divided every 4 hours for 10 to 14 days; if penicillin allergic, doxycycline 200 mg a day for 21 days.

20.6.5 Lyme Disease

Multisystem disease caused by deer tick *(Borrelia burgdorferi)*; most common arthropod-borne infection in the United States.[30] Three clinical stages: (1) early stage, characterized by a distinctive rash known as erythema migrans; (2) dissemination stage, occurs days to weeks following infection; characterized by flulike symptoms called erythema chronicum migrans, which, if left untreated, can disseminate and involve cardiac and neurologic systems. This consists of a clinical triad of meningitis, cranial neuritis, and radiculopathy.[31] It occurs in 10 to 15% of patients with stage 2 Lyme disease; (3) persistent infection, with symptoms that may not appear until weeks, months, or years after infection. Stage 3 typically involves joint pain. Other symptoms include arthritis and chronic neurologic problems, such as encephalopathy, ataxia, dementia, and neuropathy.

Diagnosis and studies: Based on history and the presence of the typical macular rash. Antibody serologies cannot be detected until ~ 3 weeks postinfection; CSF consistent with aseptic (viral) meningitis. Most laboratories use ELISA technique for diagnosis; however, due to potential for false-positives with rheumatoid arthritis, Rocky Mountain spotted fever, infectious mononucleosis, syphilis, tuberculous meningitis, and leptospirosis, if ELISA is positive, a confirmatory Western blot should be obtained.[32]

Treatment: Doxycycline 100 mg twice a day for 3 to 4 weeks. If neurologic abnormalities present, use ceftriaxone 2 g IV daily for 2 to 4 weeks.

20.6.6 Rickettsia/ Ehrlichia

Small gram-negative intracellular organisms transmitted by tick bites; can cause systemic infections that can present as encephalitis. Known as Rocky Mountain spotted fever and ehrlichiosis.

Diagnosis and studies: Clinical information is based on history of tick bite; also, specialized serological tests are available.

Treatment: Empirical treatment with doxycycline 100 mg twice a day for 10 to 14 days; in children, chloramphenicol 50 mg/kg/d divided into four doses. Mortality is 2 to 6%.

20.6.7 Amebic Encephalitis

Uniformly fatal meningoencephalitis caused by *Naegleria fowleri*; found in lakes in warm climates. It is a rapidly progressive encephalitis.

Diagnosis and studies: Based on history of swimming in warm, freshwater lakes. CSF shows bacterial or fungal meningitis picture; however, Gram's stain and culture are negative.

Imaging: MRI can show frontal lobe involvement.

Treatment: Amphotericin B IV and intrathecal tetracycline and rifampin.[33]

20.6.8 Prion Disease, Creutzfeldt–Jakob Disease (similar to "mad cow" disease)

Fatal encephalopathy characterized by rapidly progressive dementia, ataxia, and myoclonus. Also called transmissible spongiform encephalopathy. Can be inherited or acquired (ingestion of infected tissue).

Clinical presentation: Progressive dementia, fatigue, ataxia, myoclonus, tremor, rigidity, and focal neurologic deficits.

Diagnosis and studies: CSF is usually normal; EEG can show bilateral sharp waves or periodic spikes.

Imaging: No characteristic findings on CT/MRI; can show atrophy.

Treatment: None. Median survival is 5 months; 80% die in first year.

20.7 CNS Infections in HIV Patients

Forty to 60% of all patients with acquired immunodeficiency syndrome (AIDS) will develop neurologic complications related to the disease.[34] One-third of patients with HIV will have neurologic symptoms as the presenting manifestation of the disease.[35]

Most common organisms: *Toxoplasma*, primary B cell lymphoma, JC virus (causative agent for progressive multifocal leukoencephalopathy), *Cryptococcus*, and cytomegalovirus (CMV).

20.7.1 Toxoplasma gondii

Ten percent of the general population of the United States has been infected with *Toxoplasma gondii*.[36] The major reservoir is domestic cats, spread to humans by fecal–oral route. Generally asymptomatic except in the setting of severe immunosuppression, such as with advanced HIV disease when the CD4 count is < 200 or when reactivation of infection produces single or multiple abscesses in the brain parenchyma.

Clinical presentation: Headache, fever, altered level of consciousness, lethargy, focal neurologic signs. Can also present with seizures or intracerebral hemorrhage.

Differential diagnosis: Bacterial abscess, fungal abscess, parasitic infection, tumor, lymphoma, viral encephalitis, progressive multifocal leukoencephalopathy (PML), and CMV.

Diagnosis and studies: CSF analysis may be similar to that of parameningeal infection; however, there may be an elevated WBC count with neutrophilic predominance. The glucose may be normal and the protein elevated. There should be a serological test for *Toxoplasma* antibodies.

Imaging: Contrast-enhanced CT/MRI will show characteristic round, rim-enhancing lesion, single or multiple, with associated white matter edema; difficult to differentiate from tumor or other types of abscesses radiologically.

Treatment: If toxoplasmosis is suspected, start empirical therapy with pyrimethamine 200 mg orally × 1 then 75 mg/d plus sulfadiazine 1–1.5 g orally every 6 hours plus folinic acid 10–20 mg/d for 4–6 weeks after resolution of signs/symptoms. Alternate regimen: trimethoprim/sulfamethoxazole 10/50 mg/kg divided every 12 hours for 30 days. If toxoplasmosis is confirmed, then patients require suppression treatment after initial therapy: Sulfadiazine 500–1000 mg orally 4×/d plus, pyrimethamine 25–50 mg orally every 24 hours plus, folinic acid 10–25 mg orally every 24 hours. Discontinue suppression treatment if CD4 count climbs above 200 for 3 months.

Lifelong treatment for AIDS patients as primary prophylaxis: trimethoprin/sulfamethoxazole—double strength 1 tab orally every 24 hours. Follow patient clinically, and repeat imaging 10 to 14 days after starting treatment if there is no clinical or radiological response to empirical treatment. Biopsy of lesion may be required to rule out lymphoma and/or PML. Median survival is 15 months.

20.7.2 Lymphoma

Lymphoma develops in ~ 5% of patients with HIV disease.[37] It is due to Epstein–Barr virus–associated B cell type. Approximately one-third of patients will present with CNS disease.[38]

Clinical presentation: Lethargy, confusion, cognitive deficits, focal neurologic signs, seizures, and cranial nerve palsies.

Differential diagnosis: Toxoplasmosis, PML, other tumors (primary or metastatic), bacterial abscess, fungal abscess, parasitic infection, CMV, and viral encephalitis.

Diagnosis and studies: Routine laboratory tests are not usually helpful; no serological tests for identification. Diagnosis must be strongly considered in patients who do not respond to empirical treatment. For toxoplasmosis, definitive diagnosis requires biopsy.

Imaging: Contrast-enhanced CT/MRI will show white matter lesions, possibly contrast enhancement. The lesion may cross the corpus callosum.

Treatment: Chemotherapy; dexamethasone can cause tumors to "melt" away; whole brain radiotherapy. Median survival is 3 months.

20.7.3 Progressive Multifocal Leukoencephalopathy

PML is a progressive demyelinating disease, primarily seen in immunocompromised patients,[39] such as those with HIV, lymphoma, chronic lymphocytic leukemia, lupus, and diseases caused by JC virus. Antibodies to JC virus can be detected in CSF.[40,41,42]

Clinical presentation: Progressive focal neurologic deficits and cognitive decline[43,44]

Differential diagnosis: Multiple sclerosis, adrenal leukodystrophy, acute disseminated encephalomyelitis, toxoplasmosis, lymphoma, prion disease, and CMV.

Diagnosis and studies: CSF analysis usually normal. JC virus can be detected in CSF by serology and PCR. Definitive diagnosis requires biopsy, which is frequently diagnostic.

Imaging: CT/MRI shows diffuse white matter disease; does not enhance with contrast.

Treatment: There is no proven effective therapy. Median survival is 15 months.

20.7.4 Cytomegalovirus

Fifty to 80% of the general adult population in the United States has been infected; most are asymptomatic. In nonimmunocompromised adults, infection is similar clinically to mononucleosis. Seen in patients late in the course of HIV disease: CD4 count < 50; most common infection is rhinitis. Can involve the spinal cord—characterized by ascending motor weakness, areflexia, and loss of bowel/bladder function.[45] Similar to Guillain–Barré syndrome.

Clinical presentation: Progressive deterioration of mental status and cognitive function, headaches, and seizures.

Differential diagnosis: Viral encephalitis, PML, lymphoma, toxoplasmosis, parasitic infection, and prion disease.

Diagnosis and studies: CSF is essentially normal; may have elevated protein. May test serology for CMV antigen by PCR. Can also perform specific viral cultures.

Imaging: MRI can show nonspecific hyperintense signal changes on T2-weighted images and FLAIR sequences.[46]

Treatment: Ganciclovir 5 mg/kg IV every 12 hours plus foscarnet 90 mg/kg IV every 12 hours. Subsequently, treat HIV disease with antiretroviral therapy.

20.7.5 HIV Encephalopathy

Most common neurologic involvement in AIDS. Two-thirds of patients with HIV/AIDS and one-third of AIDS patients will have dementia at time of death.[47] HIV causes diffuse brain atrophy.

Clinical presentation: Altered level of consciousness, cognitive dysfunction, gait abnormalities, postural instability.

Differential diagnosis: Viral encephalitis, PML, prion disease, parasitic infection, dementia, and metabolic encephalopathy.

Diagnosis and studies: CSF is usually nondiagnostic,[48] although the patient may have a slight elevation of WBC. Glucose is normal, protein is elevated. HIV antibodies can be detected in CSF.

Imaging: CT/MRI will show generalized atrophy without specific findings. MRI may show hyperintense periventricular white matter abnormalities of T2-weighted images and FLAIR sequences.

Treatment: Antiretroviral therapy. HIV disease can also cause an AIDS-related myelopathy and cranial neuropathies.

20.8 Spinal Infections

There are three types of spinal infections: spinal epidural abscess, vertebral osteomyelitis, and diskitis.

20.8.1 Spinal Epidural Abscess

More common in elderly, immunocompromised, and IVDA.[49,50] Most common route of spread is hematogenous; most commonly located in lumbar region.

Risk factors: Osteomyelitis, diskitis, diabetes, cancer, IVDA, alcohol abuse, and chronic renal failure.[51]

Sources of infection (hematogenous): skin infection, endocarditis, bacteremia, urinary tract infection, dental abscess, respiratory infection, penetrating trauma, and psoas abscess. Can also occur from direct extension from vertebral body, disk space infection, or paraspinal/psoas abscess.[49] With hematogenous spread, abscess usually forms posteriorly in the spinal canal; if direct extension from osteomyelitis or diskitis, abscess usually forms anteriorly.[49,52] Neurologic deficits caused by epidural abscess are thought to be secondary to compression of neural elements combined with vascular thrombosis and infarction.[53,54,55]

Most common organisms: *S. aureus*, aerobic and anaerobic streptococci, *Pseudomonas*, *E. coli*, and TB (common in chronic form).[51]

Clinical presentation: Back pain, fever; associated with nerve root or spinal cord dysfunction, such as weakness, pain, and loss of bowel/bladder control.

Differential diagnosis: Spinal TB, tumor, disk herniation, spinal stenosis, multiple sclerosis, HIV, myelopathy, and spondylotic myelopathy.

Diagnosis and studies: Routine laboratory tests are not usually helpful; most common laboratory abnormality is elevated ESR.[56] Blood cultures are positive in 60% of cases.

Imaging: Contrast-enhanced MRI is modality of choice that can demonstrate fluid collection as well as the degree of spinal cord/thecal sac compression. Thorough neurologic exam and MRI can localize the affected area.

Treatment: In patients without neurologic deficits, use vancomycin 1 g IV every 12 hours, rifampin 600 mg daily, and cefotaxime 2 g IV every 8 hours for 6 to 8 weeks. Surgical evacuation is warranted if neurologic deficits are present; if surgical evacuation is done, follow with antibiotics and deescalate according to intraoperative cultures in addition to bracing when > 30 degrees upright. Bracing is recommended with or without surgery. If abscess is located posteriorly, laminectomies can be performed. If abscess is located anteriorly in the spinal canal, the patient may need corpectomy with anterior and possibly posterior stabilization. Mortality is 18 to 23%. Improvement of neurologic function postoperatively is rare.

20.8.2 Vertebral Osteomyelitis

Spinal infections account for 2 to 4% of osteomyelitis cases,[57] which is due to hematogenous spread. Fifty percent of these cases are located in the lumbar spine.[58]

Most common organisms: *S. aureus* ~ 60%,[59] gram-negative bacilli *(Pseudomonas, Proteus, E. coli),* and fungal pathogens.

Risk factors: Diabetes, chronic steroid use, dialysis, IVDA, malnutrition, malignancy, advanced age, and immunosuppression.[59,60]

Sources of infection are commonly respiratory, bacteremia, urinary tract infection, soft tissue abscess, dental abscess, and postsurgical causes (~ 2.5%).[61, 62] Spinal TB[63] has increased since the AIDS epidemic.

Clinical presentation: Localized back pain unrelated to movement or position, fever.

Differential diagnosis: Important to differentiate osteomyelitis from neoplasms.

Diagnosis and studies: Most common laboratory abnormality is elevated ESR. Blood cultures are positive in only ~ 25% of cases. CT-guided biopsy should be performed for identification of organism if blood culture is negative.[59] Open biopsy may be necessary; specimens must be sent for bacterial and fungal cultures.

Imaging: X-rays can show disk space narrowing and end plate changes. Bone scan and MRI are the most sensitive studies for identifying vertebral osteomyelitis.[64] MRI demonstrates hyperintense signal in the vertebral body on T2-weighted images.

Treatment: Antibiotic therapy for 4 weeks combined with spinal bracing. Treat with anti-TB medications for 12 months if patient has Pott's disease; also treat with spinal immobilization with bracing. Surgery is indicated if patient has neurologic deficit, spinal instability, a poor response to antibiotic therapy, or a nondiagnostic CT-guided biopsy.

20.8.3 Diskitis

Rare infection of nucleus pulposus with secondary involvement of end plate and vertebral body. Can be spontaneous or postprocedure. Risk factors are similar to those for vertebral osteomyelitis; must be differentiated from tumors that preferentially avoid the disk space.

Most common organisms: *S. aureus* (spontaneous), *S. epidermidis* (postprocedure), *Pseudomonas* (IVDA), and *E. coli.*

Clinical presentation: Localized back pain, paraspinal muscle spasm, and radicular symptoms, such as pain, weakness, and paresthesia.

Diagnosis and studies: Elevated ESR. Blood cultures are positive in ~ 50% of cases.

Imaging: X-ray can show destruction of disk space as well as end-plate irregularities. MRI can show involvement of disk space and is useful to rule out epidural abscess. CT-guided biopsy may be necessary to make definitive diagnosis.

Treatment: Similar to treatment for osteomyelitis: antibiotics (vancomycin, rifampin, cefotaxime) for 4 to 6 weeks, immobilization with brace. Surgery is rarely required.

20.9 Iatrogenic Infections

Main types: External ventricular drain (EVD)-associated ventriculitis, CSF fistula, CSF shunt infection, and postoperative wound infections.

20.9.1 EVD-Associated Ventriculitis

Infection is the most common complication associated with the use of EVDs (incidence 0–27%).[65,66,67] Prophylactic antibiotics should be directed toward gram-positive organisms.

Risk factors: Hemorrhage, neurosurgery manipulation of drainage system, and duration of use.[68]

Most common organism: *S. epidermidis*.[69]

Diagnosis and studies: CSF analysis including cell count, culture and sensitivity, Gram stain, glucose, and protein. Recent studies have shown that a temperature greater than 100.4°F was found to have the highest PPV (85%), and a WBC less than 11,000/μL demonstrated the highest negative predictive value (77%) in predicting ventriculitis up to 2 days in advance, and that routine CSF monitoring while EVD in place my not be required.[67]

Treatment: Empirical antibiotics initially, including vancomycin, as well as broad gram-negative coverage, such as ceftazidime, ciprofloxacin, gentamicin, or piperacillin/tazobactam. Adjust antibiotics based on culture and sensitivity results. May need to include intrathecal vancomycin or gentamicin, depending on culture results.

20.9.2 CSF Fistula

Three types: spontaneous, postsurgical, and posttraumatic. Two to 3% of patients with head injury developed CSF fistulas,[70] of which 70% stop spontaneously within 1 week. Common sites of leakage include mastoid air cells, frontal sinus, cribriform plate, and sphenoid sinus.

Most common organisms: *S. pneumoniae, S. aureus, P. aeruginosa,* and Enterobacteriaceae.[71]

Diagnosis and studies: CSF analysis and culture. Coronal CT with thin cuts after intrathecal contrast can be helpful for localizing leaks in the skull base.

Treatment: Elevate head of bed > 45 degrees at all times. Acetazolamide 250 mg four times a day to decrease CSF production, as well as lumbar drain, should be strongly considered. Lumbar drain provides excellent CSF diversion and allows easy access to CSF for frequent analysis. Surgical repair is indicated for persistent leaks. For infected fluid, use vancomycin 1 g IV every 8 hours with ceftazidime 2 g IV every 8 hours for 14 days, or use for 1 week after CSF normalizes. Change to nafcillin/oxacillin if not methicillin-resistant *S. aureus*. Add gentamicin, piperacillin/tazobactam, or ciprofloxacin for *Pseudomonas*.

20.9.3 Shunt Infection

Accepted infection rate is 5 to 7%.[72] There is an increased risk of seizures and mortality after infection. Fifty percent of infections are within 2 weeks, 70% within 2 months. Skin is the most common source.

Risk factors: Length of procedure and young age.

Most common organisms: *S. epidermidis*—most common, *S. aureus*, gram-negative bacilli, and *Enterococcus*.

Clinical presentation: Fever, headache, nausea, vomiting, lethargy, anorexia, irritability, and signs of shunt malfunction.

Diagnosis and studies: CSF findings are consistent with parameningeal infection (e.g., WBC mildly elevated, glucose normal to decreased, protein elevated, and Gram stain positive in 50% of cases). Culture may be negative in 40%. CT/MRI is usually not helpful for diagnosis, but when present, there may be enhancement or hyperintense signal of ependymal lining or ventriculomegaly consistent with shunt malfunction.

Treatment: Empirical antibiotics: vancomycin with or without rifampin, combined with broad gram-negative coverage; continue for 10 to 14 days or after CSF is normal for 3 days.

Specific antibiotics: *S. aureus/S. epidermidis*—IV and intrathecal vancomycin with or without rifampin; for gram-negative bacilli, use third-generation cephalosporin or aminoglycoside IV with intrathecal gentamicin.

In addition to antibiotic use, there should be removal of hardware. Most experts recommend either externalization of shunt hardware or removal of the entire shunt assembly and the additional placement of an external ventricular drain. There should be replacement of the shunt with a completely new system when CSF is sterile.

In addition, abdominal pseudocysts are a rare but important complication of ventriculoperitoneal shunt placement. Treatment of these pseudocysts is dependent on etiology, the patient's presentation, and clinical manifestations. Techniques for revision include distal repositioning of the peritoneal catheter, revision of the catheter into pleural space or right atrium, or complete removal of the shunt.[73]

20.9.4 Wound Infections

Wound infections represent a 1 to 5% risk after laminectomy.[74] The degree of infection ranges from superficial to full thickness with wound dehiscence.

Risk factors: Increasing age, diabetes, obesity, and chronic steroid use.

Most common organisms: *S. aureus.*

Clinical presentation: Pain, erythema, and purulent discharge at the incision site.

Diagnosis and studies: Wound swab, culture, and sensitivity; should include aerobic and anaerobic cultures.

Treatment: Superficial infection: use first-generation cephalosporin or anti-staphylococcal penicillin. Deep infection: use vancomycin/ceftazidime. Treat 10 to 14 days; adjust antibiotics based on culture and sensitivity results. Irrigate and drain deeper infections with antibiotic pulse irrigation, followed by tension-free closure using retention sutures.

20.10 Nosocomial Infections

Nosocomial infections account for > 20% of hospital infections.[75] The normal physical and chemical barriers are altered by trauma, surgery, endotracheal tubes, nasogastric tubes, invasive catheters, monitoring devices, and drains.

Most common infections: pneumonia, urinary tract infection, sinusitis, and bacteremia, as well as wound infections.[76]

20.10.1 Pneumonia

Pneumonia is the most common nosocomial infection in the intensive care unit.[77] There is increased incidence of pneumonia with prolonged endotracheal intubation and mechanical ventilation.

Risk factors: Endotracheal intubation and aspiration.[78]

Most common organisms: In ventilator-associated pneumonia, *S. aureus*[79]; in the neurosurgical population, *Pseudomonas,* family Enterobacteriaceae, *Acinetobacter.*[80]

Treatment: Empirical antibiotics as recommended by the American Thoracic Society: fluoroquinolone, aminoglycoside, or third-generation cephalosporin combined with antipseudomonal and anti-methicillin-resistant *S. aureus* agents.[81]

20.10.2 Urinary Tract Infection

Urinary tract infection is the second most common infection in the intensive care unit[82] and accounts for ~ 40% of all infections.[83]

Risk factors: Gender (female) and duration of catheter use.

Most common organisms: *E. coli,* proteus, *Pseudomonas,* and yeast.[84]

20.10.3 Sinusitis

Sinusitis is associated with mechanical ventilation or use of nasogastric tubes. Bacteria can reach the sinuses via facial or basilar skull fractures.

Most common organisms: *S. aureus*, gram-negative bacilli, *Pseudomonas*, and *Streptococcus*.[85] If untreated, it can lead to osteomyelitis, subdural or epidural empyemas, meningitis, or abscess.[86]

20.10.4 Bacteremia

Bacteremia represents 13% of nosocomial ICU infections; 90% are related to central venous catheters.[87] The alternative to a central venous catheter is a percutaneously inserted central catheter, which decreased the incidence of complications and infections compared with central lines.[88]

Most common organisms: *S. epidermidis*, *S. aureus*, *Pseudomonas*, and *Enterobacter*.[89]

Treatment: If bacteremia is suspected, replace the existing central venous catheter. Empirical antibiotics should include vancomycin plus broad gram-negative coverage.[89]

Case Management

The symptoms of the patient described in the case study are consistent with encephalitis or meningitis. Meningitis can be bacterial, viral, or other. Bacterial meningitis is associated with more neurologic changes; however, because there is no nuchal rigidity, meningitis is less likely than encephalitis. CSF studies are recommended as well as an MRI scan with and without contrast. The patient must be examined closely for tick bites and other changes. If there are no systemic changes, then the more likely diagnosis is *Rickettsia/Ehrlichia*. This is a small gram-negative intracellular organism transmitted by tick bites; the disease is also known as Rocky Mountain spotted fever and ehrlichiosis. The diagnosis is based on clinical information on the history of the tick bite. There may be positive specialized serological tests. Treatment is with doxycycline 100 mg twice a day for 10 to 14 days or chloramphenicol 50 mg/kg/d divided into four doses.

References

[1] Winn HR. Youman's Neurological Surgery. 6th ed. Philadelphia, PA: Elsevier; 2011

[2] Greenberg MS. Handbook of Neurosurgery. 7th ed. New York, NY: Thieme; 2010

[3] Gilbert DN, Moellening RC, eds. The Sanford Guide to Antimicrobial Therapy. 39th ed. Sperryville, VA: Antimicrobial Therapy; 2009

[4] Suarez JI. Critical Care Neurology and Neurosurgery. Totowa, NJ: Humana Press; 2004

[5] Thigpen MC, Whitney CG, Messonnier NE, et al. Emerging Infections Programs Network. Bacterial meningitis in the United States, 1998–2007. N Engl J Med. 2011; 364(21):2016–2025

[6] Ryan MW, Antonelli PJ. Pneumococcal antibiotic resistance and rates of meningitis in children. Laryngoscope. 2000; 110(6):961–964

[7] Dawson KG, Emerson JC, Burns JL. Fifteen years of experience with bacterial meningitis. Pediatr Infect Dis J. 1999; 18(9):816–822

[8] Hayden RT, Frenkel LD. More laboratory testing: greater cost but not necessarily better. Pediatr Infect Dis J. 2000; 19(4):290–292

[9] Mein J, Lum G. CSF bacterial antigen detection tests offer no advantage over Gram's stain in the diagnosis of bacterial meningitis. Pathology. 1999; 31(1):67–69

[10] Maniglia AJ, Goodwin WJ, Arnold JE, Ganz E. Intracranial abscesses secondary to nasal, sinus, and orbital infections in adults and children. Arch Otolaryngol Head Neck Surg. 1989; 115(12):1424–1429

[11] Dill SR, Cobbs CG, McDonald CK. Subdural empyema: analysis of 32 cases and review. Clin Infect Dis. 1995; 20(2):372–386

[12] Canale DJ. William Macewen and the treatment of brain abscesses: revisited after one hundred years. J Neurosurg. 1996; 84(1):133–142

[13] Nielsen H, Gyldensted C, Harmsen A. Cerebral abscess. Aetiology and pathogenesis, symptoms, diagnosis and treatment. A review of 200 cases from 1935–1976. Acta Neurol Scand. 1982; 65 (6):609–622

[14] Garvey G. Current concepts of bacterial infections of the central nervous system. Bacterial meningitis and bacterial brain abscess. J Neurosurg. 1983; 59(5):735–744

[15] Cohen DJ. Lung abscess: back for an encore? Postgrad Med. 1982; 72(1):215–218

[16] Leib SL, Tauber MG. Pathogenesis and pathophysiology of bacterial infections. In: Scheld WM, Whitley RJ, Durak DT, eds. Infections of the Central Nervous System. 3rd ed. Philadelphia, PA: Lippincott-Raven; 2004:301–304

[17] Mamelak AN, Obana WG, Flaherty JF, Rosenblum ML. Nocardial brain abscess: treatment strategies and factors influencing outcome. Neurosurgery. 1994; 35(4):622–631

[18] Desprechins B, Stadnik T, Koerts G, Shabana W, Breucq C, Osteaux M. Use of diffusion-weighted MR imaging in differential diagnosis between intracerebral necrotic tumors and cerebral abscesses. AJNR Am J Neuroradiol. 1999; 20(7):1252–1257

[19] Esiri MM. Herpes simplex encephalitis. An immunohistological study of the distribution of viral antigen within the brain. J Neurol Sci. 1982; 54(2):209–226

[20] Wheat LJ, Batteiger BE, Sathapatayavongs B. Histoplasma capsulatum infections of the central nervous system. A clinical review. Medicine (Baltimore). 1990; 69(4):244–260

[21] Vincent T, Galgiani JN, Huppert M, Salkin D. The natural history of coccidioidal meningitis: VA-Armed Forces cooperative studies, 1955–1958. Clin Infect Dis. 1993; 16(2):247–254

[22] Bouza E, Dreyer JS, Hewitt WL, Meyer RD. Coccidioidal meningitis. An analysis of thirty-one cases and review of the literature. Medicine (Baltimore). 1981; 60(3):139–172

[23] Gonyea EF. The spectrum of primary blastomycotic meningitis: a review of central nervous system blastomycosis. Ann Neurol. 1978; 3(1):26–39

[24] Zuger A, Lowy FD. Tuberculosis. In: Scheld WM, Whitley RJ, Durak DT, eds. Infections of the Central Nervous System. 2nd ed. Philadelphia, PA: Lippincott-Raven; 1997:417–443

[25] Traub M, Colchester AC, Kingsley DP, Swash M. Tuberculosis of the central nervous system. Q J Med. 1984; 53(209):81–100

[26] Barrett-Connor E. Tuberculous meningitis in adults. South Med J. 1967; 60(10):1061–1067

[27] Cohen BA. Neurologic complications in AIDS. In: Biller J, ed. Practical Neurology, 3rd edition. Philadelphia, PA: Lippincott; 2009:508–521

[28] Dastur D, Wadia NH. Spinal meningitides with radiculo-myelopathy. 2. Pathology and pathogenesis. J Neurol Sci. 1969; 8(2):261–297

[29] Arana-Iñiguez R, López-Fernández JR. Parasitosis of the nervous system, with special reference to echinococcosis. Clin Neurosurg. 1966; 14:123–144

[30] Nocton JJ, Steere AC. Lyme disease. Adv Intern Med. 1995; 40:69–117

[31] Pachner AR, Steere AC. The triad of neurologic manifestations of Lyme disease: meningitis, cranial neuritis, and radiculoneuritis. Neurology. 1985; 35(1):47–53

[32] Biller J, Cohen BA. Central nervous system infections. In: Biller J, ed. Practical Neurology, 3rd edition. Philadelphia, PA: Lippincott; 2009 :583–596

[33] Durack DT. Amebic infections. In: Scheld WM, Whitley RJ, Durak DT, eds. Infections of the Central Nervous System. 2nd ed. Philadelphia, PA: Lippincott-Raven; 1997:831–844

[34] Levy RM, Bredesen DE, Rosenblum ML. Neurological manifestations of the acquired immunodeficiency syndrome (AIDS): experience at UCSF and review of the literature. J Neurosurg. 1985; 62 (4):475–495

[35] Simpson DM, Tagliati M. Neurologic manifestations of HIV infection. Ann Intern Med. 1994; 121 (10):769–785

[36] Montoya JG, Remington JS. Toxoplasma gondii. In: Mandell GL, Bennett JE, Dolan R, eds. Principles and Practices of Infectious Disease. 5th ed. Philadelphia, PA: Churchill-Livingstone; 2000:2858–2892

[37] Jean WC, Hall WA. Management of cranial and spinal infections. Contemp Neurosurg. 1998; 20:1–10

[38] Levine AM. Epidemiology, clinical characteristics, and management of AIDS-related lymphoma. Hematol Oncol Clin North Am. 1991; 5(2):331–342

[39] Rosenblum ML, Levy RM, Bredesen DE, So YT, Wara W, Ziegler JL. Primary central nervous system lymphomas in patients with AIDS. Ann Neurol. 1988; 23 Suppl:S13–S16

[40] Koralnik IJ, Boden D, Mai VX, Lord CI, Letvin NL. JC virus DNA load in patients with and without progressive multifocal leukoencephalopathy. Neurology. 1999; 52(2):253–260

[41] McGuire D, Barhite S, Hollander H, Miles M. JC virus DNA in cerebrospinal fluid of human immunodeficiency virus-infected patients: predictive value for progressive multifocal leukoencephalopathy. Ann Neurol. 1995; 37:395–399

[42] Vago L, Cinque P, Sala E, et al. JCV-DNA and BKV-DNA in the CNS tissue and CSF of AIDS patients and normal subjects. Study of 41 cases and review of the literature. J Acquir Immune Defic Syndr Hum Retrovirol. 1996; 12(2):139–146

[43] Astrom K-E, Mancall EL, Richardson EP, Jr. Progressive multifocal leuko-encephalopathy; a hitherto unrecognized complication of chronic lymphatic leukaemia and Hodgkin's disease. Brain. 1958; 81(1):93–111

[44] Richardson EP, Jr. Progressive multifocal leukoencephalopathy. N Engl J Med. 1961; 265:815–823

[45] Eidelberg D, Sitrel A, Vogel H, Walker D, Kleefield J, Crumpacker CS, III. Progressive polyradiculopathy in acquired immune deficiency syndrome. Neurology. 1986; 36:912–916

[46] Clifford DB, Arribas JR, Storch GA, Tourtellote W, Wippold FJ. Magnetic resonance brain imaging lacks sensitivity for AIDS associated cytomegalovirus encephalitis. J Neurovirol. 1996; 2(6):397–403

[47] McArthur JC. HIV-associated CNS syndromes. In: Bellman A, ed. Director Course 140 [4/25–5/1/ 1993, St. Paul, MN]: AIDS in the Central Nervous System. New York, NY: American Academy of Neurology; 1993:5

[48] Navia BA, Jordan BD, Price RW. The AIDS dementia complex: I. Clinical features. Ann Neurol. 1986; 19(6):517–524

[49] Mackenzie AR, Laing RBS, Smith CC, Kaar GF, Smith FW. Spinal epidural abscess: the importance of early diagnosis and treatment. J Neurol Neurosurg Psychiatry. 1998; 65(2):209–212

[50] Martin RJ, Yuan HA. Neurosurgical care of spinal epidural, subdural, and intramedullary abscesses and arachnoiditis. Orthop Clin North Am. 1996; 27(1):125–136

[51] Khanna RK, Malik GM, Rock JP, Rosenblum ML. Spinal epidural abscess: evaluation of factors influencing outcome. Neurosurgery. 1996; 39(5):958–964

[52] Hlavin ML, Kaminski HJ, Ross JS, Ganz E. Spinal epidural abscess: a ten-year perspective. Neurosurgery. 1990; 27(2):177–184

[53] Obrador GT, Levenson DJ. Spinal epidural abscess in hemodialysis patients: report of three cases and review of the literature. Am J Kidney Dis. 1996; 27(1):75–83

[54] Wheeler D, Keiser P, Rigamonti D, Keay S. Medical management of spinal epidural abscesses: case report and review. Clin Infect Dis. 1992; 15(1):22–27

[55] Feldenzer JA, McKeever PE, Schaberg DR, Campbell JA, Hoff JT. The pathogenesis of spinal epidural abscess: microangiographic studies in an experimental model. J Neurosurg. 1988; 69(1):110–114

[56] Del Curling O, Jr, Gower DJ, McWhorter JM. Changing concepts in spinal epidural abscess: a report of 29 cases. Neurosurgery. 1990; 27(2):185–192

[57] Schmorl G, Junghanns H. The Human Spine: In Health and Disease. New York, NY: Grune & Stratton; 1971

[58] Khan IA, Vaccaro AR, Zlotolow DA. Management of vertebral diskitis and osteomyelitis. Orthopedics. 1999; 22(8):758–765

[59] Sapico FL. Microbiology and antimicrobial therapy of spinal infections. Orthop Clin North Am. 1996; 27(1):9–13

[60] Strausbaugh LJ. Vertebral osteomyelitis. How to differentiate it from other causes of back and neck pain. Postgrad Med. 1995; 97(6):147–148, 151–154

[61] Ozuna RM, Delamarter RB. Pyogenic vertebral osteomyelitis and postsurgical disc space infections. Orthop Clin North Am. 1996; 27(1):87–94

[62] Klein JD, Garfin SR. Nutritional status in the patient with spinal infection. Orthop Clin North Am. 1996; 27(1):33–36

[63] Broner FA, Garland DE, Zigler JE. Spinal infections in the immunocompromised host. Orthop Clin North Am. 1996; 27(1):37–46

[64] Vaccaro AR, Shah SH, Schweitzer ME, Rosenfeld JF, Cotler JM. MRI description of vertebral osteomyelitis, neoplasm, and compression fracture. Orthopedics. 1999; 22(1):67–73, quiz 74–75

[65] Alleyne CH, Jr, Hassan M, Zabramski JM. The efficacy and cost of prophylactic and perioprocedural antibiotics in patients with external ventricular drains. Neurosurgery. 2000; 47(5):1124–1127, discussion 1127–1129

[66] Khanna RK, Rosenblum ML, Rock JP, Malik GM. Prolonged external ventricular drainage with percutaneous long-tunnel ventriculostomies. J Neurosurg. 1995; 83(5):791–794

[67] Hariri O, Lawandy S, Miulli D, Farr S. Would clinically-indicated cerebral spinal fluid surveillance reliably predict external ventricular drain associated ventriculitis or is frequent routine cerebral spinal fluid surveillance necessary? In Press. Arrowhead Regional Medical Center; 2016

[68] Cummings R. Understanding external ventricular drainage. J Neurosci Nurs. 1992; 24(2):84–87

[69] Rodvold KA. Therapeutic considerations for infections caused by Staphylococcus epidermidis. Pharmacotherapy. 1988; 8(6 Pt 2):14S–18S

[70] Baltas I, Tsoulfa S, Sakellariou P, Vogas V, Fylaktakis M, Kondodimou A. Posttraumatic meningitis: bacteriology, hydrocephalus, and outcome. Neurosurgery. 1994; 35(3):422–426, discussion 426–427

[71] Hand WL, Sanford JP. Posttraumatic bacterial meningitis. Ann Intern Med. 1970; 72(6):869–874

[72] Yogev R. Cerebrospinal fluid shunt infections: a personal view. Pediatr Infect Dis. 1985; 4(2):113–118

[73] Kashyap S, Ghanchi H, Minasian T, Miulli D. Abdominal Pseudocyst as a Complication of Ventriculoperitoneal Shunt Placement: A Review of 4 Cases, Review of the Literature and Techniques for Revision. Arrowhead Regional Medical center. In Press 2016

[74] Shektman A, Granick MS, Solomon MP, Black P, Nair S. Management of infected laminectomy wounds. Neurosurgery. 1994; 35(2):307–309, discussion 309

[75] Brown R, Colodny S, Drapkin M, et al. One-day prevalence study of nosocomial infections, antibiotic usage, and selected infection control practices in adult medical/surgical ICUs in the United States [abstract]. The Fifth Annual Meeting of the Society for Healthcare Epidemiology, San Diego, CA, April 2–5, 1995. Infect Control Hosp Epidemiol April (suppl), 19955

[76] Emori TG, Gaynes RP. An overview of nosocomial infections, including the role of the microbiology laboratory. Clin Microbiol Rev. 1993; 6(4):428–442

[77] Edwards J, Jarvis W. The distribution of nosocomial infections by site and pathogen in adult and pediatric intensive care units in the United States 1986–1990. In: Program and Abstracts of the Third Decennial International Conference on Nosocomial Infections, Centers for Disease Control and the National Foundation for Infectious Diseases; Atlanta, Georgia, July 31-August 3, 1990. Abstract B19

[78] Sanderson PJ. The sources of pneumonia in ITU patients. Infect Control. 1986; 7(2) Suppl:104–106

[79] George DL. Epidemiology of nosocomial pneumonia in intensive care unit patients. Clin Chest Med. 1995; 16(1):29–44

[80] Rello J, Ausina V, Castella J, Net A, Prats G. Nosocomial respiratory tract infections in multiple trauma patients. Influence of level of consciousness with implications for therapy. Chest. 1992; 102(2):525–529

[81] American Thoracic Society. Hospital-acquired pneumonia in adults: diagnosis, assessment of severity, initial antimicrobial therapy, and preventive strategies. A consensus statement, American Thoracic Society, November 1995. Am J Respir Crit Care Med. 1996; 153:1711–1725

[82] Paradisi F, Corti G, Mangani V. Urosepsis in the critical care unit. Crit Care Clin. 1998; 14(2):165–180

[83] Weinstein RA. Epidemiology and control of nosocomial infections in adult intensive care units. Am J Med. 1991; 91 3B:179S–184S

[84] Bergen GA, Toney JF. Infection versus colonization in the critical care unit. Crit Care Clin. 1998; 14 (1):71–90

[85] Westergren V, Lundblad L, Hellquist HB, Forsum U. Ventilator-associated sinusitis: a review. Clin Infect Dis. 1998; 27(4):851–864

[86] Clayman GL, Adams GL, Paugh DR, Koopmann CF, Jr. Intracranial complications of paranasal sinusitis: a combined institutional review. Laryngoscope. 1991; 101(3):234–239

[87] Maki D. Infections due to infusion therapy. In: Bennett J, Brachman P, eds. Hospital Infections. Boston, MA: Little, Brown; 1992:849

[88] Raad I, Davis S, Becker M, et al. Low infection rate and long durability of nontunneled silastic catheters. A safe and cost-effective alternative for long-term venous access. Arch Intern Med. 1993; 153(15):1791–1796

[89] Cunha BA. Intravenous line infections. Crit Care Clin. 1998; 14(2):339–346

21 Cerebral Microdialysis in the Neurosurgical Intensive Care Unit

Jeff W. Chen, Daniella Abrams-Alexandru, and Javed Siddiqi

Abstract

While monitoring intracranial pressure is meaningful for a mechanical understanding of brain pathology, it does not provide a comprehensive picture of alternations in the brain from disease and trauma; understanding the chemical changes in the brain, as reflected in the cerebrospinal fluid and brain interstitial fluids, provides an additional (biochemical) window into brain damage and dysfunction. Cerebral microdialysis provides a nuanced approach that is relatively new to the neurosurgical intensive care unit, and not yet universally utilized due to its labor intensiveness in data collection and analysis; it is the next frontier in brain monitoring.

Keywords: beta amyloid, brain oxygenation, cerebral glutamate, dialysate, hypoglycemia, Kreb's cycle, microdialysis, perfusate, proteinomic biomarker

---

Case Presentation

A 20-year-old right-handed man was admitted to the trauma center after sustaining a traumatic brain injury in a motor vehicle collision. His best examination after resuscitation was E = 1, V = 1, M = 3, with a Glasgow Coma Scale score of 5. He had bilaterally reactive pupils. His computed tomographic scan of the head demonstrated right-sided subfrontal contusions with some surrounding edema with open perimesencephalic cisterns. A ventriculostomy was placed with initial intracranial pressure = 25 mm Hg. This decreased to 15–18 mm Hg with sedation, elevation of the head of the bed, and hypertonic saline. A Licox brain oxygenation monitor and cerebral microdialysis catheter were placed via a double-lumen bolt.

See end of chapter for Case Management.

21.1 Introduction

The cerebrospinal fluid (CSF) traditionally has been felt to be reflective of the overall biochemistry of the brain. The bulk flow of CSF through the brain, however, may follow different pathways that may not all lead to the cerebral ventricular system. The recent finding of a lymphatic system in the brain has raised questions about the relationship between the brain interstitial fluid and

composition in comparison to CSF.[1,2,3] Indeed, it is quite clear that the ventricular CSF and interstitial glucose, lactate, pyruvate, and amyloid beta levels are different.[4,5] As such, sampling the CSF for metabolic or proteinomic biomarkers of traumatic brain injury (TBI) or cerebrovascular accident may provide information that is different from the sampling of the brain interstitial fluid. Cerebral microdialysis allows the sampling of cerebral interstitial fluid and is reflective of the local milieu around the catheters.[6,7]

Cerebral microdialysis was first developed as an experimental tool. Much of the early work was pioneered by Urben Ungerstedt, who was able to collect small molecules from the brain interstitium for analysis.[8,9] The early work in the laboratory used the principles of hemodialysis and developed techniques to miniaturize the technology to enable the placement of the microdialysis membranes safely into the brain.[10,11] The microdialysis catheters have evolved and have been developed for human use. This catheter has an inner tube and an outer tube that has a semipermeable membrane at its tip. Through the inner tube is pumped the perfusate (usually artificial CSF). This perfusate exits the tip of the inner tube and goes into the outer tube. As the perfusate flows through the region of the semipermeable membrane, exchange occurs with the brain interstitium that is in contact with the semipermeable membrane. Molecules that are in higher concentration in the brain flow into the 1-cm tip of the microdialysis catheter that has the semipermeable outer membrane. The dialysate that exits is collected and analyzed.[5,12] This is depicted in ▶ Fig. 21.1. Early studies in humans analyzed the dialysate using fractionation by high-performance liquid chromatography.[13,14,15]

Cerebral microdialysis has become less of a research tool and has become a routine clinical measurement in many centers after the advent of the automated cerebral microdialysis analyzers that analyze the microdialysate for specific substances using a chemical analysis paradigm. These were approved by the U.S. Food and Drug Administration in 2005 for clinical use.[12,16] The microdialysis analyzer is now in its second generation and is the Iscus-Flex model (M Dialysis). In principle, all of the compounds that are of a higher concentration in the brain interstitium than in the perfusate may be collected and analyzed. This applies to small chemical molecules, such as glucose, as well as proteins. However, there are several considerations based on the molecular weight cutoff of the membrane. The standard microdialysis catheter available in the United States has a 20 kDa cutoff (no. 70 Microdialysis Catheter, M Dialysis). The most common analytes are glutamate, aspartate, glycerol, glucose, lactate, and pyruvate. These are also the ones that are FDA approved for analysis by the Iscus-Flex. The importance of these particular analytes will be discussed subsequently. Beta amyloid may also be isolated in the dialysate as its molecular weight is about 4.5 kDa for the ABeta 40 and ABeta 42 peptides. In contrast, the tau proteins are 49–67 kDa and may be isolated if one uses the microdialysis catheter with a 100 kDa cutoff. These catheters are currently not available except under a research protocol in the United States.[4]

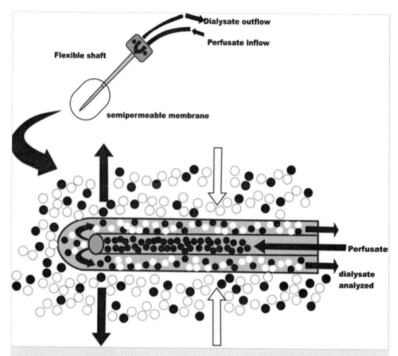

Fig. 21.1 The catheter consists of an inner tube and an outer tube with a semipermeable membrane in the tip. In the inner tube of the catheter, infused solution flows to the outer tube, which allows the exchange of extracellular substances by differences in fluid concentration. Later, the solution is collected at the external tip for biochemical analysis. (Reproduced with permission from de Lima Oliveira M, Kairalla AC, Fonoff ET, Martinez RC, Teixeira MJ, Bor-Seng-Shu E. Cerebral microdialysis in traumatic brain injury and subarachnoid hemorrhage: state of the art. Neurocritical Care 2014;21:152–162.[5])

The size of the molecule of interest as well as its charge and lipid solubility affects the ability to collect it. The ability to cross the dialysis membrane will affect the amount that is recoverable. The rate of perfusion of the dialysate will also determine the recovery of the substance. The slower the perfusion, the greater the recovery.[17] For the major biomolecules of interest that were noted above, the standard perfusion rate employed is 0.3 µL/min. This allows for adequate dialysate (18 µL) each hour to be sampled by the Iscus-Flex machine. This slow and constant perfusion is provided by a microinfusion pump.[12]

21.2 The Rationale for the Study of Cerebral Metabolites

There was a great deal of interest directed at studying the excitatory amino acids (glutamate, aspartate) with the use of cerebral microdialysis. Glutamate and aspartate levels were found to be elevated after TBI and after subarachnoid hemorrhage (SAH), indicative of tissue damage. In fact, the 2004 international consensus statement on cerebral microdialysis included recommendations to follow these analytes as indicators of brain injury and ischemia.[18,19] Glutamate levels can be followed as a marker of ischemia and also as a marker of the severity of the brain injury. Chamoun et al, in 2010, found that there were two patterns of glutamate expression in TBI. One group had the increase in glutamate with a peak at 5 days then a gradual decline. The other group had a constant increase in the glutamate levels. The first group had a lower mortality rate (17.1 vs. 39.6%) and a better 6-month functional outcome (41.2 vs. 20.7%) in comparison to the second group.[20,21] The measurement of cerebral glutamate is considered an option in cerebral microdialysis and may be useful in the estimation of prognosis.[22] Glycerol is also considered an option in the 2014 international consensus statement on cerebral microdialysis. This is a marker of cell membrane breakdown; however, it has limited specificity. Furthermore, to date, there has not been the establishment of a relationship between glycerol levels and outcome.[22]

Perhaps some of the best studied cerebral analytes are glucose, lactate, and pyruvate. These are very closely linked to each other because of their roles in the Kreb's cycle.[12] The brain has an extreme thirst for glucose because it is the main energy substrate. Low brain glucose levels (< 0.8 mM) are associated with poor outcomes. These low levels are common in TBI and SAH, largely because these injuries induce a hypermetabolic state.[23] The importance of the maintenance of the cerebral glucose became apparent with the introduction of tight glycemic control in the intensive care units. Although there were better outcomes reported with the use of tight glycemic control, the subset of patients that had worse outcomes were those with brain injuries. Tight glycemic control was defined as systemic glucose of 80–120 mg/dL (4.4–6.7 mmol/L) and intermediate as 121–180 mg/dL (6.8–10.0 mmol/L). Episodes of low cerebral glucose (< 0.7 mmol/L) were more frequent in the tight glycemic control than in the intermediate group (65% vs. 36%, $p < 0.01$).[24] Further studies have similarly demonstrated poor outcome and increased mortality with low brain glucose.[25] Thus this led to the concept of a more permissive peripheral glucose in patients with TBI or SAH.[12,24] The ability to monitor and fine tune the brain glucose by administering exogenous sources of glucose if low levels are detected by cerebral microdialysis has the potential to improve outcome. We routinely use brain glucose levels to guide us in instituting nutrition. Upper limits for brain hyperglycemia have not been determined to date. Clearly brain hypoglycemia is more detrimental than hyperglycemia.[22,24]

Lactate and pyruvate are metabolites of glucose metabolism and are closely linked with the glucose levels in the brain. If we recall the Kreb's (citric acid) cycle, glucose is broken down into pyruvate during glycolysis. When oxygen is available, the pyruvate is broken down by the citric acid cycle, generating adenosine triphosphate (ATP). When oxygen is limited, the pyruvate is converted to lactate, still generating ATP but in a more inefficient manner that consumes more glucose. This follows the pathway of anaerobic metabolism, and this is what occurs during ischemic situations.[12,26] One of the most robust and dependable markers of cerebral stress is the lactate–pyruvate ratio (LPR). When glucose is limited, the LPR increases. In ischemic/hypoxic situations, LPR also increases. Metabolic stress is generally accepted to be when the LPR > 40, although an LPR of 30–35 is concerning.[27,28] Persistently increased LPR is related to long-term frontal lobe atrophy.[28]

The common analytes and the normal values are summarized in ▶ Table 21.1. In summary, glucose and LPR are dependable, and abnormalities are reflective of cerebral ischemia or hypoxia. Common scenarios for this are TBI with increased intracranial pressure (ICP) and decreased cerebral perfusion pressure (CPP). This may also occur with cerebral vasospasm after aneurysmal SAH. The pattern seen in these situations is one of decreasing glucose and increasing LPR. Frequently, this pattern is progressive and may direct the physician to intervene to reverse the trend. For example, if one sees a trend with a decreasing glucose, increasing LPR, and increasing ICP in a patient with TBI, this might prompt early institution of hypertonic saline or early removal of a mass lesion (if it has not been removed yet). Another common example where these parameters can guide the neurosurgeon/neurointensivist is in aneurysmal SAH where the ischemia associated with cerebral vasospasm may be detected before it becomes clinically or radiographically apparent. Early institution of hypertensive therapy or augmentation of CPP with ventricular drainage may attenuate the effects of vasospasm.[19,22,29]

Table 21.1 Normal microdialysis analyte values and thresholds for investigation[22]

Analyte	Cell death	Normal	Threshold for investigation
Glucose	0.1 mM	1.7 mM	< 0.2 mM
Lactate	8.9 mM	2.9 mM	> 4 mM
Pyruvate	31 µM	166 µM	
LPR	450	23–28	> 25
Glycerol	573 µM	82 µM	
Glutamate	381 µM	16 µM	

Abbreviation: LPR, lactate–pyruvate ratio.

Note: Metabolic stress = LPR > 40.

Note: Cell death refers to values found in areas of infarction.

Note: The conversion of glucose from mmol/L to mg/dL is to divide by 0.0555.

21.3 The Nuts and Bolts of Cerebral Microdialysis

The materials listed here are needed.

From M Dialysis (Stockholm, Sweden):

- Cerebral microdialysis catheters (20 kDa cutoff—no. 70 (for direct implantation), no. 70-bolt (adapted for bolt implantation).
- Microinfusion pumps—no. 106 with syringe and battery.
- Sterile artificial CSF (purchased as premixed vials).
- Microdialysis collection vials.
- Iscus-Flex analyzer.

There have been no complications reported from the cerebral microdialysis catheter or the associated microinfusion pumps. The risks incurred are those that are inherent in the procedure to gain access to allow placement of the catheter.[16,22] There are three main ways to place the catheters: (1) directly at the time of open surgery, (2) via a burr hole or twist drill hole, (3) via a bolt that is secured to the skull. There are two different microdialysis catheters that are available, one for direct implantation and one that is adaptable to bolt technology.

Direct implantation of the catheter is done after the completion of a craniotomy. Common scenarios include a craniotomy for evacuation of subdural hematoma or craniotomy for aneurysm clipping. A stab incision is made with a no. 15 blade at the skin edge. The plastic sheath introducer is used to bring the microdialysis catheter through the skin. The plastic sheath is disengaged by unscrewing it to expose the fine microdialysis catheter (~ 0.8 mm thick). Care must be taken when handling the catheter. There is a rubber flange around the catheter at its distal end that "anchors" it to the skin in the stab incision. Fine sutures like 4–0 Nurolon are placed around this in the manner of a purse-string. This decreases significantly the risk of CSF emanating out the entry site. The tip of the microdialysis catheter is inserted into the brain via a small 1 mm corticectomy about 2 cm deep in a direction that is perpendicular to the brain surface (▶ Fig. 21.2). The remainder of the craniotomy closure is done in the standard fashion. Usually there is a sufficient gap between the bone flap and the parent skull to allow the passage of the microdialysis catheter. If not, a small passageway can be created using a Leksell rongeur. Care is taken to avoid damage to these fragile catheters during the closure of the galea aponeurosis.

The advantage of the direct implantation technique is that it is readily done at the time of surgery. The microdialysis catheter is placed into the brain under direct visualization. This minimizes the damage, and the neurosurgeon may place it more specifically. For example, there may be interest in placing the catheter just adjacent to a recently evacuated traumatic intracerebral

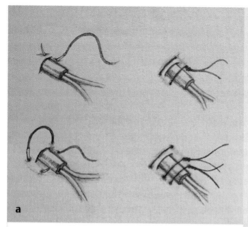

Fig. 21.2 (a) Technique for securing the tunneled microdialysis catheter to the skin using 4–0 Neurolon sutures. This prevents cerebrospinal fluid leakage around the insertion site. **(b)** Diagram demonstrating the microdialysis catheter at the insertion site at the edge of the craniotomy. The dura is closed loosely around the catheter.

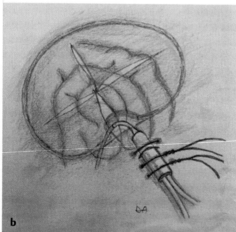

hemorrhage to target the "pericontusional" area that may be important in the generation of cerebral edema.[30] In cases of aneurysmal SAH, one may target the microdialysis catheter to an area that is in the distribution of the vessel at risk for vasospasm.[22] Some of the disadvantages include the movement of the brain relative to the catheter as the brain expands. This may lead to some fluctuations in the values obtained.

The second method is placement through a burr hole or twist drill hole. This is done in a similar manner as described earlier, wherein a stab incision is made a couple of centimeters away from the hole. The catheter is tunneled into the burr hole. It is then placed into the brain via a corticectomy. Care must be taken to ensure that the dura and pia-arachnoid are opened so that the catheter passes easily into the brain. This technique is frequently used in conjunction with a ventriculostomy. The advantage of this technique is that it takes advantage of an access point that is being done already. The disadvantage is that the space available to manipulate and place the microdialysis catheter is limited. It is very easy to damage the catheter. Furthermore, if the tip of the catheter is near the ventriculostomy track, this will lead to erroneous values as it would be reflective of injured tissue.

The cerebral microdialyis catheter may be placed via bolt technology. This offers the most rigid fixation and limits the movement of the catheters relative to the brain, thus providing for more consistent and dependable results. The usual site is at Kocher's point on the right side. If a ventricular catheter is already in place, we usually go about 1 cm anterior and lateral to the ventriculostomy site. This may be done with the double-lumen Licox bolt (Integra Lifesciences). After drilling the access twist drill hole, the dura and pia-arachnoid are opened sharply with a no. 11 blade to ensure easy passage of the fine catheters. The bolt is secured to the bone, and the microdialysis bolt catheter is passed down its lumen into the brain. The Licox oxygenation catheter is passed down the other lumen. As seen in ▶ Fig. 21.3, the Licox and microdialysis catheter tips are divergent to avoid interference between the two technologies. Recently, a new quad lumen bolt has received FDA approval. This has a similar size twist drill hole but has lumens for four different multimodal monitors (Hemedex Inc.). Typically we place an ICP catheter (Camino fiberoptic catheter,

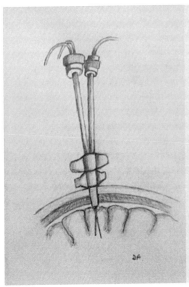

Fig. 21.3 Placement of the microdialysis catheter with a double-lumen bolt. Note the divergence of the Licox and microdialysis catheters. This is done intentionally to avoid interference in their measurements.

Integra Lifesciences), a Licox brain oxygenation catheter, a cerebral microdialysis, and a Hemedex (Hemedex Inc.) blood flow catheter down the four lumens. These catheters are divergent in the brain much as was described for the Licox double-lumen bolt.

The advantages of this method of microdialysis placement include the firm and rigid fixation obtained by the bolt. This decreases the chance of "pull-out" when the patient is moved for patient care issues. The bolt technology also provides a closed system and has a low risk of CSF leakage or infection. Furthermore, when using a double- or quad-lumen bolt, multimodal brain monitoring may be achieved. Finally, the techniques for placing the bolt are very familiar to neurosurgeons and their trainees.

21.4 From the Patient to the Analyzer

After the microdialysis catheter is implanted, the inlet is connected to the microdialysis infusion pump (M Dialysis), and the perfusion fluid is primed in the delivery syringe. We use the prepared stock artificial CSF from M Dialysis. The outlet side of the system that collects the microdialysate is connected to the small microvials. The default infusion rate is 0.3 μL/mL. This entire setup is very small, and the pump is about 4×3 cm in size. This sits in the patient's bed at the side of the head. Each hour, the bedside nurse removes the microvial that has the 18 μL of microdialysate and places it in the Iscus-Flex for analysis. Currently, the values are read off the Iscus-Flex screen and entered into the patient's electronic medical record (EMR) or printed up for a hard-copy record. Direct interfaces for the download from the Iscus-Flex to the EMR are in the process of development.

Local hospital and state regulations govern the use of the Iscus-Flex. In most institutes it is set up in a specific room in the intensive care unit, which may also house other analyzers (e.g., blood gas). It is designed as a point-of-care device and needs to pass the Clinical Laboratory Improvement Amendments regulations. Nurses who operate the analyzer need to demonstrate appropriate training and proficiency.[12] At our institute it is housed in the main clinical laboratory. The quality assurance checks and the maintenance and running of the samples are done by the laboratory staff.

21.5 Arguments for and against Cerebral Microdialysis as a Clinical Tool

Cerebral microdialysis has been shown to provide robust information about cerebral glucose and LPR. This allows the neurosurgeon/neurocritical care physician to optimize brain energy and metabolism; thus the concept of avoiding cerebral metabolic stress and cerebral ischemia even in the presence of normal ICPs.[26] The recent studies with the decompressive craniectomy trial for TBI raise the importance of the metabolic status of the injured brain in addition to the issue of ICP control.[31,32,33,34,35,36] Recent studies have demonstrated the importance of lactate and the pentose-phosphate pathways in cerebral metabolism. The concept of mitochondrial failure as detected by cerebral microdialysis in conjunction with cerebral brain oxygenation studies raises other possible pathways to attenuate brain injury pathways.[23,37,38]

Many argue that cerebral microdialysis does not improve the neurologic outcome in TBI or SAH or intracerebral hemorrhage. However, we need to point out that cerebral microdialysis is not a therapeutic tool. It provides information about the cerebral metabolic state. With the information, the clinician may tailor the treatment using the results of the multimodal brain monitoring as a guide.

Although the cerebral microdialysis analyzer has been FDA approved for over 10 years, it is not used widely in clinical applications in the United States. There is a significant amount of institutional and nursing investment that goes far beyond the capital expense of the equipment. Nursing involvement to set up, collect, and run the samples hourly requires constant education and reinforcement of microdialysis skills. Frequently, these patients with microdialysis are placed on a 1:1 status. This requires institutional resources that smaller hospital systems may not have. The invasive nature of the microdialysis has been a disincentive for many. However, with the advent of the different bolt platforms, this becomes less of an issue as these critically ill patients will usually have an ICP and Licox monitor as part of their standard treatment. The importance of multimodal brain monitoring has become more evident in recent years.[22] Finally, an argument against cerebral microdialysis is that it is very regional and only samples a small area of the brain. With careful planning and even with the placement of two catheters, it is possible to target the sampling to good brain, injured brain, or "at risk" brain. Further, the multimodal brain monitors of brain oxygenation, and cerebral blood flow provide additional confirmatory data.

21.6 Future Prospects

As we learn more about the brain metabolism, we will likely discover additional pathways different from the well-known Kreb's cycle that are important in the metabolic state of the injured brain. Future targets for therapy may be developed. Finally, the use of the 100 kDa microdialysis catheters allows the analysis of protein products in the extracellular space. Protein biomarkers such as the beta amyloid proteins and the tau proteins may shed some light on the long-term implications of TBI and stroke on dementia and Alzheimer's disease.

In particular, the CSF clearance pathways via the interstitium are likely to be important. Sampling of these pathways via cerebral microdialysis has great potential.[4,39,40]

Case Management

During the first day the patient had decreasing brain glucose to 0.8 mM with LPR increasing to 30 and increasing ICPs to the low 20 s despite increasing the Na$^+$ to 145 and continued CSF drainage (about 5 mL/h with the drainage set at 15 cm above the ear). Brain oxygenation remained stable at 30. Follow-up computed tomographic scans showed slight evolution of the subfrontal contusion with early edema. Early enteral feeding was done and the brain glucose improved to 1.2 mM and the LPR to 25. ICPs improved to the high teens. Over the next 12 hours the LPR increased to 35 and the glucose remained at about 1.2 mM. ICPs remained in the low 20 s. Because of the upward trend of the LPR and the slow increase in the ICPs, the patient underwent a right frontal craniotomy and evacuation of the subfrontal contusion. At the time of surgery the area of contused brain was clearly necrotic and under pressure. Postoperatively, the ICPs immediately decreased to 5–10 mm Hg and the LPR to 20–23, and brain glucose remained in the normal range. Postoperative computed tomographic scans demonstrated the evacuation of the high-attenuation contusion but the persisting subfrontal areas of edema. The patient was subsequently weaned off the sedation and extubated. He transitioned quickly through the step-down and brain rehabilitation units.

This provides a nice example of how the cerebral microdialysis provided information about the upward trend toward cerebral metabolic distress. Although the ICPs and CPPs were controlled with ventriculostomy and hypertonic saline, the effect of the cerebral edema on brain metabolism is seen. Although there is a reluctance to operate on the frontal lobe, the metabolic damage and the cascade of injury that exacerbates the cerebral edema can be mitigated with the surgical intervention. The normalization of the LPR suggests the reversal of the trend toward metabolic stress.

References

[1] Aspelund A, Antila S, Proulx ST, et al. A dural lymphatic vascular system that drains brain interstitial fluid and macromolecules. J Exp Med. 2015; 212(7):991–999

[2] Iliff JJ, Nedergaard M. Is there a cerebral lymphatic system? Stroke. 2013; 44(6) Suppl 1:S93–S95

[3] Iliff JJ, Wang M, Liao Y, et al. A paravascular pathway facilitates CSF flow through the brain parenchyma and the clearance of interstitial solutes, including amyloid β. Sci Transl Med. 2012; 4 (147):147ra111

[4] Tsitsopoulos PP, Marklund N. Amyloid- β Peptides and Tau Protein as Biomarkers in Cerebrospinal and Interstitial Fluid Following Traumatic Brain Injury: A Review of Experimental and Clinical Studies. Front Neurol. 2013; 4:79

[5] de Lima Oliveira M, Kairalla AC, Fonoff ET, Martinez RC, Teixeira MJ, Bor-Seng-Shu E. Cerebral microdialysis in traumatic brain injury and subarachnoid hemorrhage: state of the art. Neurocrit Care. 2014; 21(1):152–162

[6] Tisdall MM, Smith M. Cerebral microdialysis: research technique or clinical tool. Br J Anaesth. 2006; 97(1):18–25

[7] Nordström CH. Cerebral energy metabolism and microdialysis in neurocritical care. Childs Nerv Syst. 2010; 26(4):465–472

[8] Tossman U, Wieloch T, Ungerstedt U. Gamma-aminobutyric acid and taurine release in the striatum of the rat during hypoglycemic coma, studied by microdialysis. Neurosci Lett. 1985; 62 (2):231–235

[9] Vezzani A, Ungerstedt U, French ED, Schwarcz R. In vivo brain dialysis of amino acids and simultaneous EEG measurements following intrahippocampal quinolinic acid injection: evidence for a dissociation between neurochemical changes and seizures. J Neurochem. 1985; 45(2):335–344

[10] Bito L, Davson H, Levin E, Murray M, Snider N. The concentrations of free amino acids and other electrolytes in cerebrospinal fluid, in vivo dialysate of brain, and blood plasma of the dog. J Neurochem. 1966; 13(11):1057–1067

[11] Bito LZ, Davson H. Local variations in cerebrospinal fluid composition and its relationship to the composition of the extracellular fluid of the cortex. Exp Neurol. 1966; 14(3):264–280

[12] Cecil S, Chen PM, Callaway SE, Rowland SM, Adler DE, Chen JW. Traumatic brain injury: advanced multimodal neuromonitoring from theory to clinical practice. Crit Care Nurse. 2011; 31(2):25–36, quiz 37

[13] Hillered L, Hallström A, Segersvärd S, Persson L, Ungerstedt U. Dynamics of extracellular metabolites in the striatum after middle cerebral artery occlusion in the rat monitored by intracerebral microdialysis. J Cereb Blood Flow Metab. 1989; 9(5):607–616

[14] Valadka AB, Goodman JC, Gopinath SP, Uzura M, Robertson CS. Comparison of brain tissue oxygen tension to microdialysis-based measures of cerebral ischemia in fatally head-injured humans. J Neurotrauma. 1998; 15(7):509–519

[15] Goodman JC, Valadka AB, Gopinath SP, Uzura M, Robertson CS. Extracellular lactate and glucose alterations in the brain after head injury measured by microdialysis. Crit Care Med. 1999; 27 (9):1965–1973

[16] Chen JW, Rogers SL, Gombart ZJ, Adler DE, Cecil S. Implementation of cerebral microdialysis at a community-based hospital: A 5-year retrospective analysis. Surg Neurol Int. 2012; 3:57

[17] Chefer VI, Thompson AC, Zapata A, Shippenberg TS. Overview of brain microdialysis. In: Crawley JN, et al, eds. Current Protocols in Neuroscience. 2009; 47:7.1:.1–7.1.28

[18] Goodman JC, Valadka AB, Gopinath SP, Cormio M, Robertson CS. Lactate and excitatory amino acids measured by microdialysis are decreased by pentobarbital coma in head-injured patients. J Neurotrauma. 1996; 13(10):549–556

[19] Bellander BM, Cantais E, Enblad P, et al. Consensus meeting on microdialysis in neurointensive care. Intensive Care Med. 2004; 30(12):2166–2169

[20] Vespa P, Prins M, Ronne-Engstrom E, et al. Increase in extracellular glutamate caused by reduced cerebral perfusion pressure and seizures after human traumatic brain injury: a microdialysis study. J Neurosurg. 1998; 89(6):971–982

[21] Chamoun R, Suki D, Gopinath SP, Goodman JC, Robertson C. Role of extracellular glutamate measured by cerebral microdialysis in severe traumatic brain injury. J Neurosurg. 2010; 113(3):564–570

[22] Hutchinson PJ, Jalloh I, Helmy A, et al. Consensus statement from the 2014 International Microdialysis Forum. Intensive Care Med. 2015; 41(9):1517–1528

[23] Carpenter KL, Jalloh I, Hutchinson PJ. Glycolysis and the significance of lactate in traumatic brain injury. Front Neurosci. 2015; 9:112

[24] Oddo M, Schmidt JM, Carrera E, et al. Impact of tight glycemic control on cerebral glucose metabolism after severe brain injury: a microdialysis study. Crit Care Med. 2008; 36(12):3233–3238

[25] Duning T, van den Heuvel I, Dickmann A, et al. Hypoglycemia aggravates critical illness-induced neurocognitive dysfunction. Diabetes Care. 2010; 33(3):639–644

[26] Bouzat P, Sala N, Payen JF, Oddo M. Beyond intracranial pressure: optimization of cerebral blood flow, oxygen, and substrate delivery after traumatic brain injury. Ann Intensive Care. 2013; 3 (1):23

[27] Vespa P, Bergsneider M, Hattori N, et al. Metabolic crisis without brain ischemia is common after traumatic brain injury: a combined microdialysis and positron emission tomography study. J Cereb Blood Flow Metab. 2005; 25(6):763–774

[28] Marcoux J, McArthur DA, Miller C, et al. Persistent metabolic crisis as measured by elevated cerebral microdialysis lactate-pyruvate ratio predicts chronic frontal lobe brain atrophy after traumatic brain injury. Crit Care Med. 2008; 36(10):2871–2877

[29] Goodman JC, Robertson CS. Microdialysis: is it ready for prime time? Curr Opin Crit Care. 2009; 15(2):110–117

[30] Chen JW, Paff MR, Abrams-Alexandru D, Kaloostian SW. Decreasing the Cerebral Edema Associated with Traumatic Intracerebral Hemorrhages: Use of a Minimally Invasive Technique. Acta Neurochir Suppl (Wien). 2016; 121:279–284

[31] Cooper DJ, Rosenfeld JV. Does decompressive craniectomy improve outcomes in patients with diffuse traumatic brain injury? Med J Aust. 2011; 194(9):437–438

[32] Cooper DJ, Rosenfeld JV, Murray L, et al. DECRA Trial Investigators, Australian and New Zealand Intensive Care Society Clinical Trials Group. Decompressive craniectomy in diffuse traumatic brain injury. N Engl J Med. 2011; 364(16):1493–1502

[33] Cooper DJ, Rosenfeld JV, Wolfe R. DECRA investigators' response to "The future of decompressive craniectomy for diffuse traumatic brain injury" by Honeybul et al. J Neurotrauma. 2012; 29 (16):2595–2596

[34] Walcott BP, Kahle KT, Simard JM. The DECRA trial and decompressive craniectomy in diffuse traumatic brain injury: is decompression really ineffective? World Neurosurg. 2013; 79(1):80–81

[35] Iaccarino C, Schiavi P, Servadei F. Decompressive craniectomies: time to discuss not the DECRA study but the comments to the DECRA study. World Neurosurg. 2013; 79(1):78–79

[36] Kitagawa RS, Bullock MR. Lessons from the DECRA study. World Neurosurg. 2013; 79(1):82–84

[37] Jalloh I, Carpenter KL, Grice P, et al. Glycolysis and the pentose phosphate pathway after human traumatic brain injury: microdialysis studies using 1,2-(13)C2 glucose. J Cereb Blood Flow Metab. 2015; 35(1):111–120

[38] Lakshmanan R, Loo JA, Drake T, et al. Metabolic crisis after traumatic brain injury is associated with a novel microdialysis proteome. Neurocrit Care. 2010; 12(3):324–336

[39] Yang L, Kress BT, Weber HJ, et al. Evaluating glymphatic pathway function utilizing clinically relevant intrathecal infusion of CSF tracer. J Transl Med. 2013; 11:107

[40] Iliff JJ, Lee H, Yu M, et al. Brain-wide pathway for waste clearance captured by contrast-enhanced MRI. J Clin Invest. 2013; 123(3):1299–1309

22 Anticoagulation and Antiplatelet Therapy in the Neurosurgical Intensive Care Unit

Bo-Lin Liu and Javed Siddiqi

Abstract

When, and how, to manage anticoagulation and antiplatelet therapy in the neurosurgical intensive care unit (NICU) is a recurring question. All NICU patients are at risk of developing deep vein thrombosis or pulmonary embolism, but many of them also have absolute or relative contraindications for prophylactic anticoagulation or antiplatelet therapy. We review contemporary evidence-based literature on this topic and discuss our own experience and management rationales of anticoagulation and antiplatelet therapy in the NICU.

Case Presentation

A 55-year-old Caucasian male undergoes craniotomy for evacuation of a traumatic subdural hematoma and is postoperatively managed in the neurosurgical intensive care unit of a tertiary care trauma center. Neurological exam on postoperative day 7 revealed a Glasgow Coma Scale (GCS) score of 12, muscle power was 3/5 on the left upper extremity, 4/5 on the right upper extremity, and 5/5 on lower extremities bilaterally. No sensory deficit was noted. He complained of vague discomfort in his left shoulder area. Physical exam revealed left upper-extremity edema with a difference in diameter of 4 cm between upper extremities. A venous catheter was located on the left upper extremity for administration of fluids.

See end of chapter for Case Management.

22.1 Introduction

Neurotrauma, stroke (both ischemic and hemorrhagic), and postneurosurgical patients make up the majority of patients in the neurosurgical intensive care unit (NICU). Each of these three categories of patients presents complex issues about timing, and extent of, anticoagulation and/or antiplatelet prophylaxis and therapy. For example, neurointensivists commonly face the difficult issue of how to treat deep vein thrombosis (DVT) or pulmonary embolism (PE) in patients who already have acute brain hemorrhage, are immediately postop craniotomy, or have indwelling ventriculostomy catheters. Serious consideration needs to be given to when it is safe to start medications that are the standard of care for the thrombosis, while knowingly increasing the risk of exacerbating the bleed from the treatment. Dural venous sinus thrombosis is the only known condition in which the defined treatment, even in the face of intracerebral bleed, is anticoagulation; for all other conditions involving actual or potential bleeding in the brain, anticoagulation and antiplatelet prophylaxis and therapy pose known risks to the patient, mandating a deliberate and systematic treatment plan, reinforced with very clear communications with the entire treatment team and patient/family.

22.2 Indications for Anticoagulation in the NICU: Prophylaxis

22.2.1 DVT prophylaxis

Neurosurgical and neurotrauma patients are at increased risk of DVT and consequent PE. DVT may be prevalent at around 18% in the general major trauma patients without prophylaxis; however, this number skyrocketed to 54% in patients with traumatic brain injury (TBI).[1] Even in patients with isolated TBI the incidence of venous thromboembolism may be as high as 25%.[2] Several factors may account for this significant risk, such as long operating times of many procedures, prolonged bed rest, immobility related to motor deficits, as well as release of significant amounts of brain tissue thromboplastin during surgery and trauma, diuretic therapy used to reduce cerebral edema, intravascular volume losses following subarachnoid hemorrhage, and cerebral salt wasting.[3]

The 2007 guidelines for the management of severe TBI recommended the combination of mechanical and chemical (with low molecular weight heparin [LMWH] or unfractionated heparin) prophylaxis; however, in caution with an increased risk for expansion of intracranial hemorrhage (ICH).[4] Among hematomas and contusions, expansion occurs in about 38% of cases between the first and second computed tomographic (CT) scan, the risk of which is associated with the size of the initial ICH and the presence of a subarachnoid or subdural hemorrhage.[5] Venous thromboembolism prophylaxis halves the risk of DVT and PE, whereas it doubles the risk of ICH progression.[6]

Based on the latest evidence, Abdel-Aziz et al[7] refined the recommendation by following the Parkland Protocol,[8] which categorizes NICU patients into low, moderate, or high risk of spontaneous hematoma progression (thus offering some guidance on which patients can receive chemoprophylaxis relatively safely). The "low-risk" category included patients with (nonoperative) epidural or subdural hematoma < 9 mm, cerebral contusion < 2 cm, single contusion per lobe, traumatic subarachnoid hemorrhage with negative CT angiography, and intraventricular hemorrhage < 2 cm in maximum diameter. The "moderate risk" category included nonsurgical patients with a greater degree of hemorrhage than the low-risk ICH. The "high-risk" category included patients requiring craniotomy or intracranial pressure monitor. Their recommendations include the following:

- Chemoprophylaxis should be withheld for 3 days for spontaneous ICH patients, or for those with moderate or high risk for ICH progression.
- Chemoprophylaxis is reasonable when low-risk patients have not developed ICH progression within 48 hours postinjury.
- Chemoprophylaxis is acceptable after day 3 when low-risk patients develop ICH expansion within 48 hours postinjury.
- Chemoprophylaxis is reasonable on day 4 in diffuse axonal injury (DAI) patients who have not developed ICH expansion within 72 hours.
- Chemoprophylaxis should not be delayed beyond day 7, overall.
- LMWH is preferred over unfractionated heparin for lower ICH expansion.

Siddiqi and colleagues at three trauma centers in southern California have been even more aggressive with chemoprophylaxis in a subset of head injury patients when specific DVT risk factors are involved, including patient (or family) history of DVT, known significant blood loss from trauma with resulting hypotension and hypovolemia, morbid obesity, and anticipated prolonged bed rest (as for example with polytrauma or obtunded/comatose patients) (Javed Siddiqi, personal communication, May 12, 2016).

Guided by some studies in the literature,[9,10] and with good outcomes, Siddiqi and team have initiated DVT chemoprophylaxis on high-risk DVT patients as early as posttrauma day 1, but only when there is no progression of intracerebral bleeding on repeat CT scans for 24 hours.

22.3 Indications for Anticoagulation in the NICU: Treatment

22.3.1 DVT treatment

The primary objectives of DVT treatment are to prevent PE, reduce morbidity, and decrease the risk of postthrombotic syndrome. The 2012 American College of Chest Physicians (ACCP) guidelines[11] recommended that distal DVT below the knee without severe symptoms or risk for extension should be observed with serial ultrasounds for 2 weeks. Distal DVT with severe symptoms or risk for extension (including positive D-dimer, extensive DVT or close to the proximal veins, no reversible provoking factor, active cancer, previous history of blood clots, and inpatient status) and proximal DVT should be treated with anticoagulants.

The principles of anticoagulation include the following:

- Warfarin should be started on the same day as LMWH or unfractionated heparin therapy is started (Level I evidence).
- Warfarin should be overlapped with heparin for 4 to 5 days, with discontinuation around 5 to 7 days.
- Alternative medications include factor X inhibitors (such as dabigatran, rivaroxaban, apixaban, and edoxaban).
- Inferior vena cava filters (IVCFs) provide an alternative to full anticoagulation in patients at high risk for catastrophic hemorrhagic complications only during the acute phase (securing the aneurysm or 1 to 2 weeks after intracranial surgery). Full anticoagulation should be reconsidered beyond the high-risk period.
- First episode of DVT triggered by surgery should be treated with anticoagulants for 3 months, recurrent episodes should be treated for at least 12 months.

22.3.2 Treatment of Atrial Fibrillation

Atrial fibrillation (AFib) is the most common cardiac arrhythmia and is associated with a five- to sixfold increased risk of stroke.[12] It is estimated that AFib prevalence will be more than doubled by 2050 due to the aging population in the United States, which will in turn contribute to an additional 170,000 annual strokes.[13] The risk of AFib-related stroke mortality can be as high as 24% in elderly patients.

The goal of anticoagulation treatment of AFib is to reduce the risk of cardio embolic events as well as stroke. The 2011 guideline[10] for the management of patients with AFib recommended the following:

- Antithrombotic therapy is recommended for all patients with AFib except those with lone AFib or contraindications.
- Warfarin is recommended for patients without mechanical heart valves at high risk of stroke (e.g., prior thromboembolism and rheumatic mitral stenosis), and for patients with more than one moderate risk factor (e.g., age ≥ 75, hypertension, heart failure, impaired left ventricle systolic function, diabetes mellitus).
- Aspirin is recommended as an alternative for patients at low risk or those with contraindications to oral anticoagulation.
- Interruption of anticoagulation for up to 1 week without substituting heparin is reasonable for surgical or diagnostic procedure that carry a risk of bleeding.

- Antithrombotic therapy is recommended for all patients with atrial flutter as for those with AFib.

With the expectancy of a rapidly increasing number of patients with AFib, there has been a push to find alternatives to warfarin, which are more cost-effective, clinically practical, and free of frequent monitoring requirements. Recent randomized, controlled trials have confirmed the superiority of new oral anticoagulants (NOAC, including dabigatran, rivaroxaban, and apixaban) over warfarin in preventing stroke and systemic embolism as well as causing less major bleeding and ICH.[12] Therefore NOAC serves as a reasonable alternative for primary prevention of stoke in patients with AFib.

With regard to secondary prevention, the most recent consensus[14] recommended the following:

For patients with new-onset stroke ascribed to AFib, but not previously on anticoagulation treatment:
- Antiplatelet medications (aspirin or aspirin + clopidogrel) are not recommended.
- NOAC is preferred over warfarin.
- Use bleeding risk scoring to manage the modifiable risk factors and monitor the treatment course.
- Combination of warfarin + aspirin, or aspirin + clopidogrel, is only acceptable in cases associated with coronary heart disease or stenting.

For patients with ischemic or hemorrhagic stroke associated with AFib, but who are already on anticoagulation treatment:
- Switch to NOAC in patients who were taking aspirin or aspirin + clopidogrel.
- Switch to NOAC in patients who were taking warfarin, independently from the international normalized ratio.
- Start NOAC after ICH in patients who were taking antiplatelet agents or warfarin, except when absolute, transient contraindications (e.g., resumption of drug after a bleeding event, intake of aspirin, aspirin + clopidogrel, and non-steroidal anti-inflammatory drugs) or definitive contraindications (e.g., heart valvulopathy, endocarditis, severe renal insufficiency, active liver disease, and high hemorrhagic risk) are present.
- Start NOAC after gastrointestinal bleeding in patients who were taking warfarin, except when absolute, transient, or permanent contraindications are present.

It is noteworthy that for both primary and secondary prevention the contraindications to anticoagulation therapy are common but subjective. It is not uncommon that patients with reported contraindications received anticoagulants based on the judgment of benefit outweighing potential harm. Resumption of anticoagulation therapy with warfarin immediately following hospital discharge for TBI has been shown to have a net benefit in decreasing the risk of stroke (both hemorrhagic and ischemic), despite increasing the risk of other hemorrhagic events (including upper gastrointestinal bleeding, adrenal hemorrhage, and other hemorrhage).[15]

22.4 Indications for Antiplatelet Agent Use in the NICU

The risk of thromboembolic events increased in certain circumstances, including planned neuroendovascular procedures, previously placed vascular or intracranial stents, acute cardiovascular insufficiency, and so on. Therapy with anticoagulants and antiplatelet medications is crucial in such cases.

22.4.1 Prophylaxis for New Procedures

Since neuroendovascular procedures are associated with a significant risk of immediate or delayed thromboembolic and ischemic complications, perioperative antiplatelet therapy and dual or triple therapy have gained increased usage for intracranial stenting, and for stent-assisted aneurysm coiling. All these patients end up in the NICU, and current expert consensus by five academic societies in the United States (with 2007 evidence)[16] recommended the following:

- Preprocedural dual antiplatelet therapy with aspirin and clopidogrel should be given for at least 24 hours and preferably for 4 days.
- Intraprocedural anticoagulation is achieved with unfractionated heparin or bivalirudin to maintain the activated clotting time between 250 and 300 seconds.
- Postprocedural antiplatelet therapy should be started as tolerated with aspirin continued for life, and clopidogrel for at least 4 weeks.

Although intensive antithrombotic therapy reduces the risk of thromboembolic and ischemic complications, its benefit should always be balanced with the increased risk of hemorrhagic complications. For perioperative antiplatelet therapy, hemorrhagic and groin-site complications were found to be significantly higher in patients treated with three or more antiplatelet agents.[17] Acute aneurysmal subarachnoid hemorrhage secondary to fusiform or dissecting aneurysms intimately involved essential perforating arteries (e.g., vertebral artery dissecting aneurysm incorporating the posterior inferior cerebellar artery) represent an especially challenging clinical scenario because neither clipping nor coiling may be possible due to the risk to the perforating vessel(s); in this scenario, stenting may be the only practical, but less than ideal, neurointerventional option because of the necessity for dual antiplatelet therapy in the face of a fresh subarachnoid hemorrhage—in this scenario, delayed stenting (while medically minimizing the risk of aneurysm rebleed for the period of delay) may be the only neuroendovascular option, with intracranial bypass as the complex and risky surgical option to preserve flow in the perforating vessel (followed by trapping of the dissected segment).[18]

22.4.2 Treatment for Prior Conditions

The number of patients receiving chronic anticoagulant and antiplatelet medications has increased consistently during the past few years. A multidisciplinary approach is needed to optimize the perioperative management of antiplatelet therapy in patients with previously placed vascular stents. Current consensus recommended the continuation of aspirin during the perioperative period in high-risk patients with drug-eluting stents and minimization of the withdrawal time of clopidogrel.[19,20]

The ideal time to stop aspirin preoperatively remains unknown in patients with drug-eluting stents. However, it is currently a standard neurosurgical practice to continue aspirin until the day before surgery in patients with carotid artery stenosis, and then restart it in the immediate postoperative period. For patients with acute subdural hematomas who underwent emergent neurosurgery, no difference of morbidity and mortality was found related to subdural reaccumulation and the use of aspirin at the time of surgery.[21]

Eptifibatide may serve as a bridging therapy during neurosurgery when stopping clopidogrel preoperatively, taking into account the beneficial pharmacologic profile of this drug: following intravenous administration, plasma concentrations are achieved within 5 minutes, maximum inhibition of platelets occurs within 15 minutes, and steady-state concentrations are attained within 4 to 6 hours. Platelet aggregation usually returns to normal within 4 hours of discontinuing therapy.[22]

However, the current literature on the recommended time of discontinuation and restart of antiplatelet agents, as well as the safety and efficacy of such bridging medications, has not yet been assessed in prospective properly designed studies. Therefore further investigations of this therapy in various groups of neurosurgical and neurotrauma patients are warranted before it can be recommended for routine clinical use. In addition, alteration of dual antiplatelet therapy must be individualized for each patient, surgery, and institution, by weighing the risk of stent thrombosis against the risk of hemorrhagic complications.

Case Management

The presence of vague discomfort of the left shoulder and left upper-extremity edema should raise the suspicion of upper-extremity DVT. He needs to be sent to the radiology department for Doppler ultrasonography immediately, which in this case showed an 11 × 7 mm intraluminal thrombus in the distal part of the left subclavian vein. Upon diagnosis of DVT, proper management includes upper-extremity elevation and mechanical compression. Because of the recent history of craniotomy, anticoagulation with subcutaneous LMWH should not be given. The left-upper-extremity catheter should be removed as long as alternate intravenous access is available. He should also have Doppler ultrasonography repeated during the course of the management to assess the status of the flow and the thrombus. For the lower extremities, in addition to pneumatic compression, DVT chemoprophylaxis with LMWH or unfractionated heparin should have been considered after day 3 based on the status of progression of ICH on repeated CT. Safe and early mobilization after DVT is also recommended

References

[1] Geerts WH, Code KI, Jay RM, Chen E, Szalai JP. A prospective study of venous thromboembolism after major trauma. N Engl J Med. 1994; 331(24):1601–1606

[2] Denson K, Morgan D, Cunningham R, et al. Incidence of venous thromboembolism in patients with traumatic brain injury. Am J Surg. 2007; 193(3):380–383, discussion 383–384

[3] Zakaryan A. Perioperative management of neurosurgical patients receiving chronic anticoagulation therapy. Front Pharmacol. 2014; 5:64

[4] Bratton SL, Chestnut RM, Ghajar J, et al. Brain Trauma Foundation, American Association of Neurological Surgeons, Congress of Neurological Surgeons, Joint Section on Neurotrauma and Critical Care, AANS/CNS. Guidelines for the management of severe traumatic brain injury. V. Deep vein thrombosis prophylaxis. J Neurotrauma. 2007; 24 Suppl 1:S32–S36

[5] Chang EF, Meeker M, Holland MC. Acute traumatic intraparenchymal hemorrhage: risk factors for progression in the early post-injury period. Neurosurgery. 2006; 58(4):647–656, discussion 647–656

[6] Zareba P, Wu C, Agzarian J, Rodriguez D, Kearon C. Meta-analysis of randomized trials comparing combined compression and anticoagulation with either modality alone for prevention of venous thromboembolism after surgery. Br J Surg. 2014; 101(9):1053–1062

[7] Abdel-Aziz H, Dunham CM, Malik RJ, Hileman BM. Timing for deep vein thrombosis chemoprophylaxis in traumatic brain injury: an evidence-based review. Crit Care. 2015; 19:96

[8] Phelan HA. Pharmacologic venous thromboembolism prophylaxis after traumatic brain injury: a critical literature review. J Neurotrauma. 2012; 29(10):1821–1828

[9] Saadeh Y, Gohil K, Bill C, et al. Chemical venous thromboembolic prophylaxis is safe and effective for patients with traumatic brain injury when started 24 hours after the absence of hemorrhage progression on head CT. J Trauma Acute Care Surg. 2012; 73(2):426–430

[10] Phelan HA, Wolf SE, Norwood SH, et al. A randomized, double-blinded, placebo-controlled pilot trial of anticoagulation in low-risk traumatic brain injury: The Delayed Versus Early Enoxaparin Prophylaxis I (DEEP I) study. J Trauma Acute Care Surg. 2012; 73(6):1434–1441

[11] Kearon C, Akl EA, Comerota AJ, et al. American College of Chest Physicians. Antithrombotic therapy for VTE disease: Antithrombotic Therapy and Prevention of Thrombosis, 9th ed: American College of Chest Physicians Evidence-Based Clinical Practice Guidelines. Chest. 2012; 141(2) Suppl:e419S–e494S

[12] Hedna VS, Favilla CG, Guerrero WR, et al. Trends in the management of atrial fibrillation: A neurologist's perspective. J Cardiovasc Dis Res. 2012; 3(4):255–264

[13] Go AS, Hylek EM, Phillips KA, et al. Prevalence of diagnosed atrial fibrillation in adults: national implications for rhythm management and stroke prevention: the AnTicoagulation and Risk Factors in Atrial Fibrillation (ATRIA) Study. JAMA. 2001; 285(18):2370–2375

[14] Toso V. Recommendations for the use of new oral anticoagulants (NOACs) after TIA or stroke caused by atrial fibrillation (AF), after a consensus conference among Italian neurologists (the Venice group). Neurol Sci. 2014; 35(5):723–727

[15] Albrecht JS, Liu X, Baumgarten M, et al. Benefits and risks of anticoagulation resumption following traumatic brain injury. JAMA Intern Med. 2014; 174(8):1244–1251

[16] Bates ER, Babb JD, Casey DE, Jr, et al. American College of Cardiology Foundation Task Force, American Society of Interventional & Therapeutic Neuroradiology, Society for Cardiovascular Angiography and, Interventions, Society for Vascular Medicine and Biology, Society for Interventional Radiology. ACCF/SCAI/SVMB/SIR/ASITN 2007 Clinical Expert Consensus Document on carotid stenting. Vasc Med. 2007; 12(1):35–83

[17] Enomoto Y, Yoshimura S, Sakai N, et al. Current perioperative management of anticoagulant and antiplatelet use in neuroendovascular therapy: analysis of JR-NET1 and 2. Neurol Med Chir (Tokyo). 2014; 54 Suppl 2:9–16

[18] Connolly ES, Jr, Rabinstein AA, Carhuapoma JR, et al. American Heart Association Stroke Council, Council on Cardiovascular Radiology and Intervention, Council on Cardiovascular Nursing, Council on Cardiovascular Surgery and Anesthesia, Council on Clinical Cardiology. Guidelines for the management of aneurysmal subarachnoid hemorrhage: a guideline for healthcare professionals from the American Heart Association/american Stroke Association. Stroke. 2012; 43(6):1711–1737

[19] Popescu WM. Perioperative management of the patient with a coronary stent. Curr Opin Anaesthesiol. 2010; 23(1):109–115

[20] Grines CL, Bonow RO, Casey DE, Jr, et al. American Heart Association, American College of Cardiology, Society for Cardiovascular Angiography and Interventions, American College of Surgeons, American Dental Association, American College of Physicians. Prevention of premature discontinuation of dual antiplatelet therapy in patients with coronary artery stents: a science advisory from the American Heart Association, American College of Cardiology, Society for Cardiovascular Angiography and Interventions, American College of Surgeons, and American Dental Association, with representation from the American College of Physicians. J Am Coll Cardiol. 2007; 49(6):734–739

[21] Panczykowski DM, Okonkwo DO. Premorbid oral antithrombotic therapy and risk for reaccumulation, reoperation, and mortality in acute subdural hematomas. J Neurosurg. 2011; 114(1):47–52

[22] Rouine-Rapp K, McDermott MW. Perioperative management of a neurosurgical patient with a meningioma and recent coronary artery stent. J Clin Anesth. 2013; 25(3):228–231

409

23 Restraints in the Neurosurgical Intensive Care Unit Patient

Colleen Rose and Justen Watkins

Abstract

A significant proportion of patients in the neurosurgical intensive care unit are confused and agitated; some may be scared by the unfamiliar surroundings, frequent blood work, and multiple interactions with physicians and nurses they do not recognize. The pain and anxiety of this situation can leave these patients feeling highly vulnerable, and they may react with actions that are counter to their own best interests. Restraints have to be used exclusively to protect patients from self-destructive behavior, such as pulling out their lines and self-extubation, and at times to prevent them from hurting their caregivers. Important guidelines need to be followed to protect patients and caregivers, while also respecting the autonomy of the patient; accordingly, it is critical to understand the appropriate use of restraints in the intensive care unit.

Keywords: agitation, asphyxiation, chemical restraints, enclosure beds, four-point restraints, medical restraints, patient safety, psychological distress, restraints, self-extubation

Case Study

A 23-year-old Caucasian man is brought to the emergency room by police after striking his head on a concrete step while riding a skateboard unhelmeted. The patient had a brief loss of consciousness followed by severe agitation and combative behavior reported by friends. Police and Emergency Medical Service (EMS) arrived on scene to find the patient in an erratic and violent state without clear signs of trauma. EMS was unable to safely evaluate the patient. Although the patient's friends denied drug or alcohol use, the patient was subdued by police, handcuffed, and transported to the hospital. Upon arrival to the hospital the patient was helped onto a gurney and placed in four-point restraints for his safety and for the safety of hospital personnel. Minutes later the patient fell unconscious. Computed tomography of the head showed a large frontoparietal temporal epidural hematoma with a left to right 1.5 cm midline shift. The patient was taken to the operating room immediately for a left craniectomy for evacuation and decompression of the epidural hematoma; postoperatively he was combative and confused for the immediate postoperative period.

See end of chapter for Case Management.

23.1 Introduction

The neurosurgical intensive care unit (NICU) faces unique challenges when it comes to providing patient safety. Neurologic patients are often confused, impulsive, restless, and agitated. They may lack the ability to make sound judgments regarding their medical care. Frequently neurologic patients are unaware of their physical limitations. We as health care providers are confronted with the responsibility to protect our patients from physical harm, while preventing psychological distress.

Restraint reduction is the primary intent of the Joint Commission on Accreditation of Healthcare Organizations' (JCAHO) 2004 Patient Care Initiatives.[1] Centers for Medicare and Medicaid Services (CMS), formerly Health Care Financing Administration (HCFA), guidelines also focus on restraint reduction. Both institutions regard restraints and seclusion as last resort measures and encourage acute care hospitals to use them only when less restrictive means fail.

Restraint use must be guided by state and federal law as well as hospital licensing or facility accreditation requirements.

Restraint can be defined as any device or method used to restrict a person's movement, mobility, or access to one's body.[2] Medical restraint can be applied in a variety of settings for a variety of reasons. When restraint is used to promote medical treatment, such as intravenous (IV) therapy and medications; to prevent pulling lines and therapeutic tubes, such as endotracheal tubes, indwelling catheters, intracranial monitors or drains; or to prevent disturbing surgical dressings and incisions, it is considered medical restraint, no matter the hospital setting. All other alternative means of preventing the undesired behavior should be exhausted before application of restraint. By allowing patients to harm themselves by self-extubation or pulling out a subdural drain, or other medically necessary device, demonstrates a failure of patient safety.

Patient safety must be foremost when using restraints. JCAHO Sentinel Event Alert 1998 reports 20 deaths in the previous 2 years of patients in restraints.[3] These deaths had various root causes. Death by strangulation occurred in geriatric patients with vest restraints, half of whom made their way between split side rails. Forty percent of deaths occurred as a result of asphyxiation, and the remainder were due to cardiac arrest and fire (while the patient was attempting to burn off restraints). JACHO identified the following as potential contributing factors:

- Restraint of smokers.
- Restraint use with physical deformities that prevent proper application (especially vests).
- Supine position may predispose patients to aspiration.
- Prone position may predispose to suffocation.
- Not continually observing patients in restraints.

Care should be taken to decrease the risk of problems such as those listed above. All smoking supplies should be removed from the patient's belongings and environment. Visitors should be advised of smoking restrictions due to fire risk. A thorough needs assessment for a planned restraint device, considering the patient's unique physical requirements, must be carried out prior to the application. While a patient is restrained, proper positioning and observation are imperative. A nonintubated patient with an altered level of consciousness should not be restrained flat on his back due to the risk of aspiration. The head of the bed should be elevated whenever possible. Rarely will a neurologic patient need to be restrained in the prone position. If the prone position is used, the airway must be kept unobstructed at all times. The prone position is not recommended for obese, elderly, or pediatric patients.

Mindfulness of the patient's long-term immobility due to restraints is essential. Despite the described benefits of safety with restraints, the risks of immobility due to the restraints must be considered. Evidence shows that mobility is associated with improved outcomes in the ICU.[4] Frequent turning and multiple mobility sessions daily are especially essential in the restrained patient.

JCAHO's Provision of Care, Treatment and Services (PC), PC.11.10 through PC.11.100, delineate appropriate measures for restraint use in hospitals.[1] These standards establish that assessment and reassessments of the need for restraint, and alternatives to use are carried out according to hospital policy. Additionally, hospital leaders must set forth the hospital's philosophy regarding any standards for restraint use and define the situations where restraint use is allowable based on clinical evidence. Hospital policies will direct appropriate patient use of restraints. Restraints must either be ordered by a licensed independent practitioner or applied upon specific order according to a hospital-approved protocol that defines clinical criteria for use. Patients are to be monitored while in restraints, and restraint use is to be thoroughly documented in the patient's medical record according to hospital policy. The hospital works via its performance improvement process to find ways to prevent use, develop alternative measures, and improve processes to decrease the risk related to restraint use. These standards are not intended to address behavioral restraint. Restraint should never be used as a disciplinary measure.

23.2 Types of Medical Restraints

There are many different types of restraints used for medical necessity to ensure the safety of the confused, combative, and psychotic patient[5]; all of which behaviors can be found in the neurologic or neurosurgical patient. Patients with traumatic brain injury can present agitated, combative, and confused to the point where restraints must be used to ensure the safety of the patient as well as the safety of hospital staff. The choice of restraint must be considered in terms of its appropriateness for the patient. Restraints alone can cause agitation in an already confused patient and can cause deadly harm. Restraints should only be used as a last resort with the least restrictive device as possible.[6] Removal of all restraint devices should be achieved as soon as safely possible.

23.2.1 Four-Point Restraints

Four-point restraints or limb restraints are soft padded cuffs that are attached to the wrists and ankles of patients that pose a risk of harm to themselves or others. The cuffs have a strap attached that is tied to the frame of the hospital bed. Limb restraints are used on patients who are using their arms or legs to strike hospital personnel or are removing medical apparatus that is indwelling in the body. Four-point restraints heavily impair movement of all kind and will render a patient helpless in an emergency. Patients that require four-point restraints often have a hospital companion or sitter to watch them at all times. Limbs must be checked every 15 minutes to ensure proper circulation, and restraints must be removed as soon as safely possible.[6]

Physicians must be aware of the potential negative physical and psychological consequences of four-point restraints. Measures should be taken to preserve the patient's dignity and rights. The act of physically restraining a patient has both ethical and legal implications, including the potential violation of a patient's rights. Therefore, the use of four-point restraints should be a last resort after attempts to deescalate the situation have failed, and less restrictive measures have proved ineffective.

23.2.2 Limb Restraints

Limb restraints are appropriate for patients who are becoming increasingly agitated and confused and continue to try to remove necessary medical devices that would cause serious harm and a significant setback to recovery. These patients are typically found in the intensive care unit with possibly an endotracheal tube, chest tubes, halo traction, and an external ventricular device for intracranial pressure monitoring, the removal of which could be detrimental to the patient outcome. This patient would also most likely be sedated with opioids and narcotics for pain relief, which could impair a patient's awareness and orientation. Limb restraints can be found in two different types, leather, and fabric. Fabric restraints can be placed in an emergency situation by a nurse awaiting a physician order in an acute care setting; however, leather restraints must be ordered by a licensed physician who has examined the patient and deemed leather restraints necessary prior to application and the use of soft restraints must be deemed ineffective.[5]

23.2.3 Vest Restraints

Vest restraints are used to secure a patient to a bed or chair. The vest is placed on the patient, and mesh straps extending from each corner are tied to each side of the bed or together to the back of a chair. The vest restraint is used to prevent a patient from being injured by falling out of a bed or chair after numerous reminders and redirection have failed. Ensure fingers can easily slide between the patient and the vest that it has not been placed too tight. The vest should not be on so tight that the patient's midsection does not expand with inhalation.[6] The patient should always have the nurse call light within reach when in need of assistance. This type of restraint will allow the patient freedom to move around without restriction of arms or legs. Strict laws are in place that prohibit the vest from being placed with the opening to the back of the patient.[7] There have been many reported deaths from choking when the vest is applied backward. The opening of the vest must always be to the front of the patient.

23.2.4 Mitt Restraints

Mitt restraints are appropriate for a patient who is confused and impulsive and who is prone to self-injury or unintended battery, or who is prone to disrupt medical treatments by pulling tubes and catheters but can be redirected with distraction. This is a good device as it limits manual dexterity and removes the ability to remove dressings or tubes from the head or face. Confused patients often reach to touch or scratch a craniotomy site or even pull the ventriculostomy catheter. Patients can lift and move their arms but are unable to grasp or pull. Mitts can be placed on one or both hands and must be checked every 2 hours to ensure proper circulation is not compromised.[6]

23.2.5 Enclosure Beds

Enclosure beds are used when physical restraints are deemed inappropriate or ineffective, and greater freedom of movement within a "safe" environment is desired. Enclosure beds are ideal for removing the ability of the patient to get out of bed unassisted.[6] An enclosure bed has a mesh tent connected to a frame placed over a standard hospital bed. Although an enclosure bed is considered a restraint because it limits the patient's ability to get out of bed, an enclosure bed is less restrictive than other restraints. It can be implemented as an alternative when a vest restraint would create further agitation and wrist restraints are not indicated. An enclosure bed must be zipped at all times, and internal padding must be used on rigid structures.

23.2.6 Papoose Boards

Papoose Boards, originally a wood-and-leather device used by many Native American tribes to swaddle their infants and children, also known as cradle boards, are still in use in many places. A papoose board is a padded board with fabric Velcro bands that is used to limit a pediatric patient's movement during a medical procedure or examination. If a child has an acute head injury requiring sutures, washout, or examination to determine the extent of an injury, a papoose board will keep the child from flailing and causing further injury. The child will lay flat on a board in which the Velcro band wraps the child's body eliminating any movement.[8] Using a papoose board for infants and children to temporarily and safely inhibit movement is often preferable to medical sedation, which presents serious and potential risks, including death. Papoose board is preferred by some parents as an alternative to sedation. Informed consent from a parent or legal guardian is usually required prior to a papoose board being used.

23.2.7 Chemical Restraints

Chemical restraints can be used as a last resort to help control a violent situation. There are three classes of drugs used to chemically restrain a patient. Benzodiazepines, typical or classic antipsychotics, and atypical antipsychotics are usually the class of choice for patients meeting these criteria. Several options exist regarding how and when to use medication to manage agitation. The ideal chemical restraint has a rapid time of onset, regardless of the route of administration, and has few adverse effects.[9] Oral medications should be the first choice if the patient is willing to cooperate. Oral medications have a similar onset and effectiveness as their IV counterpart. If urgency is crucial, these medications can be given in an oral liquid form and quickly dissolving discs. Although IV medications act rapidly, the agitated patient may not have IV access and achieving access may be difficult and dangerous. Once the level of agitation has been determined a medication that best suits the agitation is desirable. Patients should be given medications based on their agitation level, starting with oral medications if the patient is mildly agitated to IV or IM if severely agitated. Benzodiazepines have been shown to be effective in patients with mild to moderate agitation and who are intoxicated or who will be withdrawing from alcohol or other illicit drugs. Benzodiazepines also have fewer side effects than when used in combination therapy with antipsychotic medications. The main side effects of benzodiazepines are hypotension and respiratory depression; therefore, these patients should be monitored closely.[9]

Classic or typical antipsychotics have been very effective in controlling violent behavior and acute psychosis. The two main drugs used for acute agitation and violence are haloperidol and droperidol. The major drawbacks of these medications are their adverse effects. Droperidol has been given a black box warning by the U.S. Food and Drug Administration (FDA) because it may cause QT prolongation.[10] Haloperidol received a warning from the FDA in 2008 concerning its use in the treatment of geriatric patients with dementia-related psychosis. QT prolongation can produce torsade de pointes and other cardiac arrhythmias.[11] Furthermore, typical antipsychotics are recognized for causing extrapyramidal effects. Extrapyramidal symptoms, such as tardive dyskinesia, dystonia, akathisia, torticollis, and drug-induced Parkinsonism, can occur in patients given these medications.[9] These medications have been shown to be effective in highly agitated patients; however, care must be taken with patients at risk for QT prolongation.

Pediatric usage: Haloperidol and lorazepam are the preferred agents for undifferentiated agitation in the pediatric population. The dosing of haloperidol and lorazepam is the same for oral, intramuscular, or IV administration. For children aged 6–12 years, haloperidol is dosed at 0.025–0.075 mg/kg with a maximum of 2.5 mg/dose. For the same group, lorazepam at 0.05 mg/kg with a maximum of 4 mg/dose may be used.[12]

23.3 Legal Considerations

When a decision is made to implement restraints, either physically or chemically, legal aspects must be taken into consideration. A 1982 Supreme Court Decision, *Youngberg v. Romero*, stated that "restraints are justified to protect others or self in the judgment of the health professional." Additionally, the clinician must consider the competency of the patient, which is defined as "the capacity or ability to understand the nature and effects of one's actions or decisions." Although being in the emergency department does legally imply consent to treatment, a patient does have the right to refuse a treatment course, unless the patient is deemed incompetent or a threat to himself or others.[9] If a patient displays no threat to himself or others and possesses the ability to make rational decisions, then he cannot be confined or restrained without giving his permission. If a patient is held against his will, he then has the right to charge the health professional and institution with false imprisonment and battery. Though covered by federal law, each state has its set of laws governing the rights of patients and the restriction of those rights by health care workers. Physicians must be knowledgeable of these laws and their consequences.[13]

Legal Sequels
- Failure to recognize a medical cause for agitation or assumed psychosis.
- Inadequate monitoring of vital signs after sedation.
- Failure to recognize potential lethal cardiac adverse effects from medications given.

- Failure to comply with state laws regarding patient competency and confinement.

23.4 Application of Knowledge

- Use of medical restraints should be limited to situations with appropriate clinical justification and reserved for patients at risk for self-harm, including self-extubation, pulling or disturbing medically necessary lines and tubes, and disturbing wounds and dressings, and patients that attempt to ambulate when medically unable to do so. A thorough risk assessment must be completed for all patients.
- A written order by a licensed physician is required upon initiation of restraint. A person qualified by education and experience, according to hospital policy, may initiate restraint in an emergency. The licensed physician must be notified of initiation, and the licensed physician must sign the order within 8 hours. Nurse practitioners or physician assistants may be allowed to order restraints in some institutions. Some hospitals may elect to allow application of restraints by persons qualified according to a hospital-approved protocol by state and federal law and by hospital licensing or accreditation requirements.
- The restraint order should be timed, dated, and not to exceed 24 hours. The restraint type, number of points, and reason for restraint must be included in the order. Restraints must be reordered daily after face-to-face evaluation by a licensed physician. Restraint use should be discussed in a multidisciplinary care conference at regular intervals where alternative measures are explored.
- The patient must be closely monitored. Visual observation should take place frequently, as defined by the institution. Physical and psychological needs must be attended to every 2 hours. These include skin and circulation assessment, assessment of comfort, agitation, toileting and hygiene, hydration and nutrition, and position changes with range of motion. Continuous observation should be considered for highly agitated patients as they are at increased risk for injury in spite of or resulting from restraint. Ongoing assessment of the continued need for restraint and out-of-restraint trials should also be implemented.
- The patient and family will be educated as to the reason for restraint, criteria required for release of restraint, and steps taken to maintain safety while the patient is in restraint.
- All restraint occurrences should be thoroughly documented in the medical record. Clinical justification, alternative measures, response to restraint, physician notification, patient/family education, and patient care should be recorded according to hospital policy.

- Staff should be educated regarding the hospital's restraint policies and also in the practical application of restraint. Competency should be demonstrated and maintained by in-service and skills testing at intervals specified by the policy. Education regarding the hospital's performance improvement process with respect to restraint reduction and alternatives, as well as hospital statistics compiled on restraints, should be ongoing and disseminated via unit and department meetings at regular intervals.

Important alternatives to restraint use are adequate pain relief to prevent the confused patient from disturbing a wound or dressing, allowing the patient's family to remain at the bedside to prevent or decrease anxiety and fear, and reorienting the patient frequently. Using bedside sitters to monitor the patient's behavior and prevent the patient from pulling tubes and lines or wandering may also be beneficial. Diversional activities such as games, drawing, television, and other activities may be helpful for some patients.

Case Management

Postoperatively the patient remained intubated and moderately sedated with soft restraints in place to ensure safety of the patient from removing necessary medical devices that would cause serious harm and a significant setback to recovery. In the days to follow the patient was extubated but remained confused and intermittently impulsive; he was treated with mitt restraints, and a safety companion was assigned to the bedside. Restraints were downgraded as the patient recovered; eventually the patient was released from all restraints as he made a full recovery.

References

[1] Joint Commission on Healthcare Organizations. Comprehensive Accreditation Manual for Hospitals: The Official Handbook. Oakbrook Terrace, IL: Joint Commission on Healthcare Organizations; 2014

[2] Springer G. When and How to use Restraints. Medscape http://www.medscape.com/viewarticle/838521. Accessed November 15, 2016

[3] Sentinel Event Alert. Issue 8, November 18, 1998. Updated 9/20/2010 http://www.jcaho.org/about + us/news + letters/sentinel + event + alert/print/sea_8.htm. Accessed August 31, 2015

[4] Titsworth WL, Hester J, Correia T, et al. The effect of increased mobility on morbidity in the neurointensive care unit. J Neurosurg. 2012; 116(6):1379–1388

[5] Simmons LM. Diversified Health Occupations. 7th ed. Clifton Park, NY: Delmar Cengage Learning; 2009

[6] Rose C. Choosing the Right Restraint. Am Nurse Today. 2015; 10(1):28–29

[7] Allen JE. Nursing Home Administration. New York, NY: Springer; 2003

[8] Hosey MT, UK National Clinical Guidelines in Pediatric Dentistry. UK National Clinical Guidelines in Paediatric Dentistry. Managing anxious children: the use of conscious sedation in paediatric dentistry. Int J Paediatr Dent. 2002; 12(5):359–372

[9] Mattingly BB, Kulkarni R, et al. Chemical Restraints. Updated June 3rd 2014. http:/emedicine.medscape.com/article/109717. Accessed August 31, 2015

[10] US Food and Drug Administration (FDA). Inapsine (droperidol). http://www.fda.gov/Safety/MedWatch/SafetyInformation/SafetyAlertsforHumanMedicalProducts/ucm172364.htm. Accessed September 1, 2015

[11] US Food and Drug Administration (FDA). Haldol (haloperidol injection). For Immediate Release August 2008. http://www.fda.gov/Safety/MedWatch/SafetyInformation/Safety-RelatedDrugLabelingChanges/ucm123214.htm. Accessed September 1, 2015

[12] Dorfman DH. The use of physical and chemical restraints in the pediatric emergency department. Pediatr Emerg Care. 2000; 16(5):355–360, quiz 362–363

[13] Agitated Patient in the Emergency Room. http://www.ferne.org/Lectures/agitated_patient_ED_b-bunney_saem0503.htm. Accessed September 1, 2015

24 Unique Pediatric Neurosurgical Intensive Care Unit Issues

Tanya Minasian, Daniel J. Won, and Dan E. Miulli

Abstract

Pediatric neurocritical care patients are unique, requiring a special knowledge of pediatric neurophysiology, neuropharmacology, and, of course, neuropathology. The best outcomes for patient care can be achieved with a multidisciplinary approach specifically involving the comanagement of a pediatrician. Pediatric patients have a higher cerebral blood flow requirement but a lower cerebral perfusion pressure requirement. Young pediatric patients also have a window into the brain through an open fontanelle allowing visual and palpatory inspection of intracranial pressure, which must be treated at a lower level to maintain the best outcomes. Finally, treating the pediatric patient means interacting with the family and obtaining important developmental milestone data from the parents and the use of their soothing effect.

Keywords: basal energy expenditure, child life specialist, CPP 40, dysconjugate gaze, fontanelle, high body surface to weight, multidisciplinary team, pediatric TBI guidelines

Case Presentation

A 5-year-old girl falls off a golf cart and sustains what appears to be a minor head injury. She is assessed in the emergency room by neurosurgery and found to have some memory loss and mild confusion. A computed tomographic (CT) scan of the head shows minimal frontal contusions bilaterally. She is admitted to the pediatric intensive care unit for observation, and a repeat CT scan of the head the next day. The patient deteriorates neurologically overnight, and a stat CT scan of the head shows the contusions unchanged, but significant brain edema.

See end of chapter for Case Management.

24.1 Introduction

Although many physicians treat children as "little adults," a child's physiological state is different from an adult's, both metabolically and electrophysiologically. It should also be noted that children are in a constant state of growth that disrupts their equilibrium and necessitates adjustments. For these reasons, as well as because of the variety of disease pathologies, the treatment of children, particularly in the pediatric neurosurgical intensive care unit (NICU), requires extensive training and a degree of familiarity and comfort. Comanagement of the patient with a pediatrician or intensivist is recommended.[1] Management of pediatric neurosurgical patients, especially after intracranial procedures, requires a multidisciplinary approach to ensure the best outcomes. This includes full disclosure of intraoperative events, postoperative prognosis and expectations, in addition to all potential complications expected.[2] Pediatric neurosurgical procedures, barring an emergency, should preferably be performed with a neurosurgeon well experienced in treating children. There are special neurosurgical considerations when treating the pediatric population in an intensive care situation.[3,4]

24.2 General Care Guidelines for Pediatric NICU Patients

The lack of familiarity with and misunderstanding of necessary medical treatment often frighten children and their families. Any child under the age of 16 years should be placed in the pediatric ward. Special visitation should be allowed by close family members to comfort the child. Early involvement of a child life specialist or social worker is encouraged to help with expectations and transitions, as well as to follow up on concerns. Several studies confirm the benefit of a location within the ward of a "safe haven." This is usually the playroom or family room. Within this safe haven there should be no medical conversations, patient care checks, or treatments.[5,6,7]

24.3 Intravenous Fluids and Electrolytes

Intracellular fluid, as a percentage of total body water, is ~ 30% at birth and increases to 40% by 1 year of life. Adequate fluid and electrolyte maintenance is needed for general health maintenance, as well as for recovery from neurologic injury (▶ Table 24.1).[8]

Table 24.1 Pediatric electrolyte requirements[8]

Electrolyte	Requirement
Sodium	3–4 mEq/kg/d
Potassium	2–3 mEq/kg/d
Glucose	100–200 mg/kg/h

Children have a higher body surface area to weight ratio, greater caloric expenditure, increased water losses from the skin, and a higher rate of insensible losses, leading to higher fluid requirements than adults.[9]

There are two ways to calculate baseline fluid requirements in children.[10] The "kg method" is based on the weight of the patient, as follows:

- For the first 10 kg of body weight: 100 mL/kg/d *plus.*
- For the second 10 kg of body weight: 50 mL/kg/d *plus.*
- For the weight above 20 kg: 20 mL/kg/d.

An alternative method for determining baseline intravenous (IV) fluids in children is the "meter-squared method," which is as follows:

- Maintenance fluids are 1,500 mL/m^2/d.
- Divide by 24 to get the flow rate per hour.
- To calculate the surface area, use the "rule of sixes" (see ▶ Table 24.2) or a formal body surface area chart or equation (see discussion in Nutrition section).[10]

The healthy and ideal fluid and electrolyte status of any patient is normovolemic with normal chemical balance. Of special consideration is brain injury or parenchymal edema from trauma or disease process. Like adult patients, pediatric patients with brain injury need to stay normal volemic to prevent brain edema. Sodium should stay on the high end of normal and glucose on the low end to decrease the risk of edema in patients with a broken blood–brain barrier. This rule of thumb does not hold true in endocrinological or systemic comorbidities or in spinal shock patients; these cases should treat the underlying pathology directly.[11]

Table 24.2 "Rule of Sixes" for estimating body surface area in children[10]

Weight (lb)	Body surface area (m^2)
3	0.1
6	0.2
12	0.3
18	0.4
24	0.5
30	0.6
36	0.7
42	0.8
48	0.9
60	1.0
Each additional 10 lb	Add 0.1
> 100	Treat as adult

Hyperosmolar therapy is used often in pediatric patients with traumatic brain injury (TBI). Level II evidence from pediatric TBI guidelines suggests that 3% hypertonic saline should be given at the rate of 6.5–10 mL/kg, as a continuous infusion. Level III evidence suggests the minimum dose required to maintain intracranial pressure (ICP) less than 20 to be used and to maintain serum osmolarity less than 360 mOsm. Mannitol was not recommended in these guidelines.[12]

24.4 Respiratory Maintenance

As with adults, pulmonary function and stability must be maintained in the pediatric NICU patient. Data regarding neurologic injury secondary to hypoxia in children are sparse. In general, adult guidelines should be followed, including oxygen saturation maintenance > 95% and minimum hemoglobin and hematocrit levels of 10.0 and 33.0, respectively, realizing that the normal pediatric values vary with age but are not much higher than these minimums. Children are much more sensitive to hemodynamic shifts than adults.[13,15,16]

The indications for endotracheal intubation are vast. The most obvious, of course, is respiratory distress or failure of any etiology. With pediatric NICU patients specifically, damage to the central nervous system (CNS) from infection, hemorrhage, trauma, hydrocephalus, or mass lesions can lead to the need for mechanical ventilation. Also, uncooperative patients, due to age, disease pathology, or closed head injury, may require temporary intubation to assist in ongoing care, including diagnosis, imaging, and treatment. Patients with cervical spine injuries should be intubated via an inline technique to minimize the risk of additional neurologic deficit. Those patients with possible or diagnosed facial trauma or anterior skull fractures should be intubated with direct visualization through the oral or nasal cavity as appropriate to minimize possible brain penetration, additional damage, or misplacement of the tubing.

Patients with raised ICP regardless of etiology may benefit from intubation. Care should be taken to intubate these patients, as the procedure itself may increase cerebral blood flow and subsequently ICP. Adequate sedation may help alleviate this problem. Under normal circumstances, cerebral oxygen requirements are coupled with cerebral blood flow, and are increased with temperature, activity, agitation, seizure, and injury. Blood flow will increase as the partial pressure of oxygen in arterial blood (PaO_2) falls below 60 mmHg or as the partial pressure of carbon dioxide in arterial blood ($PaCO_2$) increases. NICU patients require higher PaO_2 levels and low to normal $PaCO_2$ levels to optimize recovery. In an acute neurologic decline, a temporary period of mild hyperventilation may help minimize edema and provide the necessary time for definitive diagnostic or treatment measures, but it should never be used as maintenance treatment of elevated ICP.[13,14]

Pediatric TBI guidelines include that prophylactic hyperventilation to PCO_2 less than 30 mmHg in the first 48 hours from injury should be avoided, and if it is used then advanced neuromonitoring would be indicated to evaluate for cerebral ischemia (level III evidence).[12]

Arterial lines should be placed on all intubated patients to provide not only reliable, easily attainable blood pressure parameters but also arterial access for blood gas analysis. Arterial blood gas analysis should be performed with every ventilator adjustment, any clinical change, and as a baseline on intubated patients twice daily.

24.5 Intracranial Pressure and Cerebral Blood Flow

Cerebral perfusion pressure (CPP) is the pressure via which blood and nutrients are delivered to the brain. As ICP increases, or mean arterial pressure (MAP) decreases, the CPP will also decrease, which will ultimately decrease cerebral blood flow. Normal cerebral blood flow in adults is 50 mL/100 g/min. Gray matter blood flow is ~ 4 times higher than that of white matter. Newborn blood flow is ~ 40 mL/100 g/min. Cerebral blood flow then increases to accommodate growth and learning. By age 4, the average cerebral blood flow is 108 mL/100 g/min and can remain as high as twice that of adults until 18 years of age.[17,18,19]

An injured brain requires a fine line of adequate cerebral blood flow to maintain function, perfuse any ischemic penumbra, and heal while not increasing edema. This is where CPP plays a role. According to 2012 guidelines for acute medical management of severe TBI in infants, children, and adolescents, level III evidence suggests CPP should be kept at 40 mmHg in children with traumatic brain injury. A CPP of 40–50 mmHg can be considered, with infants maintained at the lower end and adolescents at the higher end.[12] Tight fluid control and pressors may be needed to maintain adequate MAP in the face of rising ICP to achieve this goal.

In children, it is often difficult to measure ICP. Ventriculostomies can be used as a direct measurement; however, an accurate examination can suggest elevated ICP as well. Papilledema is often a late finding of elevated ICP in children relative to adults, whereas vomiting occurs much more regularly and reliably as a predictive symptom. Assessment of fontanelles can also yield pressure data. Note that when children are lying flat or having a Valsalva maneuver, fontanelles can be bulging and firm without abnormality. However, in the sitting position, a calm child should have soft, nonbulging fontanelles; any firmness or bulge is suggestive of elevated ICP. Another useful clinical gauge of ICP is head circumference. Although head circumference abnormalities can stem from a variety of causes, they can be used to suspect intracranial pathology and possibly high ICP, particularly if augmented by other clinical findings. An estimation of ICP is 1.5 to 6.0 mm Hg in children < 2 years of age, equal to the child's age in the 2 to 15 year range, and 8 to 15 mm Hg in children and adults > 15 years old.

ICP monitoring is strongly supported in the pediatric population with severe TBI. Level III evidence from pediatric TBI guidelines suggest that for refractory ICP, addition of a lumbar drain can also be considered as long as external ventricular drain (EVD) is functional, cisterns are open, and there is no evidence of a mass lesion or shift on imaging. Studies have demonstrated that there is a frequently reported high incidence of elevated ICP in children with severe TBI and a high association of elevated ICP and poor neurologic outcome. Also, the best neurologic outcomes have been with protocol-based management of ICP. Level III evidence suggests that ICP above 20 mm Hg in the pediatric population is associated with a poor outcome. There are also limited data suggesting varying thresholds of ICP treatment: 0–24 months, 15 mm Hg should be threshold to treat; 25–96 months, 18 mm Hg; and 97–156 months: 20 mm Hg.[12]

In the pediatric NICU, ICP and CPP are treated as the fifth and sixth vital signs. Evaluation, early identification of trends, and rapid treatment can prevent additional neurologic decline and improve outcome.

24.6 Surgical Management

Level III evidence suggests that decompressive craniectomy and duraplasty should be considered in pediatric TBI patients with refractory ICP.[12]

24.7 Nutrition

States of physical and/or psychological stress change the metabolic needs of patients. Nutritional support is vital to the management and outcome of pediatric NICU patients. Most clinical research has been directed toward adult patients; however, most concepts carry over to children. In the 1960s, total parenteral nutrition (TPN) became widely used and helped to relieve the metabolic component of the systemic stress response. However, more recently, natural enteral support has been advocated to facilitate gut motility, mucosal healthiness, and natural flora preservation.[10] In particular, neonate patient data have suggested even small amounts of gastrointestinal feedings promote enterohepatic enzyme delivery, reduce mucosal atrophy, and decrease the risk of jaundice.[20,21]

Regardless of the mode of nutrition, the goal should be to maintain fluids, electrolytes, and vitamins, as well as to provide adequate calorie intake for a metabolically stressed and altered system (▶ Table 24.3, ▶ Table 24.4, ▶ Table 24.5). Some recent literature has suggested the need for an increased amount of protein, but there are conflicting views on this.[10,15] The basal energy

Table 24.3 Caloric requirements for infants and children[7]

Age (in years)	Calories (kcal/kg)
<40 weeks' gestation	80
0–1	90–120
1–7	75–90
7–12	60–75
12–18	45–60

Table 24.4 Percent change in caloric requirements in stressed conditions[7]

Percent increase in caloric requirement	Pathological condition
12	Every degree temperature > 37°C
20–30	Major surgery
40–50	Sepsis
50–100	Failure to thrive

Table 24.5 Basal metabolic rates for healthy subjects[7]

Age (years)	Males (kcal/m²/h)	Females (kcal/m²/h)
1	53	53
2–3	52	52
4–5	50	49
6–7	48	46
8–9	46	43
10–11	44	42
12–13	42	41
14–15	42	39
16–17	41	37
18–19	40	36
20–25	38	35

expenditures of patients in various states can be estimated by modified nomograms based on the Harris–Benedict formula[22] or by respirometry and indirect calorimetry. Also, hyperglycemia has been shown to increase morbidity in patients with TBI and must be avoided at all cost in the pediatric neurosurgical patient.[23]

24.8 Activity Level

The activity level of children in the NICU setting will vary depending on pathology. The general rule is to mobilize, mobilize, mobilize.

Intubated patients are the exception to this rule, as being intubated can be a traumatic state, misinterpreted by children of any age. These patients should be kept under adequate sedation and pain management. Infectious patients can increase activity within their secured environment, and bed rest patients can adjust the head of the bed. Patients with head of bed alteration limitations due to weight-bearing restrictions, drains, or underlying pathology, such as intracranial edema or spinal fluid circulation considerations, should adjust their activity within the parameters set by their condition but try to keep the head of the bed greater than 30 degrees above horizontal if safe.

Cervical collars and spinal braces, depending on the injury or baseline etiology causing the need for support, can be worn out of bed, and patients are still encouraged to increase activity. Braces should be worn snuggly and secured adequately to maximize support and minimize slipping or discomfort during activity. Some patients prefer to have a liner of gauze or a piece of material, such as a shirt, under the brace to prevent skin contact and irritation.

Activity can decrease the risk of comorbidities associated with hospitalization, including deep vein thrombosis, pulmonary embolisms, pneumonia, constipation, and pressure sores. Also, depression has been shown to be decreased among patients with out-of-bed activities and environmental changes. Environmental changes can consist of outside visits, hallway walks, wheelchair excursions, or simply a change in the furniture setup within the room.

Patients with indwelling deep tissue drains or open shunt systems should not be allowed into common areas secondary to the risk of contamination. These patients should still increase activity as tolerated, but the security of the drain system should be monitored.

24.9 Pharmacology

Injectable, oral, rectal, and transdermal medications are all used in children. Special attention is paid to dosing, preparation, delivery, and administration. Due to the lack of judgment expressed in children, IV medications are frequently used in the pediatric NICU setting to facilitate compliance and limit discomfort during administration. Dosing is usually by weight and/or therapeutic level maintenance. ▶ Table 24.6 lists several of the medications frequently used in the care of pediatric NICU patients.[24,25]

If medications require piggybacking, the suggested fluid is 0.9% normal saline. The additional osmolarity and sodium, as well as the lack of sugar, will help with edema. An exception to this is in the setting of electrolyte imbalance or endocrine pathology, whether or not related to the neurosurgical diagnosis. In these cases, a risk-to-benefit ratio as well as ease of treatment of the adverse reaction must be weighed when determining the fluid base in which to mix medication.

Table 24.6 Frequently used medications in the pediatric NICU patient[8]

Medication	Indication	Dose/Route	Miscellaneous
Acetaminophen	Pain/fever	10 mg/kg/dose PO/PR every 4–6 hours	
Acetaminophen w/codeine	Pain	1 tsp every 4 hours	For > 3 years old
Morphine (MSO₄)	Pain	0.1 mg/kg IM/SQ/IV every 1–4 hours	May raise ICP; IV not recommended in children
Midazolam	Sedation or intubation	0.2–0.7 mg/kg IV/PO/IM	
Diazepam	Sedation or intubation	0.2 mg/kg IV or PR	Maximum 30 mg IV
Lidocaine	Intubation	1.0 mg/kg IV	Dysrhythmias
Vecuronium	Relaxant, paralytic	0.1 mg/kg IV	Duration 15–30 minutes
Thiopental	Sedation	4 mg/kg IV	
Ketamine	Anesthetic, sedation	1 mg/kg IV over 1 minute; 4 mg/kg IM	10–20 minutes effect; concurrent atropine minimizes salivation
Fentanyl	Sedation	5 µg/kg IV	
Propofol	Sedation	5–50 µg/kg/min	Not recommended in children for > 12 hours
Dilantin	Anticonvulsant	Load 10 mg/kg at < 50 mg/min rate; maintenance 5 mg/kg/d	Watch levels: age dependent; can cause arrhythmias
Phenobarbital	Anticonvulsant	Load 10 mg/kg at < 60 mg/min rate; maintenance 3 mg/kg/min PO	
Phenergan	Antihistamine, antiemetic	6.25 mg PO/IV/IM/PR every 6 hours	May raise ICP
Anzemet	Antiemetic	0.35 mg/kg IV every 6 hours; 1.2 mg/kg PO every 6 hours	
Dopamine	Inotrope/pressor	2 mg/kg/min titrated to effect	Maximum 50 mg/kg/min; solution = 400 mg in 250 mL D5W
Dobutamine	Inotrope/pressor	2 µg/kg/min titrated to effect	Maximum 20 µg/kg/min; solution = 250 mg in 250 mL D5W

Abbreviations: D5 W, dextrose 5% in water; ICP, intracranial pressure; IM, intramuscularly; IV, intravenous; NICU, neurosurgical intensive care unit; PO, orally; PR, far point of accommodation; SQ, subcutaneous.

Studies have shown the most common mistake made with drug administration is carelessness in dosing because of a lack of time to recheck dosage instructions, miscalculations, or presumed familiarity with a particular drug. This problem is preventable.

Various elements of neuroanesthesia and sedation must be discussed in the pediatric population specifically. Etomidate and thiopental, for instance, have properties that allow for control of ICP. However, etomidate is less favored because it can cause adrenal suppression. Level III evidence suggests not to use propofol in the pediatric ICU setting as a sedative or for the treatment of ICP in children with severe TBI. High-dose barbiturate therapy may be used in hemodynamically stable patients with refractory ICP, despite aggressive medical and surgical management. Continuous blood pressure monitoring is required with the use of these medications to avoid precipitous drops in CPP.[12]

24.10 Temperature

With regard to hypothermia treatment in TBI patients, level II evidence suggests that moderate hypothermia for 24 hours postinjury should be avoided. However, moderate hypothermia (32–33°C) within 8 hours after severe TBI for up to 48 hours can be considered for ICP reduction, and rewarming greater than 0.5°C per hour should be avoided.[12]

24.11 Medical Imaging

There is a significant overlap between adults and children in regard to medical imaging. As a general rule, if a study is needed for diagnosis, treatment, or follow-up, then it must be done. Unnecessary studies are avoided in both subsets of patients to prevent unnecessary cost accumulation and radiation exposure, not to mention discomfort, the risk of transport, and systemic difficulties in obtaining the tests. In particular with children is the concern of radiation exposure on their developing system and bone growth. The average chest X-ray radiation exposure is 1.4 mGy, and the average head computed tomographic (CT) scan radiation exposure is 8.0 mGy. Most literature suggests adverse effects do not start occurring until after exposure to 100 mGy.[26] Young children also are usually not as cooperative and have difficulty lying still. Frequently, conscious sedation or temporary intubation is required to obtain an adequate study. This then exposes the patient to another set of risks, and the benefit-to-risk ratio needs to be clearly discussed with the legal guardians, as well as with other medical staff involved in the case. Whether sedation is required or not, it should be noted that there are risks to transporting critically ill patients to the radiology department. Risks include environmental exposure, infection, accidental line removal, systemic instability, and positional difficulties. Because of these risks, medically necessary imaging should be portable if possible and of acceptable quality; if transport to the radiology department is pertinent, all necessary studies from all disciplines should be performed during one trip to minimize risks and promote efficiency. This requires effective communication between complex multidisciplinary care plans.

In pediatric traumatic brain injury guidelines, level III evidence suggests that in the absence of neurologic deterioration or changes in ICP, routine imaging > 24 hours from injury is unnecessary.[12]

24.12 The Pediatric Neurologic Exam

Unlike adult examinations, there is no rigid normal baseline in a pediatric neurologic exam. Developmental milestones should be met sequentially and have been well documented; however, minimal timeline variations and personality trends do occur that can affect an exam at any given point.

The examiner should take into account the age of the child. The child should be placed in a comfortable setting with family present if possible. Much of the pediatric exam can be done while observing and interacting with the patient, paying close attention to facial expressions and the eyes, any verbalizations, and motor interactions. The pupils must be examined, even in uncooperative patients: no exceptions. Also, a head circumference and body weight should be documented and trends followed. The remainder of the exam can use a modified Glasgow Coma Scale format. Such standardizations help document exams reliably and reproducibly (▶ Table 24.7, ▶ Table 24.8).[27]

Table 24.7 Modified coma scale for infant[10]

Response	Score
Eye opening	
Spontaneous	4
To speech	3
To pain	2
None	1
Verbal	
Coos, babbles	5
Irritable cry	4
Cries to pain only	3
Moans to pain only	2
None	1
Motor	
Normal spontaneous movements	6
Withdraws to touch	5
Withdraws to pain	4

Table 24.7 continued

Response	Score
Abnormal flexion	3
Abnormal extension	2
None	1

Table 24.8 Children's coma scale[8,10]

Response	Score
Ocular	
Pursuit	4
EOM intact, reactive pupils	3
EOM impaired	2
EOM paralyzed, fixed pupils	1
Verbal	
Cries	3
Spontaneous respirations	2
Apneic	1
Motor	
Flexes and extends	4
Withdraws from painful stimuli	3
Hypertonic	2
Flaccid	1

Abbreviation: EOM, extraocular muscles.

During infancy, children can exhibit flexor activity while sleeping; this is a normal variant. Also, children can have asymmetric blink and dysconjugate gaze up to 6 months of age without concern. A positive plantar or Babinski's reflex can occur normally up to 1 year of age, as well as areflexia or hyperreflexia of deep tendon reflexes.

Case Management

The child described in this story has developed malignant cerebral edema syndrome, which is a phenomenon seen in children more commonly than in adults. This kind of cerebral edema can come on very rapidly and has a very high associated mortality. The child needs to be treated aggressively medically to keep cerebral perfusion pressure over 60 mm Hg and intracranial pressure under 20 mm Hg. This case also illustrates well why children with seemingly minor head injuries should be observed in the pediatric intensive care unit.

References

[1] Wexler MR, Neuman A, Umanski F, et al. A decade of experience in craniofacial surgery [in Hebrew]. Harefuah. 1992; 122(3):146–152

[2] McClain, CD, McManus ML. Intensive care risks of pediatric neurosurgery. In: Brambrink AM, Kirsch JR, eds. Essentials of Neurosurgical Anesthesia and Critical Care. New York, NY: Springer; 2012:565–573

[3] López Pisón J, Galván Manso M, Rubio Morales L, Juan Belloc S, , Ferreras Amez A, Melendo Gimeno J. Descriptive analysis of neurological disorders in the pediatric intensive care unit of a regional reference hospital [in Spanish]. An Esp Pediatr. 2000; 53(2):119–124

[4] Jones HR, Jr. Guillain-Barré syndrome: perspectives with infants and children. Semin Pediatr Neurol. 2000; 7(2):91–102

[5] Cantagrel S, Ducrocq S, Chédeville G, Marchand S. Mortality in a pediatric hospital. Six-year retrospective study [in French]. Arch Pediatr. 2000; 7(7):725–731

[6] Boldt J, Maleck W. Intensive care research in Germany–an analysis of papers in important international journals [in German]. Anasthesiol Intensivmed Notfallmed Schmerzther. 1999; 34 (9):542–548

[7] Farrell MM, Levin DL. Brain death in the pediatric patient: historical, sociological, medical, religious, cultural, legal, and ethical considerations. Crit Care Med. 1993; 21(12):1951–1965

[8] Gomella LG. Clinician's Pocket Reference. Norwalk, CT: Appleton & Lange; 1997

[9] Meyers RS. Pediatric fluid and electrolyte therapy. J Pediatr Pharmacol Ther. 2009; 14(4):204–211

[10] Fuhrman BP. Pediatric Critical Care. St Louis, MO: CV Mosby; 1998

[11] Abbate B, Donati P, Cagnoni G. Head injuries in children. Considerations on 3,715 consecutive cases [in Italian]. Minerva Pediatr. 2000; 52(11):623–628

[12] Guidelines for the Acute Medical Management of Severe Traumatic Brain Injury in Infants, Children, and Adolescents- Second Edition. Pediatr Crit Care Med 2012, 13: s1-s82. https://braintrauma.org/uploads/03/15/guidelines_pediatric2_2.pdf

[13] Smith ER, Madsen JR. Neurosurgical aspects of critical care neurology. Semin Pediatr Neurol. 2004; 11(2):169–178

[14] Smith ER, Madsen JR. Cerebral pathophysiology and critical care neurology: basic hemodynamic principles, cerebral perfusion, and intracranial pressure. Semin Pediatr Neurol. 2004; 11(2):89–104

[15] Levin DL. Pediatric Intensive Care. 2nd ed. New York, NY: Churchill Livingstone; 1997

[16] Andrews BT. Intensive Care in Neurosurgery. New York, NY: Thieme; 2003

[17] Ogawa A, Nakamura N, Sugita K, Sakurai Y, Kayama T, Wada T, Suzuki J. Regional cerebral blood flow in children–normal value and regional distribution of cerebral blood flow in childhood. No To Shinkei. 1987; 39:113–118

[18] Raimondi AJ. Pediatric Neurosurgery. New York, NY: Springer-Verlag; 1987

[19] McLaurin RL. Pediatric Neurosurgery. Philadelphia, PA: WB Saunders; 1989

[20] Merritt RJ. Cholestasis associated with total parenteral nutrition. J Pediatr Gastroenterol Nutr. 1986; 5(1):9–22

[21] Roche AF and Gussler JD. The gastrointestinal response to injury, starvation, and enteral nutrition: report of the Eighth Ross Conference on Medical Research. Columbus, OH: Ross Laboratories; 1988

[22] Harris JA, Benedict F. A Biometric Study of Basal Metabolism in Man. Washington, DC: Carnegie Institute; 1919

[23] Kochanek PM. Chapter 16. Glucose and nutrition. Pediatr Crit Care Med. 2012; 13:S68–S71– http://journals.lww.com/pccmjournal/Citation/2012/01001/Chapter_16__Glucose_and_nutrition.17.aspx

[24] Casella EB, Mângia CM. Management of acute seizure episodes and status epilepticus in children [in Portuguese]. J Pediatr (Rio J). 1999; 75 Suppl 2:S197–S206

[25] Brettfeld C, Gobrogge R, Massoud N, Munzenberger P, Nigro M, Sarnaik A. Evaluation of Ames Ser-alyzer for the therapeutic drug monitoring of phenobarbital and phenytoin. Ther Drug Monit. 1989; 11(5):612–615

[26] It's Your Health Care–Health Canada. Diagnostics x-rays and pregnancy. http://www.hc-sc.gc.ca/iyh-vsv/med/xray-radiographie_e.html. Accessed November 3, 2016

[27] Allan WC, Sobel DB. Neonatal intensive care neurology. Semin Pediatr Neurol. 2004; 11(2):119–128

25 Systemic Complications and Disease-Specific Phenomena Leading to Ischemic Injury

Hammad Ghanchi and Dan E. Miulli

Abstract

The neurointensivist is first an intensivist, trained to treat all systems of the body in the acute care setting. In addition this clinician must understand how each system affects and is affected by the brain and spinal cord. All treatment in the neurosurgical intensive care unit should be directed at preventing ischemic central nervous system injury by optimizing the other body systems to deliver the proper amount of substrate to the brain and spinal cord. The delivery of substrate must remain consistent and within parameters necessary to overcome the current injury and to prevent further injury. Thus normal parameters of perfusion, oxygenation, metabolite delivery, and physiological function should not be kept normal but must be altered to meet the altered demands of ischemic nervous system tissue and nervous tissue that is in the penumbra of the injury. Without a thorough knowledge of the nervous system just maintaining the normal physiological conditions of all other body systems may cause irreversible neurologic damage and a poor outcome.

Keywords: acidosis, anaerobic, extracted oxygen, hyperbaric oxygenation, infarction, organ dysfunction, oxygen binding capacity, Winter's formula

Case Presentation

A 69-year-old Hispanic woman undergoes craniotomy for evacuation of a traumatic subdural hematoma at a community hospital and is transferred on postoperative day 2 to a tertiary care trauma center for a higher level of care in the neurosurgical intensive care unit. At the original hospital, her abnormally high glucose level was not corrected because it was considered a normal reaction to the steroids she was being treated with "for brain swelling." She arrived at the trauma center with a Glasgow Coma Scale score of 5 and a blood pressure of 85/50. She was loaded with Dilantin at the original hospital, and started on 100 mg doses every 8 hours. No neuroimaging was sent with the patient.

See end of chapter for Case Management.

25.1 Introduction

The neurological intensive care unit (NICU) is not specific to just neurologic disease; aberrances in the normal neurologic state can lead to several systemic malfunctions. Obeying the basic principle in neurosurgery of the Monro–Kellie Doctrine, dealing with any factors that obscure the circuitry of the human body can result in altering single terminal synaptic neurotransmitter output to systemic serum hormonal fluctuations; this leads to organ dysfunction and failures and manifest as diseases commonly seen in the medical intensive care unit, along with not-so-common disease states. The most common diagnoses encountered in the NICU include strokes, intracranial hemorrhages, traumatic brain and spinal injuries, cerebral and spinal neoplasms, seizures, and postoperative neurosurgical patients. Many of these patients appear stable on admission but can quickly become the sickest patients in the hospital with a cubic millimeter displacement in neural tissue.

This chapter reviews the chief systemic complications and disease-specific phenomena most often encountered in the NICU patient along with the common treatment recommendations, and it offers recommendations to prevent their occurrence.

25.2 Ischemic Brain Injury

The human brain makes up less than 3% of the total body weight but requires around 25% of the total energy demand of the body; this metabolic rate is 3.5 times greater than that of other primates. The resting brain consumes 25–30 µmol/100 g/min of glucose and 130–180 µmol/100 g/min of oxygen. Normal cerebral blood flow (50–60 mL/100 g/min) is needed to maintain function.[1] ▶ Table 25.1 demonstrates neurologic change with reduced blood flow. Within seconds of ischemia, slowing of cortical activity is evident on electroencephalogram. This protective mechanism slightly decreases metabolic requirements, but less than 4 minutes of deprived blood flow starts to cause irreversible changes.[2] Efflux of potassium and influx of sodium and calcium due to the energy-dependent ion pump dysfunction lead to cell death. Release of glutamate, a primarily excitatory neurotransmitter, from the cell body exacerbates this process, exciting neighboring neurons in an energy-deprived environment and facilitating calcium entry into the cell, leading to further irreversible injury —known as excitotoxicity.

Responses to ischemic injuries vary in each tissue. The vasculature in the brain lacks innervation from sympathetic and parasympathetic systems; rather it is regulated by the parenchymal neurons, primarily astrocytes. The initial cellular response due to insufficient oxygen is production of lactic acid from the anaerobic metabolism of glucose; this leads to a decrease in pH. The acidic

Table 25.1 Neurologic change with reduced blood flow

Rate of cerebral blood flow (mL/100 g/min)	Neurologic change
50–60	Normal
25–30	Mild to moderate deficit; electrical impairment
16–20	Severe deficit; electrical failure
10–12	Profound deficit, ion pump failure, cytotoxic edema
<10	Metabolic failure

environment plus increasing carbon dioxide, from blood outflow, results in a right shift in the hemoglobin–oxygen dissociation curve—lessening the affinity of oxygen for hemoglobin and thus causing its release from the blood cell to the surrounding tissue. The increased carbon dioxide also causes vasodilation in an attempt to increase cerebral perfusion. Additionally, nitric oxide (NO) is produced as a vasodilator, generated by NO synthase in the endothelial cells; however, increased amounts of it can damage the blood–brain barrier, leading to further cerebral edema.[2] The end goal of uncorrected energy requirements is cell necrosis, increased cytotoxic edema, increased intracranial pressure, further injury to surrounding brain parenchyma, and eventual herniation of brain tissue.

Recovery of necrotic tissue after initial insult (primary brain injury) is futile in the central nervous system; medical and surgical efforts are aimed at the penumbra, or perilesional zone, and reducing harmful effects on the remainder of the unaffected tissue. Much of the deterioration that takes place clinically is due to secondary injury, which progresses hours to days after the initial damage. Optimizing blood pressure, brain oxygenation, cerebral perfusion pressure, and intracranial pressures is the cornerstone of successful neurologic intensive care.

25.3 Systemic Complications

25.3.1 Oxygenation

Hypoxia

The oxygen concentration in serum is the combination of oxygen bound to hemoglobin and the oxygen dissolved in plasma. It can be expressed by the following equation:

$$\text{Oxygen Content}_{\text{Serum}}\left(\frac{\text{mL}}{\text{dL}}\right) = \{1.34 \ \times [\text{Hgb}] \ \times \text{SatO}_2\}_A + \{0.003^* \ \times \text{PP}_{\text{Oxy}}\}_B.$$

The neurosurgeon does not need to memorize this equation, but a fundamental understanding of it is important for critical care. In this equation, the first bracket (A) is the oxygen content contributed by hemoglobin, and the second bracket (B) is oxygen dissolved in the serum.

a) The oxygen-binding capacity of hemoglobin (expressed in mL/g; 1 gram of hemoglobin will bind 1.34 mL of oxygen) is 1.34. One gram of hemoglobin normally binds 1.39 mL of oxygen; however, a small percentage is carboxyhemoglobin and methemoglobin so a value of 1.34 was found to be more representative. This value is multiplied by the concentration of hemoglobin and the percent of hemoglobin that is saturated (obtained from the pulse oxygenation).

b) The solubility of oxygen relies on the partial pressure of oxygen (PP_{Oxy}) and the solubility coefficient (0.003 mL/dL/mm Hg) of oxygen, which is *expressed at 37°C.

The following calculation assumes hemoglobin concentration of 15 g/dL, pulse oxygenation at 99%, partial pressure of oxygen in serum at 95 mm Hg, and body temperature of 37°C:

$$\text{Oxygen Content}_{Serum}\left(\frac{mL}{dL}\right) = \{1.34 \times [Hgb] \times SatO_2\}_A + \{0.003^* \times PP_{Oxy}\}_B.$$

$$\text{Oxygen Content}_{Arterial}\left(\frac{mL}{dL}\right) = \{1.34 \times 15 \times 0.99\}_A + \{0.003 \times 95\}_B.$$

$$\text{Oxygen Content}_{Arterial}\left(\frac{mL}{dL}\right) = \{19.9\}_A + \{0.29\}_B.$$

$$\text{Oxygen Content}_{Arterial}\left(\frac{mL}{dL}\right) = 20.2\,\frac{mL}{dL}.$$

▶ Table 25.2 is tabulated using the above equation. Given the above calculations, there is a total of about 785 mL of oxygen available in the serum. The average resting human body consumes about 250 mL/min. This means a little over 3 minutes of oxygen is available in serum, *if* 100% is released to tissue.

Table 25.2 Example of oxygen content under physiological conditions

Normal oxygen values	Serum phase	
	Arterial	Venous
Partial pressure (mmHg)	95	40
Oxygen saturation (%)	99	70
Hgb-bound oxygen (mL/dL)	19.9	14.1
Dissolved oxygen (mL/dL)	0.29	0.12
Serum oxygen content (mL/dL)	20.2	14.2
Volume (L)	1.25	3.75
Total oxygen (mL)	252	533

Note: Assumption of 5 liters normal serum volume with 25% in arterial and 75% in venous circulation.

437

Hypoxemia is defined by decreased oxygen in the serum, measured indirectly by the partial pressure of oxygen in serum. Hypoxemia can lead to *tissue hypoxia.* Cerebral hypoxia can be detrimental; loss of blood flow for 5 minutes is sufficient to cause irreversible changes. On the contrary, a similar change to cardiac myocytes requires 30 minutes.[2] Moreover, hypoxia leads to a disruption of the normal blood–brain barrier. The process of breakdown is multifactorial but is thought to be related to enhanced production of vascular endothelial growth factor, nitric oxide, and inflammatory cytokines. Experimental studies have demonstrated benefits of using simvastatin, minocycline, and melatonin in aiding with this hypoxic breakdown.[3] Avoiding a breakdown of the blood–brain barrier can reduce vasogenic edema and further aid in decreasing intracranial pressures.

After sufficient oxygenation of the blood has been achieved, the next step is oxygen delivery. The amount of oxygen delivered to tissue is dependent on the oxygen content on the serum (mL/dL) as defined earlier, multiplied by the cardiac output (CO)(L/min). Simplified, the equation is as follows:

$$D_{Oxygen} = (Oxygen\ Content_{Serum}) \times 10 \times CO.$$

A 10 multiplier is added to convert mL/dL to mL/L for the oxygen content. The average oxygen delivered is around 1,000 mL/min in the average human adult. Not all the oxygen delivered to the capillary bed is extracted; this can be calculated by comparing the oxygen content in the inflowing artery to the outflowing vein.

$$Extracted_{Oxygen} = (Oxygen\ Content_{Arterial} - Oxygen\ Content_{Venous}) \times 10 \times CO.$$

By extracting common variables, this equation is often simplified as follows:

$$Extracted_{Oxygen} = (Oxygen\ Sat_{Arterial} - Oxygen\ Sat_{Venous}) \times 13.4 \times [Hbg] \times CO.$$

Oxygen-deprived arterial blood will generally result in decreased venous oxygen content as it traverses the capillary bed. This is the principle behind measuring the venous oxygen content of the jugular vein ($SjVO_2$) in neurointensive care patients. This practice has recently been replaced by brain tissue oxygen tension ($PBtiO_2$) monitoring with intraparenchymal devices (e.g., Licox Brain Oxygen Monitoring System, Integra Neurosciences).

Hyperoxic Therapies

Hyperoxic normobaric therapy has been shown to be beneficial in the acute phase of brain injury and stroke. The most popular study was performed on patients with severe traumatic brain injury treated with 100% FIO_2, started within 6 hours, and continued for 24 hours. Intracerebral microdialysis demonstrated increased glucose and decreased glutamate and lactate levels.[4] Others have demonstrated reduction in lesion volume up to 100 mL and improved perilesional tissue oxygenation as measured by oxygen-15 positron emission tomographic scan. This was further verified by other researchers with hydrogen-magnetic resonance spectroscopy detection of N-acetylaspartate (a neuron-specific marker of mitochondrial dysfunction), which was found to be lower in the perilesional tissue with hyperoxic therapy.[5] Similarly, in patients with middle cerebral artery stroke, 40% FIO_2 as demonstrated decreased mortality and fewer complications.[6]

Hyperbaric oxygen therapy has also been tested in traumatic brain injury.[7,8,9,10] Normal atmospheric pressure at sea level is 1 ATM or 760 mm Hg. With hyperbaric treatment, up to 3 ATM of pressure is applied; this causes the oxygen content of plasma to rise from 0.3 to 6.6 mL per 100 mL of blood. Hemoglobin oxygen content is affected at a very minuscule level, not enough to be clinically significant. This would cause the above serum oxygen of 20.2 to increase to 26.5 mL/dL. The proposed benefit of this therapy is vasoconstriction; the increased oxygen content requires less blood volume to meet oxygen demands.[7] This is the same mechanism proposed for crush injuries and burns for other tissue; going back the Monro–Kellie doctrine, less blood content means decreased intracranial pressure. An average improvement of 2.68 GCS points has been found in the literature for traumatic brain injury patients treated with hyperbaric therapy.[11] It has also been shown to reduce brain inflammation in animal models.[12] Further trials are needed in human patients before this becomes standard therapy.

Ventilated Patients

In ventilated patients, common etiologies of hypoxia must be aggressively determined. To maintain adequate cerebral and systemic oxygenation, oxygen-carrying capacity, acid–base balance, and pulmonary pathologies should be determined. Some key markers that signal poor oxygenation are the alveolar-arterial gradient, lactate level, base deficit, and serum bicarbonate.

The base deficit is defined by the amount of base that must be added to 1 L of blood to raise the pH to normal (7.40). It has been used as a marker for injury severity in trauma and its normalization as a goal to reach an end point in resuscitation after acute injury.[13] Serum bicarbonate can be used in a similar manner but is less specific than base deficit, albeit easier to obtain through venous sample.[14]

In the setting of metabolic acidosis, Winter's formula is helpful in determining whether respiratory compensation in present. It is given as follows:

$$P_{CO2} = (1.5 \times [HCO_3^-]) + 8 \pm 2.$$

The patient's actual P_{CO2} is compared to the range formulated from the above equation. If the patient's P_{CO2} is higher than the range predicted by Winter's formula, then primary respiratory acidosis is also present. If the P_{CO2} is lower than the range, then primary respiratory alkalosis is present.[15] For example, if the patient presents with metabolic acidosis and is found to have a pH of 7.42 and bicarbonate of 18,

$$P_{CO2} = \left(1.5 \ \times \left[HCO_3^-\right]\right) + 8 \pm 2.$$

$$P_{CO2} = \left(1.5 \ \times 18\right) + 8 \pm 2.$$

$$P_{CO2} = \left(27\right) + 8 \pm 2.$$

$$P_{CO2} = 35 \pm 2.$$

The patient's expected P_{CO2} should be between 33 and 37 mm Hg if no instance of respiratory acidosis or alkalosis is present.

25.3.2 Anemia

Anemia is conventionally defined as a decrease in red blood cells or hemoglobin in the serum. A more valid and functional definition is a decrease in the oxygen-carrying capacity of the blood.[16] The optimal goals for hemoglobin and hematocrit values are not well established. However, observing the equation for oxygen content above, it is evident that hemoglobin plays the largest role in maintaining an adequate level of oxygenation in the blood. Patients with multisystem trauma or prolonged stays in the NICU are at greater risk of developing anemia of various etiologies. All primary sources of bleeding should be aggressively sought. Patients with blunt chest or abdominal injury should be evaluated for hemothorax and retroperitoneal bleeding, respectively. Other rare causes include medication reaction but are usually accompanied by hemolysis.

Hypoxemia is conventionally measured through partial pressure of oxygen in serum. However, as already described, hemoglobin plays a significant role in serum oxygen concentration. As shown in ▶ Table 25.3, a 50% reduction in hemoglobin (15–7.5 g/dL) results in almost equal reduction in oxygen content, whereas a 50% reduction in partial pressure (95–47.5 mm Hg) results in less than 1% change.

Table 25.3 Oxygen concentrations in different physiological conditions

Serum oxygenation	Normal	Anemia	Hypoxemia
Partial pressure (mm Hg)	95	95	47.5
Oxygen saturation (%)	99	99	99
Hgb concentration (g/dL)	15	7.5	15
Hgb-bound oxygen (mL/dL)	19.9	9.9	19.9
Dissolved oxygen (mL/dL)	0.29	0.29	0.14
Serum oxygen content (mL/dL)	20.2	10.2	20.04

Table 25.3 continued

Serum oxygenation	Normal	Anemia	Hypoxemia
Volume (L)	1.25	1.25	1.25
Total oxygen (mL)	252	128	250
Serum oxygen reduction		49%	0.01%

A normal hematocrit ranges from 40 to 54% for males and 38 to 47% for females. A hematocrit greater than 30% is generally used to optimize cerebral blood flow.[17,18] Newer studies for nonneurosurgical patients have shown evidence for adoption of conservative transfusion thresholds. One study claims to provide evidence for a transfusion threshold of 7 g/dL for head-injury patients; however, the lowest mean for the experimental arm was 9.6 g/dL and thus failed to provide significant evidence.[19] With a lack of transfusion studies specific to neurosurgery patients, when caring for the organ with the highest oxygen requirements, we recommend a more liberal approach by keeping hemoglobin concentrations greater than 10 g/dL hematocrit greater than 30% for patients with a central nervous system disease or disorder.

25.3.3 Fever versus Hyperthermia

Fever, or pyrexia, is defined as a body temperature of greater than 101°F or 38.3°C with a normal thermoregulatory system. Any condition capable of triggering an inflammatory response can cause a fever through release of cytokines, which act on the hypothalamus to elevate body temperature. Hyperthermia is the result of a defect in temperature regulation. Both result in elevated body temperatures; however, the former responds to antipyretics (like acetaminophen), whereas the latter does not.

Fever is known to develop in 30% of stroke patients within 48 hours.[20] Moreover, pyrexia in head injuries has been associated with worse outcomes.[21] In the case of head injury, fevers can originate from cerebral tissue necrosis, intracerebral hemorrhage, or even disturbance in central thermoregulation from mass effect. No matter the source, infectious causes should be aggressively sought and treated in addition to antipyretic therapy and cooling measures. One specific cause of fever seen with head injury is sympathetic storming; this phenomenon is discussed later in this chapter but should always be kept as a possible differential for fever when other workup is negative. Other possible causes to keep in mind are drug-induced fevers, transfusion reactions, and postoperative fevers.

Pyrexia is a potent vasodilator and can raise intracranial pressure and cerebral metabolic requirement for oxygen ($CMRO_2$). The increase in $CMRO_2$ is one of the primary reasons that fever should be avoided in the NICU. Moreover, increased temperature causes a decrease in hemoglobin's affinity for oxygen.

441

As discussed earlier, the goal should be to keep cerebral tissue oxygenation at the ideal levels. Untreated pyrexia will lead to hypoxia and may lead to stroke-like symptoms, which manifest as an acute change in neurologic exam. An additional consideration is to avoid shivering when getting the patient to a euthermic state; excessive shivering can lead to rhabdomyolysis.

25.3.4 Electrolyte Disturbances

Aberrant electrolytes are the most common complication seen in the NICU, occurring in 59.3% of the Traumatic Coma Data Bank register.[22] They are primarily in the category of early complications, seen from the time of admission through the first 5 days. It is therefore imperative to monitor fluid status, including total intake and output, daily body weight, and color and specific gravity of urine, to avoid unnecessary cerebral edema or volume contraction. Consideration must be made for patients on chronic diuretics, nasogastric or orogastric suction tubes, or with fever or diarrhea. Serum sodium and glucose are principally addressed due to their effects on serum osmolality (see equation below). Sodium is present intra- and extracellularly and cannot easily diffuse passively between the two compartments; observing the osmolality calculation, one can easily surmise that sodium is the major determinant of tonicity.

$$\text{Serum Osmolality}\left(\text{Normal } 275 - 295\,\frac{\text{mOsm}}{\text{kg}}\right) = 2 \times \left[\text{Na}^+\right] + \frac{[\text{BUN}]}{2.8} + \frac{[\text{Glucose}]}{18}.$$

Additionally, viscosity becomes an issue with increasing serum osmolality. When blood is flowing through capillaries that are less than $6\,\mu m$ in diameter, some smaller than an erythrocyte, hyperosmolar serum can cause a decrease in the normal cerebral blood flow. This retardation in blood flow can deprive neural tissue of essential nutrients and lead to ischemic changes if minimal metabolic requirements are not maintained.

Abnormalities in serum potassium are frequently encountered due to gastric suctioning, diarrhea, and medications. Along with correcting the underlying pathology, normal serum concentrations should be maintained. As already described, serum bicarbonate can be used as a marker for hypovolemia, especially in trauma patients. If other signs of volume depletion are present, efforts should be made to promptly correct the deficit.

25.3.5 Hyperglycemia

Glucose is vital for almost all cellular processes and is the primary source of energy for cerebral tissue. The passage of glucose is facilitated by a family of membrane transport proteins known as GLUT (glucose transporter). Many variations of these transporters exist, but GLUT1 and GLUT3 are the primary ones employed by cerebral and neuronal tissue. GLUT1 was found to be the primary transporter at the blood–brain barrier but is also found in other regions of the body. The transporter of interest is GLUT3, which is found almost exclusively in the neuronal population and has a fivefold affinity for glucose. This is thought to be the evolutionary advantage because neural tissue is the last organ you would want to deprive of energy during times of prolonged starvation. But this advantage becomes detrimental during brain injury.

Many studies have shown worse outcomes in NICU patients with poor glucose control. Hyperglycemia usually reflects a stress reaction, mediated by the sympathetic response that prevents glucose entry into nonessential fight-or-flight tissue, and can worsen outcome after traumatic brain injury, likely due to increased cerebral edema.[23,24] At the writing of this book, the GAMES trial is under way from which preliminary data have shown a continuous glyburide infusion to be associated with decreased cerebral edema.[25] Conversely, serum glucose should not be kept under tight regulation; strict regulations resulted in increased metabolic load, and cerebral microdialysis demonstrated more frequent critical reductions in glucose and elevations of lactate–pyruvate ratio.[26] We recommend blood glucose < 150 mg/dL.

A secondary effect of hyperglycemia is the transitional shift of water from the intracellular compartment into the serum. This dilutes the serum and can present as pseudohyponatremia. For every 100 mg/dL increase in glucose, there is a 1.6 mEq/L reduction in sodium. As the hyperglycemia is corrected, by the glucose shifting into cells, the water follows and autocorrects the osmolality. An inverse effect of hyperglycemia is hypercoagulability and increased serum viscosity; increased serum glucose concentrations have been shown to increase serum fibrinogen.[27] Increased serum viscosity and increased risk of thrombus formation are both detrimental complications if occurring in the cerebral vasculature; ultimately leading to ischemic injury.

25.3.6 Blood Pressure

Multiple methods to measure blood pressure exist in the NICU. Indirect methods with the pressure cuff are quick and easy. Many hospitals have transitioned from the auscultatory method to the oscillometric method, which has been shown to give more accurate measurements. Direct measurements are invasive but can give a real-time measurement. Normotension, and in some cases, hypertension, is an essential state to maintain in the NICU.

Hypotension

Patients in the NICU frequently have episodes of hypotension. In multitrauma patients, other etiologies must be entertained, necessitating examination of pulse pressure, oxygen saturation, arterial blood gases, and cardiopulmonary and abdominal compartments. In patients with severe traumatic brain injury (Glasgow Coma Scale score ≤ 8), it has been shown that a single episode of systolic blood pressure < 90 mm Hg, from injury to arrival at the hospital, doubles the mortality. In the NICU, eliminating hypotension would reduce unfavorable outcome (Glasgow Outcome Scores 1, 2, and 3) by 9.3%.[22] Additionally, patients with spinal cord injuries are prone to sustained hypotension, which, if not corrected, can lead to infarction.

To limit the effects of hypotension, the following recommendations are made:

- Patients with severe traumatic brain injury should have cerebral perfusion pressure > 50 mm Hg in most cases.
- Patients should be kept euvolemic to slightly hypervolemic, with a normal central venous pressure 6–8 mm Hg.
- Episodes of hypotension/suboptimal cerebral perfusion pressure should be treated first with fluids, then with vasopressors as necessary.

Spinal Cord Injuries and Hypotension

Patients with spinal cord injuries develop hypotension from a lack of sympathetic input to the vasculature, causing pooling and decreased return to the right heart, as well as unopposed parasympathetic tone to the heart, resulting in bradycardia. The goal of therapy is to maintain systolic blood pressure > 90 mm Hg. Moreover, studies have demonstrated using the mean arterial pressure to treat spinal cord injuries. Mean arterial pressure > 85 mm Hg is the current recommendation for acute spinal cord injuries.

The following general considerations apply to the treatment of spinal cord injuries:

- Maintain spinal precautions.
- Provide adequate oxygenation.
- Prescribe atropine for bradycardia and dopamine or norepinephrine for hypotension.
- Continue judicious fluid management.
- Watch for development of pulmonary edema.
- Start vasopressors (dopamine is the vasopressor of choice, although no difference is seen with norepinephrine).

Methylprednisolone use in spinal cord injury is controversial and not used in our practice except for specific cases. It has been associated with increased risk of infection, such as pneumonia, which increases intensive care unit days and ventilator days.[28,29] Some authors even equate it to using leeches.[30] Our practice initiates treatment for incomplete spinal cord injury to regain nerve root level function. If a patient will gain meaningful function by regaining activity at the injured nerve root level (e.g., transfer oneself from a wheelchair) then we initiate therapy. The original recommendation for it to be started within 8 hours of injury[31] is not applicable. The initial dosage is 30 mg/kg intravenous bolus over 15 minutes (rate [mL/h] = patient's weight [kg] × 1.92). After a 45-minute pause, the maintenance dose is 5.4 mg/kg/h (rate [mL/h] = weight [kg] × 0.0864). The duration of maintenance therapy depends on the timing of the initial bolus. If it is given < 3 hours from injury, maintenance steroids should be continued for 23 hours. If the initial dose is given 3 to 8 hours after injury, continue for 47 hours.[32]

Other investigational medications are naloxone, tirilazad mesylate, and lazaroid.[33,34]

Hypertension

Elevated blood pressure is of particular consequence in the NICU. Patients with unsecured aneurysms, arteriovenous malformations (AVMs), or intraparenchymal hematomas should have strict parameters for hypertension. However, hypertension associated with bradycardia and respiratory depression (Cushing's triad) is symbolic for dangerously elevated intracranial pressure and demands immediate evaluation. These symptoms may be easily missed if the patient is on a ventilator or because of autonomic instability.[35] Any sudden spike in blood pressure should warrant a neurologic exam to assess for possible impending herniation.

Intravenous Treatment of Hypertension

Nitrates, specifically nitroglycerine and nitroprusside, may elevate intracranial pressure and should not be used. They preferentially dilate peripheral vasculature, creating a cerebral steal phenomenon. Prolonged use of nitroprusside may also lead to thiocyanate toxicity.

Labetalol blocks α_1 and β_1, and β_2 receptors. It has no effect on intracranial pressure. Labetalol may be used in controlled congestive heart failure: no coronary steal effect. It is contraindicated in asthma. It should also be avoided if cocaine or methamphetamine abuse is suspected. The maximum dose is 300 mg/d. This is first line for hypertension.

Enalaprilat is an angiotensin-converting enzyme inhibitor that acts within 15 minutes. Side effects include hyperkalemia and angioedema. Up to 5 mg every 6 hours is tolerated well.

Nicardipine is a dihydropyridine calcium channel blocker that acts systemically on vascular smooth muscle to lower peripheral resistance. It has been shown to have no effect on significantly raising intracranial pressure, or increasing cerebral bleeding, and edema, but it does lower cerebral perfusion pressure.[36] It can be started as a continuous infusion at 5 mg/h and titrated up to 15 mg/h.

445

25.3.7 Thromboembolism

Deep venous thrombosis (DVT) is a common complication in the NICU. Although no hypercoagulable state is usually present, other risk factors, including endothelial damage and venous stasis, are due to immobilization or predisposing trauma. DVT may be as prevalent as 58% if no prophylaxis is used.[37] Other risk factors include spinal cord injury; pelvic, femur, or tibial fractures; surgery; blood transfusion; and older age.[37] We recommend starting nonchemical DVT prophylaxis with sequential compression devices and graded compression stockings on admission, from either the emergency room or the operating room. Timing to start chemical prophylaxis, and choice of agent, is controversial, especially for trauma. We advocate adding chemical DVT prophylaxis 24 hours after repeat imaging has shown no potential bleeding, or stabilization of previous bleeds, and the neurologic exam is steady. If prolonged immobility is expected, as in the case with complete spinal cord injury, an inferior vena cava filter should be considered.

Sequential compression stockings and low-dose unfractionated heparin have been found to decrease the incidence of thromboembolism from 8.98 to 2.9%.[38] Low-molecular-weight heparins, such as enoxaparin and fondaparinux, have shown a higher incidence of intracranial bleeds. Commonly quoted trauma studies[39] have shown no difference in the two, but a closer look at the data shows that complications arose in patients with head injuries.[40] We advocate unfractionated heparin 8,000 units subcutaneously every 8 hours due to its relatively short half-life and proven neutralization with protamine, which is questionable with low-molecular-weight heparins. Furthermore, when removing any surgical drains, heparin should be stopped for 24 hours.

25.3.8 Coagulopathy

Serologic markers for disseminated intravascular coagulation (fibrinogen split products) and degree of traumatic brain injury have been positively correlated.[41] The most common site for diffuse intravascular thrombosis is the central nervous system, often resulting in necrosis.[42] Microvascular and radiographically evident petechial hemorrhages and contusions are thought to be the result of disseminated intravascular coagulation. Coagulopathy usually presents 6–72 hours after the trauma, and its presence following traumatic brain injury has been associated as a strong predictor of in-hospital mortality.[43] The mechanism for this state is unknown. Independent risk factors for coagulopathy in isolated head injuries include a Glasgow Coma Scale score of ≤ 8, hypotension upon admission, cerebral edema, subarachnoid hemorrhage, and midline shift. The development of traumatic brain injury coagulopathy is associated with a longer intensive care unit length of stay and an almost 10-fold increased risk of death.[44]

25.3.9 Sepsis

Sepsis is diagnosed by vital signs meeting the criteria for systemic inflammatory response syndrome (SIRS) along with a source for infection. SIRS can result from a wide variety of etiologies, including infections, trauma, and stress. The criteria for the diagnosis of SIRS are heart rate > 90, temperature > 38°C or < 36°C, tachypnea > 20 breaths/minute, and white blood cell count > 12,000 cells/mm^3 or < 4,000 cells/mm^3.

Sepsis has been associated with a twofold increase in mortality in the NICU. Lungs have been identified as the most common source of infection, 93% in one study, with gram-positive organisms accounting for greater than 50% of the cases.[45] Sepsis results in a derangement of fluid balance via an array of pathologies. Insensible water loss results from elevated temperatures. Depleted intravascular volume is multifactorial, but principally due to increased microvascular permeability[46] and increased venous compliance, resulting in pooling.

Diagnosis hinges on a thorough examination of the patient and guided laboratory studies. Examination of the patient's skin for decubitus ulcers or infiltrated intravenous or central lines is crucial. Removal of all indwelling central catheters, peripheral lines, and Foley catheters with culture is paramount for removing a possible nidus of infection. A chest X-ray should be performed to evaluate for pneumonia or empyema. Blood cultures should be drawn from two different sites, and antibiotics should be started prophylactically. Arterial blood gas and lactate should also be drawn to evaluate for any pulmonary compromise and fluid status.

Initial empirical antibiotic treatment should be employed after cultures are taken. Broad-spectrum treatment with two or more antibiotics may be started and tailored once final cultures and sensitivities have returned. Aggressive hydration is also a cornerstone of treatment; initial infusion of 30 mL/kg of crystalloid therapy over a 30-minute period is recommended for septic shock which is the term when the patient is unable to maintain an adequate blood pressure due to infection. When crystalloid fluids are not adequate to maintain perfusion, norepinephrine is typically the initial vasopressor of choice. Norepinephrine has been shown to have lower short-term mortality and lower rates of arrhythmias than dopamine, which was previously used. Dopamine and vasopressin can be supplementary if needed. Endogenous vasopressin levels often spike at the initial stages of septic shock, but this results in depleted level in advanced stages of sepsis.[47] Therefore, adding low-dose vasopressin to therapy has been shown to reduce norepinephrine requirements.[48] Depending on the severity of sepsis, a cardiac output monitoring system (FloTrac sensor/Vigileo monitor, Edwards Lifesciences) is often necessary to assess fluid volume, vascular resistance, and cardiac output.

Septic encephalopathy is a disorder where the infection originates outside the central nervous system and has been reported in up to 70% of patients with sepsis. Its mechanism is poorly understood but involves the accumulation of toxins, such as ammonia, inflammatory cytokines, and bacterial endotoxins (such as lipopolysaccharide) leading to disturbances in the blood–brain barrier.[49] This in turn increases cerebral edema and causes further neurologic deterioration. Therefore, infections should be treated before they progress to sepsis to avoid further injury to NICU patients.

25.3.10 Gastrointestinal Bleed

Ulceration of the gastric mucosa is commonly seen with traumatic brain injury. The ulcers are often termed Cushing's ulcers due to Harvey Cushing having reported patients with epigastric pain, vomiting, and cerebral neoplasms. Although the mechanism is not fully understood, most experts theorize increased intracranial pressure causes excess stimulation of the vagal nerve that leads to an excess of acetylcholine released onto the gastric parietal cells. The resultant increase in gastric acidity weakens the gastric mucosa. Cerebral edema impacting the hypothalamus (vagal area located in the anterior hypothalamus) and/or brainstem (vagal nuclei) is the suspected cause of the increased vagal stimulation.[50]

Kamada et al[46] found that endoscopic evaluation of gastric mucosa demonstrates damage within the first 24 hours, with 17% of these erosions progressing to systemically significant hemorrhages. The severity of brain injury is directly related to the development of gastric bleeding.[51] Other risk factors for gastric bleeding include respiratory failure, burns > 25% body surface area, hypotension, sepsis, jaundice, peritonitis, coagulopathy, and hepatic failure. Prophylaxis includes antacids, which neutralize gastric acidity but are time consuming; histamine type 2 (H2) blockers, which block acid production but are potentially sedating and have a possible side effect of thrombocytopenia; proton pump inhibitors, which are more efficacious than blocking acid production but chronic use (> 2 weeks) has been associated with adverse effects, such as inability to wean off proton pump inhibitors, iron deficiency, and a decrease in all hematologic indexes from baseline[52]; and sucralfate, which strengthens gastric mucosa, does not alter gastrin, acid production, or pH, and produces less nosocomial pneumonia association. Proton pump inhibitors' potential to cause anemia has been the major reason we avoid its use in our NICU; instead we opt for H2 blockers and sucralfate.

25.3.11 Seizures

In those patients with severe head injury, seizures occur in ~ 15%.[17] At times seizures may be difficult to monitor in the NICU because of sedatives and paralytics. There should be a heightened clinical suspicion to detect and subsequently initiate treatment. Any acute change in neurologic exam should trigger the possibility of a seizure, even if the patient is on antiepileptic medication. A thorough neurologic exam is essential for all changes in mental status or limb paralysis. If clinically warranted, continuous electroencephalography is the method of choice for detection. Though not associated with worse morbidity or mortality, seizures can potentially impair jugular venous oxygen saturation ($SjvO_2$) if cerebral blood flow is already compromised.[46] The discharge of neurons places metabolic stress on the neural tissue and can provoke ischemic changes. Prophylaxis against posttraumatic seizures is controversial and should be discontinued after 7 days.[23,53] Patients who present with hematomas in the frontal, temporal, or parietal lobes should be placed on antiepileptics; blood's fibrotic properties make it an irritant to tissue; thus any possible irritation to the cerebral cortex increases the possibility of seizures. Moreover, an increase in intracranial pressure also lowers the threshold for firing and thus lowering the seizure threshold. Our recommendation is seizure prophylaxis for any patient with possible irritation of the cerebral cortex.

25.3.12 Paroxysmal Autonomic Instability with Dystonia or "Storming"

This is a poorly understood phenomenon that occurs after traumatic brain injury. It has also been referred to as diencephalic seizures in the literature, but no true epileptic waveforms have been described and therapeutic levels of antiepileptics have not alleviated the symptoms.[54] The name *paroxysmal autonomic instability with dystonia*, or PAID, was proposed in 2004 by Blackman et al.[35] Colloquially it is still referred to as storming. It manifests as paroxysmal changes in vital signs (e.g., fever, hypertension, tachycardia, and tachypnea) and neurologic exam (e.g., pupil size, posturing), hyperhidrosis, and excessive salivation. The most likely cause is attributed to autonomic dysfunction in the hypothalamus and/or inappropriate stimulation of the adrenal glands leading to a surge in catecholamines in the serum. These changes can take place multiple times during the day and last minutes to hours.

Many experts advocate using benzodiazepines, analgesic agents, and nonselective beta blockers. Others have reported bromocriptine, clonidine, and intrathecal baclofen to be effective. Dexmedetomidine, a centrally acting α_2 selective agonist, has been successful in our experience and supported recently in the literature[55]; presynaptic α_2 receptor stimulation blocks norepinephrine release and postsynaptic α_2 stimulation decreases sympathetic activity. In severe cases, even pentobarbital has been employed. No consensus currently exists on the exact mechanism, but we recommend starting treatment with dexmedetomidine and propranolol and then moving on to any combination of the above on a case-by-case basis.

25.4 Disease-Specific Phenomena

There is an array of diseases encountered in the neurointensive care unit. Many have specific disease complications that should be kept on the top of one's list of possible outcomes when admitting such patients. Measures should be taken to avoid the complication from occurring, and appropriate action should be taken with each specific phenomenon. All of the diseases discussed next can lead to mortality through ischemic brain injury if not corrected or properly treated.

25.4.1 Cerebral Vasospasm after Subarachnoid Hemorrhage

Mechanical narrowing or spasm of the lumen of cerebral vessels results in decreased blood flow, leading to ischemia and infarction. It is most commonly seen after aneurysmal subarachnoid hemorrhage (SAH), but it is also seen after traumatic SAH, intraventricular hemorrhage, and SAH of unknown etiology. It is the most significant cause of morbidity and mortality in patients surviving the initial aneurysm rupture. There are two components: clinical vasospasm (delayed ischemic neurologic deficit) and radiographic vasospasm. Radiographic vasospasm has a high incidence, up to 80%, but does not become clinical vasospasm until onset of ischemic injury to the cerebral tissue, about 55% of the time.[56]

Characteristics of Vasospasm

Vasospasms decrease blood flow to the brain and thus result in strokelike symptoms. The onset of cerebral vasospasm (CVS) almost never occurs before the third day after SAH and typically will have a peak incidence between days 6 and 10. Clinical spasm is usually resolved by the end of the second week posthemorrhage, although the onset can occur as late as day 21.

Radiographic CVSs are seen in 30 to 80% of angiograms,[57,58] as opposed to clinical spasms, which are seen in ~ 20 to 55% of patients after SAH. Radiographic spasm may occur in the absence of clinical spasm and vice versa (i.e., patients may have a small vessel spasm, causing neurologic deficit, but an angiogram may not be able to detect it). Mild CVSs are usually reversible, whereas severe CVSs can result in permanent deficits and death in 7% of patients. CVSs that occur early are associated with the worst neurologic deficits.

In 1980, Fisher et al[59] revealed a correlation between the thickness of the subarachnoid blood on CT scan and the risk of developing CVS. Patients classified as Fisher III (localized clot and/or vertical layer > 1 mm thick within the subarachnoid space) are at greatest risk of developing symptomatic CVS.

Twenty-three of the 24 patients in Fisher et al's study who were grade III developed clinical CVS.

Diagnosis of Vasospasm

Diagnosis of vasospasm is primarily clinical, but it can be confirmed and monitored with various radiological and neurodiagnostic tests. Clinical CVS in the anterior cerebral artery territory is more common than that of the middle cerebral artery.

Clinical signs:
- Worsening headache.
- Confusion/altered level of consciousness.
- Meningismus.
- Focal neurological deficit.

Methods of diagnosis:
- Transcranial Doppler (TCD)—least invasive, no radiation.
- Computed tomographic angiography (CTA).
- Magnetic resonance angiography (MRA).
- Xenon-enhanced computed tomography (CT perfusion).
- Digital subtraction angiography (DSA)—gold standard, most invasive.

Transcranial Doppler (TCD) ultrasound is the most used method of diagnosing and monitoring clinical CVSs. It measures blood velocity in major intracranial arteries (ICAs), which is used to determine if there may be arterial narrowing. Not only the actual velocity but also the relationship between the relative velocity of the ICAs and the velocity of flow in the internal carotid artery is important. This relationship is referred to as the Lindegaard ratio. It is commonly used to express the difference in velocity between the middle cerebral artery and the ICAs, but it is also used in velocity measurements of all large intracranial vessels. The Lindegaard ratio may help to distinguish vasospasm from hyperemia.[60]

Another option for visualizing spasm is computed tomographic angiography (CTA) of the head. It is a relatively quick way to look at the major vessels and diagnose spasm by comparing the caliber of the vessels. The only major shortcoming of this technique is the requirement of contrast administration; renal failure patients are not able to use this imaging modality. A contrastless option is available with magnetic resonance angiography (MRA) employing the time of flight technique. This modality requires more time but provides higher temporal resolution. In contrast, the CTA provides higher spatial resolution and able to provide a better overall picture to diagnose vasospasm. With the development of newer 3 tesla magnets and possibly adding gadolinium contrast, MRA spatial resolution is comparable to that of CTA.

451

Digital subtraction angiography (DSA) is the gold standard for visualizing the vessels of the brain. It also provides the opportunity for treatment through intra-arterial infusions. This is the most invasive procedure to diagnose vasospasm. Intra-arterial vasodilators can be infused as well as balloon angioplasty for mechanical dilatation (see below).

Xenon 133, xenon computed tomography, single-photon emission computed tomography, and positron emission tomography are among the other methods used to detect low-flow arterial states. However, these may not be routinely available at many institutions, and they may not be practical for daily or frequent use. TCD ultrasound is less time consuming, less costly, and can be used daily to monitor CVS and its response to treatment. CTAs can quickly provide a better overall picture of the cerebral vascular anatomy and aid in the confirmed diagnosis of vasospasm.

Treatment of Vasospasm

Treatment of CVS is aimed at preventing and reversing ischemic insults. Hypovolemia can hasten the onset of CVS, and spasm can be lessened or prevented by ensuring that post-SAH patients are adequately hydrated. Early surgery for clipping of aneurysms can allow for more aggressive hyperdynamic therapy and can also allow for removal of cisternal clots, reducing the incidence of CVS. The primary issue with vasospasm is decreased cerebral perfusion, which leads to lack of oxygen and glucose to neuronal tissues.

Currently, the use of nimodipine as a neuroprotectant and, alternatively, nicardipine has been found to offer protection by improving blood rheology, preventing calcium influx into injured cells, and acting as an antiplatelet aggregator. Additionally, patients chronically on statins, pravastatin and simvastatin, at admission were found to have better outcomes with SAH with reduced vasospasm; prospective studies have given controversial results.[61] The Simvastatin in Aneurysmal Subarachnoid Hemorrhage trial in 2014 found no benefit with the use of simvastatin in the acute phase.[62] Further studies are still being performed.

Hyperdynamic, or "triple-H," (hypertensive, hypervolemic, and hemodilution) therapy is the mainstay of treatment in patients with surgically or endovascularly treated aneurysms. A mild form of this type of therapy can be used in unsecured aneurysms, but it may cause the aneurysm to rerupture. Hyperdynamic therapy should not be started if there is a new cerebral hemorrhage, a new large infarct, or severe cerebral edema.[63]

Some experts advocate starting therapy prior to the onset of CVS to combat the common occurrence of hypovolemia in patients with SAH.[64] In a randomized, controlled trial, Lennihan et al[65] found that the prevention of hypovolemia rather than the promotion of hypervolemia was critical in the prevention of cerebral ischemia. Induction of hypervolemia can be done with isotonic/hypertonic crystalloids and with colloids (albumin) or blood.

After the ruptured aneurysms have been clipped or coiled, the neurosurgeon has greater freedom to use certain medicines to raise blood pressure. Vasopressors can be used to augment blood pressure to improve cerebral perfusion. In this approach, increase blood pressure in 10 to 15% increments until neurologic function shows improvement. This may require increasing systolic blood pressure to 240 mm Hg or mean arterial pressure to 150 mm Hg (for clipped aneurysms). Wean pressors upon improvement and allow blood pressure to fall to sustain an acceptable neurologic function. Targets for central venous pressure are 6 to 8 mm Hg; pulmonary capillary wedge pressure, 16 to 18 mm Hg.

Once a patient has evidence of symptomatic vasospasm, he or she should be treated with hyperdynamic therapy for at least 14 days or until symptoms resolve and there is no angiographic evidence of vasospasm. Complications of triple-H therapy include exacerbation of cerebral edema, pulmonary edema, intracerebral hemorrhage (ICH), worsened infarctions, rebleeding of unsecured aneurysms, myocardial infarction, and problems related to pulmonary artery catheter.

Transluminal Balloon Angioplasty

Transluminal balloon angioplasty allows the neurosurgeon to direct mechanical opening of a vessel using neuroendovascular techniques. It is reserved for patients with clinical vasospasm not improving using hyperdynamic therapy and with radiographic evidence of vasospasm. The best results are seen if the procedure is done within 24 hours of neurologic decline.[66,67,68,69] Up to 70% of patients can have clinical and lasting improvement.

Angioplasty should be avoided if there is a new cerebral hemorrhage or a large area of infarction because of the risk of reperfusion injury. Furthermore, angioplasty, if clinical and radiological benefits do not persist, may need to be repeated.

Endovascular use of intra-arterial nicardipine has shown some improvement in clinical vasospasm; however, the clinical benefits are short-lived. It is helpful in placing angioplasty balloons and in treating vessels inaccessible to angioplasty catheters.

Recent investigations measuring cerebral lactate to pyruvate ratios and brain tissue oxygen tension before and after balloon angioplasty show data that may be able to provide an early diagnosis of CVS and allow monitoring of threatened cerebral tissue regions.[70]

Recognizing signs of vasospasm can head off potential compromise in cerebral blood flow. Ischemic injury that takes place during vasospasm is similar to an embolic stroke; if vasospasm is detected radiographically, steps should be taken to prevent delayed cerebral ischemia. This can lead to early brain injury with increased intracranial pressures, which will further impede cerebral blood flow, and progress to further cytotoxic edema through apoptosis and necrosis.

25.4.2 Cerebral Salt Wasting Syndrome and Subarachnoid Hemorrhage

Hyponatremia is a frequent finding in the NICU patient, and it can be a common cause of neurologic deterioration in a patient with aneurysmal SAH, especially in anterior communicating artery aneurysms. In the 1950s, when the condition was first described, NICU patients with hyponatremia were initially thought to have cerebral salt wasting (CSW); but as the description of the syndrome of inappropriate antidiuretic hormone (SIADH) became more popular later in that decade, CSW fell out of favor, and many hyponatremic patients with CSW were treated with fluid restriction.[71] CSW is associated with hyponatremia and extracellular volume depletion. Harrigan[72] summarized the evidence in favor of CSW as follows:

1. A negative salt balance is present with hyponatremia in many patients with intracranial disease.
2. These patients were found to be volume depleted, which is incompatible with SIADH.
3. They improved with volume and salt replacement.

Clinical manifestations of hyponatremia include confusion, lethargy, seizures, and coma. It is likely that both humoral and neural mechanisms are involved in the renal wasting of sodium. Atrial natriuretic factor involvement is likely, but it does not appear to be the primary factor. No solid laboratory studies are available to reliably distinguish SIADH and CSW. In fact, laboratory tests may be identical.

Findings in Cerebral Salt Wasting

Laboratory findings include the following:
- Hyponatremia.
- Elevated urine sodium.
- Increased blood urea nitrogen/creatinine ratio.
- Serum osmolality normal or increased.
- Hematocrit normal or increased.
- Serum uric acid normal.

Clinical findings include the following:
- Central venous pressure decreased (<6 cm)
- Pulmonary capillary wedge pressure decreased (<8 mm Hg).
- Negative salt balance.
- Decreased plasma volume (<35 mL/kg).
- Signs and symptoms of dehydration.
- Decreased weight and orthostatic hypotension.

Treatment of Cerebral Salt Wasting

It is crucial to make a correct diagnosis because treatment plans for CSW and SIADH are opposite. Patients with cerebral injury who are already hypovolemic will be at greater risk of ischemia and infarction. In one study, the administration of normal saline 50 mL/kg/d and oral salt 12 g/d was shown to be effective in restoring serum within 3 days.[73] Three percent saline is also used for severe hyponatremia, especially if the patient is symptomatic. Correction of sodium should occur no faster than 0.5 to 1.0 mEq/L/h, and maximum correction should not exceed 20 mEq/L in the first 48 hours. Correct initially to a serum sodium level of 130 to 134 mEq/L and the remainder of the salt deficit over 1 or 2 days. Hyponatremia also lowers the serum osmolality, which results in increased shift of fluid into the intraparenchymal and intracellular compartments (discussed earlier in this chapter). In a neurosurgical patient, it is essential to keep the patient euvolemic iso-osmolar, or slightly hyperosmolar, or prevent unneeded increases in intracranial pressure.

25.4.3 Hyperdynamic Syndrome after Carotid Endarterectomy

Hyperdynamic syndrome, also known as reperfusion syndrome, following carotid endarterectomy (CEA) occurs in ~0.3 to 1.0% of patients, and usually >24 hours after surgery. The pathophysiology is similar to reperfusion injury after an ischemic stroke; increase in ipsilateral blood flow greater than the metabolic demand. Chronic hypoperfusion leads to production of vasodilatory substances such as carbon dioxide and nitric oxide. These are known to cause endothelial dysfunction in the chronic state.[74] Restoration of normal blood flow causes breakdown of the blood–brain barrier and thus can lead to vasogenic edema and increased intracranial pressures.[75,76]

Heralding signs and symptoms include ipsilateral frontal headache within the first week (better with sitting), focal motor seizures that are characteristically difficult to control,[77] and etiology thought to be the return of blood flow to areas previously rendered chronically ischemic and with poor autoregulation.[78,79] Care must be taken to admit these patients to the NICU and control hypertension rather than medical intensive care unit for purely seizure management.

Risk factors for hyperdynamic syndrome include the following:

- Carotid stenosis > 90%.
- Poor collateral hemispheric flow.
- Contralateral carotid occlusion.
- Evidence of ipsilateral chronic hypoperfusion.
- Pre- and postoperative hypertension.
- Preexisting ipsilateral cerebral infarction (especially recent).
- Preoperative anticoagulation or antiplatelet treatment.

CT Findings of hyperdynamic syndrome may show mild edema, petechial hemorrhages, and ICH ipsilateral to the side of the CEA.

25.4.4 Intracerebral Hemorrhage after Carotid Endarterectomy

ICH is the most catastrophic complication of the hyperperfusion syndrome. It occurs in ~ 0.5 to 0.7% of patients after CEA and accounts for ~ 20% of perioperative strokes. In one study, all ICHs occurred between days 1 and 10 postprocedure.[80] The cause of ICH is most likely the blood–brain barrier being overcome by a rapid increase in the cerebral blood flow that occurs after CEA. The mortality is ~ 30%, with the highest risk factor appearing to be relief of high-grade stenosis.

Treatment of ICH after CEA

Once ICH is seen, stop all anticoagulation, and control blood pressure. If ICH is accompanied by mass effect and progressive deficit, and there is an accessible lesion, a craniotomy should be performed with evacuation of the hematoma.

In general, neurologic deficit within the first 12 hours after CEA is almost always due to thromboembolic phenomena from the CEA site. The CEA site should be urgently reexplored. However, deficits occurring 12 to 24 hours after CEA could be from hyperperfusion syndrome and should be investigated with noncontrasted computed tomography of the brain and cerebral angiography. Anticoagulation or antiplatelet therapy in the latter group of patients could result in catastrophic consequences if started prior to knowing if there is an ICH.

25.4.5 Arteriovenous Malformations and Rebleeding

Cerebral AVMs can be treated by open surgical resection, radiosurgically, endovascularly, or a combination of the three. Depending on the size and flow characteristics, there can be various degrees of adjacent brain vascular steal, hemorrhage, chronic hypoperfusion, and low-grade ischemia.

The most common cause for postoperative ICH after AVM surgery is retained AVM, which needs to be meticulously searched for. However, hemorrhagic complications can occur after total extirpation of cerebral AVMs.[81,82,83,84,85,86,87, 88,89,90,91,92,93] AVMs that are large and with the highest flow rates are at greatest risk. The incidence is 0.01 to 0.10%.

There are two theories to explain rebleeding. The normal perfusion pressure breakthrough theory, as outlined by Spetzler et al[83] in 1978, says that chronic hypoperfusion leads to impaired autoregulation around the AVM; after excision, the return of normal pressure causes local hyperemia and capillary leakage. The occlusive hyperemia theory, first proposed by al-Rodhan et al[90] in 1993, maintains that the obstruction of the venous outflow system of adjacent brain causes passive hyperemia and a stagnant arterial flow in the former AVM feeders.

Exact pathophysiological and hemodynamic mechanisms are not fully understood, and it is likely that combinations of the above theories in conjunction with a yet unidentified mechanism are at play.

The treatment of ICH after fully resected AVM surgery may require evacuation of ICH, careful blood pressure management, and antiedema medication. Adequate hydration and blood volume are required since dehydration can promote further venous thrombosis. Serum hematocrit < 35 is recommended. If the patient is in poor neurologic condition, a barbiturate coma may be helpful by globally reducing blood flow and allowing the normal brain to develop normal autoregulation.

25.5 Conclusion

One common trait with the above systemic complications is the end-resultant ischemic injury to the brain. Eighty percent of patients who die after traumatic brain injury have evidence of cerebral ischemia.[1] The main goal of the neurosurgeon in the NICU is to prevent systemic complications and provide the brain with the optimal milieu to heal. Patients are intubated due to the inability to protect their airway because this would cause hypoxemia resulting in global tissue hypoxia; in the human body, the tissue most sensitive to hypoxia is the neural tissue. As explained before, more than 3–4 minutes of hypoxemia can lead to cerebral ischemia. This would lead to global ischemia, resulting in inflammation and cytotoxic edema and eventual brain death.

One of the primary goals of neurosurgery is decompression of neural tissue to alleviate mass effect by nonneural components or neoplasms. However, inability to provide the neural tissue with its essential nutrients results in cytotoxic edema, which causes swelling of the neural tissue from within. Neural tissue is extremely sensitive to inadequate nutrient supply; thus all efforts should be made to create the optimal environment and ultimately prevent ischemic stroke. Many tools are at the disposal of the neurosurgeon to monitor intracerebral pressures, brain tissue oxygenation, and brain metabolic needs; these must be used and appropriate measures taken to ensure the best outcomes for our patients.

Case Management

The surgical evacuation of the subdural hematoma is only the beginning of the sophisticated management of this patient. She needs to have her steroids discontinued immediately, as they have no role in traumatic brain injury. She should have a repeat computed tomographic head scan to get a good baseline of her intracranial picture, and because her Glasgow Coma Scale score is 8 or less, she will need a ventriculostomy/intracranial pressure monitor inserted after confirmation that she is not coagulopathic. It is essential that her hypotension be corrected because it is associated with a poor prognosis. As hyperglycemia can be damaging to the brain, using an insulin drip, her glucose level should be corrected to an ideal level of < 150 mg/dL. After a Dilantin level is sent, the patient should be continued on 100 mg Dilantin every 8 hours for a total of 7 days. The patient will need aggressive cerebral partial pressure management, serial computed tomographic head imaging, and close follow-up of her electrolyte levels.

References

[1] Tan C, Khurana VG, Benarroch EE, Meyer FB. Cerebral blood flow and metabolism and cerebral ischemia. In: Winn HR, ed. Youmans Neurological Surgery. 6th ed. Philadelphia, PA: Saunders Elsevier; 2011:3537–3562

[2] Lee J-M, Grabb MC, Zipfel GJ, Choi DW. Brain tissue responses to ischemia. J Clin Invest. 2000; 106 (6):723–731

[3] Kaur C, Ling EA. Blood brain barrier in hypoxic-ischemic conditions. Curr Neurovasc Res. 2008; 5 (1):71–81

[4] Tolias CM, Reinert M, Seiler R, Gilman C, Scharf A, Bullock MR. Normobaric hyperoxia–induced improvement in cerebral metabolism and reduction in intracranial pressure in patients with severe head injury: a prospective historical cohort-matched study. J Neurosurg. 2004; 101 (3):435–444

[5] Signoretti S, Marmarou A, Aygok GA, Fatouros PP, Portella G, Bullock RM. Assessment of mitochondrial impairment in traumatic brain injury using high-resolution proton magnetic resonance spectroscopy. J Neurosurg. 2008; 108(1):42–52

[6] Chiu EH, Liu CS, Tan TY, Chang KC. Venturi mask adjuvant oxygen therapy in severe acute ischemic stroke. Arch Neurol. 2006; 63(5):741–744

[7] Palzur E, Vlodavsky E, Mulla H, Arieli R, Feinsod M, Soustiel JF. Hyperbaric oxygen therapy for reduction of secondary brain damage in head injury: an animal model of brain contusion. J Neurotrauma. 2004; 21(1):41–48

[8] Singhal AB, Benner T, Roccatagliata L, et al. A pilot study of normobaric oxygen therapy in acute ischemic stroke. Stroke. 2005; 36(4):797–802

[9] Nortje J, Coles JP, Timofeev I, et al. Effect of hyperoxia on regional oxygenation and metabolism after severe traumatic brain injury: preliminary findings. Crit Care Med. 2008; 36(1):273–281

[10] Menzel M, Doppenberg EM, Zauner A, Soukup J, Reinert MM, Bullock R. Increased inspired oxygen concentration as a factor in improved brain tissue oxygenation and tissue lactate levels after severe human head injury. J Neurosurg. 1999; 91(1):1–10

[11] Bennett MH, Trytko B, Jonker B. Hyperbaric oxygen therapy for the adjunctive treatment of traumatic brain injury. Cochrane Database Syst Rev. 2012; 12:CD004609

[12] Vlodavsky E, Palzur E, Soustiel JF. Hyperbaric oxygen therapy reduces neuroinflammation and expression of matrix metalloproteinase-9 in the rat model of traumatic brain injury. Neuropathol Appl Neurobiol. 2006; 32(1):40–50

[13] Ibrahim I, Chor WP, Chue KM, et al. Is arterial base deficit still a useful prognostic marker in trauma? A systematic review. Am J Emerg Med. 2016; 34(3):626–635

[14] Martin MJ, FitzSullivan E, Salim A, Berne TV, Towfigh S. Use of serum bicarbonate measurement in place of arterial base deficit in the surgical intensive care unit. Arch Surg. 2005; 140(8):745–751

[15] Hasan A. The analysis of blood gases. Handbook of Blood Gas/Acid–Base Interpretation. London, UK: Springer; 2013:253–266

[16] Rodak BF. Hematology: Clinical Principles and Applications. 3rd ed. Philadelphia, PA: Saunders; 2007:220

[17] Jennett B. Early traumatic epilepsy. Incidence and significance after nonmissile injuries. Arch Neurol. 1974; 30(5):394–398

[18] Kumar MA. Red blood cell transfusion in the neurological ICU. Neurotherapeutics. 2012; 9(1):56–64

[19] Robertson CS, Hannay HJ, Yamal JM, et al. Epo Severe TBI Trial Investigators. Effect of erythropoietin and transfusion threshold on neurological recovery after traumatic brain injury: a randomized clinical trial. JAMA. 2014; 312(1):36–47

[20] Jauch EC, Saver JL, Adams HP, Jr, et al. American Heart Association Stroke Council, Council on Cardiovascular Nursing, Council on Peripheral Vascular Disease, Council on Clinical Cardiology. Guidelines for the early management of patients with acute ischemic stroke: a guideline for healthcare professionals from the American Heart Association/American Stroke Association. Stroke. 2013; 44(3):870–947

[21] Jones PA, Andrews PJ, Midgley S, et al. Measuring the burden of secondary insults in head-injured patients during intensive care. J Neurosurg Anesthesiol. 1994; 6(1):4–14

[22] Temkin NR, Dikmen SS, Wilensky AJ, Keihm J, Chabal S, Winn HR. A randomized, double-blind study of phenytoin for the prevention of post-traumatic seizures. N Engl J Med. 1990; 323 (8):497–502

[23] Cherian L, Goodman JC, Robertson CS. Hyperglycemia increases brain injury caused by secondary ischemia after cortical impact injury in rats. Crit Care Med. 1997; 25(8):1378–1383

[24] Cherian L, Hannay HJ, Vagner G, Goodman JC, Contant CF, Robertson CS. Hyperglycemia increases neurological damage and behavioral deficits from post-traumatic secondary ischemic insults. J Neurotrauma. 1998; 15(5):307–321

[25] Sheth KN, Elm JJ, Beslow LA, Sze GK, Kimberly WT. Glyburide Advantage in Malignant Edema and Stroke (GAMES-RP) Trial: Rationale and Design. Neurocrit Care. 2016; 24(1):132–139

[26] Sulter G, Elting JW, Maurits N, Luijckx GJ, De Keyser J. Acetylsalicylic acid and acetaminophen to combat elevated body temperature in acute ischemic stroke. Cerebrovasc Dis. 2004; 17(2–3):118–122

459

[27] Lemkes BA, Hermanides J, Devries JH, Holleman F, Meijers JCM, Hoekstra JBL. Hyperglycemia: a prothrombotic factor? J Thromb Haemost. 2010; 8(8):1663–1669

[28] Braun SR, Levin AB, Clark KL. Role of corticosteroids in the development of pneumonia in mechanically ventilated head-trauma victims. Crit Care Med. 1986; 14(3):198–201

[29] Born JD, Albert A, Hans P, Bonnal J. Relative prognostic value of best motor response and brain stem reflexes in patients with severe head injury. Neurosurgery. 1985; 16(5):595–601

[30] Cheung V, Hoshide R, Bansal V, Kasper E, Chen CC. Methylprednisolone in the management of spinal cord injuries: Lessons from randomized, controlled trials. Surg Neurol Int. 2015; 6:142

[31] Driks MR, Craven DE, Celli BR, et al. Nosocomial pneumonia in intubated patients given sucralfate as compared with antacids or histamine type 2 blockers. The role of gastric colonization. N Engl J Med. 1987; 317(22):1376–1382

[32] Bracken MB, Shepard MJ, Collins WF, et al. A randomized, controlled trial of methylprednisolone or naloxone in the treatment of acute spinal-cord injury. Results of the Second National Acute Spinal Cord Injury Study. N Engl J Med. 1990; 322(20):1405–1411

[33] Bracken MB, Shepard MS, Holford TR, et al. Administration of methylprednisolone for 24 or 48 hours or tirilizad mesylate for 48 hours in the treatment of acute spinal cord injury. Results of the Third National Acute Spinal Cord Injury Randomized Controlled Trial. National Acute Spinal Cord Injury Study. JAMA. 1997; 277:1597–1604

[34] Kunihara T, Sasaki S, Shiiya N, et al. Lazaroid reduces production of IL-8 and IL-1 receptor antagonist in ischemic spinal cord injury. Ann Thorac Surg. 2000; 69(3):792–798

[35] Blackman JA, Patrick PD, Buck ML, Rust RS, Jr. Paroxysmal autonomic instability with dystonia after brain injury. Arch Neurol. 2004; 61(3):321–328

[36] Nishiyama T, Yokoyama T, Matsukawa T, Hanaoka K. Continuous nicardipine infusion to control blood pressure after evacuation of acute cerebral hemorrhage. Can J Anaesth. 2000; 47(12):1196–1201

[37] Geerts WH, Code KI, Jay RM, Chen E, Szalai JP. A prospective study of venous thromboembolism after major trauma. N Engl J Med. 1994; 331(24):1601–1606

[38] Nurmohamed MT, van Riel AM, Henkens CM, et al. Low molecular weight heparin and compression stockings in the prevention of venous thromboembolism in neurosurgery. Thromb Haemost. 1996; 75(2):233–238

[39] Geerts WH, Jay RM, Code KI, et al. A comparison of low-dose heparin with low-molecular-weight heparin as prophylaxis against venous thromboembolism after major trauma. N Engl J Med. 1996; 335(10):701–707

[40] Connolly ES, Mocco J. Enoxaparin in neurosurgical patients. N Engl J Med. 1998; 339(22):1639–1640

[41] Kaufman HH, Hui KS, Mattson JC, et al. Clinicopathological correlations of disseminated intravascular coagulation in patients with head injury. Neurosurgery. 1984; 15(1):34–42

[42] Hinshaw LB. Sepsis/septic shock: participation of the microcirculation: an abbreviated review. Crit Care Med. 1996; 24(6):1072–1078

[43] Chhabra G, Sharma S, Subramanian A, Agrawal D, Sinha S, Mukhopadhyay AK. Coagulopathy as prognostic marker in acute traumatic brain injury. J Emerg Trauma Shock. 2013; 6(3):180–185

[44] Talving P, Benfield R, Hadjizacharia P, Inaba K, Chan LS, Demetriades D. Coagulopathy in severe traumatic brain injury: a prospective study. J Trauma. 2009; 66(1):55–61, discussion 61–62

[45] Berger B, Gumbinger C, Steiner T, Sykora M. Epidemiologic features, risk factors, and outcome of sepsis in stroke patients treated on a neurologic intensive care unit. J Crit Care. 2014; 29(2):241–248

[46] Kamada T, Fusamoto H, Kawano S, Noguchi M, Hiramatsu K. Gastrointestinal bleeding following head injury: a clinical study of 433 cases. J Trauma. 1977; 17(1):44–47

[47] Sharshar T, Blanchard A, Paillard M, Raphael JC, Gajdos P, Annane D. Circulating vasopressin levels in septic shock. Crit Care Med. 2003; 31(6):1752–1758

[48] Russell JA, Walley KR, Singer J, et al. VASST Investigators. Vasopressin versus norepinephrine infusion in patients with septic shock. N Engl J Med. 2008; 358(9):877–887

[49] Ziaja M. Septic encephalopathy. Curr Neurol Neurosci Rep. 2013; 13(10):383

[50] Kemp WJ, Bashir A, Dababneh H, Cohen-Gadol AA. Cushing's ulcer: Further reflections. Asian J Neurosurg. 2015; 10(2):87–94

[51] Brain Trauma Foundation, American Association of Neurological Surgeons, and Joint Section on Neurotrauma and Critical Care. Role of antiseizure prophylaxis following head injury. J Neurotrauma. 2000; 17(6–7):549–553

[52] Sarzynski E, Puttarajappa C, Xie Y, Grover M, Laird-Fick H. Association between proton pump inhibitor use and anemia: a retrospective cohort study. Dig Dis Sci. 2011; 56(8):2349–2353

[53] Piek J, Chesnut RM, Marshall LF, et al. Extracranial complications of severe head injury. J Neurosurg. 1992; 77(6):901–907

[54] Boeve BF, Wijdicks EF, Benarroch EE, Schmidt KD. Paroxysmal sympathetic storms ("diencephalic seizures") after severe diffuse axonal head injury. Mayo Clin Proc. 1998; 73(2):148–152

[55] Goddeau RP, Jr, Silverman SB, Sims JR. Dexmedetomidine for the treatment of paroxysmal autonomic instability with dystonia. Neurocrit Care. 2007; 7(3):217–220

[56] Ali Mahmoud AM. Postaneurysmal subarachnoid hemorrhage vasospasm: a review of the incidence of radiographic and clinical vasospasm. Egypt J Neurol Psychiat Neurosurg. 2015; 52:172–175

[57] Kassell NF, Sasaki T, Colohan AR, Nazar G. Cerebral vasospasm following aneurysmal subarachnoid hemorrhage. Stroke. 1985; 16:562–572

[58] Heros R, Zervas NT, Varsos V. Cerebral vasospasm after subarachnoid hemorrhage: an update. Ann Neurol. 1983; 14:599–608

[59] Fisher CM, Kistler JP, Davis JM. Relation of cerebral vasospasm to subarachnoid hemorrhage visualized by computerized tomographic scanning. Neurosurgery. 1980; 6:1–9

[60] Grosset DG, Straiton J, McDonald I, Cockburn M, Bullock R. Use of transcranial Doppler sonography to predict development of a delayed ischemic deficit after subarachnoid hemorrhage. J Neurosurg. 1993; 78(2):183–187

[61] Su S-H, Xu W, Hai J, Wu YF, Yu F. Effects of statins-use for patients with aneurysmal subarachnoid hemorrhage: a meta-analysis of randomized controlled trials. Sci Rep. 2014; 4:4573

[62] Kirkpatrick PJ, Turner CL, Smith C, Hutchinson PJ, Murray GD, STASH Collaborators. Simvastatin in aneurysmal subarachnoid haemorrhage (STASH): a multicentre randomised phase 3 trial. Lancet Neurol. 2014; 13(7):666–675

[63] Shimoda M, Oda S, Tsugane R, Sato O. Intracranial complications of hypervolemic therapy in patients with a delayed ischemic deficit attributed to vasospasm. J Neurosurg. 1993; 78(3):423–429

[64] Solomon RA, Fink ME, Lennihan L. Early aneurysm surgery and prophylactic hypervolemic hypertensive therapy for the treatment of aneurysmal subarachnoid hemorrhage. Neurosurgery. 1988; 23(6):699–704

[65] Lennihan L, Mayer SA, Fink ME, et al. Effect of hypervolemic therapy on cerebral blood flow after subarachnoid hemorrhage: a randomized trial. Stroke. 2000; 31:383–391

[66] Newell DW, Eskridge JM, Mayberg MR, Grady MS, Winn HR. Angioplasty for the treatment of symptomatic vasospasm following subarachnoid hemorrhage. J Neurosurg. 1989; 71:654–660

[67] Polin RS, Coenen V, Hansen C, et al. Efficacy of transluminal angioplasty for the management of symptomatic cerebral vasospasm following aneurysmal subarachnoid hemorrhage. J Neurosurg. 2000; 92:284–290

[68] Bejjani GK, Bank WO, Olan WJ, Sekhar LN. The efficacy and safety of angioplasty for cerebral vasospasm after subarachnoid hemorrhage. Neurosurgery. 1998; 42:979–986

[69] Rosenwasser RH, Armonda RA, Thomas JE, Benitez RP, Gannon PM, Harrop J. Therapeutic modalities for the management of cerebral vasospasm: timing of endovascular options. Neurosurgery. 1999; 44(5):975–979, discussion 979–980

[70] Hoelper BM, Hoffman E, Sporleder R, Soldner F,, Behr R. Transluminal balloon angioplasty improves brain tissue oxygenation and metabolism in severe vasospasm after : case report. Neurosurgery. 2003; 52:970–974

[71] Cort JH. Cerebral salt wasting. Lancet. 1954; 266(6815):752–754

[72] Harrigan MR. Cerebral salt wasting syndrome: a review. Neurosurgery. 1996; 38(1):152–160

[73] Sivakumar V, Rajshekhar V, Chandy MJ. Management of neurosurgical patients with hyponatremia and natriuresis. Neurosurgery. 1994; 34(2):269–274, discussion 274

[74] Sekhon LH, Morgan MK, Spence I. Normal perfusion pressure breakthrough: the role of capillaries. J Neurosurg. 1997; 86(3):519–524

[75] Vespa P, McArthur DL, Stein N, et al. Tight glycemic control increases metabolic distress in traumatic brain injury: a randomized controlled within-subjects trial. Crit Care Med. 2012; 40 (6):1923–1929

[76] Hosoda K, Kawaguchi T, Shibata Y, et al. Cerebral vasoreactivity and internal carotid artery flow help to identify patients at risk for hyperfusion after carotid endarterectomy. Stroke. 2001; 32 (7):1567–1573

[77] Kieburtz K, Ricotta JJ, Moxley RT, III. Seizures following carotid endarterectomy. Arch Neurol. 1990; 47(5):568–570

[78] Riles TS, Imparato AM, Jacobowitz GR, et al. The cause of perioperative stroke after carotid endarterectomy. J Vasc Surg. 1994; 19(2):206–214, discussion 215–216

[79] Pomposelli FB, Lamparello PJ, Riles TS, Craighead CC, Giangola G, Imparato AM. Intracranial hemorrhage after carotid endarterectomy. J Vasc Surg. 1988; 7(2):248–255

[80] Sundt TM. Occlusive Cerebrovascular Disease. Philadelphia, PA: WB Saunders; 1987

[81] Batjer HH, Devous MD, Seibert GB, Purdy PD, Bonte FJ. Intracranial arteriovenous malformation: relationship between clinical factors and surgical complications. Neurosurgery. 1989; 24:75–79

[82] Batjer HH, Devous MD, Meyer YJ, Purdy PD, Samson DS. Cerebrovascular hemodynamics in arteriovenous malformation complicated by normal perfusion pressure breakthrough. Neurosurgery. 1988; 22:503–509

[83] Spetzler RF, Wilson CB, Weinstein P, Mehdorn M, Townsend J, Telles D. Normal perfusion pressure breakthrough theory. Clin Neurosurg. 1978; 25:651–672

[84] Spetzler RF, Hargraves RW, McCormick PW, Zabramski JM, Flom RA, Zimmerman RS. Relationship of perfusion pressure and size to risk of hemorrhage from arteriovenous malformations. J Neurosurg. 1992; 76:918–923

[85] Batjer HH, Purdy PD, Giller CA, Samson DS. Evidence of redistribution of cerebral blood flow during treatment for an intracranial arteriovenous malformation. Neurosurgery. 1989; 25:599–605

[86] Morgan MK, Johnston IH, Hallinan TM,, Weber NC. Complications of surgery for arteriovenous malformations of the brain. J Neurosurg. 1993; 78:176–182

[87] Sekhon LHS, Morgan MK, Spence I. Normal perfusion pressure breakthrough: the role of capillaries. J Neurosurg. 1997; 86(3):519–524

[88] Pollock BE. Occlusive hyperemia: a radiosurgical phenomenon? Neurosurgery. 2000; 47(5):1178–1182, discussion 1183–1184

[89] Schaller C, Urbach H, Schramm J, Meyer B. Role of venous drainage in cerebral arteriovenous malformation surgery, as related to the development of postoperative hyperperfusion injury. Neurosurgery. 2002; 51:921–929

[90] al-Rodhan NRF, Sundt TM, Piepgras DG, Nichols DA, Rüfenacht D, Stevens LN. Occlusive hyperemia: a theory for the hemodynamic complications following resection of intracerebral arteriovenous malformation. J Neurosurg. 1993; 78:167–175

[91] Young WL, Pile-Spellman J, Prohovnik I, Kader A, Stein BM. Evidence for adaptive autoregulatory displacement in hypotensive cortical territories adjacent to arteriovenous malformations. Neurosurgery. 1994; 34:601–611

[92] Young WL, Kader A, Orstein E, et al. Cerebral hyperemia after arteriovenous malformation resection is related to "breakthrough" complications but not to feeding artery pressure. Neurosurgery. 1996; 38:1085–1095

[93] Roost DV, Schramm J. What factors are related to impairment of cerebrovascular reserve before and after arteriovenous malformation resection? A cerebral blood flow study using xenon-enhanced computed tomography. Neurosurgery. 2001; 48:709–717

26 Acute Ischemic Stroke

Robert J. Claycomb, Luis T. Arangua, Vladimir Adriano Cortez, Glenn Fischberg, and Javed Siddiqi

Abstract

Approximately 87% of all strokes are ischemic (vs. hemorrhagic). Because of the brain's privileged status in receiving a disproportionately high share of cardiac output, it is also the most vulnerable to focal or global cerebral ischemia, which is often the final common pathway of many different forms of brain damage. Rapid diagnosis of cerebral ischemia is critical because "time is brain," rendering prompt medical therapy or intervention the best hope for a good prognosis. This chapter reviews the current state of the art for acute ischemic stroke therapy, which includes intravenous thrombolytics and intra-arterial endovascular therapies, such as thrombectomy; it reviews the latest evidence in favor of these therapies.

Keywords: atrial fibrillation, global aphasia, hyperlipidemia, ischemia, lentiform nucleus, NIH stroke scale, thrombectomy, thrombolysis, wake-up stroke

Case Study

A 62-year-old woman with a history of atrial fibrillation, type 2 diabetes, hypertension, and hyperlipidemia had acute onset of right arm weakness and "problems speaking" while eating dinner at a family gathering. Within 30 minutes of the onset of symptoms, she was evaluated in a local emergency room. She was noted to have a blood pressure of 217/105. Her neurologic exam was notable for global aphasia, left-sided gaze preference, severe right facial droop, labial dysarthria, right arm hemiplegia, and right leg hemiparesis correlating with a National Institutes of Health Stroke Scale score of 19. Noncontrasted computed tomography (CT) of the head revealed a hyperdense proximal segment of the left middle cerebral artery (M1 segment) and mild sulcal effacement of the left frontoparietal lobes, effacement of the left caudate head and lentiform nucleus, and no evidence of hemorrhage. A CT arteriogram of the head and neck, performed 45 minutes after symptom onset, revealed no opacification of the left middle cerebral artery distal to the midportion of the M1 segment.

See end of chapter for Case Management.

26.1 Triage and Initial Management

Despite ongoing efforts aimed to minimize the risk of acute ischemic stroke (AIS), it still remains the fourth leading cause of death and one of the greatest causes of disability in the United States. Because the brain is highly sensitive to ischemia, it is not surprising that the overall outcome is highly dependent on the management of the patient within the first few hours after the first symptoms of AIS. The main goal within the first hour after presentation to the emergency department is to confirm the diagnosis of AIS and to determine the patient's eligibility for intravenous (IV) thrombolysis and other therapies. This process begins outside the hospital.

Emergency medical services should transport patients with signs and symptoms of AIS to the "highest level of care available within the shortest period of time."[1] Upon arrival to the emergency department, several processes should happen quickly and in parallel (▶ Table 26.1). A basic evaluation of the patient's airway, breathing, and circulation should be performed as well as a focused neurologic assessment to determine the presence and severity of new neurologic deficits. At this time, the patient should be placed on a cardiac monitor with frequent blood pressure monitoring, placed on supplemental oxygen for a saturation of at least 94%, positioned supine, and IV fluids should be started and lab work drawn. Contemporaneously, a focused medical history should be obtained. This rapid interview should concentrate on when the patient's symptoms first occurred, if known, or when the patient was last seen without the current deficits. The interview should also focus on elements of the medical history that may exclude the use of IV thrombolytics (▶ Table 26.2). Also during this initial evaluation, a noncontrasted computed tomographic (CT) scan of the head should be performed and immediately evaluated, specifically for intracranial hemorrhage, which would be a contraindication for IV thrombolysis.

Table 26.1 Rapid initial evaluation of acute ischemic stroke patients[1]

Parameter	Time
Door to ED physician evaluation	≤ 10 minutes
Door to stroke team	≤ 15 minutes
Door to start of CT	≤ 25 minutes
Door to CT interpretation	≤ 45 minutes
Door to IV tPA	≤ 60 minutes
Door to admission to stroke unit	≤ 180 minutes

Abbreviations: CT, computed tomography; ED, emergency department; IV, intravenous; tPA, tissue plasminogen activator.

26.2 Administration of Thrombolytics

The use of IV thrombolytics, specifically tissue plasminogen activator (tPA), has been widely studied and considered to be the mainstay of initial AIS treatment.[1,3,4] To safely administer tPA, there should be no contraindications (▶ Table 26.2), and the patient's blood pressure should be below 185/110 mm Hg. Once tPA is administered, the blood pressure should be maintained below 180/105, which is typically achieved by IV antihypertensive medications (e.g., labetalol and nicardipine). Recently, the American Heart Association (AHA) guidelines for the administration of tPA have been liberalized, and some medical conditions that initially precluded the use of tPA have been determined to carry minimal risk of adverse events and therefore have been eliminated from the list of contraindications (▶ Table 26.3).[5] In most circumstances, given the low risk of adverse outcomes described in stroke mimics, additional confirmatory or ancillary testing, such as magnetic resonance imaging (MRI) of the brain, CT angiography, and perfusion studies should not delay treatment with tPA.[1,6,7]

Table 26.2 Absolute contraindications for tPA use in the setting of acute stroke[2]

Current intracranial hemorrhage
Subarachnoid hemorrhage
Active internal bleeding
Intracranial/intraspinal surgery or serious head trauma within 3 months
Presence of intracranial conditions that may increase risk of bleeding
Bleeding diathesis
Current severe, uncontrolled hypertension

Table 26.3 Selected recommendations from the revised inclusion and exclusion criteria for the use of intravenous (IV) tissue plasminogen activator (tPA)[5]

Recommendation	Class; level of evidence
IV tPA is safe and can be effective in AIS patients > 80 years of age presenting between 3 and 4.5 hours after symptoms onset[a]	Class IIa; level of evidence B
IV tPA appears safe and beneficial in AIS patients taking warfarin but with an INR ≤ 1.7 presenting between 3 and 4.5 hours after symptoms onset[a]	Class IIb; level of evidence B
The benefit of IV tPA is uncertain in AIS patients with NIHSS > 25 presenting between 3 and 4.5 hours after symptoms onset[a]	Class IIb; level of evidence B
IV tPA may be safe and effective in AIS patients with a previous stroke and diabetes presenting between 3 and 4.5 hours after symptoms onset[a]	Class IIb; level of evidence C

(continued)

465

Table 26.3 continued

Recommendation	Class; level of evidence
IV tPA may be considered in pregnancy	Class IIb; level of evidence C
IV tPA may be considered after major surgery within 14 days if the benefits outweigh the risks	Class IIb; level of evidence C
IV tPA is reasonable after NSTEMI, STEMI involving right or inferior myocardium	Class IIa; level of evidence C
IV tPA may be reasonable after STEMI involving left anterior myocardium	Class IIb; level of evidence C
IV tPA may be reasonable in the setting of a severe/disabling AIS and acute pericarditis or known left ventricular thrombus	Class IIb; level of evidence C
IV tPA is reasonable in the setting of known small (≤ 10 mm) unruptured, unsecured aneurysms	Class IIa; level of evidence C
IV tPA may be considered in the setting of a severe/disabling AIS and known AVM	Class IIb; level of evidence C
IV tPA is probably recommended with AIS patients with known extra-axial neoplasms	Class IIa; level of evidence C
IV tPA is reasonable in AIS patients presenting with a seizure if the deficits are not entirely due to postictal phenomenon	Class IIa; level of evidence C
IV tPA is reasonable within 7 days of dural puncture	Class IIb; level of evidence C

Abbreviations: AIS, acute ischemic stroke; AVM, arteriovenous malformation; NIHSS, National Institutes of Health Stroke Scale; NSTEMI, non-ST segment elevation myocardial infarction; ST, ST segment is the flat, isoelectric section of the ECG between the end of the S wave (the J point) and the beginning of the T wave; STEMI, ST segment elevation myocardial infarction.

[a] These recommendations clarify the use of tPA within the expanded time window described in the ECASS II trial.[4]

26.3 Use of Intra-arterial Therapies

Endovascular treatment of AIS is now thought to be the standard of care for carefully selected patients after a series of studies published in 2015.[8,9,10,11,12] Patients that may benefit from endovascular therapy with a stent retriever will usually have moderate to severe deficits (i.e., National Institutes of Health Stroke Scale [NIHSS] score ≥ 6) due to an occlusion of the internal carotid artery or proximal M1 segment and has access to an institution that can begin the procedure (i.e., groin puncture) within 6 hours of symptom onset if all the criteria are met[12] (▶ Table 26.4). While IV tPA use is the preferred initial treatment of AIS, endovascular therapies may still be beneficial in carefully selected patients when there is a contraindication to tPA.[12] Those patients undergoing endovascular treatment, regardless of tPA use, should still be monitored closely

Table 26.4 Criteria for endovascular therapy[12]

Patients *should* receive endovascular treatment with a stent retriever if *all* of the following criteria are met:

Prestroke modified Rankin Scale of 0 or 1

Received tPA within 4.5 hours of symptoms onset

Stroke caused by ICA or proximal M1 occlusion

Age ≥ 18 years old

NIHSS score of ≥ 6

ASPECTS of ≥ 6
Treatment can be initiated within 6 hours of symptoms onset

Abbreviations: ASPECTS, Alberta Stroke Program Early CT score; ICA internal carotid artery, NIHSS, National Institutes of Health Stroke Scale; tPA, tissue plasminogen activator.

in an intensive care unit (ICU) setting.[12] Patients in whom IV tPA is contraindicated remain candidates for thrombectomy with use of a stent retriever or aspiration device. In practice, in those patients not receiving IV tPA, and at the discretion of the interventionalist, intra-arterial (IA) tPA is sometimes used alone or in combination with thrombectomy devices, particularly as a salvage technique. Mechanical thrombectomy following IV tPA or in combination with IA tPA has been demonstrated to be safe. Combination use of adjunctive glycoprotein GP IIB/IIIA inhibitors, such as abciximab, with concomitant use of tPA and thrombectomy, however, has been demonstrated to increase the risk of intracerebral hemorrhage (ICH), particularly asymptomatic subarachnoid hemorrhage (SAH) in patients presenting with more severe stroke and at a longer time window from stroke onset. However, in some selected cases the benefit may outweigh the risk.

26.4 Intensive Care Unit Management of Acute Ischemic Stroke

Admission to an ICU typically occurs after tPA administration, IA intervention, or when the stroke involves a large territory so these patients can be monitored closely. One of the parameters that is closely monitored is blood pressure. Typically, most oral antihypertensive medications are discontinued or, in the case of beta-blockers, continued at a reduced dose (to avoid rebound tachycardia).[1,13] During this time, dramatic fluctuations of blood pressure should be avoided, and IV agents are commonly used. Within the first 24 hours after IV thrombolysis, the blood pressure is typically held below 180/105 mm Hg to balance the risk of reperfusion-associated hemorrhage with the need to optimize collateral circulation if thrombolysis was incomplete.[1,5] In the setting of

IA intervention, blood pressure goals are typically lower, and there is no clear consensus or guidelines; however, a blood pressure goal of less than 160/100 mm Hg is reasonable.[1] If an AIS patient did not receive IV thrombolysis or mechanical intervention, higher blood pressure goals (e.g., <220/110 mm Hg) can be used to maximize collateral circulation.[1] After the first 24 hours, blood pressure management should be specifically tailored to the individual patient. There are no clear guidelines, and there are conflicting studies regarding the optimal timing and extent of blood pressure reduction.[14,15, 16,17,18,19] Other factors, such as intra- or extracranial arterial stenosis, post-stroke hemorrhage, cardiac ischemia, and volume status, can significantly influence the management of blood pressure reduction. When these medical issues require more aggressive blood pressure lowering, systolic blood pressure can be lowered by 15% per day while the patient's neurological status is frequently assessed.[1]

Current guidelines do specifically recommend thrombectomy (if initiated within 6 hours) for anterior circulation occlusions of the internal carotid artery (ICA) and the proximal M1. The guidelines do not specifically recommend, but they state that it may be reasonable to attempt, thrombectomy using stent retrievers on more distal M2 /M3, anterior cerebral artery (ACA), or posterior circulation occlusions.[12] Endovascular interventions involving these locations are left to the discretion of the interventionalist. In practice, interventionalists will frequently extend patient eligibility windows beyond the recommended 6 hours if perfusion studies demonstrate a salvageable penumbra with a relatively small infarcted core based on either CT perfusion or MR perfusion/diffusion mismatch studies. For posterior circulation strokes where outcomes may be particularly devastating, many interventionalists will extend eligibility windows up to 12–24 hours based on perfusion studies indicating a salvageable penumbra.

In cases of wake-up strokes where time of stroke onset is not known and generally taken to be the last time the patient was known well, often placing the patient outside the time window for IV tPA, neither IV nor IA tPA is currently recommended. Some studies looking at wake-up strokes have demonstrated in certain selected patients with appropriate MR diffusion and flair sequence profiles that IV tPA may be safely administered.[20] Prior studies looking at thrombectomy in wake-up strokes have demonstrated mixed results; however, current studies are under way looking at the safety of mechanical thrombectomy based on advanced imaging profiles using perfusion studies.[21, 22,23] Currently some interventionalists will use advanced imaging modalities, such as computed tomography angiogram (CTA) or computed tomography perfusion (CTP) or MRI to select patients demonstrating a salvageable penumbra with a small-core infarct to offer endovascular therapies.

Cerebral edema due to large-territory strokes can complicate the management of the AIS in the ICU. Standard measures to reduce the risk of cerebral edema should be employed, such as keeping the head of the bed elevated to 30 degrees, avoiding hypo-osmotic fluids, recognizing and treating hyponatremia, correcting hyperthermia and hyperglycemia, and minimizing hypoxia and hypercarbia.[1] If cerebral edema begins to cause increased intracranial pressure (ICP), standard management of ICP should be employed (see Chapter 13).

In some cases of acute ischemic stroke, and the associated subset who may progress to hemorrhagic conversion, decompressive surgery may be effective and lifesaving. In large cerebellar infarcts, craniectomy for decompression may be lifesaving to avoid herniation and brainstem compression.[24,25,26] Since the posterior fossa is a relatively small compartment, where increasing infarction, edema, or hemorrhagic conversion can rapidly cause life-threatening neurological decline, the neurosurgeons should be aware of such patients in case of a need for surgical intervention with craniectomy and/or hematoma evacuation. Supratentorially, decompressive craniectomy for large cerebral infarcts (e.g. due to malignant middle cerebral artery [MCA] infarct) remains controversial, but the procedure may be lifesaving; however, patients and families need to understand that the patient will typically have severe disability because the underlying damage from the infarct will not be reversed from the craniectomy.[1,27,28] The decision to proceed with decompression will need to be individualized.[1] Delayed ICH can also complicate large-territory infarctions, and this may lead to possible surgical intervention for hematoma evacuation as a lifesaving measure.

Also, while the patient is in the ICU, secondary prevention of AIS should be considered. If the patient did not receive IV thrombolytic therapy, aspirin (325 mg) should be administered within the first 24 to 48 hours from stroke onset.[1] The use of clopidogrel in this setting has not yet been established.[1] If the patient did receive thrombolytic therapy, aspirin should be administered 24 hours after initiation of IV tPA unless there is a clear contraindication.[1] Anticoagulation for secondary prevention in the setting of AIS should be tailored to the individual patient. The risk of recurrent stroke will need to be carefully weighed against the risk of hemorrhagic conversion.[1] Investigations to determine the etiology of the stroke should also be initiated early in the patient course while still in the ICU setting.

Lastly, optimal medical treatment of the patient's other comorbid conditions should be aggressively managed.[1] For example, hyperglycemia should be aggressively controlled because poststroke hyperglycemia is independently associated with poorer outcomes and a higher incidence of symptomatic ICH.[1,29,30,31,32] Fever and concurrent infection also need to be treated because these are also associated with poor outcome in AIS patients.[1,33,34,35,36]

Case Management

After the completion of the CT arteriogram, the patient was brought back to the emergency department. Her repeated blood pressure was 199/105, and her exam was unchanged and notable for a severe left MCA syndrome. After a quick discussion with the patient's family, they consented to the use of tPA. The patient received 20 mg labetalol IV, which minimally affected her blood pressure. A nicardipine drip was started and titrated to 5 mg/h, resulting in a blood pressure of 175/95. Intravenous tPA was administered at a dosage of 0.9 mg/kg, with 10% given over 1 minute and the remainder administered over the next hour approximately 65 minutes after onset of symptoms. The patient was then taken to the interventional suite, and after two attempts, full recanalization of the left MCA territory was achieved. Immediately after the procedure, she was able to lift her arm and respond appropriately to simple commands. Her ICU course was complicated by aspiration pneumonia treated with IV antibiotics, and severe hyperglycemia requiring an insulin drip. She was discharged 7 days after onset of symptoms with a mild receptive aphasia and minimal loss of dexterity of the right hand with instructions to start warfarin.

References

[1] Jauch EC, Saver JL, Adams HP, Jr, et al. American Heart Association Stroke Council, Council on Cardiovascular Nursing, Council on Peripheral Vascular Disease, Council on Clinical Cardiology. Guidelines for the early management of patients with acute ischemic stroke: a guideline for healthcare professionals from the American Heart Association/American Stroke Association. Stroke. 2013; 44(3):870–947

[2] Activase [prescribing information]. South San Francisco, C.G., Inc.; 2015 https://www.activase.com/

[3] Tissue plasminogen activator for acute ischemic stroke. The National Institute of Neurological Disorders and Stroke rt-PA Stroke Study Group. N Engl J Med. 1995; 333(24):1581–1587

[4] Hacke W, Kaste M, Bluhmki E, et al. ECASS Investigators. Thrombolysis with alteplase 3 to 4.5 hours after acute ischemic stroke. N Engl J Med. 2008; 359(13):1317–1329

[5] Demaerschalk BM, Kleindorfer DO, Adeoye OM, et al. American Heart Association Stroke Council and Council on Epidemiology and Prevention. Scientific Rationale for the Inclusion and Exclusion Criteria for Intravenous Alteplase in Acute Ischemic Stroke: A Statement for Healthcare Professionals From the American Heart Association/American Stroke Association. Stroke. 2016; 47(2):581–641

[6] Winkler DT, Fluri F, Fuhr P, et al. Thrombolysis in stroke mimics: frequency, clinical characteristics, and outcome. Stroke. 2009; 40(4):1522–1525

[7] Chernyshev OY, Martin-Schild S, Albright KC, et al. Safety of tPA in stroke mimics and neuroimaging-negative cerebral ischemia. Neurology. 2010; 74(17):1340–1345

[8] Berkhemer OA, Fransen PS, Beumer D, et al. MR CLEAN Investigators. A randomized trial of intra-arterial treatment for acute ischemic stroke. N Engl J Med. 2015; 372(1):11–20

[9] Campbell BC, Mitchell PJ, EXTEND-IA Investigators. Endovascular therapy for ischemic stroke. N Engl J Med. 2015; 372(24):2365–2366

[10] Saver JL, Goyal M, Bonafe A, et al. SWIFT PRIME Investigators. Solitaire™ with the Intention for Thrombectomy as Primary Endovascular Treatment for Acute Ischemic Stroke (SWIFT PRIME) trial: protocol for a randomized, controlled, multicenter study comparing the Solitaire revascularization device with IV tPA with IV tPA alone in acute ischemic stroke. Int J Stroke. 2015; 10 (3):439–448

[11] Goyal M, Demchuk AM, Menon BK, et al. ESCAPE Trial Investigators. Randomized assessment of rapid endovascular treatment of ischemic stroke. N Engl J Med. 2015; 372(11):1019–1030

[12] Powers WJ, Derdeyn CP, Biller J, et al. American Heart Association Stroke Council. 2015 American Heart Association/American Stroke Association Focused Update of the 2013 Guidelines for the Early Management of Patients With Acute Ischemic Stroke Regarding Endovascular Treatment: A Guideline for Healthcare Professionals From the American Heart Association/American Stroke Association. Stroke. 2015; 46(10):3020–3035

[13] Karachalios GN, Charalabopoulos A, Papalimneou V, et al. Withdrawal syndrome following cessation of antihypertensive drug therapy. Int J Clin Pract. 2005; 59(5):562–570

[14] Castillo J, Leira R, García MM, Serena J, Blanco M, Dávalos A. Blood pressure decrease during the acute phase of ischemic stroke is associated with brain injury and poor stroke outcome. Stroke. 2004; 35(2):520–526

[15] Boreas AM, Lodder J, Kessels F, de Leeuw PW, Troost J. Prognostic value of blood pressure in acute stroke. J Hum Hypertens. 2002; 16(2):111–116

[16] Chamorro A, Vila N, Ascaso C, Elices E, Schonewille W, Blanc R. Blood pressure and functional recovery in acute ischemic stroke. Stroke. 1998; 29(9):1850–1853

[17] Jensen MB, Yoo B, Clarke WR, Davis PH, Adams HR, Jr. Blood pressure as an independent prognostic factor in acute ischemic stroke. Can J Neurol Sci. 2006; 33(1):34–38

[18] Oliveira-Filho J, Silva SC, Trabuco CC, Pedreira BB, Sousa EU, Bacellar A. Detrimental effect of blood pressure reduction in the first 24 hours of acute stroke onset. Neurology. 2003; 61(8):1047–1051

[19] Ritter MA, Kimmeyer P, Heuschmann PU, et al. Blood pressure threshold violations in the first 24 hours after admission for acute stroke: frequency, timing, predictors, and impact on clinical outcome. Stroke. 2009; 40(2):462–468

[20] Schwamm LH, et al. IV Alteplase in MR-selected patients with stroke of Unknown onet is safe and feasible: results of multicenter MR Witness Trial. ISC; 2016; Abstract LB23 https://professional. heart.org/idc/groups/ahamah-public/@wcm/@sop/@scon/documents/downloadable/ ucm_481857.pdf

[21] Stampfl S, Ringleb PA, Haehnel S, et al. Recanalization with stent-retriever devices in patients with wake-up stroke. AJNR Am J Neuroradiol. 2013; 34(5):1040–1043

[22] Mokin M, Kan P, Sivakanthan S, et al. Endovascular therapy of wake-up strokes in the modern era of stent retriever thrombectomy. J Neurointerv Surg. 2016; 8(3):240–243

[23] Clinical Trial NCT02142283; Trevo and Medical Management versus Medical Management Alon in Wake up and late Presenting Strokes (DAWN) https://clinicaltrials.gov/ct2/show/NCT02142283

[24] Horwitz NH, Ludolph C. Acute obstructive hydrocephalus caused by cerebellar infarction. Treatment alternatives. Surg Neurol. 1983; 20(1):13–19

[25] Hornig CR, Rust DS, Busse O, Jauss M, Laun A. Space-occupying cerebellar infarction. Clinical course and prognosis. Stroke. 1994; 25(2):372–374

[26] Chen HJ, Lee TC, Wei CP. Treatment of cerebellar infarction by decompressive suboccipital craniectomy. Stroke. 1992; 23(7):957–961

[27] Vahedi K, Hofmeijer J, Juettler E, et al. DECIMAL, DESTINY, and HAMLET investigators. Early decompressive surgery in malignant infarction of the middle cerebral artery: a pooled analysis of three randomised controlled trials. Lancet Neurol. 2007; 6(3):215–222

[28] Foerch C, Lang JM, Krause J, et al. Functional impairment, disability, and quality of life outcome after decompressive hemicraniectomy in malignant middle cerebral artery infarction. J Neurosurg. 2004; 101(2):248–254

[29] Baird TA, Parsons MW, Phan T, et al. Persistent poststroke hyperglycemia is independently associated with infarct expansion and worse clinical outcome. Stroke. 2003; 34(9):2208–2214

[30] Cucchiara B, Tanne D, Levine SR, Demchuk AM, Kasner S. A risk score to predict intracranial hemorrhage after recombinant tissue plasminogen activator for acute ischemic stroke. J Stroke Cerebrovasc Dis. 2008; 17(6):331–333

[31] Demchuk AM, Tanne D, Hill MD, et al. mMulticentre tPA Stroke Survey Group. Predictors of good outcome after intravenous tPA for acute ischemic stroke. Neurology. 2001; 57(3):474–480

[32] Pundik S, McWilliams-Dunnigan L, Blackham KL, et al. Older age does not increase risk of hemorrhagic complications after intravenous and/or intra-arterial thrombolysis for acute stroke. J Stroke Cerebrovasc Dis. 2008; 17(5):266–272

[33] Greer DM, Funk SE, Reaven NL, Ouzounelli M, Uman GC. Impact of fever on outcome in patients with stroke and neurologic injury: a comprehensive meta-analysis. Stroke. 2008; 39(11):3029–3035

[34] Prasad K, Krishnan PR. Fever is associated with doubling of odds of short-term mortality in ischemic stroke: an updated meta-analysis. Acta Neurol Scand. 2010; 122(6):404–408

[35] Castillo J, Dávalos A, Marrugat J, Noya M. Timing for fever-related brain damage in acute ischemic stroke. Stroke. 1998; 29(12):2455–2460

[36] Azzimondi G, Bassein L, Nonino F, et al. Fever in acute stroke worsens prognosis. A prospective study. Stroke. 1995; 26(11):2040–2043

27 Brain Death

Omid R. Hariri and Dan E. Miulli

Abstract
It is difficult for the neurointensivist, who has attempted without hesitation and with all available measures to save and restore brain function, to accept a loss of all brain function and the loss of that patient. When such time does occur the neurointensivist should be the clinician to perform the final neurological examination, including an apnea test, which is in itself the determination of the loss of life. Brain death is the irreversible and complete cessation of all brain and brainstem function. All interfering factors that may suppress brain or brainstem function must be excluded. As the process progresses toward pronouncing a person dead by neurologic examination, there should be extensive family communication. One consolation to pronouncing the person dead by neurologic exam is that other organs are usually available to help other lives.

Keywords: cold calorics, complete cessation, complete neurological exam, corneal reflex, fixed dilated pupils, irreversible, no toxicity, Uniform Brain Death Act

Case Presentation

A 72-year-old woman presented with acute loss of consciousness while sitting in a chair at home. Her workup included a computed tomographic scan of the head that demonstrated a complete left hemispheric infarction, causing mass effect, and 2 cm of midline shift. She was admitted to the neurosurgical intensive care unit, where she was intubated. Her temperature was 32.8°C/91°F, blood pressure 90/45, and heart rate 65. Her neurologic exam demonstrated no response to pain, her pupils were 8 mm and nonreactive, and there were no corneal, cough, nor gag reflexes. The family wanted to know about the patient's prognosis and if she was "dead."

See end of chapter for Case Management.

27.1 History of Death Policy

Individually, states determine the definition of death, as do countries. In the 1950s, medical advancements that included mechanical ventilation made it possible to keep some vital organs viable. The hope delivered by transplant surgeons, and their ability to restore vital organs to patients dying from similar organ failure, led to brain death as a declaration of death. Death can also be characterized as somatic death, which is the complete cessation of cardiac and respiratory function. In 1970, the first statute determining death in all circumstances was passed. In 1978, the National Conference of Commissioners on Uniform State Laws completed the Uniform Brain Death Act. In 1980, the same commission drafted the Uniform Determination of Death Act, which is the basis for the majority of death laws in the United States. The Death Act of 1980 sets the general legal standard for determining death, but not the medical criteria for doing so. The medical profession remains free to formulate acceptable medical practices and to utilize new biomedical knowledge, diagnostic tests, and equipment.[1,2,3,4,5,6]

27.2 Definition of Death

According to the Death Act of 1980, for death to be declared, "The entire brain must cease to function, irreversibly." The "entire brain" includes the brainstem and the neocortex. This definition takes into consideration anencephaly, a condition in which an infant is born with the anatomical lack of most cerebral hemispheres but with a functioning brainstem. Such an infant is considered alive.[7] Although the Death Act of 1980 established the criterion for death, the definition did not address diagnostic tests. This provided the medical and legal profession flexibility to develop diagnostic procedures while leaving the door open for disagreement and the need for judicial review. In 1981, the President's Commission for the Study of Ethical Problems in Medicine and Biomedical and Behavioral Research developed standards for the determination of brain death, which, with some modifications, are adhered to worldwide.[3,8]

The consensus on death declaration by way of lack of brain function must include three mandatory parts: (1) there must be no brain and no brainstem function—the person must be apneic; (2) the etiology must be known and irreversible; and (3) there must be no confounding factors. The following is an example of a state law, the State of California Health and Safety Code, Section 7184:

A person who is declared brain dead is legally and physiologically dead. An individual who has sustained either (1) irreversible cessation of circulatory and respiratory functions, or (2) irreversible cessation of all functions of the entire brain, including the brainstem, is dead.

A determination of brain death must be made in accordance with accepted medical standards. In 42 states, one licensed physician is required (in a few states, the physician's representative can declare brain death); in the 8 other states, two licensed physicians are required. Hospital bylaws usually provide for criteria to pronounce death by means of a neurologic exam and may add qualifications. In most guidelines, the physician who declares a patient dead can be any licensed physician knowledgeable of and comfortable with performing a detailed neurologic exam and familiar with the procedures to declare someone dead. Uniformly, the licensed physician does not have to be a neurologist or a neurosurgeon. The only ethical consideration should be that the physician is not the transplant surgeon, because this may appear as a conflict of interest.

In 48 states, family permission is not required prior to performing a brain death exam. Only in New York and New Jersey can families object for religious reasons.[8]

The opposing opinion to the Death Act is that the entire body must not function for the declaration of death. When there is cardiac and pulmonary deterioration, which is the criterion for somatic death, an artificial and mechanical support can take over until a new heart and lung(s) are transplanted. The result will be an individual who, after recovery, may resume his or her life. However, after the brain ceases to function, there are no machines that can take over until transplantation. In the future, if transplantation were to occur, the result would be a different person lacking the memories and physical abilities, as well as lacking the hope, love, caring, and spirit, that resided in the brain in the unique individual that died. In essence, the other brain that was being transplanted was simply acquiring a new body.

27.3 Initial Criteria

To pronounce a person dead, there must be evidence of irreversible brain damage. The examining licensed physician must personally review the computed tomographic (CT) or magnetic resonance imaging (MRI) scan; it must be consistent with an irreversible condition incompatible with life, such as sustained negative cerebral perfusion pressure, massive stroke, lack of gray–white junction, edema, shift, and multiple other conditions. To proceed with a complete neurologic exam for pronouncing the patient dead, there must be hemodynamic stability; the patient cannot be arresting. It is not unusual for pupils to be fixed and dilated immediately after resuscitation. This nonresponsive brain condition can also be seen during seizures, when abnormal brain activity is impeding functional interaction. To declare death, a patient can be on multiple vasopressors.

There are major prerequisites, outlined by American Academy of Neurology, 2012, that must be met before considering a valid neurologic exam for the purpose of declaring a patient dead. Coma must be irreversible and the cause known. Moreover, neuroimaging should explain the coma. The body should have a systolic blood pressure > 100 mm Hg. The patient cannot be under the effects of a skeletal muscle paralytic (electrical stimulation if paralytics used), and all central nervous system depressant drug effect must be absent (if indicated a toxicology screen must be performed and if barbiturates were given, the serum level must be < 10 micrograms/mL). The body core temperature must be normothermic or mild hypothermic (core temperature > 36°C). Below 28°C, there is loss of brainstem reflexes.[1,4,9] In a trauma center, it is not unusual to see hypothermia in patients, such as snow skiers, the winter homeless, addicts, and cold-acclimatized patients who have ingested opioids, barbiturates, benzodiazepines, phenothiazines, tricyclic antidepressants, and lithium, or patients on a hypothermia protocol after cardiac arrest.[10,11] Furthermore, there can be no severe acid–base, electrolyte, or endocrine abnormality.

Patients can be declared legally dead if they have ingested drugs; however, the licensed physician has to certify and document that the patient is not toxic on drugs and that the drugs are not preventing brainstem function and are not causing coma. Even in the case of overdose, the pupillary reflex is preserved. However, medications can cause almost any side effects, and there are anecdotal reports that tricyclic antidepressants can mimic brain death. When drug ingestion is suspected, do not rush to pronounce death; instead, wait and investigate. Attempt to discover which drug was used, and before proceeding with the neurologic exam, observe the patient for at least 4 or 5 times the excretion half-life, assuming there is no half-life prolongation due to additional organ dysfunction. Some guidelines provide for specific drugs.[1,12] Excessive intake of alcohol would delay the performance of a death-determining exam. Alcohol (EtOH)–valid levels for brain death determinations are < 800 to 1,500 mg/dL, whereas the legal intoxication level is 80 to 100 mg/dL.[1] With certain suspected drug and medication ingestion, antidotes may be administered. However, if a medication is being prescribed to reduce the cerebral metabolic rate for oxygenation ($CMRO_2$) or if it is necessary to protect the brain in some form, the benefits of giving the antidote for benzodiazepine overdose must outweigh the risks, for example, when administering flumazenil it should be divided, first giving the dose as 0.2 mg intravenous (IV), then giving 0.3 mg. When opioid overdose is suspected, administer naloxone 0.2 to 2.0 mg IV. Additional therapeutic cerebral protectant medications are barbiturates, used to reduce increased intracranial pressure (ICP), and $CMRO_2$ by inhibiting brain activity, placing the patient in a medication-induced coma. The clinical diagnosis of brain death can still be made after stopping the medication if the serum levels are less than the therapeutic range. In most laboratories, the level would be < 5 to 15 µg/mL. This is below the level required for burst suppression, 50 µg/mL. When a drug or poison cannot be quantified but seems highly likely from history, one should not make the diagnosis of brain death.

One criterion for death pronouncement is the consideration of altering neurologic status due to drugs' effect on metabolism. The same consideration of pure systemic abnormalities must also be made; the systemic abnormality must not be causing the coma or loss of brainstem reflexes. Severe abnormalities, such as hypoglycemia or hyperglycemia, hyponatremia, hypernatremia, hypothyroidism, panhypopituitarism, or Addison's disease, may decrease the level of consciousness and confuse the neurologic examination, but a complete loss of brainstem reflexes is seldom observed. The licensed physician must once again document that the systemic abnormalities are not the cause of coma.[1]

27.4 Brain Death Exam

Only after the initial criteria are met can the licensed physician proceed with the neurologic exam. The exam documents the function of the cerebral hemispheres and the brainstem. It will not assess the entire or specific function of the basal ganglia, thalamus, or cerebral cortices. To assume a lack of functional cerebral hemispheres, the patient must be in a coma. An often touted but rare clinical condition that, by exam, may mimic complete and irreversible lack of entire brain function is a severe locked-in syndrome, when there is profound damage to the brainstem, with the exception of the ascending reticular activating system (ARAS), and intact cerebral hemisphere function. This circumstance is rare and may be excluded easily in most instances. The history, physical, radiological, and physiological review should argue against this condition. The less severe locked-in syndrome is produced by ischemic or hemorrhagic destruction to the descending motor pathways, the corticospinal and corticobulbar tracts of the basis pontis (ventral pons), and the reticular formation of the pontine tegmentum, sparing the ARAS. It is a pure motor paresis, sparing the sensory pathways. In this somewhat less severe condition, the patient still retains vertical eye and eyelid movements. If there is true concern about either type of locked-in syndrome in which the person is conscious but cannot move or breathe, electroencephalography (EEG) can be performed to determine the function of the cerebral hemispheres.[13]

The main test of cortical, and basal ganglia function is conscious interaction and conscious reaction to painful stimuli. Pain reaction does occur without consciousness in brainstem and spinal reflexes. Although brainstem reflexes negate death, pronouncement by detailed neurologic exam can occur if spinal reflexes are present. A viable spinal cord is not an exclusion of death; a person could have spinal cord function, such as spinal reflexes, and still be dead.

In examining consciousness, the physician must determine if the patient makes any sound. Next, the physician must determine if the patient will open his or her eyes to name, touch, or painful stimuli. The examiner must then determine if the patient follows commands, localizes to pain, withdraws to pain, or has decorticate or decerebrate response to pain. Simply applying pinpricks to the body is not an appropriate stimulation of pain. Pressure on the supraorbital nerve positioned on the medial aspect of the eyebrow ridge is the best place to test for motor response to pain. It can also be elicited with temporomandibular joint compression. Additionally, peripheral stimulation, such as nail bed pressure, may elicit a spinal reflex instead of a central response, often confusing the exam. A spinal reflex is a stereotypical repetitive, nonsustained movement that is usually monosynaptic. A withdrawal brainstem response is more complex because of additional inputs. The difference between high-level withdrawal response and decorticate reflex or spinal reflex can be determined by applying pain to the medial upper arm. The withdrawal response will usually be to abduct the arm away from the chest, whereas the reflex will be to adduct the arm toward the chest. A nonreflex conscious pain response demonstrates some integrity of the spine–brainstem–thalamus–cortical basal ganglion pathway. If there is decreased input from the cerebral hemispheres, decreased input through the cortical spinal tract, a functioning rubrospinal tract, and motor flexor of the distal limb, inhibition of extensor muscles becomes dominant, resulting in decorticate activity.

If there is disruption between the superior colliculi (anterior quadrigeminal bodies) or the decussation of the rubrospinal pathway, the rostral portion of the vestibular nuclei, pain stimulation becomes the major response of the vestibulospinal tract. This results in extensor tone to motor neurons innervating the neck, back, and limbs, and inhibition of flexion of the trunk and limbs. Since the track is uncrossed, the decerebrate activity occurs on the same side of the lesion. Spinal cord responses in addition to the stereotypical repetitive, nonsustained movement at the site of stimulation may also be seen as a slow response in the extremities, brief flexion of the fingers, or minimal eyelid deviation.

As the detailed neurologic exam proceeds down from the cerebral cortex and diencephalons, the function of the midbrain and the nuclei of cranial nerve (CN) II and CN III is probed. The physician examines these structures, testing the pupillary reflex using a bright flashlight, first directed into one pupil so that it hits the retina, and then into the other. Dilated pupils are > 4 mm, and asymmetric pupils are > 1 mm different. Pupils that are asymmetrical and small are usually a sign of midbrain or pontine injury in a living person. Always err on the side of caution and on the side of life. If orbital or papillary inspection is hampered, use a magnifying glass. This reflex of sensory and autonomic motor response can demonstrate activity even if the patient has been chemically paralyzed.

The corneal reflex indicates the integrity of the midpons, cranial nerve (CN) V sensory component, and CN VII motor component. It is performed by touching the cornea away from the pupil with a cotton-tipped applicator and observing a blink response. The blink may be slight; however, any movement is an indicator of function and life. For this test, do not use a paper towel, piece of paper, or any material that may be abrasive to the cornea.

Next, the midbrain to lower pons is tested, investigating the oculovestibular reflex by injecting ice water into the external auditory canal that is known to have an intact unobstructed tympanic membrane. The physician observes the eye movement while stimulating the vestibular system. First, elevate the head to 30 degrees to allow maximum stimulation of the horizontal canal. Then inject 30 to 50 cc of ice water into the external auditory canal and watch 30 seconds or more for the slow movement to the side of the cold-water stimulus. In coma, the quick nystagmus is lost, and the slow component to the side of the cold-water stimulus remains. If there is no brainstem reflex, the eyes will not move. Test one side, wait 5 minutes, then test the other. Testing the other side too soon after the first will inhibit the slow component to the side of the cold-water stimulus. This tests the CN III, VI, and VIII, the medial longitudinal fasciculus (MLF), the paramedian pontine reticular formation (PPRF), and the lower pons. Similar information can be obtained during the oculocephalic reflex. However, if spinal cord injury is suspected, do not perform the test. The oculocephalic reflex is observed while turning the patient's head. Fast turning of the head to both sides should not produce any eye movement; however, conjunctival swelling sometimes makes this difficult to elicit. This is referred to as the doll's eyes reflex because the patient's eyes, like the painted eyes of a doll, stay fixed forward without movement. This reflex tests the similar components of the oculovestibular reflex: CN III, VI, and VIII; MLF; PPRF; and lower pons.

A cough response should be attempted using a suction catheter inserted into the endotracheal tube and advanced to the level of the carina, followed by deep suctioning to test lower brainstem or medulla function. Do not just move the endotracheal tube. The simple stimulation of the gag reflex is a variable test, as it can be blunted by medication and normal physiology. This test, in which there is a cough or sensation, then elevation of the uvula, monitors the function of CN V, IX, and X and the medulla.

Certain movements are seen in the dead body and do not denote brainstem function. There can be spinal reflex spontaneous movements of the head and limbs; respiratory-like spinal reflex movements of the shoulders, back, and intercostal muscles without tidal volumes; and deep tendon reflexes, superficial abdominal reflexes, triple flexion response, Babinski's reflex, and other spinal reflexes due to stimulation from acidosis or other means. There can also be spinal autonomic responses, such as tachycardia, sudden increases in blood pressure, blushing, and sweating. There does not have to be the need for blood pressure control, nor does diabetes insipidus have to be present.[14,15]

27.4.1 Irreversibility

It is advised to have two licensed physicians perform the detailed neurologic exam, as is the requirement in eight states. However, it may not be practical in some settings. It should be determined before the first physician examines the patient whether there is any question that the injury is reversible or not. The

CT scan or MRI must be reviewed and be consistent with an irreversible condition incompatible with life, such as sustained negative cerebral perfusion pressure, massive stroke, lack of gray–white junction, edema, shift, and multiple other conditions. If there is a question about irreversibility, then wait some time before the second neurologic exam is performed. Four or more hours is an arbitrary time to wait in an adult; some municipalities wait longer, and in other countries the wait can extend into days. Another licensed physician can repeat the neurologic exam immediately if there is no question about irreversibility, and if required by law, bylaws, or conscience. Once again, it is practical in some instances to have only one detailed neurologic exam to pronounce brain death.

27.4.2 Apnea Test

After the final detailed neurologic exam, the hallmark of brain death should be performed: the apnea test. Do not perform it before the first detailed neurologic exam. Instead, the apnea test can be performed with the first of two detailed neurologic exams or with the second. It does not have to be performed twice, even in states where two licensed physicians are required to certify death by detailed exam. When a second exam is required, the physician must verify the results of any previous apnea test. It is often practical to perform the apnea test with the first of two required detailed neurologic exams if there is no additional requirement for a waiting period. However, the apnea test may produce a period of relative hypotension or hypoxia, which, with a condition of uncertainty in which the patient may still be alive, is detrimental. Therefore, optimally, the apnea test should be performed with the second detailed neurologic exam (▶ Table 27.1).

The apnea exam tests the reticular formation of the caudal medulla. The strongest human drive is to breathe, and the living human will breathe if the by-product of metabolism, CO_2, increases above a certain threshold. Only rarely will the individual not breathe at mildly elevated CO_2 levels, such as a minority with chronic obstructive pulmonary disease (COPD) who function normally

Table 27.1 Apnea test to declare death[1,2,3,4,5,6,7,8]

Requirements to do test	When to perform
One required physician and neurologic exam	At the end of the detailed neurologic exam
Two required physicians and neurologic exams, no waiting period or waiting period	At the end of the second neurologic exam. It is acceptable for the second exam to follow the first immediately if there is no reason for a waiting period. Pronouncement of death occurs when second exam is completed.

with increased CO_2. Although the drive to breathe occurs earlier with hypoxia and later with acidosis, the most reliable drive to determine a lack of brainstem function is a rise in CO_2. Acidosis will drive respiration; however, the blood–brain barrier is not as permeable to hydrogen ions as it is to CO_2 gas. Therefore, the microenvironment of the medulla is most responsive to escalating CO_2 gas, and brain death is determined by apnea due to the rise of CO_2 above the threshold. Brain death is not determined by hypoxemic or acidemic apnea.

Do not perform the apnea test unless the criteria to proceed with death declaration by neurologic examination have been met; there can be no effect of paralytics, no toxic effects of drugs, and, specific to the apnea test, no high spinal cord injury to prevent ventilation. Before performing the last part of the neurologic exam, the apnea test to investigate the reticular formation of the caudal medulla, the patient must meet additional criteria. The patient should be normothermic, with a core temperature of 35.0 to 36.5°C or 95 to 97°F. The warmer the body, the quicker the CO_2 will rise. If the body is colder, the apnea test will take longer, leading to possible hypoxia or hemodynamic instability. However, do not attempt to make the patient hyperthermic, a condition that will increase $CMRO_2$ should the patient be alive. There should be no hypotension; the systolic blood pressure (SBP) should be greater than 90 mm Hg, although hypotension using 90 mm Hg is an arbitrary number. Young, small women and smaller children have blood pressures normally < 90 mm Hg. To decrease the time required off the ventilator, which increases the chance of O_2 desaturation leading to hypotension and cardiac instability, the partial pressure of CO_2 (PCO_2) should be normal, 35 to 45 mm Hg by arterial blood gases (ABGs). If COPD is suspected, start with a PCO_2 60 mm Hg or higher. Before beginning the apnea test, the fluids should be running wide open. Vasopressors should be running or hanging and connected to the IV line and able to be given within seconds. SBP in the average adult should be as close to 120 mm Hg as possible but not < 90 mm Hg. Vasopressors should be increased as necessary. There should be pulse oximetry, and it should be maintained at 100% to start and without hypoxia throughout the test. The blood pressure and vitals should be monitored continuously; however, if no arterial line has been inserted, monitor the blood pressure with a cuff every minute. Monitoring blood pressure less often will only lead to the arrest of cardiac and pulmonary systems, with the resultant prolonged resuscitation of a patient who would have possibly been pronounced dead 10 minutes later. Hypotension is usually due to acidosis from decreased oxygenation or perfusion. Therefore, high temporary concentrations of O_2 and a hypervolemic state are necessary. If hypotension cannot be controlled, a blood gas should be drawn immediately and the remaining time aborted until measures can be taken to control loss of blood pressure.

The apnea test will measure the ability of the body to take a breath in response to increasing blood CO_2 (PCO_2). The PCO_2 will rise 3 to 6 mm Hg per minute depending on circulation and temperature. Some authors state that PCO_2 will rise 2 to 8 mm Hg; however, these are unusual conditions. The target PCO_2 is 60 mm Hg on an ABG test, although some municipalities use 55 mm Hg. When the patient has COPD, not only should the PCO_2 rise above 60 mm Hg, it must rise at least 20 mm Hg above baseline to prevent any false diagnosis of brain death. To facilitate the levels of CO_2, the ventilator should be adjusted in the COPD patient who is known to be a CO_2 retainer; begin with a PCO_2 of 60 mm Hg before the apnea test. After the increased baseline of 60 mm Hg or higher, the PCO_2 should be allowed to rise at least 20 mm Hg[4,16,17,18,19,20] Additional concerns may be that the patient has absolutely no CO_2 drive, another unusual condition. Under those circumstances, a cerebral blood flow study should be ordered to confirm the complete absence of brain and brainstem blood flow.

In an attempt to ensure that the apnea test does not lead to cardiac arrest, or that a surviving person does not suffer further injury from hypoxia or ischemia, preoxygenate the patient for 8–10 minutes with 100% O_2 to eliminate the nitrogen stores, hyperoxygenate tissue to maintain organ viability, and prevent hypotension and cardiac instability. The patient may still develop acidosis during the apnea test from increased CO_2 levels; however, this can be minimized with excellent fluid flow, oxygenation, and blood pressure.

After hyperoxygenation, disconnect the ventilator while maintaining a superadequate O_2 source using a catheter, such as a nasal cannula with the nostril insert cut off, placed at the carina delivering O_2 at 6 L/min or higher. The alternative is to keep the patient on the ventilator, stopping the breaths administered while maintaining positive pressure support at 10 mm Hg. Be careful: some ventilators have an automatic backup that will deliver 0.5 to 1.0 breath/min; this fail-safe mechanism must be turned off. Furthermore, the licensed physician must not depend on the ventilator measuring the breaths; instead, he or she must observe the rise and fall of the chest, if present. If using the nasal cannula in the endotracheal tube, verify that both cannulas are at or before the end of the tube. Verify the length before insertion. If the cannulas are too long, they may oxygenate only one lung, and the nasal cannulas may get stuck; neither condition will be known initially. Furthermore, guarantee that there is enough room between the endotracheal tube and the catheter for O_2 to escape so there is no pressure buildup and pneumothorax. The person will be temporarily off the ventilator ~ 8 to 10 minutes, based on the pretesting PCO_2 level. Under optimal conditions of temperature and blood pressure, after the 10 minutes of apnea multiplied by ~ 3 mm Hg of arterial CO_2 rise per minute, there should be 30 mm Hg rise from baseline PCO_2 toward the desired target value of 60 mm Hg. During the apnea test, the licensed physician must be present. The apnea test is the last part of the neurologic exam. The physician must observe the abdomen and chest for movements. If there are no movements after 10 minutes, then a new blood gas is drawn. When the arterial blood PCO_2 has reached at least 60 mm Hg, or at least 60 mm Hg plus 20 mm Hg above the patient's elevated normal baseline, if there is a suspected CO_2 retainer, then the apnea test is positive, and the person is pronounced dead. If the PCO_2 has not reached 60 mm Hg on the ABG test, or has not gone 20 mm Hg higher than the minimum 60 mm Hg starting baseline in the CO_2 retainer, the test must be repeated for longer times.

When initial neurologic brain death testing criteria have been met, when there is demonstrated irreversible loss of brain function, when confounding factors are known to not be responsible for coma and absent brainstem function, and when a detailed neurologic exam is completed, including an apnea test, that demonstrates absent brain and brainstem function and reflexes, the clinical diagnosis of death can be made. The patient is pronounced at the time the final detailed neurologic exam and positive apnea test are concluded.

The apnea test procedure involves the following steps:
- Disconnect the ventilator, or turn the ventilator to pressure support only, and disconnect the backup breath.
- Start the timer.
- Place the nasal cannulas with nasal inserts into the endotracheal tube only up to the end of the tube. Be sure that both nasal cannulas slide into the tube without getting stuck and that air is escaping.
- Place one hand on the patient's chest, observe, and listen for breath.
- Check blood pressure readings every minute or continuously by ABG. In the average adult, keep as close to 120 mm Hg as possible.
- Check pulse oximetry reading every minute or continuously.
- Be able to increase fluids quickly.
- Be able to increase vasopressors quickly.
- If too hypoxic, abort the test.
- If too hypotensive, abort the test.
- If there are too many cardiac arrhythmias, abort the test.
- After 10 minutes, obtain ABG, place the patient back on the ventilator, and document the time.

27.4.3 Confirmatory Test

A confirmatory test is not needed in adults. The neurologic exam that includes the apnea test must document the lack of brain and brainstem function, must document irreversibility, and must document a lack of confounding factors, such as hypothermia and drugs. Only if the entire neurologic exam and complete repeated exam, if applicable, including the apnea test, cannot be performed or is not valid is a confirmatory test required. A confirmatory test cannot replace the apnea test portion of the neurologic exam but is performed when the apnea test or other part of the neurologic test cannot be achieved successfully. It is rare that the patient will not tolerate the apnea test if the above precautions are followed.

If a confirmatory test is mandated, a cerebral angiogram should be performed. The angiogram must include visualization of all remaining anterior and posterior circulation. To diagnose death, there must be no intracerebral filling of the carotid, basilar, or vertebral artery from where it enters the skull. Only the lack of intracerebral arterial circulation needs to be documented. There can be a patent external carotid circulation and delayed filling of the superior sagittal sinus.

EEG does not detect brainstem function and cannot be the sole test to pronounce death. Electrocerebral silence does not exclude the possibility of reversible coma; however, multiple EEGs over an extended time, such as 24 hours, in the absence of medication- or metabolic-induced electrocerebral silence, correlate with a lack of cerebral function. EEG is not the gold standard for diagnosis of brain death, and it does not replace the apnea test, but it is used occasionally. When performing an EEG, there should be no electrical activity during at least 30 minutes of recording. The recording must adhere to the minimum technical standards of the American Clinical Neurophysiology Society (ACNS; formerly the American Electroencephalographic Society)[21] for EEG recording in suspected brain death. The guidelines include a 16- or 18-channel EEG instrument, with scalp electrodes at least 10 cm apart. The inter-electrode impedances should be between 100 and 10,000 ohms. There should be no activity over 2 μV/mm (better determined at 1 μV/mm) for 30 minutes. The high-frequency filter setting should be at 30 Hz, and the low-frequency setting should not be below 1 Hz. There should be no EEG reactivity to intense somatosensory or audiovisual stimuli.[21,22] If cerebral angiography is not performed, and EEG has to be relied on for confirmation of death, then EEG and repeat EEGs should be combined with brainstem auditory evoked responses (BAERs) to at least examine the brain and brainstem. Both electrical tests have characteristics that can lead to misinterpretation.

Transcranial Doppler (TCD) ultrasonography is now being entertained to assist in the confirmation of brain death. The TCD probe should be placed at the temporal bone above the zygomatic arch or the vertebrobasilar arteries through the suboccipital transcranial window. There should be insonation of at least three separate vessels on each side demonstrating the equivalent findings. However, 10% of people have no temporal insonation windows. Therefore, the initial absence of TCD signal cannot be interpreted as consistent with brain death. TCD utilization must produce a signal at all tested vessels demonstrating small systolic peaks in early systole with a lack of diastolic flow. The posterior cerebral artery (PCA) is usually the first to change, with the middle cerebral artery (MCA) being the last. Other criteria include the pulsatility index, which will be above 2.0 globally, indicating very high vascular resistance associated with greatly increased ICP. If the TCD reveals oscillating flow through the intracranial arteries, then brain death is more certain. Except for oscillating flow, all other criteria can be seen in pentobarbital coma. However, TCD does not detect brainstem flow or flow through small vessels, and it must not be used as meeting criteria to pronounce death.[23,27]

Single-photon emission computed tomography (SPECT) measures brain uptake activity using radiolabeled amphetamine or radionuclide scan using IV technetium 99 m hexamethylpropyleneamineoxime (Tc 99m-HMPAO).[28] Tc 99m-HMPAO adequately reflects brain activity and has been used for the determination of brain death. The isotope needs to be injected within 30 minutes of reconstitution and reveals initial dynamic flow images. Then there are important static images of 500,000 counts at several time intervals recorded immediately, between 30 and 60 minutes, and at 2 hours. Tc 99m-HMPAO static images are adequate for demonstrating the posterior fossa and brainstem.[29] During evaluation, there should be no uptake of isotope in intra-cerebral parenchyma; however, there may be activity in the external carotid circulation that will demonstrate a hollow skull. To have a valid test, correct IV injection needs to be confirmed with additional liver images demonstrating uptake. By comparison to conventional technetium agents, Tc 99m-HMPAO is not dependent on bolus quality and allows evaluation of the posterior fossa and brainstem.[30] The Tc 99m-HMPAO scan is portable, less expensive, and does not require intra-arterial injection.

27.5 Brain Death Exam in Children

Before beginning with an examination as part of the declaration of death, the child must meet the initial criteria of irreversibility, no hypothermia, hypotension, or hypoglycemia, and no medications or metabolic changes that would cause coma or loss of brainstem reflexes. The difficult neurologic exam must be completed twice. The nervous system of the newborn is different from the adult because certain physiological functions may not have been developed. However, the same detailed neurologic exam, including the apnea test, must be performed twice. The detailed neurologic exam must be performed before and after the observation period, and the apnea test must be performed only with the second exam.[31]

Some brainstem reflexes are developed late. In children, the pupillary response to light is obtainable only after week 32 of gestation. The grasp response is obtainable after week 36 of gestation. Most importantly, the last part of the detailed neurologic exam, the apnea response to a PCO_2 stimulus, can only be elicited after 33 weeks of gestation. Therefore, in children there need to be additional criteria mandated for the brain death examination. There is a mandatory observation period in children, and the observation is age dependent. The complete neurologic exam must be completed before and after the observation period. For children ages 8 days to 2 months, the observation period is 48 hours. For ages 2 months to 12 months, the observation period is 24 hours. For ages 12 months and older, the observation period is 12 hours. An infant must be at least 8 days old to be evaluated for clinical brain death.[31,32,33,34,35]

27.5.1 Children's Confirmatory Test

Because the complete neurologic and repeat neurologic exams after the appropriate observation period may not be reliable, as the functions tested may not have developed, confirmatory tests are mandatory. A cerebral angiogram is the gold standard. EEG should be performed in accordance with ACNS[21] standards, adjusting the 10 cm interelectrode distance proportional to the head circumference. Because children < 1 year old can survive longer periods of electrocerebral silence without cerebral death, EEGs must be repeated. In children ages 8 days to 2 months, there should be two EEGs and two complete neurologic exams (including an apnea test), 48 hours apart. Two EEGs and complete neurologic exams 24 hours apart or the combination of two complete neurologic examinations 24 hours apart, an EEG showing electrocortical silence, and a Tc 99m-HMPAO radionuclide test showing no cerebral uptake are required in children ages 2 months to 1 year, the rationale being that, in addition to the complete neurologic exams, the radionuclide scan will demonstrate no metabolic brain activity, as well as no electrical activity. Some criteria state that the waiting period is not necessary in children ages 2 months to 1 year if there is a complete neurologic exam, an EEG showing electrocortical silence, and a Tc 99m-HMPAO radionuclide test demonstrating no cerebral uptake. Children's brains demonstrate an ability to recover substantial function after much more significant damage than do adult brains; therefore, the observation period is longer. It remains questionable why the cerebral arteriogram as the sole test has not been incorporated into published criteria for pediatric brain death.

27.6 After the Declaration of Brain Death

Brain death is dead. According to Youngner et al, "First and foremost, brain death is irreversible. Patients who are brain dead have permanently lost the capacity to think, be aware of self or surroundings, experience, or communicate with others."[36]

Death must be recorded in the medical record chart when the complete neurologic exam, including the apnea test, is finished. The brain dead patient does not remain alive only to die once the ventilator is removed; the person is dead. There is no need for a physician to return to the body and pronounce the body dead again when the heart stops beating. Death is at the time of the completed full neurologic exam; it is not recorded as the time when the body is removed from the organ-supporting ventilator or when cardiopulmonary function ends.

Health care workers must not state that a patient will be kept alive on the ventilator until organs are recovered. The patient is not alive; only the organs are supported with ventilation. After death is pronounced, the ventilator is turned off if no organs are being donated. The family can visit with the body after removal of the remaining organ support. They should be notified that the patient is dead. The family will naturally ask about the beating heart and should be told that the brain, which contains the memories, activities, joys, love, kindness, and spirit of life, has died and will not return; only the body remains. The heart will continue to beat for an unknown length of time, and most of the organs will function if given support; however, the person is gone. The hospital staff policy must address the length of time that the body can remain in the NICU after the declaration of brain death until a decision about organ donation or until the ventilator is stopped. This short period lasting minutes to a few hours should be offered to allow grieving to begin but should not be so long as to provide false hope. Allowing many hours or, worse, days for out-of-state relatives to visit is not in the best interest of the family. An unusually long length of time only prolongs the family's agony and inhibits the healing process.

After the declaration of death, when there is no decision to donate organs, the ventilator is discontinued. During this time until minutes after complete cessation of cardiac function, there may be acidosis, ischemia, and a sympathetic surge. This surge can trigger multiple simultaneous muscle contractions leading to opening of the eyes, elevation of the arms, and sitting up. This is called the Lazarus syndrome. Therefore, the family should be counseled should they decide to remain with the body from the time of ventilator discontinuation and extubation until removal to the morgue.

27.7 Organ Donation

Sometimes the body remains in the NICU while the family decides if the dead individual had wanted to donate organs. It is best for the family to discuss the gift of organ donation with the organ donation workers prior to death.[37,38,39] The organ donation agency should be contacted anytime the patient has a Glasgow Coma Scale score of 5 or less. The agency could then decide if the individual meets the criteria for donation. If questions from the family arise about organ donation prior to the arrival of organ donation workers, the family may be asked about the wishes of the patient. If the patient is pronounced dead by a complete neurologic exam and the family has consented on behalf of the individual to organ donation, the ventilator continues, and the care of the body should be turned over to the organ transplant agency. The agency coordinators will assume care, write orders, and attempt to maintain the adult parameters of $PO_2 > 100$ mm Hg, SBP > 100 mm Hg, and PCO_2 35 to 45 mm Hg.

Case Management

The patient described in the case study is hypothermic and cannot meet initial criteria to be declared brain dead. The patient must be warmed slowly, must not be comatose from medication, must not be hypoglycemic, and must not have severe metabolic abnormalities that would cause coma and loss of brain-stem reflexes. If the initial criteria are met and there is an irreversible lesion on CT scan, then the licensed physician may proceed with a brain death exam.

References

[1] Wijdicks EFM. Determining brain death in adults. Neurology. 1995; 45(5):1003–1011

[2] A definition of irreversible coma. Report of the Ad Hoc Committee of the Harvard Medical School to Examine the Definition of Brain Death. JAMA. 1968; 205(6):337–340

[3] Guidelines for the determination of death. Report of the medical consultants on the diagnosis of death to the President's Commission for the Study of Ethical Problems in Medicine and Biomedical Behavioral Research. JAMA. 1981; 246(19):2184–2186

[4] The Quality Standards Subcommittee of the American Academy of Neurology. Practice parameters for determining brain death in adults (summary statement). Neurology. 1995; 45:1012–1014

[5] Wijdicks EF. The diagnosis of brain death. N Engl J Med. 2001; 344(16):1215–1221

[6] Curry PD, Bion JF. The diagnosis and management of brain death. Curr Anaesth Crit Care. 1994; 5 (1):36–40

[7] The Medical Task Force on Anencephaly. The infant with anencephaly. N Engl J Med. 1990; 322 (10):669–674

[8] Wijdicks EFM. Brain death worldwide: accepted fact but no global consensus in diagnostic criteria. Neurology. 2002; 58(1):20–25

[9] Byrne PA, Nilges RG. The brain stem in brain death: a critical review. Issues Law Med. 1993; 9 (1):3–21

[10] Danzl DF, Pozos RS. Accidental hypothermia. N Engl J Med. 1994; 331(26):1756–1760

[11] Gilbert M, Busund R, Skagseth A, Nilsen PA, Solbø JP. Resuscitation from accidental hypothermia of 13.7 degrees C with circulatory arrest [letter]. Lancet. 2000; 355(9201):375–376

[12] Kennedy M, Kiloh N. Drugs and brain death. Drug Saf. 1996; 14(3):171–180

[13] Patterson JR, Grabois M. Locked-in syndrome: a review of 139 cases. Stroke. 1986; 17(4):758–764

[14] Ropper AH. Unusual spontaneous movements in brain-dead patients. Neurology. 1984; 34 (8):1089–1092

[15] Saposnik G, Bueri JA, Mauriño J, Saizar R, Garretto NS. Spontaneous and reflex movements in brain death. Neurology. 2000; 54(1):221–223

[16] Marks SJ, Zisfein J. Apneic oxygenation in apnea tests for brain death. A controlled trial. Arch Neurol. 1990; 47(10):1066–1068

[17] Benzel EC, Gross CD, Hadden TA, Kesterson L, Landreneau MD. The apnea test for the determination of brain death. J Neurosurg. 1989; 71(2):191–194

[18] Benzel EC, Mashburn JP, Conrad S, Modling D. Apnea testing for the determination of brain death: a modified protocol. Technical note. J Neurosurg. 1992; 76(6):1029–1031

[19] Belsh JM, Blatt R, Schiffman PL. Apnea testing in brain death. Arch Intern Med. 1986; 146 (12):2385–2388

[20] van Donselaar CA, Meerwaldt JD, van Gijn J. Apnoea testing to confirm brain death in clinical practice. J Neurol Neurosurg Psychiatry. 1986; 49(9):1071–1073

[21] American Electroencephalographic Society. Guideline three: minimum technical standards for EEG recording in suspected cerebral death. J Clin Neurophysiol. 1994; 11(1):10–13

[22] Silverman D, Saunders MG, Schwab RS, Masland RL. Cerebral death and the electroencephalogram. Report of the ad hoc committee of the American Electroencephalographic Society on EEG Criteria for determination of cerebral death. JAMA. 1969; 209(10):1505–1510

[23] Assessment: transcranial Doppler. Report of the American Academy of Neurology, Therapeutics and Technology Assessment Subcommittee. Neurology. 1990; 40(4):680–681

[24] Payen DM, Lamer C, Pilorget A, Moreau T, Beloucif S, Echter E. Evaluation of pulsed Doppler common carotid blood flow as a noninvasive method for brain death diagnosis: a prospective study. Anesthesiology. 1990; 72(2):222–229

[25] Petty GW, Mohr JP, Pedley TA, et al. The role of transcranial Doppler in confirming brain death: sensitivity, specificity, and suggestions for performance and interpretation. Neurology. 1990; 40 (2):300–303

[26] Jalili M, Crade M, Davis AL. Carotid blood-flow velocity changes detected by Doppler ultrasound in determination of brain death in children. A preliminary report. Clin Pediatr (Phila). 1994; 33 (11):669–674

[27] Newell DW. Transcranial Doppler measurements. New Horiz. 1995; 3(3):423–430

[28] Bonetti MG, Ciritella P, Valle G, Perrone E. 99mTc HM-PAO brain perfusion SPECT in brain death. Neuroradiology. 1995; 37(5):365–369

[29] de la Riva A, González FM, Llamas-Elvira JM, et al. Diagnosis of brain death: superiority of perfusion studies with 99Tcm-HMPAO over conventional radionuclide cerebral angiography. Br J Radiol. 1992; 65(772):289–294

[30] Laurin NR, Driedger AA, Hurwitz GA, et al. Cerebral perfusion imaging with technetium-99 m HM-PAO in brain death and severe central nervous system injury. J Nucl Med. 1989; 30 (10):1627–1635

[31] American Academy of Pediatrics Task Force on Brain Death in Children. Report of special Task Force. Guidelines for the determination of brain death in children. Pediatrics. 1987; 80(2):298–300

[32] Ashwal S, Schneider S. Brain death in children: Part I. Pediatr Neurol. 1987; 3(1):5–11

[33] Ashwal S, Schneider S. Brain death in children: Part II. Pediatr Neurol. 1987; 3(2):69–77

[34] Ashwal S. Brain death in the newborn. Current perspectives. Clin Perinatol. 1997; 24(4):859–882

[35] Bernat JL. A defense of the whole-brain concept of death. Hastings Cent Rep. 1998; 28(2):14–23

[36] Youngner SJ, Landefeld CS, Coulton CJ, Juknialis BW, Leary M. 'Brain death' and organ retrieval. A cross-sectional survey of knowledge and concepts among health professionals. JAMA. 1989; 261 (15):2205–2210

[37] Franz HG, DeJong W, Wolfe SM, et al. Explaining brain death: a critical feature of the donation process. J Transpl Coord. 1997; 7(1):14–21

[38] Chabalewski F, Norris MK. The gift of life: talking to families about organ and tissue donation. Am J Nurs. 1994; 94(6):28–33

[39] Medicare and Medicaid programs; hospital conditions of participation; provider agreements and supplier approval. 62 Federal Register 1997;42 CFR Part 482. https://www.gpo.gov/fdsys/pkg/FR-2006-11-27/pdf/E6-19957.pdf

28 Family Communication

Mark Krel and Dan E. Miulli

Abstract

No other facet of medicine is as difficult for the neurointensivist as communication. Sometimes communication occurs with the patient but more frequently it takes place with the family members. There have been many articles and books written about communication; however, Shannon's book on the mathematical theory of communication from 1949 discussed that, at its basic elements, there is a source that produces a message, a transmitter of the message through a channel to a receiver, which transforms the message for whom the message was intended. Each part and step can be influenced; therefore the health care worker should realize the importance of gathering the data, empathizing with and respecting the individuals in the relationship and the redundancy and reconditioning of the information. The neurointensivist being part of a team should be aware that, to achieve the best patient experience, other members of the health care team, such as the palliative care team, can provide resources and support not available through other areas in order to improve the quality of life of the patient.

Keywords: body language, empathy, exchange information, gather data, relationships, respect, Shannon's theory, tone of voice

Case Presentation

As the neurosurgeon on call, you are called to the emergency room to see a patient who presented having been found down by his family. The emergency medicine (EM) provider tells you that the patient was intubated for decreased Glasgow Coma Scale (GCS) score as he was GCS score 8 on arrival with briskly reactive pupils. On questioning the EM provider for the patient's medical record number and name you realize it is a patient you have previously operated on twice to remove recurrent glioblastoma multiforme tumors from the left sylvian region. At his last clinic visit, you recall that the patient had speech difficulties as well as right-sided weakness and recurrent seizures currently managed with Dilantin and Keppra. Given your familiarity with the patient and his disease process, you start heading for the emergency room anticipating the difficult conversation you will have with the patient and his family.

See end of chapter for Case Management.

28.1 Introduction

Care of the neurosurgical intensive care unit (NICU) patient is more than managing the clinical situation. There are numerous areas that are just as important and must be attended to, particularly communication. Communication should not be left for health care workers to learn on their own; it must be part of the neurosurgical curriculum. The recommendations in this section have been developed over time, using the expertise of countless clinicians.

This chapter outlines the definition of communication in the NICU setting, along with the goals of communication and its role in relationship building. It offers suggestions on dealing with barriers to communication, including hostile patients and their families. Scenarios are presented depicting challenges in communication between medical and allied health professionals and NICU patients and their families. Additionally, circumstances requiring specialized protocols for communications are discussed.

28.2 Definition of Communication

The broadest definition of communication in this setting is the exchange of information between and among physicians doing neurocritical care, their colleagues, multidisciplinary health care specialists, and patients and their families.[1]

Physicians cannot function in the NICU outside the bounds of their relationships with staff. The physicians and the multidisciplinary staff of caregivers in the hospital are one unit in a dyad. The cohesiveness of that unit and its ability to converge on a goal in an organized battle array are a matter of planning, dedication, mutual respect, and practice.

Regardless of the patient's level of consciousness and capacity, the patient cannot be managed and communication cannot be said to occur if the available family members are not taken into account.[2] The patient and his or her family are the other unit in the dyad. The cohesiveness of this unit is subject to patterns of functioning that began before the crisis centered attention on the patient and will continue, in some manner, irrespective of the patient's outcome.

The narrow scope of communication for this section is the exchange between physicians and the patient and his or her family. This is the familiar stage for the relationship between the dyads. Communication encompasses all manner of conveying information, but this section will focus on verbal communication and unspoken behaviors that convey feelings encountered during conversations.

The milieu in which the communication occurs, that is, the medical setting, the emergency room, and the NICU, indelibly colors the information conveyed, how it is remembered, and how it is used to make decisions both for patients/families and physicians/health care teams.[3]

Communication does not occur in a vacuum. The doctor–patient relationship is the basis for communication. The patient and his or her family give and receive information in the context of this relationship, extended to include all of the health care team.

28.3 Goals of Communication

Communication can be said to be achieved when the patient/family and physicians/health care team create a dialogue between each other for the patient's sake in which questions are asked and answered truthfully, wisely, and respectfully, and the unanswerable questions are acknowledged with compassion, patience, and trust. One-sided conveyance of information devoid of human context may, in some circumstances, seem necessary and appropriate, even if painful, but it is not communication unless it is acknowledged and assimilated.

The goal of communication is fundamentally the exchange of information that might lead to saving the patient's life or salvaging the disabled patient from ruin, but this goal is accomplished or derailed by the quality of the relationship that develops between patient/family and physicians/health care team as a result of the quality of their communication.

It is not enough to know what has happened or will happen or to be able to say it out loud. The quality of each party's contribution to communication depends as much on presentation, timing, delivery, and receptivity to feedback as it does on the accuracy of the factual data presented.[1,2,4,5]

If no one is pausing to listen, then speech is meaningless, regardless of its content. Silence can be the ultimate in communication if it is shared. ▶ Table 28.1 and ▶ Table 28.2 outline the premises underlying communication and the type of information needed by the patient and his or her family. ▶ Table 28.3 lists the three main sources of stress—the environment, the patient, and family factors.

Table 28.1 Premises underlying communication between the health care team and patients and their families[1,6]

All communication is filled with concerns for the risks of death or disability.
A common vocabulary, shared context, and shared set of expectations between physicians and patients and their families must be crafted, not assumed.
Medically logical priorities are unlikely to match family priorities.
Opinions concerning goals, values, and quality of life must be explored, not assumed.
Trust and respect between physicians and patients and their family have to be reciprocal; they must be earned and returned.
Communication begins with the first staff member the patient and his or her family sees: there is no second chance to make a first impression.

Table 28.2 Patient situation preventing meaningful communication[3]

Loss of identity/loss of control/altered future/dependency
Coma
Paralysis
Death

Table 28.3 Sources of stress for NICU patients and their families[3,6,7,8,9,10,11]

Environment

Unfamiliar sights/sounds, unfamiliar activities and fast pace, isolation, separation, waiting, friction with staff/changing staff assignments, communication failures and delays, hunger/thirst, sleep deprivation, hygiene, lack of privacy, no place to store things

Patient

Altered appearance of patient by trauma, disease, or surgery; unfamiliar behavior of patient; unfamiliar tests and procedures, loss of identity; loss of recognition by family; concerns about the future

Family factors

Siblings'/other family members' demands, parental role revision, conflicts for control between spouses and parents, role revisions within the family, career concerns, travel concerns, financial stresses, geographic distance from support systems, discharge planning, future family economic and support issues

28.4 The Relay of Information

Before any information can be communicated, primary to even the message itself, communication theory dictates that there is a hierarchy of factors that must be met appropriately for the context of conversation. Primary to all, from Shannon's theory, is the source of information. This element of communication is that which drives the rest. The source of information in the context of our discussion must be premised in objective findings including imaging, laboratory investigation, objective physical findings, and, to some degree, clinical acumen and experience.

Next is the sender. This is the person doing the delivery of information. In Aristotelian communication theory, this was referred to as the orator or speaker. If the sender is available, affable, and authoritative, there is a higher likelihood that the message will be assimilated. Conversely, if the sender is brusque, speaks at a level above the understanding of his or her audience, or does not communicate the right message with the right source, the message will be lost.

The subsequent level of hierarchy is the channel. This, according to Shannon's theory of communication is merely the medium used to transmit the signal from the transmitter to the receiver. Specifically, this means that the channel can be anything from nonverbal cues to direct verbal communication inclusive of telephone conversations, e-mail, text messages, letters, and the like. The exact selection of the channel, however, becomes critically dependent on the message, which will be addressed shortly. The receiver, as mentioned previously, is not, in point of fact, the person or persons to whom the sender wishes to convey information in the form of the message—this would be the destination. The receiver is an intermediate step between the channel and the destination that performs the inverse function of the sender insofar as it decodes and reconstructs the message for the destination. In the framework of health information delivery and family communication this may be the appointed family representative, a translator, a trusted nurse, a member of a palliative care team, or others who might facilitate transmission.

Last there are the concepts of feedback and positive and negative entropic elements. Without feedback that necessarily proceeds in the reverse of the original missive along the communication pathway, the source and sender cannot know what, if anything, or how much of the message is understood and accepted by the patient or family. Entropy, as is accepted from the laws of thermodynamics and readily adapted for communication, is the natural state of affairs, and therefore communication has an affinity toward entropy. Without strong guidance from the source and sender as well as aid from the receiver, the message will be garbled and misinterpreted or lost altogether. To summarize, by Shannon's theory, the components of effective communication are the source, sender, channel, receiver, destination, message, feedback, and positive/negative entropy. Each piece of this hierarchical approach to communication must be addressed in order for the message to be successfully delivered to its appropriate destination.

28.5 Factors Affecting How Information Is Transmitted and Received

Communicating with the patient and family begins and grows by getting to know them. This applies to the health care team as much as it relates to the patient and his or her family.

Data gathering that may hold the key to reaching a patient or family member begins on the first meeting, is supported by the impressions and information gathered by the remainder of the health care team, and continues to expand as the relationship with the patient and family deepens. Some considerations to assist with data gathering should be documented in the nurse's intake sheet. ▶ Table 28.4 outlines the basic information that should be gathered in the first meeting. ▶ Table 28.5 lists the positive and negative coping mechanisms that can be anticipated. ▶ Table 28.6 and ▶ Table 28.7 give examples of charged words and behaviors, respectively.

Table 28.4 Initial family information to gather[1]

Coping mechanisms the physicians want to encourage versus coping strategies patient/ family already use

Health and emotional condition that the patient/family arrives in, including the presence of family members with disabilities

Patient's/family's immediate resources for self-care (psychological, social, monetary, and access to transportation)

Socioeconomic and educational background of patient/family

Cultural and religious precepts/prejudices/preconceptions

Availability, dedication, proximity, and strength of extended support system, including sympathetic employers

Chemical dependency of both patient and family members, including tobacco

Table 28.5 Coping mechanisms the family is likely to use

Positive	Negative
Leaning on others for support	Clinging to the patient/refusing to leave the bedside
Reliving the events that led to the crisis	Probing events/questioning information/ intellectualizing
Acting strong and competent	Putting on a show of confidence and strength
Blaming themselves or others	Focusing on trivial issues to avoid greater issues
Comparing their plight to those in worse straits (relief)	Exaggerating their circumstances to see themselves as heroes or martyrs
Rehearsing for death	Clinging to inappropriate hope

Table 28.6 Words that can be misunderstood

Death/dying	Coma	Disability
Dependence	Consciousness	Paralysis
Pain/suffering	Communicate	Rehabilitation
Anxiety/fear	Control	Vision/hearing/speech

Table 28.7 Charged behaviors that take on enhanced significance for patients and their families

Behavior	Significance
Looking	Eye contact or equivalent denotes focus, connectiveness, attentiveness, respect
Listening	Nodding, facial expressions, taking notes (and looking up) denote receptiveness
Touching	Refraining from examining or touching or carrying out other activities while listening denotes focus and implies that what is being heard matters to the one listening
Posture/ position	Sitting down and taking steps to ensure privacy or to protect the conversation from interruption indicate commitment to listening and receptiveness to what is said; standing implies a time limit unless it is at the bedside

28.6 Techniques for Dealing with the Hostile Patient/Family

Appropriate professionals should address any threat of violence and make preliminary efforts to resolve the conflict. The physician may be dealing with the aftermath of others' interventions or with patient's or family members' refusal to proceed with needed care/procedures. ▶ Table 28.8 outlines actions and suggested approaches to dealing with the hostile patient or family members.

Table 28.8 Approaches to dealing with hostile patients and their families

Action	Patient and family present	Family present without patient
Act quickly	Find out precipitating factors from others first; call for help if violence is threatened.	Same; delegate other commitments quickly to limit interruptions.
Find privacy	If the patient is stable, unite the angry patient or family members with < 10 key family members.	If patient cannot be included, unite < 10 key family members separately in a private place.
Enlist support	Have another health care professional present while defusing hostility.	Have a staff member listen in; enlist key family members to assist.
Acknowledge the anger, then redirect to focus on the patient	Opening ploy acknowledges the stressor, validates the patient's or family's feelings without admitting fault, then diverts attention back to the patient.	Indicate willingness to deal with the trigger for the hostility after the patient/family has been updated and the patient's acute needs are addressed.
Avoid the quarrel	Use nonverbal cues to give impression of openness. Use words to confirm your authority and dedication to the patient's critical medical needs.	Same. Postpone issues not directly related to the patient's survival (e.g., visitation) to be handled as promptly as possible by others more appropriate to the task.
Commit the time; leave an impression of focus, competence, and caring	Limit discussion of what provoked the hostility to information gathering. Defer negotiation about those circumstances to appropriate channels. Avoid making promises or "bribing." Lead by example, away from hostility and away from unreasonable demands.	Detach from the problem, not the people. Display willingness to incorporate their concerns into how things are done (without agreeing to favors/ privileges that are not your purview to permit).

28.7 Barriers to Communication

Language differences can cause many problems in communication, both with patients and with their families. This should be addressed by hospital policy using available translators/services in the hospital, the community, or the Internet before the communication problem arises. Communicating via signs and single words by health care providers unfamiliar with a patient's native language may be all that is possible in a crisis, but this practice is to be avoided and never accepted as a habit. Furthermore, the provider must be cognizant of the stages a patient must pass through to cope with devastating news. One of the most classical stratifications of the grieving process is the Kübler–Ross model outlined below.

1. Denial. In this stage, the patient and/or family will react with disbelief and either cling to false hope in careless or vague statements made by any member of the care team. They may also simply disbelieve what has been told to them.

2. Anger. Once denial has run its course or has proved futile, the next Kübler–Ross stage of grieving involves frustration and oftentimes lashing out. Typically, this is directed at proximate individuals, including not only the care team, but the patient's own loved ones, or the loved ones may be angry with the patient for life choices that have led to the situation in which the patient now exists.

3. Bargaining. The third Kübler–Ross stage involves the notion that an individual can negotiate avoidance of grief. In this stage, the griever will often attempt to exchange a reformed lifestyle for an extension of life.

4. Depression. This is occasionally the most evident stage of grieving, but not necessarily so. In this stage, the griever will often refuse visitors, spend much of his or her time being mournful and sullen, and may become silent and, thereby, incommunicative.

5. Acceptance. The final Kübler–Ross stage of grieving in which the individual embraces either inevitable mortality or an immutable future. Anecdotally, it is often seen that the dying individual precedes the survivors in this state. This state is often accompanied by a calm, introspective insight and stable emotions. It is in this state, perhaps obviously, that the griever is most receptive to communication by the health care and ancillary teams.

The chronic absence of family members for meetings may be addressed by social workers and discharge planners; in a crisis, law enforcement agencies may need to be contacted. The hospital should have protocols to facilitate two-physician consent for emergency procedures. This should include involvement of social services and hospital administrators for documentation purposes.

In some cases, families impose demands for special favors that present unique challenges to hospital staff and social services. Physicians can become part of the problem if they make promises to the family that others must cope with keeping. "Bribes" and "rule bending" for patients and families reinforce the family's worst fears about the severity of illness and undermine the family's confidence in the health care team to solve the patient's difficulties. Nothing is as reassuring as "business as usual."

28.8 Challenges in Communication: Scenarios

There are certain situations that reveal the challenges to communication between health care workers and NICU patients and their families. ▶ Table 28.9, ▶ Table 28.10, ▶ Table 28.11, ▶ Table 28.12, ▶ Table 28.13, and ▶ Table 28.14 offer practical applications of communication skills. ▶ Table 28.9 gives pointers on what to expect at the first meeting between the physician and the patient's family. ▶ Table 28.10 presents the scenario of a patient's death and what the medical team can do to ease the situation. ▶ Table 28.11 gives the case of a patient presenting in decompensation. ▶ Table 28.12 offers suggestions on possible interventions when a patient arrives unstable and worsens. ▶ Table 28.13 distinguishes among situations in which needs are not being met and gives basic suggestions on how to meet those varied needs. Finally, ▶ Table 28.14 addresses the situation in which a patient's recovery is prolonged by further complications.

Table 28.9 Initial meeting between the health care team and the patient and his or her family[5]

The doctor says. . .	The patient/ family hears. . .
The doctor approaches the family and engages the attention of all before speaking.	Something important is about to be said by a person of authority who cares about whether he or she is heard.
The doctor introduces him- or herself by name and demands the identities of his or her audience, sets the stage for a family spokesperson to emerge, or appoints one.	Distinguishing who is listening and the physician's relation to the patient is a way of acknowledging authority in the family and can be seen as respect; where there is already dissension, this may polarize family members.
The doctor summarizes the patient's state (two sentences) and interrupts him- or herself to gather baseline data, enlarges on the patient's likely diagnosis and prognosis, then opens the floor to questions. *OR*	Family will infer that crisis is under control and will respond to overture to tell about the patient and themselves in ways depending on their level of stress and past functioning as a family.
The doctor launches into a summary of the patient's status and current, emergent needs, postpones questions, gets consents for ongoing procedures, indicates what is likely to occur shortly, and leaves. *OR*	Family will infer that patient's crisis is not contained. If vocabulary is kept simple and the choices offered are straightforward, the family may accept data at face value. If the family hears condescension or is culturally

Table 28.9 continued

The doctor says. . .	The patient/ family hears. . .
	or historically conditioned to expect neglect and exploitation, the family may be angered.
The doctor summarizes the patient's status, current needs, and likely progress; introduces other staff members who will report to the family; estimates when the family can see the patient, gets consents for needed procedures; and departs. *OR*	Same as above, but the family is likely to respond positively to the promise of ongoing reports by people that the physician approves and the hope of seeing the patient at some specified time in the future.
The doctor or representative uses terminology that the family cannot comprehend, does not introduce or condone liaison personnel, and leaves without ascertaining if he or she has been understood.	Family may assume that the patient's crisis is so severe the physician or representative has no time for them or that the physician does not care about them or the patient. Families with past trust issues may become hostile. Families will conjecture and reinforce erroneous assumptions to cover knowledge deficits.

Table 28.10 Communication approaches when the patient dies[5]

The family sees. . .	The medical team sees. . .	Possible interventions
Family arrives after the patient is pronounced dead. Family confronts outcome with shock.	The patient is assessed, and appropriate management is offered. Physicians and staff disperse to care for others. Appropriate agencies are contacted.	Emergency room liaison personnel succor family while waiting for physicians to return to the scene; the family sees the patient after being updated and after staff has prepared the patient for viewing.
Family members arrive during resuscitation but are denied access to the patient. They confront the outcome with shock and rage.	The patient is assessed, and appropriate management is offered. Liaison personnel are not present to facilitate involving family, or a communication failure occurs, so the team is unaware that the family has arrived, or the family's presence is deemed unwise.	Best case: Physicians and liaison personnel meet the family first, re-create events, answer the answerable, and empathize with the loss. Referrals to appropriate agencies are made. Worst case: Family members are exposed to the dead patient without preparation and without ready access to those best able to explain what happened.
Family arrives during resuscitation and has access to the bedside before the pa-	Constraints imposed by the family's presence do not excessively hinder a prac-	Ideally, staff liaison is continuously present and attends to the family's needs

(continued)

Table 28.10 continued

The family sees. . .	The medical team sees. . .	Possible interventions
tient dies. Family is exposed to the resuscitation process. They confront the outcome with varying degrees of shock.	ticed team. Resuscitation proceeds with all team members performing as best as possible.	while preventing interference with resuscitation efforts. Worst case: Family members intrude, pose a threat to resuscitation providers, affect the outcome of the resuscitation, and due to a lack of medical knowledge believe that something was done wrong, blames the health care team and destroys the relationship.

Table 28.11 Communication approaches when the patient presents in decompensation[5]

The patient/family sees. . .	The medical team sees. . .	Possible interventions
Catastrophic injury/illness make shocking changes in self or loved one.	Disease or trauma impacts on patient's immediate chances of sustaining life.	Staff and physicians share a duty to describe what they see, what they want to change, and how they will go about it.
Assessment and resuscitation look chaotic to the already frightened family and patient.	Systematic application of protocols by a professional team working under pressure	As above. Use "Good/better/ not as good" to update and avoid statistics or interrupting care to explain. Use liaison personnel.
Initial damage and uncertain progress in self or loved one inspire fear of lethality or permanent disability.	Results of examinations, indicating diagnosis, current status, response to treatment, and ultimate prognosis, are obvious.	As above. Ask family for opinions, then counter with accuracy. Give frequent updates, and quickly introduce senior physicians and staff.
Family has one person or a few people who appear in charge and worth listening to.	A hierarchy of authority is based on training and skill set; many are capable of providing information.	Team defers to leader, and leader reinforces confidence in team.
Unexplained delays/unexpected changes in plans/ inadequate explanations seem evasive.	Resuscitation is carried forward in a setting where many compete for the same resources and the attention of the same staff.	Avoid excuses; explain delays as soon as possible. Provide reassurance. Staff should give family a role in supporting the patient.

Table 28.12 Communication approaches when the patient arrives unstable and worsens[3,5,6,7,8,9,10,11]

The patient/ family sees	The medical team sees...	Possible interventions
Limited access of the patient to his or her family is offered.	An unstable patient is isolated for his or her protection.	The health care team repeatedly explains to, empathizes with, but always protects the patient.
Strangers converge and do inexplicable or painful things to the patient.	Necessary procedures are done to preserve life by people who should but may not identify their purposes to the family.	Physicians respond with increased opportunity for the family to vent and for doctors to update. The team shares the opportunity to assess pain control needs with the family.
Contradictory information or no information is conveyed to the family; the "wrong" person is contacted, making the information conveyed suspect; information conveyed is too technical to be absorbed; communication with a recognized authority is too sparse or contaminated by the family's hostility; and individual dynamics foster denial.	Confusion follows when caregivers fail to communicate with each other; when individuals communicate who incorrectly assume a common knowledge base; when information changes as it passes between staff or family members; when the patient deteriorates so rapidly that it is impossible to adequately prepare and sustain the family. The foregoing is exacerbated by preexisting family dysfunction and socioeconomic or cultural considerations. Further complications from unrelated stressors are imposed on the staff.	Impromptu multidisciplinary rounds with available staff and key family members are done so that "everybody is heard and everyone hears the same thing." A family spokesperson and team spokespersons are identified. Referrals are made to appropriate support specialists. Ongoing multidisciplinary rounds are made with the family present, and increased scheduled opportunities are provided for the family to connect with attending physicians. The chain of command is reinforced. Physicians validate the staff.

Table 28.13 Communication approaches when needs are not being met[5]

The patient/ family sees. . .	The medical team sees. . .	Possible interventions
Emotional needs are not being met.	Lack of leadership, failure to accommodate between specialists, lack of team cooperation.	Same as in ▶ Table 28.12, but increase the frequency of family updates.
	Staff members recognize the probable grim outcome and distance themselves from patient/family; the	

(continued)

Table 28.13 continued

The patient/ family sees. . .	The medical team sees. . .	Possible interventions
	staff withdraws from the increasingly dependent, demanding family; the family exhausts the staff's emotional reserve.	
Physical needs are not being met.	The hospital is unable to provide food, sleeping accommodations, and privacy to meet family demands, whether appropriate or not.	Emphasize role of authority figures in all disciplines. Physicians in authority must demonstrate confidence in bedside caregivers.
Spiritual needs are not being met.	Staff lacks direction and cohesiveness; gives the impression of lost hope, lost motivation, or dissension among themselves; is unable to hide the same from the family; and is exacerbated as the family spirals out of control.	The health care team must meet separately to support themselves, cope with the looming loss of the patient on their own terms, and recover lost momentum in dealing with the patient's and family's crises.
Patient and family are dissatisfied regardless of the outcome.	Physicians and staff caregivers are dissatisfied regardless of the outcome.	Social services representatives appeal for funds to sustain an indigent family in crisis. The family is counseled regarding available resources. The hospital regains a limit-setting role for the safety of patients and staff. The family is treated with respect but with appropriate limit setting. Physicians lead by example, supporting both the team and the family realistically. Focus groups, including physicians, are appointed to alleviate any remaining tensions and to help participants learn from the experience.

Table 28.14 Communication approaches when a patient's recovery is prolonged by further complications[5]

The patient/family sees. . .	The medical team sees. . .	Possible interventions
The patient/family is dissatisfied with the patient's rate of improvement and/or prolonged NICU stay due to complications.	The patient's and family's reserves are depleted emotionally, physically, spiritually, and financially.	Physicians insist on and staff facilitate a "timeout" for the family.
The family "settles in," regaining some control and predictability in their lives measured in the services they can convince others to provide. Family looks to find fault or place blame: something is owed them because "this shouldn't have happened in the first place" and "why can't this be over?"	A dependent relationship becomes ingrained. The family is perceived as ungrateful and increasingly demanding because they assume ongoing privileges granted earlier when the patient was more acute, or because they manipulate relationships that divide the staff, or because they impose preferences on patient care that increase staff work, or because they require reassurance very frequently or at inappropriate or inconvenient times.	Senior staff chair multidisciplinary meeting first without, then with, the family to address the new structure with new privileges, new responsibilities, and new roles for family members. Physician involvement is key to helping predict patient progress and to better assist bedside caregivers in redefining the family's relationship with the health care team.
"Someone is not telling us something."	Staff perceives that communication is treated with suspicion, that the family exploits any discrepancies in communicated content or communication delivery, that there may be dissension in the family; that the delay in good news is leading staff to avoid confrontation and perpetuating the family's impression that they are being left out	
"Something finally gets better."	Best case: Events lead senior nursing staff and physicians to resume a leadership role, confirm	

(continued)

Table 28.14 continued

The patient/family sees. . .	The medical team sees. . .	Possible interventions
	patient's status and progress in unambiguous terms, set limits on special privileges demanded by the family in supportive fashion, and recover mutual respect.	
"Something gets worse."	Worst case: Whether or not the patient worsens, the family attitude worsens, the family withdraws or behaves with hostility toward the staff, and the hospital administration steps in to arbitrate.	

Table 28.15 Perspective: what patients and their families need from physicians and nurses

Honesty: tell the truth; tell it when you know it; admit it when you don't

Predictability, dependability, availability

Compassion

Open-mindedness and a willingness to learn

Knowledge, wisdom, and a willingness to teach

Skill

The role of physicians and the health care team in relationship building with NICU patients and their families can be complicated. ▶ Table 28.15 lists what is needed of physicians and nursing staff from the perspective of the patient and family. These needs should be the focus of the health care team.

28.9 The Health Care Team

It would be ideal if physicians and nurses could meet all of the needs of patients and their families. In real life, though, no one can be all things to all patients at all times. Physicians and other members of the health care team, working together, can create a composite, well-orchestrated program to fulfill the needs of most people. ▶ Table 28.16 and ▶ Table 28.17 address the team approach to communication.

Table 28.16 Communications: it takes a team

Foundation	The team approach is hierarchical, discriminatory, and privileged.
Authority	The chain of command begins with the attending neuro- or trauma surgeon, descends through resident physicians, ramifies through physician consultants, and burgeons to involve nurses, respiratory therapists, and specialists and technicians of ancillary disciplines, inclusive of appropriate hierarchies per discipline.
Sourcing for dissemination	The NICU team sets the tone and controls the flow of information through all contributing health care providers by making sure that the information they want communicated is disseminated to the health care providers with the greatest, most frequent access to the patient. Daily rounds are done with nursing staff. A chart or phone contact is kept with consulting physicians.
Choreography for emergencies	Communication during resuscitation should begin via trained liaison personnel who educate and support families per protocol and by rote according to stages of resuscitation identified by the resuscitating physicians.
Postresuscitation	There should be impromptu, frequent meetings between neurosurgeons, consultants, and family at bedside or with nursing staff, including ongoing support from liaison personnel.
Routine care program	Daily updating of staff and family will be by bedside rounds with nursing and multidisciplinary meetings that involve the neurosurgeons, physician consultants, nurses, respiratory therapists, rehabilitation and other services, the patient, and his or her family.

Table 28.17 Team approach to communication

Individual members represent the team; the team incorporates all; what each one says should reflect what the team is conveying as a unit.

Information disseminated by team members should conform in content and implication: the patient/family should not get mixed or conflicting messages.

The ultimate resource should be the primary physician service; dissension should be shared within the team, not the patient or the patient's family.

Substantive information conveyed should be restricted by scope of practice. Any team member should be able to convey empathy and concern.

When confronted with a question he or she cannot answer, the team member should admit it and refer the question to the appropriate resource.

All team members owe mutual respect and respect for the team as a whole; promoting confidence in the team is the job of every team member.

It is the responsibility of the primary service, from attending physician to intern, to establish the credibility and importance of the entire network of health care providers in the critical care setting as sources of information for the patient and family.

Nurses need to hear what the family hears. At least daily, the physicians guiding minute-to-minute care in the unit should define, with the chief bedside caregivers, the content to be shared with the family by all health care team members. Nurses will choose how to transmit information according to gravity and complexity of data and by competency of the communicating caregiver, and share the responsibility with respiratory therapists and others. Ideally, there will be planned (weekly) and impromptu multidisciplinary rounds, with and without the patient and family in attendance, in which the team as a whole assimilates and adapts to the patient's changing condition, then formulates a presentation to share the information with the family.

Nurses, therapists, and others with the greatest access to the patient and family have the burden of ongoing education and minute-by-minute reinforcement of information already provided to the patient/family. Nurses and others with bedside care responsibilities will not act as independent entities but as contributing members of an organized whole whose opinions will be assimilated into the overall plan discussed with the patient/family.

All health care providers should feedback patient-related information to the primary physician team and wait for the team's directions regarding sharing that data with the patient/family.

The burden of telling all and the responsibility for coordinating and ameliorating the patient's/family's exposure to dissenting opinions are privileges earned by the primary team of physicians through their responsiveness to new data, new questions, and new concerns brought to their attention by their physician consultants, by nurses, and by all other representatives of caregiving disciplines contributing to the patient's ultimate outcome.

The burden of absorbing and acting on the implications of the patient's current and future status belongs to the patient and family: the greatest gift the medical team may offer is to influence how that burden is conferred (▶ Table 28.18, ▶ Table 28.19).

Be prepared to supply family members with a frame of reference to help them assimilate the information they are about to receive. Reinforce that frame of reference as a foundation for continuing communication throughout the patient's course of treatment (▶ Table 28.20, ▶ Table 28.21, ▶ Table 28.22, ▶ Table 28.23).

Table 28.18 Practitioners who should be incorporated into the health care team

Discipline	Sphere of influence
Physicians	Ultimate information source; center for assimilation of new data from other disciplines; the "authority" that the patient/family will recognize.
Nurses (and trained liaison personnel)	Ultimate implementers of any treatment plan; ultimate disseminators of information because of their greater access to patients and families; primary resource for monitoring; the first and the last to touch the patient and family; the "authority" that the patient and family needs to recognize.
Therapists: respiratory, physical, occupational, speech, nutritional, and, to a lesser degree, technical specialists throughout the hospital	More limited scope of access and practice but convey information relevant to their areas of concern; the harbingers of change in the patient's condition, the "authority" that the patient and family will look to for new hope.
Social workers, case workers, discharge planners, child life specialists, clergy, hospital administrators	Ultimate implementers of plans that hinge on family participation; the authorities that patients look to for their future and families look to for support.

Table 28.19 Communication approaches assuming patient/family duress[1,3,6,7,8,9,10,11]

Assume the patient/ family at risk for. . .	What the health care team member can do
Fear and anxiety leading to preformed conclusions.	Be prepared with appropriate facts.
Attention spans that are likely to be short.	Watch for wandering; redirect if needed; be brief.
Poor retention of information.	Repeat what matters most and confirm that it is heard.
Distraction by side issues. Having a secondary agenda focused on comfort, security, and control over their immediate surroundings.	Ask questions that refocus attention. Leave time to address appropriate concerns. Show you care. If needed, set the stage for limiting inappropriate requests.

Table 28.20 Making a frame of reference

Begin by describing the patient's baseline appearance to him- or herself and the family in simple, easy-to-remember words. Use the primary survey of resuscitation but in layperson's terms.

Tell the family how you make an assessment (what characteristics and in what order) and what changes would indicate improvement or deterioration. Point to features of the patient that the family can see for themselves.

Introduce the family to medical terms they are likely to hear. Use all of what you've taught them to update the family whenever you get a chance.

Table 28.21 Establishing a relationship[5]

The gulf between patient/family and health care team	Bridging the gulf
Assume ignorance of proper use of medical terms.	Avoid medical terms, or define them every time.
Expect a demand for statistics regarding outcome. Assume pre-conceptions about status.	Clearly state that statistics refer to population, then explain what they tell us about the patient. As simply as possible, explain what parameters are assessed and what conclusions have been made concerning the patient's status; set the stage for the future use of labels *good*, *better*, *worse*, and *unchanged*, and avoid discussing numeric values or monitored data that can frighten family members if they misinterpret them. Avoid the word *stable*.
Assume a need to "do something."	Validate the family's roles as historians, as assistants in ongoing assessments, and as decision makers.
Assume a need to find hope, whether you see it or not.	Remind family members that "everyone knows what normal looks like" and that if something they think is an improvement is real, it will be evident in time.

Table 28.22 Situations requiring special communication obtaining informed consent

Physicians and nurses should know departmental policy and apply it.
The patient/family should know from the outset that the purpose of the update is to obtain consent for a procedure needed to save the patient's life/restore functioning/ hasten recovery, etc.
Initial approach to the patient/family will be to update them on the patient's progress.
The need for the procedure should be apparent to the patient/family from the update. A description of the procedure, including use of visual aids, if available, should follow.
The specific benefits that will be mentioned in consent documents should be discussed next.
A discussion of possible ill effects from the procedure should follow departmental policy and should be comprehensive, but they should be presented in the context of how likely the patient is to experience these difficulties. Patient discomfort should be addressed, including consent for conscious sedation, if needed.
Patient and family need to know where the procedure will be done, when it will be done, who will do it, how long it will take, and what the arrangements will be to update the patient/family after it is done.
Always remind the patient/family that there are "no guarantees."

It is assumed that all appropriate medical workup has been done to confirm the diagnoses and prognoses leading to this decision point. For purposes of this discussion, it is assumed that there is no advanced directive, no living will, and no written documentation of the patient's wishes. The approach to the family is then predicated on agreement or acceptance that withdrawal of support or withholding cardiopulmonary resuscitation (CPR) seems ethical, legal, reasonable, respectful, and compassionate to the members of the health care team. It is assumed that all proceedings will be in keeping with hospital policies regarding bioethics committees, and so on. If consent is sought to withhold resuscitation or deny CPR, the procedure with the family then follows the pattern outlined in ▶ Table 28.24.

Table 28.23 Situations requiring special communication: withdrawal of support/do not resuscitate[6,7,8,12,13,14,15]

Patient status	Examples
Illness or trauma has led imminently and unavoidably to a terminal condition.	Intracranial hypertension after severe head trauma
Criteria are met for irreversible coma.	Head injury, near-drowning, asphyxia, stroke
Incurable, progressive illness exists entailing intractable suffering and unacceptable quality of life.	Lou Gehrig's disease, multiple sclerosis
Illness or trauma has led to such severe disability with such poor quality of life that there is no reason to continue artificial means to prolong life or resuscitate from cardiac arrest.	End-stage pulmonary disease in a profoundly brain-damaged patient, as seen in ventricular hemorrhage due to prematurity; brain tumor; stroke; near-drowning

Table 28.24 A protocol for obtaining consent to withdraw support or withhold CPR

A team of doctors, nurses, therapists, social workers, clergy, and so on, discusses the case in advance and arranges to meet with the family as a group. (Some or all of the team members should attend. Do not send only one person.)

The family is approached by a representative of the group to make an appointment to discuss the consent, with the family arranging for appropriate attendance of its members.

The physician reviews the patient's case, including the factors leading to the present discussion.

The family and health care team discuss the implications of the patient's history.

The health care team solicits the family's feelings about the patient's likely outcome, about death and dying in general, about what they think the patient would want, about what they would want for themselves, and about how they will want to remember their actions and decisions 10 years in the future.

The health care team answers questions about what the patient will feel and do if support is withdrawn or resuscitation is denied, the mechanics of the process, and how it will appear to the family. The hospital's documentation for consent for DNR status, including the options to choose some but not all aspects of resuscitation, can be discussed with the family at this point. The family's wishes on how withdrawal of support should be conducted, whom they wish to have present, and so on, can also be discussed now.

The family is given a time frame in which to carry on the discussion in privacy and return a decision. Meetings are arranged and repeated with appropriate/selected members of the health care team until the family delivers a decision.

Abbreviations: CPR, cardiopulmonary resuscitation; DNR, do not resuscitate.

A patient who is declared "brain dead" per protocol (see Chapter 27) is removed from life support because he or she is dead. While no consent is legally necessary to do the brain death exam, or to remove the patient from life supports, if at all possible, it is empowering for a lengthy family discussion about the brain death exam to take place, or at the minimum to be informed of it in advance, so they can be psychologically prepared for the outcome; this also gives them a chance to understand that if the patient is found to be brain dead, the next logical step is to discontinue artificial supports, such as the ventilator. The family should be informed with all possible compassion and sensitivity of the brain death exam and its meaning; the timing of the brain death examination, and consequent discontinuation of artificial supports, should accommodate family wishes within reason.

28.10 The Role of the Palliative Care Team[6,7,8,9, 12,13,14,15]

When a patient and the patient's family reaches a point in medical and surgical therapy where the patient's quality of life begins to be affected by the treatment as well as the disease process, the palliative care team is able to provide a plethora of services to the patient and family that the neurosurgeon, in isolation, cannot. These services include assistance and streamlining the care of the chronically diseased and end-of-life patient, providing an impartial third-party bridge to help facilitate the communication and partnership of the health care team and the patient and to allow the patient to participate in the formation of the health care plan, involving the patient and the family in planning care and therapeutic goals, and helping the patient to believe that he or she is both empowered to- and has the ultimate responsibility for his or her well-being. In many cases, the physician is seen as the "captain of the ship," but in the case of transitional life care, the physician becomes an equal member of the team. This team includes nurses, social workers, case managers, clergy, and physicians.

It is important to note that the role of the palliative care team is not to assume the care of the patient, but only to assist should other health care workers request it. The palliative care team helps to recognize recurring symptoms of the patient and ensure they are brought to the attention of the health care team, to facilitate the patient in reaching his or her satisfaction goals, to bridge communication between the patient and the health care team and ensure that the patient's decisions are heard and understood by the health care team, and to assist with discharge planning, inpatient needs, outpatient needs, hospice, funding, and follow-up palliative care. In point of fact, in today's patient-satisfaction-driven health care milieu, the palliative care team directly helps chronically diseased patients and patients approaching end of life to be satisfied with their health care. In this sense, the palliative care team is an indispensable aid for both the patient and family as well as for the health care team. Palliative care maximizes the quality of life for the patient and the family. They are meant to be involved as soon as a terminal diagnosis is made so that the family can be assisted in feeling comfortable with further treatment and care—whether radiation therapy, chemotherapy, surgical therapy, or even no therapy is selected. They assist the family in realizing and sorting through these options and in what the next steps are when these options fail.

In the performance of their assigned function, the palliative care team improves the quality of life of patients and their families; improves communication; helps to prevent and relieve suffering; and identifies, assesses, and treats pain as well as physical, psychosocial, and spiritual problems. While it goes without saying that those of us who have answered the calling to the health care fields innately seek to help our fellow humans, we must remain humble in our pursuit of our craft and recognize that no neurosurgeon is an island. Although we certainly have a vast expertise in our field of study, it is imperative that we seek to do what is best for our patients. In this perspective, the palliative care team can facilitate the care regarding the four primary aspects of overall well-being as outlined here.

1. Physical well-being and symptom control.
   - Functional ability.
   - Strength and fatigue.
   - Sleep and rest.
   - Nausea.
   - Appetite.
   - Constipation.
   - Pain.
2. Psychological well-being.
   - Anxiety.
   - Depression.
   - Enjoyment and leisure.
   - Distress caused by pain.
   - Happiness.
   - Fear.
   - Cognition and attention.
3. Social well-being.
   - Financial burden.
   - Caregiver burden.
   - Roles and relationships.
   - Affection and sexual function.
   - Appearance.

4. Spiritual well-being.
   • Hope.
   • Meaning.
   • Suffering.
   • Religiosity.

With regard to this extensive list of equally crucial facets of well-being, the palliative care team will work to create a plan to address all of these needs on behalf of the patient and his or her family. They are trained to assess what the patient and family know and how much they want to know. In this way, they facilitate the dissemination of information bidirectionally between the family and the health care team. They will also help to ensure that the family and patient's needs are met in terms of long-term-care planning and in ensuring that all necessary contacts are made, appointments booked, and needs met. Again, this directly increases the patient's and his or her family's direct satisfaction with the care received in the most dire of circumstances.

Finally, the last part of palliative care is hospice care. Surveys at our institution indicate that patients tend to overwhelming prefer to die at home, with 67% preferring this over 18% preferring an in-hospital death and 15% preferring another location. Even then, those that prefer a death away from home prefer this not for their own sake, but because they hope to avoid burdening their family and caregivers with the effort and expense of home care and final needs. The hospice phase of palliative care begins when death is expected (in the state of California, for example, this is when death is expected within 6 months) and is involved in the last phase of care. Typically, this is carried out outside of the hospital. The hospice phase of palliative care provides medical support services, limited emotional support, and limited spiritual resources for those in the last stage of life. Additionally, hospice can help family members manage the practical details and emotional challenges of caring for a dying loved one. The hospice team can prepare and support the family and patient for impending death outside of the hospital environment. This indispensable team facilitates communication between the health care team and the patient and family with regard to patient and family wishes, the patient's health status, realistic goals of care, and the appropriate role of the physician and interdisciplinary care team. Certainly, the neurosurgeon can pronounce a grave prognosis, but it is critical to remember that, once this news is delivered, oftentimes, the patient and family will not be able to hear or process anything else that is said and, in truth, despite appearances, may not have even understood the gravity of the pronouncement. It is paramount for the neurosurgeon to understand that what the patient experiences is not what onlookers see. As such, when the resources of a palliative care team and a hospice care team are available, they ought be brought to bear for maximizing the care and satisfaction of the patient and family.

Returning to the case presented at the beginning of this section, magnetic resonance imaging, with and without contrast, of the patient's brain indicates a recurrent mass in the area of the previous resection. Given the patient's clinical history, you know it is likely to be a recurrent glioblastoma multiforme. As this is now a third recurrence, and the palliative care team has already been involved in the care planning and family communication with this patient, you call the hospital palliative care liaison, who meets you at the emergency department with the emergency medicine provider. The three of you discuss your clinical impression of the scan as well as the patient's current presentation. Certainly, the patient's prognosis is poor at this time given the recurrence of an aggressive malignancy, and the three of you, as representatives of a larger team, go to speak with the patient and his family. You explain his condition, the unlikeliness of a meaningful long-term functional recover, as well as possible therapeutic options. The palliative care representative provides emotional, psychological, and spiritual support to the visibly shaken family members and further discusses with them the treatment options as well as potential measures to enhance the patient's comfort. The patient's wife produces a Physician Orders for Life Sustaining Treatment (POLST) form that had previously been signed by the patient and his primary care physician. In it, the patient had made his wishes clear that he would not want aggressive surgical intervention in the case of a recurrent malignancy with poor prognosis. The palliative care representative discusses this with the family, and the family tearfully voices their appreciation for all the care that has been provided to the patient up to this point. Arrangements are then made for the patient to be placed in hospice care, and the palliative care representative arranges for a home hospital bed, home oxygen, and home intravenous infusion pumps. The hospice care team arranges for intravenous pain medications to keep the patient comfortable.

The patient is discharged home with these arrangements made, and the palliative care team makes follow-up calls to the patient's family to check in on them. The family requests contact with clergy who can pay a home visit to the patient. Three weeks later, on a subsequent follow-up call, they are informed that the patient has passed away peacefully, at home, surrounded by his family and dearest loved ones. Two weeks after that, when reviewing your mail, you find a greeting card. On opening it, you find a heartfelt note of sincere appreciation from the family for not only the medical care and clinical acumen you brought to bear in the care of their departed loved one, but more importantly, for the frank care and compassion that you showed, along with the palliative care and hospice care teams in facilitating the patient's peaceful passing after having struggled with his devastating illness.

28.11 Conclusion

No illness or injury carries a greater potential for loss of one's identity and perspective on one's environment than injury or illness of the brain or spinal cord. A patient whose critical illness arises from damage of the central nervous system is a person at risk of dying, but also at risk of never being the person he or she was again, or at risk of never being the person he or she could have been. Every interchange between the physician and patient or the patient's family in this setting will be overshadowed by these implications. Attempts by the physician or layperson to focus on any finite detail and exclude the greater context is likely to lead to confusion and friction between and among physicians, other health care providers, family members, and the patient.

The physicians trying to save the patient's life and preserve his or her abilities have a duty to explain what they are doing, why, and what is likely to happen next as best they can. The duty is shared with the remainder of the health care team to a degree in keeping with the potential to affect the outcome that accompanies their skills, knowledge, or authority. All share the complementary duty to acknowledge, process, and respond to what the patient and family express after they hear what the prognosis and progress are likely to be.

Case Management

The patient and his or her family have a duty to provide a history that will help delineate the cause of the patient's catastrophe, and they have a duty to convey what the patient was like before his or her illness or injury occurred. Most of all, they have an obligation to listen, process what they hear, and provide feedback on what they have heard. Ultimately, they will be responsible for coping with the aftermath, including death or disability.

Neither the physicians nor the patient and his or her family will see the patient's illness in the same context. It is up to the physicians and the team of health care providers surrounding and supporting the patient's care to bridge the gap in understanding between themselves and the patient/family.

The patient and family are one: the patient's crisis separates him or her from the life to which medical care endeavors to return the patient. This goal cannot be accomplished unless the context of the patient's life before his or her crisis is fully appreciated.

References

[1] Shannon C. The Mathematical Theory of Communication. Urbana: University of Illinois Press; 1949

[2] Koerner AF, Fitzpatrick MA. Toward a theory of family communication. Commun Theory. 2002; 12 (1):70–91

[3] Kodali S, Stametz R, Clarke D, et al. Implementing family communication pathway in neurosurgical patients in an intensive care unit. Palliat Support Care. 2015; 13(4):961–967

[4] Koerner FA, Mary Anne F. Understanding family communication patterns and family functioning: The roles of conversation orientation and conformity orientation. Annals of the International Communication Association. 2002; 26(1):36–65

[5] Ritchie LD, Fitzpatrick MA. Family communication patterns measuring intrapersonal perceptions of interpersonal relationships. Communic Res. 1990; 17(4):523–544

[6] Curtis JR, White DB. Practical guidance for evidence-based ICU family conferences. Chest. 2008; 134(4):835–843

[7] Curtis JR, Patrick DL, Shannon SE, Treece PD, Engelberg RA, Rubenfeld GD. The family conference as a focus to improve communication about end-of-life care in the intensive care unit: opportunities for improvement. Crit Care Med. 2001; 29(2) Suppl:N26–N33

[8] Gries CJ, Curtis JR, Wall RJ, Engelberg RA. Family member satisfaction with end-of-life decision making in the ICU. Chest. 2008; 133(3):704–712

[9] Nelson JE, Mulkerin CM, Adams LL, Pronovost PJ. Improving comfort and communication in the ICU: a practical new tool for palliative care performance measurement and feedback. Qual Saf Health Care. 2006; 15(4):264–271

[10] Pronovost P, Berenholtz S, Dorman T, Lipsett PA, Simmonds T, Haraden C. Improving communication in the ICU using daily goals. J Crit Care. 2003; 18(2):71–75

[11] Shaw DJ, Davidson JE, Smilde RI, Sondoozi T, Agan D. Multidisciplinary team training to enhance family communication in the ICU. Crit Care Med. 2014; 42(2):265–271

[12] Ciemins EL, Brant J, Kersten D, Mullette E, Dickerson D. A qualitative analysis of patient and family perspectives of palliative care. J Palliat Med. 2015; 18(3):282–285

[13] Curtis JR, Engelberg RA, Wenrich MD, et al. Studying communication about end-of-life care during the ICU family conference: development of a framework. J Crit Care. 2002; 17(3):147–160

[14] Fitzpatrick MA, Ritchie LD. Communication schemata within the family. Hum Commun Res. 1994; 20(3):275–301

[15] Keeley MP. Family Communication at the End of Life. J Fam Commun. 2016; 16(3):189–1–97

29 Spiritual Care of the Neurosurgical Intensive Care Unit Patient and Family

John Spitalieri, Marc Billings, and Javed Siddiqi

Abstract

With all the high-tech equipment, monitoring, and imaging in the neurosurgical intensive care unit (NICU), there are occasions when the patient and family need more support than can be provided by the neurointensivist and nursing staff. Offering spiritual care in the face of the suffering patient and family, in concert with conventional medical and surgical interventions, is a necessary part of any NICU. We discuss the patient and family needs in the spiritual realm and emphasize its role in healing.

Keywords: compassion, covenant, faith, grief counseling, mourning, spirituality, suffering

Case Study

A Muslim family is concerned about issues of organ donation for their loved one, who has suffered an irreversible brain injury. The family is seeking spiritual guidance on this topic.

See end of chapter for Case Management.

29.1 Initial Encounter with the Neurocritical Care Unit

There can be no more completely upsetting and frightening event than to find that a loved one has become critically ill or severely injured and has been taken to the hospital and admitted to the intensive care unit. Suddenly, everything that was stable before has now changed, and the question of our own mortality, as well as that of our loved one, is brought to the forefront. What may have started off as a normal day has had a surrealistic change. Expressed thoughts begin to echo: "This can't be happening, there must be a mistake, either you have the wrong family or the wrong patient, or the wrong diagnoses." Inevitably, the truth starts sinking in as the physical and emotional pain associated with loss and separation takes hold. These are the times when many questions are asked, and few pleasant or satisfying answers are given. The emotional strength of a family is put to task, and they begin to search for solace and understanding.

29.2 The Role of the Neuroscience Team

During the initial meeting with the patient and family, the neurointensivist is invariably sharing bad news with individuals who have usually never met him or her before—this is the nature of acute care medicine, which brings the patient, family, and neurointensivist together due to some health tragedy. The patient and family feel especially vulnerable in the early phases of the doctor–patient, and doctor–family relationship, and this is the time when building trust, offering hope, and nourishing spirituality are most important.

While many neurosurgical intensive care unit (NICU) patients go on to have good outcomes, the primary mission of the NICU physician and team is to rescue the patient from secondary injuries, while also healing the stressed family by a demonstration of genuine caring and compassion. The neuroscience team meets the patients as they come into the hospital and then adopts them. The neuroscience team becomes part of the patient's life as the patient goes from the initial computed tomographic (CT) scan, and then directly to the operating room or NICU. The patients are followed daily, not merely seen once a day, but cared for continuously as each patient becomes the mission of the neuroscience team until he or she goes home, is transferred to a rehabilitation facility, or passes away. When these patients leave the hospital their care is not ended; the amount of care changes slightly, becoming surpassed by the care provided to patients that remain in the hospital. The neuroscience team is committed to each and every patient, providing each with the optimal care. However, given similar circumstances some patients do better than others.

29.3 Family Support

The common denominator for those who do well is support from family. If a patient's injury or illness is too great, then their destiny is out of the health care provider's hands. While sharing in the patients' lives, regardless of outcome, the neuroscience team can make the experience more comfortable and less harsh. There are ways to identify the suffering of patients and their families, and to help with major life transitions, such as recovery, permanent disability, and death. Perhaps addressing the spiritual needs of patients and families could hold another modality of treatment that needs to be explored. At the heart of the spiritual distress of the sick and dying is suffering, and this spiritual distress is often not addressed adequately.[1,2,3,4,5,6,7,8] Health care providers have taken on a responsibility to relieve physical pain and suffering; this duty should also include spiritual suffering.

Even though spirituality is becoming more recognized and accepted as a part of treatment, not many established guidelines exist for physicians in the NICU for inquiring about the spirituality of patients and families.[9,10,11,12,13,14] In fact, a recent survey of top-selling neurology textbooks showed minimal guidelines for the care of patients at the end of life and in the NICU. Additionally, none of the textbooks had a chapter on end-of-life care.[14] There is a need to discuss the approaches for inquiring about patients' and families' spirituality, the importance of spirituality in medical decision making, the role suffering takes with patients, and the effects on health care. Those requirements must be tailored to patients in the NICU.

29.4 Neurosurgical Intensive Care Unit Setting

Unique experiences associated with a stay in the NICU include round-the-clock observation with frequent neurologic exams, intracranial pressure monitoring, electroencephalography, and frequent trips to the CT or MRI scanners. Families will see their loved ones on complete life support with the monitors and machines making their own special noises. This can be very frightening and overwhelming to families whose last memory of their loved one was someone walking and talking. Immediately, the stress level of families is high, and the neuroscience team must be watchful for the signs of that stress. At this time the different teams should introduce themselves and identify the family spokesperson. Also, the current patient's condition and overall plan should be discussed. These conversations should not include the jargon of the neuroscientist; rather time should be taken to explain the situation in simple, concise, and accurate terms.

29.5 Spirituality

Spirituality has been defined as "that which allows a person to experience transcendent meaning in life. This is often expressed as a relationship with God, but it can also be about nature, art, music, family, or community—whatever beliefs and values give a person a sense of meaning and purpose in life."[13] Many people identify themselves as being spiritual.[7,8,9] People feel that on some level their life has meaning and purpose. Illness and injury can cause a threat to the individual's spirituality.[7,9] Patients admitted to an ICU may not even have the strength or ability to care for themselves, even on the most basic levels; their focus may be entirely on survival. The meaning and purpose of their life may be lost to them, leading to emotional distress in the sick and dying, as well as in their families. At this time spiritual counseling can benefit patients and families the most by allowing them to express their concerns for the future while at the same time helping them cope with their suffering.[8,11]

Patients and families may subscribe to the words of David in the Twenty-third Psalm and think that goodness and mercy will follow them always. They do not think of the possibility of bad things happening to them. Or they may think that once bad things do happen, a miracle will occur that will deliver them from their suffering. It is human nature to have hope, and hope affects patient health.[8] Hope, as explained by Buchman, "is a form of trust in the future, and is often deeply ensconced in a religious cultural matrix."[13] As an extension of this hope, the neuroscientist enters into a relationship with the patient that commits the physician to doing the most to return the patient to a state of health. This relationship takes on the properties of a covenant, and includes shared hope, shared risk, and mutual respect.[13]

The era is approaching where spirituality is having more clinical relevance, for example, when coping with illness and death. Patients and families are basing decisions on their religious beliefs.[4,7,8] Medical science is still uncertain if spirituality has an effect on health, but several sources are investigating the psycho-neuro-immuno axis and how spirituality and religion can be a factor in treatment of those who are critically ill or critically injured.[1,4] This involves the personal concerns of patients. Some patients' concerns involve only their faith in a god and the pursuit of heaven. Others are most concerned with interpersonal relationships with families and friends. These things are intangible, but they give hope and reassurance to those who are so troubled. Spirituality, in whatever form it takes, gives people meaning and purpose in life.[4,7]

In addressing purpose and meaning, large gains can be made with small efforts by health care providers. For all of the complex treatments of a patient's illness, there does not have to be a complex course for spiritual treatment. Even simply providing access to spiritually oriented activity can be uplifting to individuals and can also help in healing. Recent studies show that for families who had recent deaths and are mourning, adding religious support in the form of scriptural readings along with standard grief counseling can assist these families to recover sooner from their mourning than if they are only given grief counseling.[4] Allowing families freedom to seek solace in scripture can reintroduce purpose and meaning when personal values are skewed by grief. This once again illustrates the importance of addressing the spiritual needs of families in critical care situations.

29.6 Spiritual History

In the pursuit of patients' health and alleviation from suffering, spirituality needs to be constantly addressed, not just once at the beginning or ending of care. The patient's and family's spirituality should be brought up from time to time during continued care. It is important to ask questions about spirituality to help understand and anticipate patients' needs. Although inquiries should be welcomed, health care professionals should be careful not to impose their own beliefs; this is best achieved by keeping an open mind to varying cultures and religions. Also, respecting a patient's and family's wishes and values, especially when it comes to end-of-life matters, will help with this goal. Ask if a patient wants a visit from the chaplain, do not wait for the patient to inquire because they may be unsure whom to ask or how.

Health care providers may feel odd discussing spiritual matters, or they may think that these types of discussions are out of the scope of treatment. Some may feel this would be getting too personal with their patients or that the questions may be interpreted as prying. Numerous studies are showing that these questions are actually welcomed by patients and families, and that they also help the patient–family–doctor relationship.[4,6,7,12,13] In fact, many patients describe themselves as being religious but also report that, the majority of the time, their doctor has not asked questions regarding spirituality as it pertains to medical decision making.[4] The health care giver should also be on the lookout for certain phrases that imply spiritual influence in their patients and families. Patients who speak of being blessed or tortured may actually be giving clues to their religious nature.[7]

In essence, it is helpful to take a spiritual history of the patient and family. Like most other aspects of the patient's history, there are aids for the efficient gathering of the spiritual history. A screening tool, developed by Puchalski, helps the health care provider explore the spirituality of patients and families. The acronym FICA is used to ask about a patient's faith (F), the importance of their faith (I), if they identify with a community of faith (C), and how they wish health care providers to address spiritual issues (A).[13]

Other questions that are helpful and comforting include those related to hopes and expectations and fears of the near future that are centered on issues of palliative care and end-of-life issues. These particular types of questions are actually aimed at the spiritual suffering of patients and their families.[4]

Suggested screening questions that can be used during the spiritual assessment include the following[7]:

- Do you consider yourself a religious or spiritual person?
- What sustains your hope?
- Do you have religious or spiritual beliefs that help you through difficulty?
- What gives your life meaning?
- How important is your faith or belief in your life?
- Does your faith influence your feeling about your illness? Your surgery?
- Do you see any possible conflicts between your health care and your beliefs?
- Do you belong to a community of faith?
- Is there a group of people particularly important to you?
- How is your faith working for you today?

29.7 The Role of Health Care Providers

Nurses have the most exposure to patients and families and form bonds with them that can be utilized to elicit communication and cultural information. Nurses are the ambassadors relaying information between individuals in the patient–family–doctor relationship.[4,10,15,16] "When patient, family, and caregivers share common perceptions and goals, this particular role is often simplified to that of translator, ensuring that communication is timely, accurate, and consistent. In contrast, when the perceptions and goals are dissonant, the brokerage role often requires nurses to assume additional responsibilities of arbitration and diplomacy."[4]

29.8 Suffering

In an attempt to identify the subtleties of suffering, Hinshaw describes four domains of pain as (1) physical pain, (2) psychological or emotional pain, (3) social pain (pain associated with fear of separation from loved ones), and (4) spiritual pain.[9] These are four areas of potential suffering for patients in the NICU, and integral to the patient's treatment is the easing of their suffering no matter what form it takes.[5] Physicians strive to alleviate the pain and suffering of patients. What may prove daunting to the health care provider is effectively treating spiritual pain when encountered because it is not identified and often health care workers are ill prepared to treat this type of suffering when it is discovered. Health care providers have to identify the forms of distress and suffering in their patients and families to provide well-rounded care.[9]

Research is showing that a patient's spirituality can play an important role in ameliorating the sequelae of severe illness.[2] Spiritual suffering is ever present in the sick and dying, and, if not looked for, it will not be recognized when it manifests itself.[5,7] Those who suffer spiritually may be losing hope, may be losing the meaning of their life and self-worth, and may be doing this in silence and unnecessarily.[7] Much of the patient's suffering begins with worry about an uncertain future. For example, patients fear their physical and emotional symptoms may become too much to bear.[5] Also, families do not want their loved one to suffer and often inquire about pain medications, specifically asking the dosing and frequency of administration. Key to this is understanding that suffering is different from patient to patient; what causes suffering in one patient may not be a cause of suffering in another.[5]

Suffering is a state of distress that can occur in all patients, but this distress is even more severe when it occurs in ICU patients. Patients suffer when they feel their integrity and autonomy are threatened and that their end is near. This is easily understood when considering the thoughts of a patient on a ventilator, when they have intravenous lines and electrical leads all over their

521

body. This is frightening to patients and their families. Patients will continue to suffer until the threat is ended or their integrity is restored.[5,9] It is part of the physician's duty to restore a patient's sense of autonomy and to calm their fear in order to reduce their suffering.

29.9 Comforting the Patient

A goal of treatment is comfort. The level of pain is assessed on a regular basis and is rated on a scale of 0 to10 to help quantify the amount of pain a patient is in. Pain medication and sedation are used to help make patients more comfortable and give them relief from their physical symptoms. Doctors and nurses try to use the least amount necessary to alleviate patients' symptoms so as to not overmedicate the patient, which could potentially mask the neurologic exam. At times, especially in patients who are intubated, sedation is kept so high as to make the patient unresponsive. Intubated patients with severe head injuries may be unresponsive regardless of the level of sedation. This may be upsetting to family members, and it is therefore important to reassure them of the necessity for treatment as well as the quantity of treatment. Using narcotics and sedation for pain management may be insufficient to relieve all of a patient's suffering. These medicines can help control physical suffering of the severely injured or terminally ill, but it may not relieve all of their suffering.[9]

Addressing the issues of suffering may allow patients to feel that they are regaining some control over their condition and empower them to ease their own suffering.[4] A 0–10 scale can also be adapted for stress and worry. Patients and families can be asked simple and direct questions to diagnose sources of pain, such as, Are you suffering? What are your concerns and fears? What is it that worries you the most?[5] Even just the simple effort of asking the questions and listening to the answers can help to alleviate suffering.[5,9]

29.10 Prayer and Clergy

There are specialists in the hospital who routinely handle spiritual and religious aspects of patient care. The hospital chaplains are sources of guidance, comfort, and support to the critically ill and their families. There will often be requests for chaplain and prayer services for the ill. Many families believe in the power of prayer.[4,8,13] There are chapels for families to go and reflect, and chaplains are available in every hospital. Clergy are also available from communities. Pastoral care is an integral part of health care facilities. Hospitals offer patients the spiritual services of prayer, sacraments, a listening presence, and assistance in dealing with the emotions and questions that come with sickness. This is provided for both patients and families. Experienced staff chaplains offer sacraments, assist with spiritual care regardless of faith or religious tradition, strive to visit inpatients and make outpatient visits upon request, and will notify a patient's own pastor upon request. The masses turn to their religious leader for comfort and hope when they are troubled. There are many times that health care is not enough for restoring health. This should be presented to the families succinctly and directly so there will be no misunderstanding. Respectfully and in a supportive manner, patients must be permitted to express their spirituality.[4,8,13]

29.11 Closure

Physicians are aware that, ultimately, no matter what collective efforts are taken, patients sometimes die. Those who are terminally ill may die in weeks to years; those who are critically injured may die in minutes to days. Yet there is still potential for healing in the face of death, for both patient and family, and even for the health care provider.[11] Healing does take place during the process of dying when families gather and can find some meaning of their loved one's life. Important factors in this process include hope, reconciliation, and assurance that suffering and pain will be controlled for the patient.[9,11,16] If a critically injured or ill patient still has his or her faculties, assurance of not being abandoned and that pain and suffering will be treated and minimized is comforting.[9] Frequently, family members and patients feel the need for forgiveness or reconciliation, which can be facilitated or mediated by chaplains.[9,16] As a patient's death approaches, health care providers can shift their priorities from sustaining life to bringing comfort.[16] As for the terminally ill patients, hospice offers death with dignity and assists with the change in priority to comfort.[9] Hospice can also comfort the dying in knowing they will not be a burden to their loved ones and that their life and suffering will not be prolonged.[16]

29.12 Suggestions for Families

It is important to remember that, although NICU patients may not be able to respond to a voice or touch, they may still be able to hear and feel. Families should be encouraged to talk to their loved ones, hold their hand, and let them know they are loved. This gives comfort to family members by restoring some sense of control, allowing them to contribute to their loved one's comfort. It is also important to help orient patients by telling them who is holding their hand, what day it is, and to update them on the current events of the family. It is best to encourage the family members to maintain a "good news only" policy, not to relay any distressing news or information. It is appropriate to withhold information about the foreclosure on the house or a favorite pet running away. Health care providers should remind families feeling too emotional to take a break from visiting. Family members should always be informed that there are chaplains available for them and the patient.

29.13 Suggestions for NICU Physicians

Spirituality is hard to quantify or qualify. Who is to say how families should react or to what extent they should show emotion? Who can predict how health care providers will respond when placed in similar situations? Patients and their families may not be able to comprehend the new and undesirable realities forced upon them, or understand the limitations of modern medicine. For these reasons, health care providers are obligated, as soothers, to be serene and understanding. The physician must explain in detail the complexities involving the patients' state of health and the level of care being presented.

"Because it can be particularly important to patients with terminal or chronic diagnoses, the support of hope should fall within the clinical purview of the skilled physician. In times of severe disabling illness, hope maybe mediated through ritual, meditation, music, prayer, traditional sacred narratives, or other inspirational readings. Spiritual care in hospice skillfully redirects hope toward caring relationships and higher meaning."[4]

Physicians should not pass judgment on patients or their families when it comes to spiritual issues, nor should they try to persuade anyone to change or subscribe to their own beliefs. Physicians should not form opinions or prejudices.[7,16] Remember to ask often about the importance of faith, any religious issues, and how the team of care givers can help with these issues.[7] Despite all the technology in the NICU, often the most valuable thing the neurointensivist can do for the patient and family is to hold a hand and offer a kind word, acknowledging distress and helplessness. If asked by families to join them in prayer, the neurointensivist should consider it his or her obligation to participate as much as possible, irrespective of the religion of the patient, and irrespective of the physician's own personal beliefs. Indeed, by holding hands with the patient's loved ones, and bowing one's head in silent prayer, the physician acknowledges the sanctity of each human life, and soul, and lives the creed summarized well in the words of one of our coauthors: "service is the highest form of worship" (J. Siddiqi, pers. comm.).

The following "Principles Guiding Care at the End of Life" were developed by the American College of Surgeons Committee on Ethics and were approved by the Board of Regents at its February 1998 meeting[17]:

- Respect the dignity of both patient and caregivers.
- Be sensitive to and respectful of the patient's and family's wishes.
- Use the most appropriate measures that are consistent with the choices of the patient or the patient's legal surrogate.
- Ensure alleviation of pain and management of other physical symptoms.

- Recognize, assess, and address psychological, social, and spiritual problems.
- Ensure appropriate continuity of care by the patient's primary and/or specialist physician.
- Provide access to therapies that may realistically be expected to improve the patient's quality of life.
- Provide access to appropriate palliative care and hospice care.
- Respect the patient's right to refuse treatment.
- Recognize the physician's responsibility to forgo treatments that are futile.

29.14 Conclusion

Spirituality and the assessment of a patient's spirituality are becoming important features in the care of patients in the NICU. Health care providers must adopt the duty to ease spiritual suffering for patients and their families. Very simple questions can be asked, and the mere asking can show patients a level of compassion in a highly mechanized, alien, and somewhat frightening environment as the NICU. Health care providers can bring surcease from suffering to persons in need with timely attentiveness to these details.

Case Management

Compassion and empathy are basic human values that should be transparent in all interactions with patients and their families in the NICU. In this situation, involvement of any Muslim physicians taking care of the patient may be of some comfort to the family; alternatively, the discussion of the patient's condition with family friends who may be physicians sometimes helps them understand the complexity of the situation. Perhaps most importantly, the NICU team should invite local clergy from the patient's religion to comfort the family, to help them with difficult spiritual decisions, and to say any prayers that may be appropriate. While involvement of the NICU team in final rites for the patient would be at the discretion of the family, and of the individual doctor or nurse, there should be emphasis on the fact that human dignity, and appreciation of the family's loss, are essential to the care of the patient at this time of tragedy for this family.

References

[1] Baggs JG. Intensive care unit use and collaboration between nurses and physicians. Heart Lung. 1989; 18(4):332–338
[2] Baggs JG, Schmitt MH, Mushlin AI, Eldredge DH, Oakes D, Hutson AD. Nurse-physician collaboration and satisfaction with the decision-making process in three critical care units. Am J Crit Care. 1997; 6(5):393–399

[3] Bull Am Coll Surg. 1998; 83(4)

[4] Buchman TG, Cassell J, Ray SE, Wax ML. Who should manage the dying patient?: Rescue, shame, and the surgical ICU dilemma. J Am Coll Surg. 2002; 194(5):665–673

[5] Cassell EJ. Diagnosing suffering: a perspective. Ann Intern Med. 1999; 131(7):531–534

[6] Cassel EJ. The nature of suffering and the goals of medicine. N Engl J Med. 1982; 306(11):639–645

[7] Dunn GP. Patient assessment in palliative care: how to see the "big picture" and what to do when "there is no more we can do". J Am Coll Surg. 2001; 193(5):565–573

[8] Ehman JW, Ott BB, Short TH, Ciampa RC, Hansen-Flaschen J. Do patients want physicians to inquire about their spiritual or religious beliefs if they become gravely ill? Arch Intern Med. 1999; 159(15):1803–1806

[9] Hinshaw DB. The spiritual needs of the dying patient. J Am Coll Surg. 2002; 195(4):565–568, discussion 568–569

[10] Jezewski MA. Do-not-resuscitate status: conflict and culture brokering in critical care units. Heart Lung. 1994; 23(6):458–465

[11] Parker-Oliver D. Redefining hope for the terminally ill. Am J Hosp Palliat Care. 2002; 19(2):115–120

[12] Post SG, Puchalski CM, Larson DB. Physicians and patient spirituality: professional boundaries, competency, and ethics. Ann Intern Med. 2000; 132(7):578–583

[13] Puchalski C, Romer AL. Taking a spiritual history allows clinicians to understand patients more fully. J Palliat Med. 2000; 3(1):129–137

[14] Rabow MW, Fair JM, Hardie GE, McPhee SJ. An evaluation of the end-of-life care content in leading neurology textbooks. Neurology. 2000; 55(6):893–894

[15] Simpson SH. Reconnecting: the experiences of nurses caring for hopelessly ill patients in intensive care. Intensive Crit Care Nurs. 1997; 13(4):189–197

[16] Singer PA, Martin DK, Kelner M. Quality end-of-life care: patients' perspectives. JAMA. 1999; 281 (2):163–168

[17] The following "Principles Guiding Care at the End of Life" were developed by the American College of Surgeons Committee on Ethics and were approved by the Board of Regents at its February 1998 meeting. http://www.journalacs.org/article/S1072-7515(05)00093-1/abstract

30 Medical-Legal Issues in the Neurosurgical Intensive Care Unit

Bailey Zampella, Dan E. Miulli, Silvio Hoshek, Rosalinda Menoni, and Yancey Beamer

Abstract

The central nervous system is the unique person. Through it come memories, emotions, function, social, and spiritual structure. As such, any damage to it changes the person more than damage to any other body system. Therefore, the neurointensivist has the highest medical-legal risk, which can be mitigated by creating an atmosphere of security, confidence, and respectfulness through a caring and professional multidisciplinary team approach. The primary goals should include an effort to minimize confusion and doubt through many health care providers working in unison to provide a free flow of communication and education that is documented in numerous areas of the medical record.

Keywords: communication, consent, documentation, interpretation, patient dignity, professional, self-determination, teamwork

Case Presentation

The police bring into the emergency room an adult Asian man, seemingly in his 40s, who was detained for wandering the streets partially clothed and confused. He is initially placed on a psychiatric 72-hour hold as a result of a mental disorder. While in the emergency room, the patient is observed having complex repetitive movements prior to a grand mal seizure. The patient is taken to the radiology department for a computed tomographic (CT) scan. In the meantime, the police produce his passport, indicating that he is most likely a visitor from China. The CT scan reveals a left temporal lobe lesion with edema. The patient awakens after the seizure; he is deaf and appears to be acting appropriately, but no one, including the telephone translation service, speaks his dialect. What should be the next steps taken by the hospital and the neurosurgical intensive care unit?

See end of chapter for Case Management.

30.1 Introduction

Neurologists and neurosurgeons attempt to treat the systems of the body that make the individual a unique person. If a person suffers almost any permanent neurologic deficit, he or she is usually changed forever. The person may not be able to hold the same employment position, make the same income, or relate to his or her family; be an interacting family member, caregiver, or productive member of society. Or the person may die. Not only does the patient change, but the patient's family and dynamics change. Therefore, neurologists and neurosurgeons continually face health care situations that put them at the highest medical-legal risks.

Being admitted to the neurosurgical intensive care unit (NICU) may indeed be an intense and tumultuous time for the patient and his or her loved ones. This is especially true if an emergency trip to the hospital was necessary as opposed to being part of an elective procedure. It is therefore of paramount importance to create an atmosphere of security, confidence, and respectfulness through caring, multidisciplinary professionalism. The primary goals should include an effort to minimize confusion and doubt during this very stressful period while providing a free flow of communication and education. This is best achieved through a holistic team approach, which clearly identifies all treating members of the team and their individual areas of expertise. Most important is communication. During the period of patient and family stress, physicians and other health care workers must remain close and unified. They must not back away because of difficulties in care, in family dynamics, or with patients and families relating to the situation. This is even more necessary if complications have arisen.

30.2 Health Care Teamwork

All health care workers must present a united front for the patient and family. There must be clear communication about diagnosis, prognosis, and care from all team members involved in patient care. It is the physician's responsibility to discuss the patient's condition with the nurse, the primary patient advocate. It is the nurse's responsibility to ask any questions so that he or she may understand all the care provided. It becomes severely problematic when the nurse dismisses or belittles any treatment options. If such a situation exists, then changing the lead health care provider should be discussed with the charge nurse and care transferred. Patients and their families, although under great emotional and physical stress, can perceive the discord and will turn that discord into frustration with and a lack of confidence in the health care provided. This situation can lead to medical-legal claims.

At times, patients in the NICU require care from multiple specialties. Although mandatory, it once again provides an opportunity for confusion in communication to patients and their families. The members of the health care delivery team may include trauma service, orthopedists, surgical subspecialists, intensivists, internists, pulmonologists, neurologists, infectious disease specialists, and physiatrists. The hierarchy within the ranks of a service should be delineated as well, appropriately identifying residents, physicians' assistants, and attending physicians. Besides the doctors involved in the patient's care, the patient and/or the family should be able to recognize the nursing staff, respiratory therapists, social workers, dietitians, clinical pharmacists, clergy, and therapists from the physical, occupational, and speech services. The best care of the patient involves much input and coordination; everyone should be of one mind and plan. Such coordination is accomplished through the guidance of regularly scheduled interdisciplinary meetings, during which information is updated and shared so that daily treatment plans can be formulated.

30.3 Health Care Workers–Patient/Family Communication

Most legal claims result from a lack or misunderstanding of information. Most patients state that they were not told about an unexpected outcome. This can be defended only by careful communication in the presence of a witness and documentation in the medical record. Health care witnesses need to be present when a physician discusses any planned procedures. The situation for the patient and family is complex, with emotions often drawing concentration away from discussions. Especially when discussing emergent procedures, it is common that the patient and/or family is not retaining all the information being explained due to the stressful situation. In most circumstances, the primary service should discuss the coordinated care with the patient and family, often relying on attendance by a consultant. In the NICU, the captain of the team is usually the neurosurgeon, who should be the primary spokesperson, unless deferring to the expertise of another colleague individually or in a conference setting. References to colleagues and ancillary staff should always be made with professional decorum in mind, as a misinterpretation may undermine the credibility of the unit.

The key to achieving the primary objective of an environment of trust and security is the demonstration of regard for preserving the patient's dignity and displaying sensitivity and compassion while making time for daily briefings, particularly when the news is discouraging. It is vital to verify that successful communication has been accomplished. This can be quite challenging when attempting to convey the complexity of the natural history of a disease process or the risks and benefits of an intervention to patients and families from various cultural and socioeconomic backgrounds. The communication to the patient and family must be that the team recognizes the importance of their participation in the treatment plan and eventual outcome. It is especially important for the physician and health care team to speak in terms that the patient and the family understand. Oftentimes, we as physicians use medical terms that the layperson may not understand. During this time it is important to make sure everyone involved understands. This can be demonstrated by asking the patient and/or family members to use their own words to describe the conversation and ask any clarifying questions.

The patient and family must pick a spokesperson for the group, the main contact for the patient and family. Patients and family members will not understand everything told to them. As expected, they will absorb what they understand most. Every person has a different background, and therefore the information that he or she takes away from any conversation will be different. If each person communicates at separate times with the NICU staff, there will be numerous interpretations of what has been told. When that interpretation is transmitted among the family, there will be opportunities for discrepancies. These discrepancies will be turned into stress, hostility, and lack of confidence in the health care team.

During conferences and discussions with the patient and his or her family, it is necessary not only to convey information but to educate. Many people are visually oriented and benefit from seeing pertinent radiographic studies, such as X-rays, computed tomographic (CT) and magnetic resonance imaging (MRI) scans, and angiograms, while encouraging and soliciting questions. At times, patients and families overcome with shock and grief understandably hesitate to ask questions; they should then be invited to write down questions for the next discussion. The importance of establishing and maintaining this rapport cannot be overstated; it can prove to be sustaining, even in the face of a bad outcome or inevitable complications. Striving to create and maintain this type of atmosphere may actually foster trust and may prevent the formation of misunderstandings and misgivings that lead to discontent and possibly litigation.

30.3.1 Documentation

Detailed documentation of all discussions with patients and their families should always be noted in the medical record, preferably dictated because that comes with an electronic time and date in the electronic medical record (EMR). This is strongly recommended in addition to any institutional forms requiring signature. The presence of a witness, preferably the patient's nurse, for discussion of care and signing of any legal documents is advisable.

Despite best efforts, certain situations involving consent, advanced directives, right to privacy, abuse, and declaration of death may require additional diligence lest they lead to polarization or true confrontation. Should such situations occur, the risk management officer must be informed immediately.

Documentation of communication can be in the form of handwritten notes, collaborating nurses and ancillary staff notes, dictations, hospital forms, and, more recently, EMRs. Each one should document that communication took place and note any additional members of the health care team present during said interaction. Each member of the NICU team must learn to communicate and exist in harmony, not only with patients but also with other members of the team. Physicians cannot and should not stand alone. The duty of the NICU team is to eliminate shame, encourage hope, communicate with respectful, unselfish caring about any emotions, and by logic, build bonds, and teach and inspire others to feel the same. People are different; however, differences build a better and stronger world. The NICU team must ask for opinions and try to empathize with what others are feeling.

With the introduction of the EMR, documentation in real time has become more convenient for both the physician and the nursing staff. Documentation of medications and when they were administered is readily available for the physician and nursing staff to view. This allows for clarification and less miscommunication between team members. In addition, the EMR also allows for physician documentation of any conversations with the patient and/or family members in one location that can easily be accessed by any health care team member. It is important that all health care professionals document any interaction they had with the patient or family as soon as it occurs. The advantage of the EMR is that, whenever the documentation is entered, it allows all team members to see the time and date of said occurrence and does not allow backdating of an interaction. Documentation in the EMR by the nursing staff is also available and is readily accessible for users to view. This can allow for corroboration among health care team members if an important interaction has occurred.

30.3.2 Obtaining Consent

Consent is communication about and understanding of a treatment that the health care team is providing to the patient. It is not just about surgery but about many treatments, such as central or arterial line placements, blood transfusions, ventriculostomy, chest and feeding tubes, and other tube and ostomy procedures. According to the California Hospital Association,

Every competent adult has the fundamental right of self-determination over his or her body and property. Individuals who are unable to exercise this right, such as minors or incompetent adults, have the right to be represented by another who will protect their interests and preserve their basic rights.[1]

It is paramount that the physician providing the proposed care discuss and obtain consent. Only the health care provider can know what information is material to the decision making of the patient (▶ Table 30.1).[2,3,4]

Table 30.1 Medical issues of consent[2,3,4]

Issue	Description, who determines or who consents
Implied consent in a medical emergency	Patient unable to consent; no surrogate available; no evidence that patient or surrogate would refuse the treatment; patient would consent if able.
Capacity	Patient's ability to understand nature and consequences of decision, to make and communicate a decision, and to understand its significant benefits, risks, and alternatives. Unless otherwise specified in a written advanced health care directive, the primary physician should make the determination that a patient lacks capacity.
Incompetence	Judicial determination; person lacks the capacity to perform a specific act, needs a conservator to make those individual decisions; consent deferred to other surrogate decision makers. A family member or significant other is the most common surrogate.
Nonconsent	Patient refuses recommended care. The patient has a right to know the consequences of refusing care so that the refusal is also informed. The physician has a duty to inform the patient of the risks of refusing to undergo a recommended simple and common procedure. A court order should be considered if motives are suspect.
Emancipated minor	Married or divorced, active duty with U.S. military, and 14 years of age and older by court order.
Self-sufficient minors	15 years of age or older, living separate and apart from parents, and managing own financial affairs. Providers can notify parents if not dealing with sensitive services, such as reproductive services, sexual assault, rape care and treatment, infectious reportable conditions, and some select behavioral health issues.
Minors	Consent obtained from adult parent or legal guardian, such as either of married biological parents, adoptive parents, a divorced parent with legal custody, or unmarried parents (the father may have to prove paternity if the mother disputes his role). Parents under 18 years of age still have capacity. Other possible consent givers include foster parents, same-sex partners, registered domestic partners, stepparents, grandparents, surrogate parents, and a temporary party with delegated authority, such as a coach or camp director.

When a neurosurgical intervention is performed with implied consent, it is important to discuss the treatment with the patient, if capacity is restored, and with the family as soon as identification of next of kin is established.

The patient and family must understand the risks, benefits, and alternatives to the treatment, as well as the sequelae of the perioperative period. In reference to the initial intervention, this may include infection, rebleeding, further neurologic deterioration, and the need for reintervention. The inherent risks should not be trivialized. The physician must also discuss the nature and goals of alternatives or specific adjunctive medical treatment regimens, such as medications that have known side effects or complications. A dictated example of supratentorial surgery follows:

The risks and benefits of craniotomy for tumor resection have been discussed with the patient and family in extensive detail. I mentioned diagnosis and decompression as the major benefits. I emphasized that risks of surgery include, but are not limited to, bleeding, infection, [cerebrospinal] leak, stroke, seizure, cognitive deficits, speech problems, bowel/bladder dysfunction, visual deficits and/or diplopia, hemiplegia, and death. Any possible risk may occur. There may be additional pain, and the current pain may not resolve. General risks of pneumonia, [urinary tract infection], [deep venous thrombosis], cardiac arrhythmias, and pulmonary embolus were also discussed. The possibilities of incomplete resection, no benefit, repeat surgery, and need for adjuvant therapies such as radiation and/or chemotherapy were discussed. The seriousness of the patient's condition, and of the planned intervention, was emphasized. I answered all questions and explained it was not possible to foresee all possible complications or adverse outcomes. No guarantees were given. Patient and family wished to proceed with surgery. (Javed Siddiqi, personal communication.)

30.4 Reporting Abuse

Reporting child, elder, and domestic abuse and violent crime is mandated by state and federal statutes. Legally mandated reporters can be criminally or civilly liable for failing to report suspected abuse. The penalties can be 6 months of incarceration or a fine of $1,000. Any legally mandated reporter has immunity when making a report. Confidentiality laws do not apply in suspected abuse cases. The statutory duty to report supersedes the confidentiality privilege.

30.5 Recording Accidents

When accidents or mistakes happen that result in adverse outcomes, report them to the patient, family, and hospital administration immediately.

When incidents happen, fill out an incident report that is meant to be a confidential communication within the hospital. The report is intended solely to be transmitted to the hospital attorneys for their information and their use in the preparation, investigation, and defense of the health care worker in litigation or potential litigation. It should not be photocopied or made part of the medical record or referenced in the medical record. The incident report should contain a one-sentence summary, a description of the type of incident, including where it occurred, who was involved, any witnesses, contributing factors, the severity of the outcome, what changes could be made to reduce the risk in the future, analysis and actions taken, who completed the form, departmental manager review, and quality assurance review. The form should be completed within 24 hours.

30.5.1 Seizure

Seizures may occur in the setting of either primary or secondary disease processes. As there are many types of seizure disorders, it is important to identify the type of seizure and understand what may be the underlying cause of the seizure before the appropriate medication can be administered.

When a patient is actively seizing, it is important that the first health care team member present notifies a physician as quickly as possible; whether this be the emergency room physician, intensivist, neurologist, or neurosurgeon. Generalized seizures have the potential to compromise the patient's airway. Most seizures will cease spontaneously within 2 minutes, and the administration of a benzodiazepine or other antiepileptic medication is not necessary. However, the patient should have immediately available intravenous (IV) access in case the seizure does not cease on its own. Once the acute seizure subsides, it again is a multidisciplinary effort of multiple specialties to understand the cause of the seizure and the best way to treat it.

Newly diagnosed seizures can have many psychosocial effects on a patient. Seizures may lead to a loss of independence, ability to drive and return to work, among other aspects of a patient's life. The Americans with Disabilities Act (ADA), which was amended by the ADA Amendments Act of 2008 (ADAAA), is a federal law that prohibits discrimination against qualified individuals with disabilities.[5] The ADA requires employers to provide adjustments or modifications to enable applicants and employees with disabilities to enjoy equal employment opportunities.[5] Patients may return to work when both they and their physician who is managing the antiepileptic medication feel that the seizures are under control. In addition, driving restrictions for individuals with seizure disorder are still controversial. Due to limited data on driving risk and epilepsy, the restrictions imposed are often based on rather arbitrary standards. The seizure-free interval is the most common standard used to assess a patient's driving risk. Longer seizure-free intervals (>6–12 months) are typically associated with reduced risk of seizure-related accidents. However, different states and countries have different seizure-free interval requirements for licensure[6] (▶ Table 30.2).

Table 30.2 Driving and epilepsy: regulations and practices of U.S. states in 2001

State	Seizure-free restrictions, months	Physician liable for driving recommendations
Alabama	6	No
Alaska	6	Yes
Arizona	3	No
Arkansas	12	Yes
California	3, 6, or 12	Yes
Colorado	None	No
Connecticut	3	Yes
District of Columbia	12	Yes
Delaware	None	No
Florida	24	No
Georgia	12	No
Hawaii	None	Yes
Idaho	None	No
Illinois	None	No
Indiana	None	Yes
Iowa	6	No
Kansas	6	No
Kentucky	3	No
Louisiana	6	No
Maine	3	No
Maryland	3	No
Massachusetts	6	Yes
Michigan	6	Yes
Minnesota	6	No
Mississippi	12	No
Missouri	6	No
Montana	None	No
Nebraska	3	Yes
Nevada	3	Yes
New Hampshire	12	Yes
New Jersey	12	Yes
New Mexico	12	No

(continued)

Table 30.2 continued

State	Seizure-free restrictions, months	Physician liable for driving recommendations
New York	12	No
North Carolina	6–12	No
North Dakota	6	No
Ohio	None	No
Oklahoma	12	No
Oregon	6	Yes
Pennsylvania	6	No
Rhode Island	None	No
South Carolina	6	No
South Dakota	12	Yes
Tennessee	6	Yes
Texas	6	No
Utah	3	Yes
Vermont	None	Yes
Virginia	6	No
Washington	6	Yes
West Virginia	12	No
Wisconsin	3	No
Wyoming	3	Yes

30.6 Components of a Lawsuit

For a lawsuit to be successfully completed and neglect proven, four areas have to be involved in the conduct between two parties:

1. There must be duty between individuals.
2. There must have been breach of duty by violation of the standard of care as determined by a reasonable physician.
3. There must be injury due to breach of duty.
4. There must be proximate cause.

Once all parts have been proven, the case is settled or judgment is made. Most physicians will be sued at least once in their career. Medical malpractice cases flooded the U.S. court system by the 1930s, and such suits have continued unabated. The cultural, social, ethical, and economic system determines the probability of a lawsuit; however, communication between the doctor and the patient/family is paramount. The lead physician and the NICU team must be united and must communicate and educate patients and their families.

The time in the NICU is emotional and stressful. Those emotions can either be soothed by the NICU team or manipulated and twisted. There are individuals who tend to prey on the emotions of others, inventing or reestablishing baseline emotional confusion. Adding more energy to them, reigniting smoldering emotions renews the intensity that may have dissipated. These individuals may even fabricate new emotions for the patient and family, based on their interpretation of a previous foundation. Thus plaintiffs' cases are generated by creating an emotional response. To prevent this, empathize, communicate, teach, and console.

One exception to consent being voluntary is found in the mental health acts that specify that a person can be involuntarily held and transported, assessed, and admitted for up to 72 hours for mental health evaluation and treatment if, as a result of a mental disorder, the person is a danger to himself, a danger to others, or gravely disabled. A related provision[7] provides that any physician providing emergency services to a patient shall not be civilly or criminally liable for detaining the patient (without consent) for up to 8 hours, pending transportation to a mental health facility.

An exception to the aforementioned rule stating that the primary physician determines capacity was ruled on by the California Supreme Court,[8] which found that in the case of a patient on an involuntary 72-hour hold who refuses medication, the determination of capacity shall be made pursuant to a judicial proceeding.

Case Management

The psychiatry and neurosurgery departments are consulted. The Chinese consulate provides an interpreter, and the patient's history and physical examination are completed. No dysfunction in understanding is present using equipment for the hearing impaired. The patient is assessed to have the capacity to consent for medical care, comprehending the risks and benefits germane to the options of treatment. The patient is offered craniotomy for diagnosis and excision of the lesion. The risks and benefits are communicated thoroughly through the official interpreter. All steps are documented in the medical record, including the participation by the interpreter. The patient is amenable and undergoes surgery to excise the lesion. The postoperative course of treatment is uneventful, and he returns home.

References

[1] California Hospital Association. Consent Manual. 43rd ed. Sacramento, CA: California Hospital Association; 2016 www.calhospital.org/consent

[2] Cobbs v Grant, 8 Cal 3d (1972)

[3] Truman v Thomas, 27 Cal 3d 285 (1980)

[4] California Probate Code sections 4658, 4657, 4609, http://leginfo.legislature.ca.gov/faces/codes_displaySection.xhtml?lawCode=PROB&sectionNum=4658

[5] U.S. Equal Employment Opportunity Commission. Americans with Disabilities Act (ADA); 2008 https://www.eeoc.gov/laws/types/disability.cfm

[6] Up-To-Date: Driving Restrictions for Patients with Seizure and Epilepsy. February 12, 2015 http://www.uptodate.com/contents/driving-restrictions-for-patients-with-seizures-and-epilepsy

[7] Health and Safety Code 1799.111http://leginfo.legislature.ca.gov/faces/codes_displaySection.xhtml?lawCode=HSC&sectionNum=1799.111

[8] Riese v St. Mary's Hospital and Medical Center, 259 Cal 2d 698 (1989)

31 Discharge Planning for the Neurosurgical Intensive Care Unit Patient

Dan E. Miulli, Jacob Bernstein, and Paula Snyder

Abstract
Discharge planning should begin at admission, taking into consideration the patient's disease, health care needs, ability to recover in the short and long term, family support, finances, insurance, and social support. Many times the patient will not be able to return home immediately after hospitalization or ever, and the complex process to provide discharge planning requires unusually long periods of negotiation between the case manager, social workers, and many others. Working with the physiatrist, physical therapist, occupational therapist, and others can facilitate the patient's transfer to a rehabilitation center.

Keywords: family meeting, functional capacity, insurance, LTAC, physical therapy, rehabilitation, resources, skilled nursing facility

Case Presentation

A 17-year-old boy presents to the trauma bay with a self-inflicted gunshot wound to the head and is found to have a Glasgow Coma Scale score of 4 T. The patient is found to have left-sided traumatic subarachnoid hemorrhage, subdural hematoma, and intraparenchymal hemorrhage (IPH). The patient is emergently taken to the operating room for a left decompressive craniectomy. Postoperatively, the patient remains in critical condition.

See end of chapter for Case Management.

31.1 Introduction

The complexity of the neurosurgical intensive care unit (NICU) patient often leads to an equally complex, and frustrating, process for discharge planning. The old adage of starting discharge planning upon admission is particularly relevant to the NICU patient, where multisystem injuries and issues often exist that require specialized care outside the hospital setting. In general, discharge planning out of the NICU involves the following categories:
1. Discharge to the floor for stable, alert, and awake patients, followed by discharge to home, rehabilitation, or skilled nursing facilities.

2. Discharge to an NICU step-down unit for nonventilated patients, followed by discharge to the floor, home, rehabilitation, or skilled nursing facilities.
3. Discharge straight from the NICU to long-term acute care (LTAC) facilities for ventilated and severely disabled patients.

The functional capacity of the neurosurgical patient may be significantly decreased because of cognitive and/or physical impairments related to traumatic brain injury, spinal cord injury, hemorrhagic stroke, brain tumors, and so forth. These patients may have tracheostomy or gastrostomy tubes and limited or no bowel or bladder control. They may be at increased risk for injury due to cognitive impairment, recent memory deficits, and judgment and impulse control issues and may require constant supervision. Most inpatient rehabilitation programs require that the patient be able to participate in at least 3 hours of therapy each day. Some patients with complex medical problems may not be able to tolerate intensive rehabilitation; others may be medically stable but may not be able to participate in intensive rehabilitation due to the severity of their neurologic injury. Many of these patients may need subacute rehabilitation or skilled nursing with less intensive physical therapy. Generally, the more severe the injury or the longer the NICU/hospital stay, the longer the recovery period and the greater the need for more intensive rehabilitation or long-term care. Patients with only cognitive impairments may not qualify for inpatient rehabilitation.

Early identification of the patient's resources, community resources and outpatient rehabilitation programs, home situation and adaptability, and family support system is imperative for patients not meeting inpatient rehabilitation criteria. Patients rehabilitated on an outpatient basis will need careful evaluation and planning by the multidisciplinary team. Identification of caregivers among a patient's family and friends is essential to a smooth discharge plan. Other areas to be assessed include (1) where outpatient therapies will be received; (2) transportation availability to and from therapies and physician visits; (3) whether home therapy is needed and, if so, whether it is covered by insurance; (4) evaluation of the home environment to identify needs for assistive devices, such as a hospital bed, commode, and shower chair, as well as supplies (for tracheotomy care, feedings, etc.).

The nurse/case manager, in concert with the multidisciplinary team, assesses the anticipated needs of the patient for discharge. The team usually consists of the nurse, physician, physiatrist, physical therapist, occupational therapist, speech pathologist, dietitian, respiratory therapist, and social worker, along with the patient and his or her family. Each team member has a specific area of responsibility related to discharge planning. Areas of particular concern when evaluating a patient for potential rehabilitation needs include motor dysfunction, alteration in sensory perception, altered communication patterns, behavioral issues, altered respiratory function, cranial nerve impairment, and cognitive impairment (▶ Table 31.1, ▶ Table 31.2, ▶ Table 31.3).[1]

Table 31.1 Evaluating patients for potential rehabilitation needs[1]

Alteration	Associated with/demonstrated by
Alteration in motor function	Associated with spinal cord injury, traumatic brain injury, and stroke resulting in paresis, paralysis, incoordination, apraxia, spasticity, and abnormal reflexes
Alteration in sensory perception	Blindness and visual disturbances and defects, loss or disturbance in pain, temperature, and pressure perception, position sense, agnosia
Altered communication patterns	Receptive, expressive, and global dysphasias, aphasia, motor dysphasia
Alteration in behavior	Demonstrated by mood disturbances, depression, poor impulse control, disinhibition, anger, aggressive behavior
Alteration in cranial nerve function	Swallowing and speech defects, ptosis, diplopia, disruption of taste, smell, hearing, cranial nerve (CN) VII palsy
Alteration in cognitive function	Confusion, altered level of consciousness, impaired memory, judgment, concentration, problem solving, higher thought processes

Table 31.2 Potential discharge destinations based on diagnosis and/or deficit[1]

Condition/situation	Discharge destination
Spinal cord injury (SCI)	Acute rehabilitation
Stroke with hemiplegia	Acute rehabilitation
Brain injury with paresis, paralysis, apraxia, ataxia, inability to ambulate	Acute rehabilitation vs. skilled nursing facility with physical therapy vs. home with outpatient therapy
Ventilator dependent (excluding SCI)	Subacute placement with rehabilitation/physical therapy
Persistent vegetative state	Skilled nursing facility vs. subacute facility
Mild cognitive impairment	Home with outpatient therapy
Moderate cognitive impairment	Acute rehabilitation vs. home with outpatient therapy
Severe cognitive impairment	Acute rehabilitation vs. skilled nursing facility
Sensory impairment: blindness	Acute rehabilitation
Communication deficits: aphasia, dysphasia	Home with outpatient therapy
Behavioral issues	Home with outpatient therapy and supervision vs. skilled nursing facility

Table 31.3 Team member responsibilities for discharge and rehabilitation planning[1]

Team member	Initial assessment	Eligibility and needs evaluation	Environmental assessment	Patient and family education
Case manager	Communicates with insurance/HMO	Determines covered services and rehabilitation options	Communicates with potential rehabilitation facilities	Educates patient and family regarding treatment and discharge plan
Social worker	Family support system and home resources	Determines covered services and rehabilitation options; assists in applications for funding	Communicates with potential rehabilitation facilities	Educates patient and family regarding treatment and discharge plan
Physician	Assesses medical needs and stability	Assesses prognosis for recovery		Educates patient and family regarding treatment and discharge plan
Physical therapist	Assesses physical limitations and functional capacity	Recommendation re: need for assistive devices and ongoing therapy	Explores home environment and related needs	Educates patient and family regarding treatment and discharge plan
Occupational therapist	Assesses physical limitations and functional capacity	Recommendation re: need for assistive devices and ongoing therapy	Explores home environment and related needs	Educates patient and family regarding treatment and discharge plan
Speech pathologist	Assesses cognitive and physical limitations as related to speech, swallowing, and cognition and functional capacity	Recommendation re: need for assistive devices and ongoing therapy	Explores home environment and related needs	Educates patient and family regarding treatment and discharge plan
Dietitian	Assesses nutritional status and physical limitations	Recommends nutritional program based on assessed needs		Educates patient and family regarding treatment and discharge plan

Table 31.3 continued

Team member	Initial assessment	Eligibility and needs evaluation	Environmental assessment	Patient and family education
Respiratory therapist	Assesses respiratory status and associated needs	Recommends respiratory program based on assessed needs		Educates patient and family regarding treatment and discharge plan
Physiatrist	Assesses physical, cognitive, and social needs and limitations	Designs patient-specific medical and rehabilitation program	Facilitates entry into appropriate rehabilitation program	Educates patient and family regarding treatment and discharge plan
Nurse	Assesses physical, cognitive, and social needs and limitations	Communicates perceived need to appropriate team members	Coordinates care and activities of team members	Educates patient and family regarding treatment and discharge plan

Abbreviation: HMO, health maintenance organization.

31.2 Implications

Determining discharge destination early in the acute hospital phase can facilitate treatment decisions, resource allocation, family education, and counseling. It enables families and discharge planners to choose appropriate posthospital facilities (▶ Table 31.4)[2] or prepare the home environment. Case management increases patient and family understanding of posthospital needs and promotes the family's ability to meet those needs confidently. It also decreases the length of hospital stay and costs.

Case Management

The patient subsequently stabilized and improved to a GCS score of 10 T and underwent placement of a tracheostomy and percutaneous endoscopic gastrostomy (PEG) tube. The patient was assessed by case managers immediately upon admission, as well as respiratory therapists, physical therapists, occupational therapists, speech therapists, and dietitians. It was deemed that the patient was a candidate for long-term acute hospital placement for continual tube feeding, ventilator management and weaning, further skilled nursing care, physical therapy, occupational therapy, and cognitive/speech therapy.

Table 31.4 Comparing the different discharge destinations

Destination	What is it?	Requirements	Purpose	Therapy (PT/ST/OT)
Outpatient	Patient lives at home and travels to therapy appointments	Patient medically stable to be discharged home and can take care of self at home	To aid in patient's recovery from illness/injury	Physical therapy, occupational therapy, or speech therapy 2–5 days per week
Home based	Patient lives at home but needs full-time or part-time assistance	Patient medically stable to be discharged home but not able to fully be independent or has some skilled nursing need	To assist in patient's recovery and provide aid and/or skilled nursing care (wound care, IV antibiotic therapy via PICC, IV/PEG tube feedings, etc.) till patient able to fully care for him-/herself	Physical therapy, occupational therapy, or speech therapy 2–5 days per week
Acute rehab	An inpatient rehabilitation hospital for patients with traumatic injuries, debilitating diseases, or certain postsurgical patients who will benefit from an intensive multidisciplinary rehabilitation approach	Patient needs to be medically stable and physically able to participate in 3 hours of therapy per day	To assist in recovery and for the patient to return home	3 hours of therapy per day based on patient's needs, 5–7 days per week
Subacute rehab	An inpatient rehabilitation hospital for patients with traumatic injuries, debilitating diseases, or certain postsurgical patients who will benefit from a multidisciplinary rehabilitation approach but cannot tolerate an extensive therapy	Patients who are medically stable but are not able to tolerate the amount of therapy provided in acute rehab	To assist in recovery and for patient to get strong enough for acute rehab or discharge home	Therapy less than 3 hours per day 3–5 days per week

Table 31.4 continued

Desti-nation	What is it?	Requirements	Purpose	Therapy (PT/ST/OT)
	regimen such as in acute rehab			
Long-term acute care hospital	A hospital specializing in treating patients requiring extended hospitalization with an average length of stay > 25 days	Patient requiring prolonged hospitalization with multiple medical problems requiring skilled medical and nursing care (antibiotic therapy, ventilator management, wound care, tube feeding, etc.) and daily physician visits	Goal is recovery to subacute or acute rehab, stabilization of medical issues in transport to long-term care or skilled nursing facility	Less than 3 hours per day and 5–6 days per week
Skilled nursing facility	An inpatient facility that provides care for patients who require intense skilled medical care	Patient requiring skilled medical care such as wound care, PEG feedings, chronic O_2, therapy, dialysis, diabetes monitoring. Cognitively impaired, cognitively + physically impaired, physically impaired. Do not require daily physician visits.	Short-term vs. long-term stay depending on severity of medical conditions	One hour a day

Abbreviations: IV, intravenous; OT, occupational therapy; PEG, percutaneous endoscopic gastrostomy; PICC, peripherally inserted central catheter; PT, physical therapy; ST, speech therapy.

References

[1] Barker E. Neuroscience Nursing: A Spectrum of Care. 2nd ed. St. Louis, MO: CV Mosby; 2002
[2] Association of Rehabilitation Nurses. Description of Rehabilitation Settings. 18 May 2016. www.rehabnurse.org/pdf/PRNavigatingRehabSettings.pdf

545

Index

Index

548

Index

Q

R

Index